HIV Prevention

with Latinos

HIV PREVENTION WITH LATINOS
THEORY, RESEARCH, AND PRACTICE

Edited by Kurt C. Organista

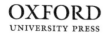
OXFORD
UNIVERSITY PRESS

OXFORD
UNIVERSITY PRESS

Oxford University Press, Inc., publishes works that further
Oxford University's objective of excellence
in research, scholarship, and education.

Oxford   New York
Auckland   Cape Town   Dar es Salaam   Hong Kong   Karachi
Kuala Lumpur   Madrid   Melbourne   Mexico City   Nairobi
New Delhi   Shanghai   Taipei   Toronto

With offices in
Argentina   Austria   Brazil   Chile   Czech Republic   France   Greece
Guatemala   Hungary   Italy   Japan   Poland   Portugal   Singapore
South Korea   Switzerland   Thailand   Turkey   Ukraine   Vietnam

Published by Oxford University Press, Inc.
198 Madison Avenue, New York, New York 10016
www.oup.com

Oxford is a registered trademark of Oxford University Press

Library of Congress Cataloging-in-Publication Data

HIV prevention with Latinos : theory, research, and practice / edited by Kurt C. Organista.
    p. cm.
Includes bibliographical references and index.
ISBN 978-0-19-976430-3 (pbk. : alk. paper) 1. Hispanic Americans—Health and hygiene.
2. AIDS (Disease)—United States—Prevention. 3. Reproductive health—Latin America.
4. Reproductive health—United States—History. I. Organista, Kurt C.
RA644.A25H5938 2012
362.196'9792008968073—dc23   2011047203

135798642
Printed in the United States of America
on acid-free paper

To every member of our extended Latino family and community, who are made healthier through our full recognition, respect, acceptance, and care.

Contents

Section One Theorizing HIV Risk in Latinos at the Intersection of Sexual Health, Culture, Poverty, and Minority Status

Section Two Illuminating Complex Dimensions of HIV Risk in Diverse Latino Populations, Environments, and Situations

Section Three Best and Promising HIV Prevention Interventions with Diverse Latino Populations, Locations, and Situations

Foreword

Latinos are the fastest growing ethnic minority in the United States. Understanding this diverse community's cultural, behavioral, economic, and environmental experiences from a public health perspective is vital to improving the health of the nation. The HIV epidemic is a serious public health issue in the Latino community and has affected it disproportionately.

After three decades of seeking to understand, treat, and prevent HIV transmission in the United States, social scientists, clinicians, public health professionals, policy makers, and advocates have, at last, a comprehensive treatise on HIV prevention in the Latino community.

Vitally important research, compiled by editor and contributor Kurt C. Organista, Ph.D., in his *HIV Prevention with Latinos: Theory, Research, and Practice,* comes at a time when the color of the domestic epidemic continues to change. According to the Centers for Disease Prevention and Control, Latinos accounted for 20% of new infections in 2009 while representing approximately 16% of the U.S. population.

Professor Organista's deep commitment to interdisciplinary and community-based research is demonstrated in this masterfully culled collection of research from academicians of various disciplines across the country. Collectively they provide a rich, culturally nuanced, understanding of factors that are often given cursory and stereotypical attention in the HIV/AIDS literature. His scholarly study of migrant day labor workers concisely and insightfully provides the structural cohesion for the entire body of work.

Researchers examine critical sexual identities that are taboo within the broader society and even more so within the Latino community. A former student of Professor Organista offers pioneering work on the embedded HIV risks associated with transexuality and sheds light on the many precarious social margins within which this population survives. Another research team explores the situational contexts of bisexuality in the Latino community. This population is often perilously overlooked in prevention efforts that target "men who have sex with men."

A case study by nursing researchers of Latino labor migrants working in New Orleans post Katrina dramatically depicts important learnings about behavioral and clinical aspects of Latino migrants while interfacing with a new receiving community. As U.S. Latinos continue to migrate throughout the south, this research is timely and highly relevant to public health and health care providers in regions that have not historically been home to large Latino communities.

Thanks to Professor Organista, his colleagues, and their research teams, the HIV/AIDS epidemic in the Latino community can no longer be set aside by a lack of culturally relevant research. They have collectively brought a new sensibility to the conversation within the Latino family, new tools to community-based educators, and a rigorously designed cultural framework for all of us in public health to apply to HIV and other sexually transmitted disease prevention efforts. This state-of-the art research sets a new bar for program design and community-based efforts and should inspire all of us to continue to learn about how the diverse Latino cultural milieus can effect better health and social outcomes for this youthful and growing demographic.

"We should acknowledge differences, we should greet differences, until differences makes no difference anymore."

Dr. Adela Allen

Sandra R. Hernandez, M.D.
CEO of the San Francisco Foundation
and former director of public health
San Francisco, California

Acknowledgments

The honor of doing HIV prevention work with Latinos over the past twenty years has acquainted me with some of the most extraordinary human beings across the country at the intersection of research, practice, administration, community activism and advocacy, compromised health, and death. Mentors who have been central to my development as an HIV prevention researcher include Dr. Barbara Marín from the very beginning, Dr. Rafael Díaz present in the careers of so many Latino scholars, and Dr. Alex Kral who generously taught me the culture of NIH-level grant writing. Special thanks to Maura Roessner, my editor while at Oxford University Press, who supported this book project one hundred percent. Closer to home, heartfelt thanks to my lovely wife, Dr. Pamela Balls Organista, and daughters, Zena Laura and Zara Luz, for their recognition, respect, acceptance, and care.

Contributors

Carmen Albizu-García
Department of Health Services
  Administration and
Center for Evaluation and
  Socio-medical Research
Graduate School of Public Health
University of Puerto Rico
San Juan, Puerto Rico

Hortensia Amaro
Bouvé College of Health Sciences and
  Institute on Urban Health Research
Northeastern University
Boston, Massachusetts

Sonya G. Arreola
Urban Health Program
Research Triangle Institute,
  International
San Francisco, California

George Ayala
Global Forum on MSM & HIV
  (MSMGF)
Oakland, California

Jose Bauermeister
School of Public Health
University of Michigan
Ann Arbor, Michigan

Fernanda T. Bianchi
Department of Psychology
George Washington University
Washington, District of Columbia

Héctor Carrillo
Department of Sociology and Gender
  Studies Program

Northwestern University
Evanston, Illinois

Lina Cherfas
Capacity Building Assistance Program
  Manager
Latino Commission on AIDS
New York, New York

Megan Comfort
Urban Health Program
RTI International
San Francisco, California

Lisa de Saxe Zerden
University of North Carolina
  Chapel Hill
School of Social Work
Chapel Hill, North Carolina

Rafael M. Díaz
Cesar E. Chávez Institute
San Francisco State University
San Francisco, California

Frank Galvan
Bienestar Human Services, Inc.
Los Angeles, California

Vincent Guilamo-Ramos
Silver School of Social Work
New York University
New York, New York

Diana Hernández
Department of Sociomedical Sciences
Columbia University
New York, New York

Jennifer S. Hirsch
Department of Sociomedical Sciences
Mailman School of Public Health
Columbia University
New York, New York

JoAnne Keatley
Center of Excellence for Transgender Health
University of California, San Francisco
San Francisco, California

Patricia Kissinger
Department of Epidemiology
School of Public Health and Tropical Medicine
Tulane University
New Orleans, Louisiana

Alex H. Kral
Research Triangle Institute, International
San Francisco, California

Lisa M. Kuhns
Children's Memorial Hospital
Chicago, Illinois

Haiyan Li
Children's Memorial Hospital
Chicago, Illinois

Lena Lundgren
School of Social Work
Center for Addictions Research and Services
Boston University
Boston, Massachusetts

Luz Marillis López
School of Social Work
Boston University
Boston, Massachusetts

Carlos Molina III
Political Science and Legal Studies
University of California, Berkeley
Berkeley, California

Miguel Muñoz-Laboy
Department of Sociomedical Sciences
Columbia University
New York, New York

Torsten B. Neilands
Department of Medicine
University of California, San Francisco
San Francisco, California

Kurt C. Organista
School of Social Welfare
University of California, Berkeley
Berkeley, California

Thomas M. Painter
Division of HIV/AIDS Prevention
National Center for HIV/AIDS Viral Hepatitis, STD, and TB Prevention
Centers for Disease Control and Prevention
Atlanta, Georgia

Paul J. Poppen
Department of Psychology
George Washington University
Washington, District of Columbia

James Quesada
Department of Anthropology
California State University San Francisco
San Francisco, California

Anita Raj
Division of Global Public Health
Department of Medicine
University of California, San Diego
San Diego, California
and
Department of Medicine
Section of General Internal Medicine
Clinical Addiction Research and Education
Boston University School of Medicine/ Boston Medical Center
Boston, Massachusetts

Jesus Ramirez-Valles
UIC School of Public Health
University of Illinois-Chicago
Chicago, Illinois

Carol A. Reisen
Department of Psychology
George Washington University
Washington, District of Columbia

Scott D. Rhodes
Department of Social Sciences and
    Health Policy
Wake Forest School of Medicine
Winston-Salem, North Carolina

Britt Rios-Ellis
National Council of La Raza/California
    State University
Long Beach, Center for Latino
    Community Health
Long Beach, California

Edgar Rivera Colón
Department of Sociomedical Sciences
Mailman School of Public Health
Columbia University
New York, New York

Timoteo Rodriguez
Department of Anthropology
University of California, Berkeley
Berkeley, California

Sheilla Rodríguez-Madera
Social Sciences and Criminal Justice
    Department
University of Puerto Rico at Carolina
Carolina, Puerto Rico

Jorge Sánchez
Cesar E. Chávez Institute
San Francisco State University
San Francisco, California

Fernando M. Sañudo
Health Promotion Center
Vista Community Clinic
Vista, California

Kurt Schroeder
Cesar E. Chávez Institute
San Francisco State University
San Francisco, California

Michele G. Shedlin
College of Nursing
New York University
New York, New York

Monica D. Ulibarri
Department of Psychiatry
University of California,
    San Diego
San Diego, California

Nelson Varas-Díaz
Center for the Study of Social
    Differences and
Health Graduate School of
    Social Work
University of Puerto Rico
San Juan, Puerto Rico

Emily Vasquez
Department of Sociomedical
    Sciences
Mailman School of Public Health
Columbia University
New York, New York

Miriam Y. Vega
Vice President
Latino Commission on AIDS
New York, New York

Antonia M. Villarruel
School of Nursing
University of Michigan
Ann Arbor, Michigan

Paula A. Worby
Multicultural Institute
Berkeley, California

Maria Cecilia Zea
Department of Psychology
George Washington University
Washington, District of Columbia

Introduction
Kurt C. Organista, Ph.D., Editor

It is often said that the HIV virus knows no borders and does not discriminate because it is an equal opportunity infector. But although this makes sense from a biomedical perspective, even the most cursory examination of infection patterns in the United States leads us to the opposite conclusion: HIV, the virus that causes AIDS, appears to discriminate against the most vulnerable and stigmatized minority populations in society. That is, according to the Centers for Disease Control and Prevention (CDC) (2005), about 75% of AIDS cases in men in the United States are among men who have sex with men (MSM), whereas 50% and 20% of AIDS cases occur in African Americans and Latinos, respectively, despite the fact that these two populations comprise only 13% and 15% of the population, respectively. A breakdown by gender shows that women are primarily infected by male partners, and the rates for women of color are astounding with African-American women 20 times, and Latinas 5 times, more likely to become infected than their white female counterparts. And although research on transgendered people is still scarce, the little that exists indicates alarmingly high rates of HIV infection in male-to-female transgendered people: between 8% and 78%!

But although it would be preposterous to conclude that the HIV virus is homophobic, racist, sexist, or transphobic, we can conclude that HIV/AIDS infection patterns mirror patterns of inequality in the United States on the basis of sexual orientation, race and ethnicity, gender, and gender identity. That is, members of these particular groupings of people are structurally vulnerable to a vast array of socioeconomic, psychosocial, and health disparities, of which HIV/AIDS is one of many serious risks.

Purpose. The purpose of this unique and overdue book project is manifold, with the core goal of disseminating current and original thinking, research, and writing about the growing problem of HIV/AIDS in Latinos in the United States. As such, the book includes some of the most innovative *theorizing* about HIV/AIDS in its social, environmental, and cultural contexts; informative *research* that illuminates various dimensions of HIV risk across various Latino groups and situations; and best and promising *prevention interventions* for decreasing HIV risk in U.S. Latinos at individual, community, and larger structural-environmental levels.

Audience. Addressing Latino psychosocial and health problems requires specialized background knowledge and skills to enhance the awareness and cultural sensitivity of health and social service agencies and providers, researchers, and students in training. The book is intended as a resource and reference for Latino-serving agencies and professionals, the growing number of Latino-focused HIV prevention researchers, and graduate students in helping professions such as public health, mental health, social welfare, and allied fields interested in this topic area.

Background. The problem of HIV/AIDS in U.S. Latinos is a serious and growing one, located at the dynamic and complex intersection of sexual health and behavior, poverty, culture, race/ethnicity, and minority status. As such, HIV/AIDS is both a social and health problem affecting, to various degrees, subgroups of Latinos differing along the lines of gender and gender identity, sexual orientation, age, or immigration status. Because vulnerability to HIV/AIDS increases with stigmatized and discriminated minority status, conflated with low socioeconomic status, it requires us to think comprehensively about structural-environmental, social, and cultural factors that frame the risk for HIV as well as prevention. Such a contextual approach casts HIV/AIDS, as well as our prevention efforts, within broader social, political, and cultural contexts by connecting the roles of macrosocial and environmental forces with formal and informal institutional practices contributing to HIV risk and barriers to effective solutions at individual, community, and societal levels.

BOOK PROJECT ORGANIZATION AND CONTRIBUTIONS

The book is organized around three classic academic domains: Theory, Research, and Practice, because we now have a critical mass of scholars, ongoing research, and published literature to compile such an important presentation of work.

Section I

The book's first major section, *Theorizing HIV Risk in Latinos at the Intersection of Sexual Health, Culture, Poverty, and Minority Status*, contains six chapters by preeminent scholars whose work expands our thinking about the complex causes of HIV risk and needed prevention efforts with various Latino populations. The opening chapter by the editor and his research colleagues features an innovative structural-environmental (SE) model of HIV risk and prevention in Latino day laborers. Chapter 1 serves as an overarching frame for all subsequent chapters, each of which examines its topic in relation to an SE analysis of risk and prevention with Latinos. More needed focus on the context of risk and prevention is reflected in the other five chapters in the book's initial theory-driven section. In Chapter 2, Dr. Jesus Ramirez-Valles and colleagues test their theory that LGBT Latinos can decrease personal HIV risk through HIV/AIDS activism and greater community participation and connectedness. Dr. Héctor Carrillo (Chapter 3) presents a transnational framework for thinking about HIV risk and sexual health by considering Latino migrations and related changes in sexual cultures. The issue of gendered HIV risk in Latinas is revisited by Hortensia Amaro and colleagues, Drs. Monica D. Ulibarri and Anita Raj, in Chapter 4, in which they update Amaro's classic 1995 *American Psychologist* article, "Love, Sex, Power: Considering Women's Realities in HIV Prevention." With regard to HIV prevention with Latino migrant laborers in new growth communities, in Chapter 5 Dr. Scott D. Rhodes illustrates how invaluable community-based participatory research (CBPR) methods are in clarifying links between migrant labor, problem drinking, masculinity, and sexual risk taking, and how especially helpful CBPR is for non-Latino researchers working in Latino communities. Finally, the book's first section ends with Dr. Jennifer S. Hirsch and Emily Vasquez (Chapter 6) drawing upon over 15 years of ethnographic research with Mexican immigrants, on both sides of the border, to describe ways in which migration policy, housing availability, urban development policies, U.S. health insurance reform, enforcement of occupational safety and health regulations, the gendered organization of the U.S. labor market, and how changing patterns of consumption by middle-class Americans are all part of the broader context of HIV risk for Mexican and Latino labor migrants. Germane to this book project, Hirsch argues that the limited impact of most individual and behavioral prevention interventions and the need for scalability demand addressing public health problems at the population level.

Section II

The book's second section, *Illuminating Complex Dimensions of HIV Risk in Diverse Latino Populations, Environments, and Situations*, is made up of eight chapters, each designed to elucidate significant dimensions of HIV risk in various Latino populations and locations. For example, three chapters focus on Latino men who have sex with men (MSM), who continue to bear the major burden of HIV/AIDS among Latinos in the United States. Chapter 7, by Dr. Rafael M. Díaz and colleagues, provides us with a current review of the literature on risk and prevention in Latino MSM, with an emphasis on the roles of inequality and discrimination. Similarly, Chapter 8, by Dr. George Ayala, reports on a mixed-methods analysis of various forms of social discrimination and HIV risk in the lives of Latino and African American MSM. In Chapter 9, Dr. Zea and colleagues also employ mixed research methods to study the situational context of risk and protection in the sexual encounters of MSM among newer Latino groups such as Dominicans, Columbians, and Brazilians. Dr. Rivera Cólon and colleagues, in Chapter 10, provide us with a fascinating study of bisexual male sex markets in New York City, a population and topic too infrequently broached in the Latino HIV literature. Similarly, Latina transgender women and their particular set of risk and prevention-related circumstances are the focus of Chapter 11, by Dr. Frank Galvan and JoAnne Keatley. That Latinos unfortunately continue to fill the ranks of prisons and the criminal justice system in America makes Chapter 12, by Megan Comfort and colleagues, both urgent and innovative for beginning to think about risk and prevention in the context of the prison with its porous boundaries with the Latino community. A fascinating qualitative study by Drs. Rodríguez-Madera and Varas-Díaz gives us rare insights into the lives of serodiscordant heterosexual Puerto Rican couples in Chapter 13. At the end of the book's second section, Drs. Patricia Kissinger and Michelle G. Shedlin describe HIV risk and prevention in mostly Central American migrant day laborers in post-Katrina New Orleans, with an emphasis on the risk networks they encounter and comprise in a new Latino-receiving region of the country (Chapter 14).

Section III

The third and final major section of the book, *Best and Promising HIV Prevention Interventions with Diverse Latino Populations, Locations, and Situations*, contains five chapters that illustrate innovative prevention interventions with some of the most vulnerable and understudied Latino subgroups along the lines of age (youth), gender (girls and women), and occupational status (farmworkers and urban day laborers). Few research and writing publications on HIV and Latinos focus on evidence-based or promising prevention interventions. Thus, the five chapters that make up this final section of the book project are precious contributions.

Drawing upon years of pioneering research and direct service provision, Drs. Antonia M. Villarruel, Vincent Guilamo-Ramos, and Jose Bauermeister describe HIV risk and prevention within an ecodevelopmental perspective to consider both developmentally appropriate and contextually sensitive ways of understanding and reducing HIV risk in young Latinos (Chapter 15). In Chapter 16, Dr. Britt Rios-Ellis describes how she and her research team have broken the silence by facilitating urgently needed dialogue between Latina mothers and adolescent daughters about HIV risk and prevention, and sex more generally, facilitated by the use of *promotoras* and community-based participatory research methods. In Chapter 17, Dr. Miriam Y. Vega and Lina Cherfas provide a timely review and critique of three federally funded community-based outcome studies to prevent HIV in Mexican and Puerto Rican women in three different regions of the country. In Chapter 18, Dr. Painter and colleagues review three published case studies of HIV prevention interventions with both rural farmworkers and urban-based day laborers. And finally, Drs. Lisa de Saxe Zerden, Luz Marilis López, and Lena Lundgren, in Chapter 19, review the literature on the extremely urgent topic of HIV prevention with Puerto Rican injection drug users, one of the most affected groups of Latinos in America.

Most book projects are a labor of love for editors and authors, and this one has been even more than that: after two decades of doing HIV prevention research with Mexican/Latino labor migrants, avidly learning about Latino HIV risk and prevention more generally from my colleagues in the field, and also getting to know, both professionally and personally, most of the committed and caring scholars in the field, I am especially gratified to facilitate the development and dissemination of this timely if not overdue book project. My editor at Oxford University Press, Maura Roessner, was consistently committed and helpful to the project, and all of the authors were exceptionally receptive and responsive to the process. All of the above lifts my confidence that together we will continue to prevent unnecessary suffering and death, partly through the collection of theory, research, and practice-oriented contributions to this book, and partly by inviting Latino and Latino-interested scholars, service providers, persons affected, and other community members to articulate why we believe risk happens in our Latino communities, and the many ways we believe it can (and will) be prevented.

HIV Prevention
with Latinos

Section I
Theorizing HIV Risk in Latinos at the Intersection of Sexual Health, Culture, Poverty, and Minority Status

1 The Urgent Need for Structural-Environmental Models of HIV Risk and Prevention in U.S. Latino Populations

The Case of Migrant Day Laborers

Kurt C. Organista, Paula A. Worby, James Quesada, Alex H. Kral, Rafael M. Díaz, Torsten B. Neilands, and Sonya G. Arreola

INTRODUCTION

"But sometimes it is difficult to get work and then the desperation, the loneliness that one finds in this country! . . . Sometimes you have no friends, nobody to talk with. You are all alone . . ."
–(Organista et al., 2006)

"There are guys who lose morale, you understand? The only thing they do is drink, smoke marijuana. Why? To forget, you know, to forget a little while that they have problems because everyone has a bunch of problems—pay the rent, pay the bills, send money to Mexico."
–(Worby, 2007)

". . . The issue of women and sex—like family and longing for home—is at the heart of most conversations on the [day labor site street] corner . . ."
–(Ordoñze, 2010)

The purpose of this opening chapter by the book editor and his research colleagues is to provide direction for an urgently needed paradigm shift in HIV prevention science by articulating a broader and more comprehensive model of HIV risk and prevention for U.S. Latino populations. This model, termed *structural-environmental* (SE), is designed to contextualize behavioral risk for HIV by considering the relations between structurally induced *environmental* factors (i.e., living and working conditions), their *individual* level impacts (e.g., mental and physical health), and *behavioral* HIV risk, as mediated by *situational* factors frequently encountered by members of various Latino populations and subgroups. In other words, both vulnerability and resilience to HIV transmission are not simply a matter of behavior but also of situational factors that make up the context that facilitates or inhibits specific risk behaviors. Such situational factors (e.g., interpersonal, economic, alcohol, and substance related) dynamically interact with individual factors (e.g., psychological distress, self-efficacy) to produce varying levels of risk. In turn, situational and individual factors are a function of environmental factors that are produced and reproduced by structural factors operating at the macrosocietal level. A concrete example is evidenced by labor markets structured so that predominantly undocumented and low-paid workers comprise the core work force. In turn, the behavioral choices of such workers are shaped by limited social networks and resources to which they have access.

The major advantage of an SE analysis is that it allows us to shift our attention from solely individual risk behaviors to situations that heighten risk, as well as the living and working conditions that reproduce these risky situations frequently encountered by members of a particular Latino population. And although somewhat abstract, figuring out the key SE factors related to HIV risk and prevention is facilitated by focusing on a particular population of Latinos within a particular geography and social setting. Thus although the SE model described in this chapter is intended to be applied to U.S. Latinos generally, it is illustrated with Latino migrant day laborers (LMDLs) in the San Francisco Bay Area as the case study. Migrant laborers such as farmworkers and day laborers in particular are a population of interest given the high identification of their occupations with Latinos, the multiple ways such workers are marginalized in society, and the availability and unrealized potential of community and culture-based resources that could improve their health and well being, and in particular decrease their chances of HIV risk and related psychosocial and health problems.

LATINO MIGRANT DAY LABORERS

HIV risk behaviors among LMDLs and the hardships they face are well documented. However, there is little research linking how the former is shaped by the latter or how interventions at structural-environmental levels could potentially influence individual behavior. This chapter attempts to describe the SE context of sexual HIV risk in LMDLs, emphasizing alcohol-related situations as a mediator of the relation between environmental and individual factors and sexual risk behavior. The sections below (1) define LMDLs, (2) review the literature on HIV risk and alcohol use in Latino labor migrants in general, and (3) review the literature on environmental, individual, and situational factors that contribute to alcohol-related sexual HIV risk.

Valenzuela (2003) notes that although the U.S. Bureau of Labor Statistics has tried to document the prevalence of day labor, no standardized definition exists. His research documents the day labor market that is characterized by informal or nonstandard work performed mostly by poor foreign-born Latino migrant men who congregate in "open air" markets (e.g., street corners) to solicit temporary work. In their 2005 National Day Labor Survey (NDLS), Valenzuela, Theodore, Melendez, and Gonzalez (2006) estimated that on any given day over 117,000 day laborers were seeking work or working in the United States. Day laborers were found predominantly in the West (42%), followed by the East (23%), Southwest (18%), South (12%), and Midwest (4%). Although a few centers have emerged to help support LMDLs, 80% seek work at informal hiring sites where they are employed mostly by homeowners/renters (49%) and construction contractors (43%) to perform construction, landscaping and gardening, painting, roofing, and drywall installation. The NDLS confirms that LMDLs are almost all male, predominantly born in Mexico (59%) and Central America (28%), and that most are undocumented (75%), with U.S. citizens comprising only 7%. In California, the number of undocumented LMDLs is presumed to be higher; in Valenzuela's 1999 (2000) survey of 481 male LMDLs in California, he found that they were predominantly Mexican (77%) and Central American (20%), that 84% were undocumented, 53% had been in the United States for less than 5 years, they were 34 years of age on average, that 50% had a spouse or partner, and that they had 7 years of education on average. Thus, we define day laborers as predominantly foreign-born, Spanish-speaking, undocumented, male Latinos performing day labor as a main source of income.

RISK FOR HIV AND PROBLEM DRINKING IN LATINO LABOR MIGRANTS IN GENERAL

Reviews of the literature on male Latino labor migrants, of which day laborers are a subgroup, and their HIV risk (Organista & Balls Organista, 1997; Organista et al., 2004) and alcohol use (Worby & Organista, 2007), document high numbers of sex partners in the United States, sex with female sex workers, sex between men, low levels of condom use, high levels of sexually transmitted diseases (STDs), and high levels of drinking that cooccur with sexual activity. Comprehensive data are lacking given that risk surveillance data are scarce, but no study to date has documented a high prevalence or incidence of HIV among the Latino labor migrant population. However, numerous HIV risk factors and behaviors, as well as impoverished migrant-related living and working conditions, suggest that if HIV or other STDs were to enter the sexual networks of particular groups of labor migrants, the likelihood of an epidemic would be high. For example, an outbreak of chancroid among 266 Latino labor migrants was reported during a 2-year period at a California STD clinic as compared to zero cases the year prior (Blackmore et al., 1985). It was concluded that these men were having sex with the same six infected female sex workers.

Results from the first multistage probability survey of migration on the U.S.–Mexico border also found no HIV infection in over 1000 migrants administered the oral HIV antibody test (Martínez-Donate et al., 2005). However, the second report from this survey ($N = 1606$) documented HIV risk behaviors in four migrant subgroups: undocumented deportees, voluntary returnees from the United States, arrivals to the border from other parts of the border region, and arrivals from sending Mexican communities farther from the border: Unprotected heterosexual relations with regular and casual partners, including sex workers, were found in all four migrant groups (Rangel et al., 2006). Sex with injection drug users, sex workers, and multiple partners was higher in migrants returning from the United States and in those from other border regions as compared to migrants from sending communities in Mexico en route to the United States. This suggests that there are characteristics of the particular environments encountered by migrants in the United States or in border regions that are facilitating risk behaviors or otherwise heightening risk.

Borges et al. (2009) found a similar pattern of greater risk for alcohol and substance use, including risk for substance use disorders, in migrants returning from the United States as compared to their nonmigrant counterparts, in a cross-sectional survey of three urban areas in Northern Mexico that included large border cities such as Tijuana and Ciudad Juarez. Correlates of substance use in migrants included length of time in the United States, experience of discrimination, and working in the service sector and in agricultural labor.

Missing from the literature is any examination of how migration-related environments, especially those in the United States, contribute to risk. One small survey of 102 LMDLs in the San Francisco Bay Area documents alcohol-related sexual HIV risk: over half the men were sexually active with women, evenly divided into regular sex partners (including spouses) and one-time-only sex partners (including sex workers) (Organista & Kubo, 2005). Participants generally did not carry condoms, knowledge of condom use was poor, and actual use was infrequent. High proportions of alcohol use and binge drinking that cooccur with sexual activities were reported. Although LMDLs in this study reported no HIV infection, a third reported a history of STDs, similar to the 40% prevalence reported by 290 LMDLs also surveyed in a subsequent study (Ehrlich et al., 2007). These lifetime prevalence of STDs contrast with the only point prevalence assessment in LMDLs by Wong et al. (2003), who screened a San Francisco sample and found one positive syphilis diagnosis (0.4%) among the 235 screened, one (0.5%) case of gonorrhea, and seven (3.5%) cases of Chlamydia among the 198 screened for these two conditions. A study of 180 LMDLs in post-Hurricane Katrina New Orleans similarly found five positive cases of Chlamydia (2.8%), but also a 10% proportion of self-reported history of HIV (Kissinger et al., 2008). Although not derived through testing, the latter is the highest proportion of HIV infection in LMDLs reported to date. With regard to risk factors, this New Orleans sample reported high proportions of drinking during the past week (75%), including binge drinking in two-thirds of those reporting drinking. Nearly 75% reported sexual activity with high-risk partners, mostly with female sex workers, with 50% reporting inconsistent condom use. The above studies suggest that sexual risk in LMDLs is related to migration-related environmental circumstances most likely mediated by participation in alcohol-related situations. Predominantly Honduran day laborers in New Orleans are revisited in Chapter 14 in which Kissinger and Shedlin share findings from their analysis of risk networks in this new Latino immigrant growth setting.

The prevalence of alcohol use or problem drinking has rarely been documented for LMDLs specifically. The above cited survey of 102 LMDLs in the Bay Area found that seven beers was the average number of drinks per sitting, with a weekly average of more than 16 drinks, and that sexual relations typically cooccurred with drinking (Organista & Kubo, 2005). Walter et al. (2004) conducted an ethnographic study of 40 LMDLs in San Francisco, including injured workers, and found that substance abuse and dependence accompanied injury, depression, anxiety, and *nervios* [nerves]. Epidemiological research has documented alcohol use among Mexican-origin farmworkers in California. The Mexican American Population Prevalence Survey (MAPPS) assessed diagnosable mental disorders in Fresno County, California, in 3012 Mexican-origin urban and rural men and women, more than half of them Mexicans that migrated as adults to work in the United States ($N = 1,576$). The MAPPS also included an additional sample made up only of farmworkers ($N = 1001$) (Alderete et al., 2000; Finch et al., 2003; Vega et al., 1998). These MAPPS data show that among the 500 male farmworkers, almost 10% had a lifetime prevalence of alcohol dependency or abuse (Alderete et al., 2000). Another MAPPS report by Finch et al. (2003), examining the 1576 Mexican male and female adults that had migrated to work in the United States, found that those reporting discrimination at work had higher proportions of alcohol abuse and dependence than those not reporting this problem. Although an imperfect proxy for LMDLs, research on Latino farmworkers provides insight into risk for LMDLs given the overlap in harsh migration-related living and working conditions.

Ethnographic studies of Mexican farmworkers in migrant camps in the 1990s documented high volume consumption on weekends: in a migrant housing center in Northern California, the mean consumption was 10 beers per individual per episode, with a range from 6 to 24 beers (Alaniz, 1994). Survey research on a Mexico-based sample of men that had worked in U.S. agriculture found 13% to be heavy drinkers, consuming alcohol 6–7 days per week for a total average of 21 drinks per week (Mines et al., 2001). The above suggests an urgent need to document relations between work-related factors and alcohol-related situations linked to HIV risk, by combining ethnographic and quantitative methods to develop SE models of risk and resilience in Latino labor migrant populations.

DEFINING THE STRUCTURAL-ENVIRONMENTAL CONTEXT OF BEHAVIORAL HIV RISK IN LMDLs

Gaps in the literature include a compelling lack of information about the context of risk, or how SE factors, such as the harsh living and working conditions that characterize labor migration, are related to situations that place LMDLs at alcohol-related sexual HIV risk. In this section, we review the literature on migration-related environmental factors and consequent psychological distress in Latino labor migrants that we believe constitute a preliminary list of environmental, including structural and situational, and individual factors connected to alcohol-related sexual HIV risk in need of further research.

Environmental Factors

Work-Related Stress

Given the primacy of working and earning money in the lives of LMDLs, it is imperative that we study how stressful working conditions relate to psychological distress and risk for alcohol-related sexual HIV. Data from the NDLS (Valenzuela et al., 2006) showed that day labor pays poorly because work instability results in volatile monthly earnings. At the time of that study, monthly earnings ranged from $1400 a month during peak periods to below $500 during bad months. Valenzuela et al. (2006) calculate that it is unlikely that annual incomes exceeded $15,000, a figure not only below the federal poverty threshold, but an amount further eroded by the economic downturn that continued through the end of the 2000–2010 decade. NDLS findings also show that LMDLs commonly suffer employer abuses such as wage theft (almost 50% reported at least one experience with being underpaid or unpaid) and being denied food and water breaks.

Results from the survey of 102 LMDLs in the San Francisco Bay Area (Organista & Kubo, 2005) found that day laborers' primary concerns centered on unemployment, underemployment, and lack of money. Work injury also needs to be studied given its prevalence and impact on earnings and mental health. For example, 20% of NDLS participants reported work-related injuries with most receiving no medical attention (Valenzuela et al., 2006). An ethnographic study in San Francisco of LMDLs found chronic anxiety about the potential for injury given work characterized by inadequate safety equipment, lack of training, yet economic pressures to take dangerous chances. Interestingly, when injury occurred, it was usually internalized as a personal failure to fulfill one's role as a man and provider for one's family, thus leading to shame and depression that inhibited communication with families (Walter et al., 2002). Rhodes et al. (2009) also reported threats to masculinity resulting from economic hardship and not being able to send money home in migrant workers in the Southeastern United States engaging in risky behaviors. Chapter 5 features more work by Scott Rhodes who uses community-based participatory research methods to link alcohol, masculinity, and sexual risk taking in Northern Carolina.

Prolonged Separation from Home and Family

Months and even years of painful separation from home and family has become the norm for Latino labor migrants. For example, qualitative interviews with 75 farmworkers found that separation from friends and family was the most commonly perceived stressor, followed by rigid work demands, unpredictable work, uprooting/frequent moves, little money for family/living in poverty/receiving poor pay, and poor housing. Separation from home and family has become exacerbated over the past 15 years with the advent of restrictive immigration and border control policies making it so difficult, dangerous, and expensive to cross the border that migrants now remain far longer in the United States than desired (Massey et al., 2002). In a small qualitative study of nine migrant men in the Southeastern United States, Rhodes et al. (2009) found that alcohol and sexual risk behaviors were partly attributed to feeling distant from home and family and powerless to do much about it given extremely restrictive border control.

Substandard Housing and Homelessness

Descriptions of labor migrant housing are consistent in depicting substandard living conditions in labor camps and farms with makeshift housing or none at all. Housing for day laborers frequently consists of single rooms in boarding houses, apartments, or garages that are overcrowded with other workers pooling resources to cover expenses or each charged separate rent by property owners interested in maximizing profit (Quesada, 1999). Substandard housing and the constant threat of homelessness potentially are related to problem drinking and risky sex and represent compelling environmental factors that warrant exploration. For example, Denner, Organista, Dupree, and Thrush (2005) studied a sample of marginally housed and homeless Latino migrants in Northern California and found high levels of risk: 28% injection drug users, 21% engaged in sex work, and 27% MSM with inconsistent protection. A study specific to the phenomenon of day laborers being solicited on the street by men wanting to pay for sex uncovered the frequency with which day laborers in Los Angeles were approached, and documented that at least some turn to this option as a way to make money or gain other resources (Galvan et al., 2008).

Social Stigma, Discrimination, and Isolation

The experiences of stigma and discrimination related to being an undocumented Latino need to be studied for their probable relation to alienation and isolation. NDLS findings show that 20% of LMDLs report being insulted by merchants, and 15% report being refused services by local businesses. LMDLs in the NDLS also reported being arrested (9%) and cited by police (11%) while searching for work. After economic concerns, "sadness" and "racism" were the next most frequently encountered problems reported by Bay Area LMDLs (Organista & Kubo, 2005). Sixty percent of New York City undocumented Mexican immigrants in a recent study (N = 505) reported experiencing discrimination; 25% of the sample had participated in day labor in the previous 6 months (Nandi et al., 2008). The intensity of stigma related to being undocumented or an "illegal alien," as it is commonly referred to, continues to intensify unabated.

Lack of Social, Recreational, and Romantic Outlets

High proportions of unprotected sex with female sex workers among Latino labor migrants in the United States are well documented. For example, Organista et al. (1997) found that 44% of 342 Mexican migrants reported sex with sex workers in the United States, married as well as single men. In a small HIV prevention study with LMDLs, men reported the frequent need to relieve the desire for sex with female sex workers and being frequently being solicited by them (Organista et al., 2006). Such sexual relations appear to be common among labor migrants yet the specifics of how LMDLs succumb to or resist such risky sex, or why they use or do not use protection, need to be studied. Furthermore, LMDLs in the same prevention study (Organista et al., 2006) also expressed a desire for romantic relationships with *amantes* [lovers], but also noted that being undocumented and not knowing local social and cultural protocols inhibit pursuing such relationships and exacerbate sexual frustration.

Individual Factors

Desesperación [Desperation]

In the aforementioned survey of 102 LMDLs in the Bay Area (Organista et al., 2006), it was found that frequent unemployment and underemployment can result in a state of distress that some referred to as *desesperación* [desperation]. Participants described *desesperación* as interfering with their main goals of working to send money home, and as leading to participation in *vicios* [vices] such as excessive drinking, occasional drug use, and sex with female sex workers. Latino migrants in New York used the term *desesperación* to describe frustration resulting from social isolation and not knowing local laws or acceptable behavior (Shedlin et al., 2005, 2006). To explore how this seemingly culture-based form of distress results from harsh migration-related factors, and how it is linked to alcohol-related sexual HIV risk, careful inquiry into its meaning is needed (e.g., during participant observation and in-depth ethnographic interviews). In research currently underway, we are trying to determine if a construct of *desesperación* can be developed that is distinct from other forms of psychological distress that can be included in our SE model.

Psychological Distress

A pair of small studies, focusing on stress and coping in Mexican farmworkers, link migrant-related stressors to psychological distress. The first study examined farm work-related predictors of depression and anxiety in 45 farmworkers and found that 38% met the cut off for depression while 30% met the cut off for anxiety as compared to normative scores of 20% and 16%, respectively, in the general population

(Hovey & Magaña, 2000). In this study, anxiety and depression were predicted by acculturative stress (stressful experiences related to the immigrant experience), low control over the decision to live a migrant farmworker lifestyle, poor social support, family dysfunction, low self-esteem, and low religiosity. The second study of 75 farmworkers found that the most commonly perceived stressors were separation from friends/family, rigid work demands, unpredictable work, uprooting, low money for family/living in poverty/receiving poor pay, and poor housing (Magaña & Hovey, 2003). Anxiety was predicted by rigid work demands and poor housing while depression was predicted by rigid work demands and little money for family.

High rates of major depression and anxiety disorders in farmworkers were also documented in the MAPPS. Both male and female farmworkers had a high lifetime prevalence of mood (7.2% and 6.7%, respectively) and anxiety disorders (15.1% and 12.9%, respectively) (Alderete et al., 2000). These proportions are higher than those of Mexico-based counterparts and the gender pattern contradicts U.S. population studies that consistently document greater mood and anxiety disorders in women versus men, thus implicating the stress of a migratory lifestyle on farmworker men. Muñoz-Laboy, Hirsch, and Quispe-Lazaro (2009) studied loneliness in 50 Mexican migrant workers in New York City and found that it strongly correlated with sexual risk behaviors. Over a third of the sample reported high levels of loneliness and ethnographic observations revealed loneliness to be a dominant theme with which the men coped either by going to bars and dance halls or to church. With regard to sexual risk taking, it was concluded that loneliness can engender an indifference to health that we find consistent with the "I don't care any more" attitude of LMDLs connecting *desesperación* to problem drinking and sexual risk taking.

Deeper insight into the stress of being separated from families is provided by a study of 60 male Latino farmworkers in North Carolina, each with a wife and children in their country of origin, in which it was found that symptoms of anxiety were related to the ambivalence inherent in trying to support one's family financially while feeling irresponsible as an absent husband and father (Grzywacz et al., 2006). When farmworkers in this study were asked how they coped with separation from home/family, they reported calling family on the phone and writing letters. However, it is not known how frequent and effective such forms of coping were for the farmworkers in the study or for LMDLs for whom the above stressors are highly relevant and warrant further exploration.

Resilience

While distress in Latino labor migrants is well documented, how some cope effectively with migration-related environmental stressors has not been documented. Thus, there is a considerable need to study resilience in LMDLs, with regard to the environmental factors listed above, by exploring it at environmental (e.g., community and culture-based formal and informal supports), individual (e.g., English proficiency, marketable work skills, social networks), and situational levels (e.g., coping with stress).

Situational Factors That Mediate the Relation between Environmental and Individual Factors: The Role of Alcohol

Research on alcohol-related situations associated with sexual HIV risk has been extremely limited. Our previous research with LMDLs shows that average number of drinks per week (i.e., 16) and per sitting (i.e., 7) are high and co-occur with sexual relations (Organista & Kubo, 2005). We also found that stress related to lack of work can prompt an attitude of "I don't care anymore" leading to heavy drinking or drug use (Organista et al., 2006). Research also documents the day laborers' explanation of heavy alcohol use as a reaction to insufficient work and economic woes, sometimes leading to monthly binges (Walter, 2000; Worby, 2007). A review of the literature on alcohol use in Latino labor migrants shows that illicit substance use appears to be less of an issue relative to alcohol (Worby & Organista, 2007), although such patterns could change rapidly in an urban environment where low-cost illicit drugs may penetrate new groups of consumers among the urban poor (Hernández et al., 2009). Thus, while alcohol is the primary substance consumed among Latino labor migrants, there is also need to study illicit substance use to further identify the mediation effects of substance-related situations in the relation between sexual HIV risk and environmental and individual factors.

TOWARD THE DEVELOPMENT OF A STRUCTURAL-ENVIRONMENTAL MODEL OF HIV RISK AND PREVENTION IN LMDLs

The role of environmental factors and consequent psychological distress in the production of alcohol-related sexual HIV risk in Latino labor migrants appears considerable, yet no such theoretical perspective or prevention effort has been developed. A review of the literature on HIV prevention with Mexican labor migrants (Organista et al., 2004) found only four small studies of individual behavioral risk, and concludes that that there is urgent need for models that transcend a sole focus on the behavioral science model of HIV risk and prevention. A review of the literature on alcohol use in Latino labor migrants found only a few brief descriptions of programs addressing this issue, all of which lacked evaluation (Worby & Organista, 2007).

Our SE model of alcohol-related sexual HIV risk in LMDLs situates individual risk within harsh living and working conditions that produce psychological distress, which in turn increases participation in alcohol-related situations in which safer sex is difficult to practice. Two highly relevant models of HIV causation and prevention inform our SE model. The first is a descriptive social-ecological model by Sweat and Dennison (1995) that uses labor migrants as the example with which to illustrate how individual level factors are embedded within environmental and structural levels (see Table 1.1). This model helped us to frame and articulate many of the risk and prevention factors at different levels that we have studied in LMDLs. The model also helps visualize which factors might cut across levels and which are the most feasible to study and alter through interventions. For example, the following socio-ecological levels defined by Sweat and Dennison are applied to labor migrants in ways consistent with our research with this population: (1) *superstructural factors* refer to macrosocial and political arrangements, resources, and power differences that result in unequal advantages between groups both within the United States as well as between the United States and Latino migrant-sending countries. In this sense, structural vulnerability in Mexican labor migrants is rooted in the contradiction between increasingly restrictive U.S. immigration policies despite increasingly open integration of the United States and Mexican economies as formalized by the North American Free Trade Agreement (NAFTA) treaty of 1994. That is, unprecedented U.S. economic penetration into Mexico exacerbates regional economic instability and displaces hundreds of thousands of workers, propelling labor migration to the United States (Massey et al., 2002); (2) *structural* factors involve laws, social policies, and standard ways of operating (e.g., predominance of undocumented workers in certain industries and occupations, ineligibility for social services, persecutory laws); (3) *environmental* factors include harsh living and working conditions (e.g., underemployment, separation from home/family, inadequate housing); and (4) *individual* factors include how the environment is experienced and acted upon (e.g., psychological distress, stigma and discrimination, few outlets for romantic and sexual human companionship, maladaptive and resilient coping responses). Jennifer S. Hirsch and Emily Vasquez also articulate a multisectorial approach to understanding HIV risk and prevention in Mexican immigrants in Chapter 6.

Implicit in Table 1.1 are linkages between multiple levels of HIV causation and prevention, most directly between environmental and individual levels or precisely

Table 1.1 Levels of Causation for HIV Incidence

Definition	Examples	Change Mechanism
Macrosocial and political arrangements, resources, and power differences that result in unequal advantages	Economic underdevelopment, declining agricultural economy, poverty, sexism, homophobia, Western domination, imperialism	National and international social movements, revolution, land redistribution, war, empowerment of disenfranchised populations
Laws, policies, and standard operating procedures	Unregulated commercial sex, bachelor wage system, no family housing required at worksites, lack of human rights laws, no financial support for social services	Legislative lobbying, civil and human rights activism, boycotts, constitutional and legal reform, voting, political pressure, structural adjustment policies by international donors
Individual living conditions, resources and opportunities, recognition of individual, structural and superstructural factors	Work camps with many single men and few women, few condoms, high prevalence of HIV/sexually transmitted disease, family far away, few job opportunities, few social services, failing agricultural economy, industrialization and urbanization	Community organization, provision of social services, legal action, unionization, enforcement of laws
How the environment is experienced and acted upon by individuals	Loneliness, boredom, lack of knowledge, low risk perception, sexual urges, moral values, perceived self-efficacy, perceived locus of control	Education, provision of information, improved self-efficacy, rewards and punishment, counseling

From: Sweat and Denison (1995). Reproduced with permission from Lippincott Williams & Wilkins.

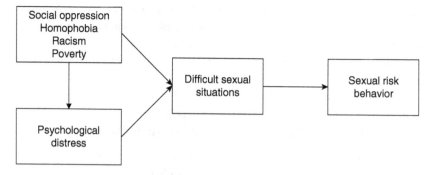

FIGURE 1.1 Model on the effects of social oppression on HIV sexual risk behavior. From Diaz et al. (2004, p. 257). Reproduced with permission from the American Psychological Association.

those closest to our ability to research. By studying factors that mediate the relation between environmental and individual factors, we can make explicit situational factors not detailed in Table 1.1 that link these factors in unique ways for LMDLs.

Another informative framework is Rafael Diaz's empirically derived model (Diaz et al., 2004), demonstrating sexual HIV risk in predominantly immigrant Latino men who have sex with men (MSM) who face many of the same social and environmental conditions as LMDLs (i.e., poverty, migration, social stigma, and discrimination). In fact, Diaz's model demonstrated that various forms of oppression lead to psychological distress that increased sexual HIV risk by increasing participation in substance-related situations that undermined safer sex (see Figure 1.1). Although we expect environmental, individual, and situational factors to differ for LMDLs (e.g., greater alcohol than substance-related situations), the basic associations demonstrated in Diaz's model are precisely those that need to be studied with other Latino populations. Thus, Diaz's model provides evidence that contextual models of HIV risk and prevention can be developed and tested with marginalized Latino populations (see Chapter 7 by Diaz and colleagues for an updated review of the literature on inequality, discrimination, and HIV risk in Latino gay men).

Analogous to Diaz's model, we posit a model of sexual HIV risk in LMDLs that shows how harsh migration-related environmental factors (e.g., work-related stress) result in psychological distress that increases participation in alcohol-related situations in which it is difficult to practice safer sex.

Pushing the Envelope of Contemporary HIV Prevention Science

Our continuing overreliance on behavioral models of HIV risk and prevention can be remedied by pushing the envelope of current prevention science by developing and testing SE models that articulate key environmental, individual, and situational factors related to HIV risk in different Latino populations. Through rigorous research, SE model development and testing can help us more precisely articulate SE vulnerability for Latino groups and subgroups struggling with HIV prevention. Such research provides a rare opportunity for Latino communities, including those directly affected by HIV risk, to test out and refine population-specific theories and models of risk and prevention, thereby using research to facilitate knowledge generation and prevention implications in Latino communities. In the case of LMDLs, an SE model such as the one proposed below has the potential to inform recommendations for feasible and acceptable SE interventions to decrease alcohol-related sexual HIV risk by making migration-related environments less harsh and psychologically distressing, and by marshalling the community and cultural-based resources necessary to buffer stress and enable better coping with HIV risk at the individual level.

A STRUCTURAL-ENVIRONMENTAL MODEL OF ALCOHOL-RELATED SEXUAL HIV RISK IN LMDLs

In research underway by us we plan to develop and test an SE model of alcohol-related sexual HIV risk and prevention in LMDLs that explores how harsh migration-related environmental factors (e.g., work-related poverty, separation from home/family) can result in distress at the individual level (e.g., *desesperación*, loneliness, boredom) that can increase participation in a variety of risky alcohol-related situations in which it is difficult to practice safer sexual behavior (see Figure 1.2). Although we conceptualize the structural vulnerability of Latino labor migrants as rooted in migration-related superstructural and structural factors as defined and illustrated by Sweat and Dennison (see Table 1.1), such macrolevel factors require macrolevel analysis and interventions (e.g., immigration, labor, and global economic policy reform) beyond the reach of community-level interventions. However, it is feasible to study the harsh migration-related environments that are reproduced by structural factors, how such environments are experienced and acted upon at the individual level, and how specific environmental-level and individual-level factors combine to result in HIV risk or resilience in a specific population (LMDLs) and geographic setting (e.g., San Francisco Bay Area).

Missing from Sweat and Dennison's model is any description of which key environmental and individual factors, separately or combined, result in behavioral risk and resilience. Also missing is attention to the situational contexts in which environmental and individual factors dynamically interact and relate to risk and or resilience. Thus the proposed model draws upon Diaz's empirical model of substance-related sexual HIV risk in predominantly immigrant Latino MSM in which it was demonstrated that oppressive factors in the social environment can lead to psychological distress, which in turn increased sexual risk by increasing participation in substance use-related situations in which it was difficult to practice

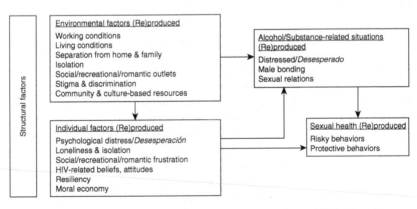

FIGURE 1.2 Structural-environmental model of alcohol-related sexual HIV risk and prevention in LMDLs.

safe sex (see Figure 1.1). Analogously, the proposed model posits that the relations between sexual HIV risk outcome and environmental and individual explanatory factors are mediated by participation in primarily alcohol-related, and secondarily substance-related, situations in which safer sex is less likely (Figure 1.2).

Although it is beyond the scope of this chapter to describe detailed research methods, the design follows a mixed methods approach that deploys qualitative and quantitative methods both sequentially and concurrently. To develop and test our SE model, the research plan includes a first phase of data collection through extensive participant observation ethnography, including in-depth interviews with a purposive sample of LMDLs with the major objective of providing thick, rich descriptions of the constructs that will populate our model (i.e., mostly a mix of those variables listed in the model and some yet to emerge). Such qualitative data are necessary to inform the development of the quantitative survey instrument needed to empirically test the theoretical SE model.

To make the cross-sectional study sufficiently robust, the survey will be administered to a large enough sample of LMDLs (e.g., 300) that will be recruited using time-location sampling (TLS) at all active outdoor day laborer hiring sites in the cities of San Francisco and Berkeley. Methods to classify the sizes of each hiring site and how to use time intervals within which to randomly sample participants will be based on the sampling techniques used by Valenzuela et al. (2006) in the NDLS. The results of empirical model testing combined with ongoing qualitative research will generate recommendations for SE prevention interventions, including possibly scaling-up existing community and culture-based resources and activities that LMDLs find helpful, with the potential to reduce risk by making migrant environments less harsh and distressing, and by enhancing coping at the individual level with alcohol-related situations in which sexual HIV risk can be difficult to avoid.

The outcome variables, independent variables (environmental and individual), and mediating (situational) variables suggested by the model and to be explored through the proposed research project are shown in Figure 1.2 and are as follows.

Sexual Risk Outcome Variables

Sexual risk outcome will be assessed using already developed and culturally appropriate behavioral measures of sexual HIV risk with analyses focused primarily on four behavioral outcomes: (1) any unprotected vaginal sex in the past 6 months, (2) any unprotected anal sex in the past 6 months, (3) sex immediately following alcohol consumption in the past 6 months, and (4) more than one sexual partner in the past 6 months. These behavioral outcomes focus specifically on risk behaviors that may cause transmission of HIV/STDs and are common to epidemiological research. The 6-month timeframe allows adequate recall of sexual behaviors without affecting accuracy, and is the standard used in this research area. Sexual behaviors will be queried by partner type (steady, paying, casual/anonymous).

Independent Variables

Environmental: (1) Work-related stress due to unemployment and underemployment, as well as the threat of physical injury, all related to psychological distress (Walter et al., 2004, 2002), (2) separation from home/family shown in the literature to be related to psychological distress in Latino farmworkers (Hovey & Magaña, 2003; Magana & Hovey, 2003; Organista et al., 2004) and multiple sex partners including sex workers (Duke & Gómez Carpinteiro, 2009; Viadro & Earp, 2000), (3) substandard housing and homelessness related to risk for HIV and alcohol and substance use in farmworkers (Denner et al., 2005), (4) social stigma and discrimination as documented in the NDLS (Valenzuela et al., 2006), and (5) lack of social/recreational/romantic outlets related to risky sex with sex workers on the part of LMDLs (Organista et al., 2006) and Latino labor migrants generally (Organista et al., 1997, 2004).

Individual: (1) *Desesperación* or what appears to be a culture-bound syndrome related to an "I don't care anymore" attitude leading to careless participation in risk taking with alcohol, drugs, and unprotected sex with sex workers in LMDLs (Organista et al., 2006), and also related to feeling socially isolated in urban-based Latino labor migrants in general (Shedlin et al., 2006), and (2) psychological distress found to be related to insecurity about too little work and the threat of work injury in LMDLs, and to separation from home/family in farmworkers (Hovey & Magaña, 2000; Magana & Hovey, 2003). We will explore undocumented factors such as resilience, frustration from lack of social, recreational, and romantic outlets, as well as how the stigma of being undocumented is experienced.

Mediating Situational Variables

The following risky alcohol-related situations will be examined along with others emerging from the ethnography for their potential role in mediating the relation between the above independent and sexual risk outcome variables: (1) drinking in response to psychological distress and negative mood states, (2) drinking as a way of male bonding, and (3) drinking with easy access to sex partners such as sex workers, other men, and transgendered persons. In a model as complex as the one proposed, statistical methods such as structural equation modeling represents an appropriate choice of assessing the significance of relations between all of the above categories of variables, with special emphasis on testing our hypothesis that involvement in alcohol-related situations mediates the relation between environmental and individual level factors and sexual risk outcome. Given the potential mediating effects of illicit substances in our model, we plan to measure those most associated with LMDLs: cocaine, methamphetamine, and heroin measured by frequency of use and quantity ingested within the past 30-day period. Not only will the testing and development of the SE model deepen our understanding of the complex, multilevel context of HIV risk, but the results of such a model can also be used to make strong recommendations for SE prevention interventions aimed not at individual behaviors, but at living and working conditions that reproduce risk situations that compete with individual level prevention knowledge, skills, and intentions.

IMPLICATIONS FOR STRUCTURAL-ENVIRONMENTAL PREVENTION INTERVENTIONS FOR LMDLs

We believe that Latino community and culture-based resources that decrease the harshness of migration-related living and working conditions, and their psychologically distressing impacts, have the potential to also decrease participation in and/or improve individual coping with alcohol-related risky sexual situations frequently encountered by LMDLs. Furthermore, the proposed research on SE model development and testing has the potential to help us identify what is, is not, and could be effective in preventing HIV in LMDLs. That is, model results could help inform strong recommendations for SE prevention interventions. For example, such recommendations could include scaling-up existing community and culture-based resources, endorsed by LMDLs as helpful by making them more widely available and systematically implemented, as well as replicating them in other locations as needed. Furthermore, results of the proposed study could also shed new insights into supporting individual level efforts that LMDLs use successfully to prevent HIV risk and problem drinking.

Below are several possible examples of SE HIV prevention interventions, divided into community and culture based, that seem to mitigate the negative environmental and individual level factors listed in our model, and that will be fleshed out by our proposed study. It is worth noting here that when grant reviewers read such examples of interventions for SE prevention in our proposal, they accuse our research team of knowing in advance what we were planning to explore in our SE model development and testing. The reviewers were half right in the sense that we do have a good sense, after years of research, of the kinds of community-based and culture-based resources that seem to protect these men from engaging in risky situations reproduced by structurally induced harsh environmental conditions. On the other hand, our hunches need to be rigorously researched and we fully expect to find implications for other SE recommendations that we have not yet anticipated.

While separated into community-based and culture-based SE prevention interventions below, we envision both types as overlapping and mutually enforcing, and as part of a health engendering socioecological environment that our proposed model attempts to capture for the particular Latino population and geographic location under study.

Community-Based Resources

Sanctuary Cities

At the macrostructural city-wide level, cities offering some sort of "sanctuary" for immigrants, such as those in the San Francisco Bay Area, represent a broad way of mitigating harsh social and physical environments and reducing individual level distress related to stigma, discrimination, and persecution. Sanctuary in these situations generally refers to policies either ignoring (i.e., not asking about) immigration status by police or in determining eligibility for certain services, but in addition may mandate that police not cooperate with federal agents pursuing individuals only because of their immigration status. Providing an umbrella humane social policy approach such as this offers some basic measures of safety (i.e., removing certain fears about police) and support (i.e., access to basic human and social services). We need only consider how the specter of SB1070 in Arizona, a law passed by voters in 2010 to give police unprecedented power to stop anyone suspected of being undocumented, could exacerbate the already distressing living and working conditions for LMDLs and other undocumented people in that state. Among the invaluable community-based resources available to LMDLs, especially in sanctuary cities, are day labor centers discussed below.

Migrant Day Laborer Centers

Migrant day labor centers, originally designed to help organize street corner and other outdoor work pick up sites, take different forms, but mostly have evolved over the years to provide LMDLs with a number of ways to satisfy basic needs and provide services such as English language instruction, vocational skills, and negotiating on behalf of workers for fair wages, recovery of unpaid wages, etc. Of course, such centers or similar programs cannot exist in city environments hostile to labor migrants (e.g., day labor centers have been outlawed in Arizona), underscoring the multiple socioecological levels involved in LMDL well being, distress, and vulnerability to risk.

Communication with Home and Family

Distributing phone cards or increasing phone access to increase communication with family and friends back home in Mexico or Central America could help decrease the loneliness and stress of separation from loved ones (Worby, 2007). Arranging virtual visits with family by using Skype or webcams to provide teleconferencing between migrants locally in the United States and their loved ones in countries of origin could further help to reinforce the central migrant goal of progressing on behalf of one's family, and hence taking care of one's self for the sake of the family. Ironically, such communication might happen least when it is needed most because LMDL feel shame for not being able to earn enough money to send home or because they are experiencing other kinds of problems such as problem drinking and its many negative consequences (Duke & Gómez-Carpinteiro, 2009).

Improve Basic Housing

Although potentially more complex to address, creative efforts to improve inadequate housing and diminish the risk for homelessness have tremendous potential to decrease distress and could act indirectly to curtail behaviors such as excessive drinking. For example, it has been reported that when high numbers of men share the same room or small apartment, they often cope with boredom and fear of apprehension by remaining indoors after work and taking turns buying cases of beer to pass the time (Worby & Organista, 2007). Conversely, dignified housing and the flexibility to choose roommates who are like-minded can reinforce some men's efforts to pursue and maintain practices that promote their health.

Promote Organizing for Worker and Human Rights

Involvement in political activism aimed at reducing the stigma and discrimination related to being an undocumented worker in the United States (e.g., national May 1st rallies by Latino immigrants protesting Congress' proposed bill to make lack of documentation a felony) as well as for promoting basic worker rights (e.g., fair wages, unionizing activities) represents proactive ways that day laborers and other migrant workers have advocated on their own behalf, sometimes improving working and living conditions, as well as uniting in activism for a just cause (Bacon, 2008).

Culture-Based Resources

Soccer

Weekly soccer games have been organized by a few LMDL-serving community agencies as a way of providing these men with a healthy recreational outlet that reduces loneliness, isolation, and boredom, and provides them with a culturally familiar and enjoyable way of bonding with fellow workers. The Multicultural Institute, operating day laborer programs in Berkeley and Redwood City, CA, provides weekly Friday afternoon games, along with lunch and other activities, in part as a way of preventing weekend binges among some men unsuccessful at securing work that day. Rhodes et al. (2009) list soccer leagues as a community strength noting that in the Southeastern United States they are sometimes organized by family networks and hometown-based associations.

Music

In his book, *Illegal people: How globalization creates migration and criminalizes immigrants*, David Bacon (2008) documents the emergence of a day laborer band in Los Angeles in response to the hard living and working conditions, including mistreatment, experienced by LMDLs in that city. He cites the following lyrics among others (p. 119):

I'm going to sing you a story, friends that will make you cry,
How one day in front of K-Mart la migra came down on us,
Sent by the sheriff of this very same place. . .
We don't understand why, we don't know the reason,
Why these is so much discrimination against us.
In the end we'll wind up in the same grave.

This culture-based form of messaging through a traditional Latino entertainment medium is part of a long tradition in Mexican/Latino and other cultures throughout the world. Such musical messaging is part historical documentation, part protest, with the potential to validate often unarticulated experiences of stigma and social injustice. More specific to HIV prevention, the authors have also listened to performances by an LA-based Mariachi group that actually wrote a song about HIV risk and prevention in migrant workers.

Theatre

Teatro or political Chicano street theater has been a staple of the Chicano movement in the United States since the 1960s where it grew out of the farmworker moment with the birth of Luis Valdez' *El Teatro Campesino* [The Farmworker Theater], performing original *actos* about important issues of the day affecting Latino communities. Bacon (2008) discusses the play, *The curse of the day laborers*, which grew out of the improvisation of Los Angeles day laborers to depict hostile residents near a work pickup site who put a curse on the workers in the person of a sheriff notorious for hassling the men. In the play, the curse is eventually lifted by a local *curandera* [Mexican folk doctor]. Popular theater has also been used to communicate information about HIV prevention in a way that transforms the performers through the production process while also creating public health messages that are easily assimilated.

Religion

As research summarized in Worby and Organista (2007) indicates, religious practices support some migrants' strategies to reduce alcohol use and regulate their behavior in other ways. Having a place to be (church services or bible study groups), receiving social support from a religious network, and choosing religious traditions stressing and supporting abstinence from activities considered "vices" are examples of how church communities can alter a local environment for their participants. A Catholic folk tradition, known as *juramentos* (pledges), is a culture-based method for swearing off alcohol, drugs, or other activities for a specific period of time (García & González, 2009). In addition to the perceived help to commit to abstinence, demonstrating that one is *jurado* (has taken such a pledge) can be a mechanism to mitigate peer pressure among Latino labor migrants, which otherwise can be a powerful social element to drink even for those concerned about their drinking or determined not to drink. In an example cited by research by one of the authors, a man initially refuses to drink with his roommates but following their coercive teasing, "What? Are you too good to drink with me?" would often end up having at least one drink (Worby, 2007). In the same study, showing a *juramento* card, provided by local priests and parishes, was mentioned as a way to say no to alcohol and have that decision be respected.

CONCLUSIONS

In conclusion, the SE model advocated in this chapter represents an effort to think more comprehensively or through a socioecological framework about the complex contexts of Latino HIV risk and prevention for various Latino groups struggling with this. This model advocates conceptualizing HIV risk as a *structural vulnerability* or as risk embedded within the dynamic interplay of key environmental, individual, situational, and sexual risk outcome factors. Although this chapter illustrates the SE model with LMDLs as the particular case study, the model is intended to be comprehensive enough to be applied to almost any U.S. Latino group under study. For example, Rafael Diaz's pioneering research on Latino MSM included a variation of our proposed model that empirically demonstrated that the harsh environments typically experienced by Latino MSM frequently produced psychological distress, which in turn increased their participation in risky substance-related sexual situations. Hence the SE model proposed here is broad enough to be used to help Latino communities and researchers theorize, assess, and identify the key contextual elements of HIV risk and prevention for the Latino group served and under study.

An important motivation for using a multilevel analysis in research is the goal of shifting interventions away from approaches using strictly individual behavior change given the disappointing record of many such interventions (Smedley & Syme, 2000). Structural interventions, on the other hand, according to Blankenship and colleagues (2000), aim to "locate the sources of public-health problems in factors in the social, economic and political environments that shape and constrain individual, community, and societal health outcomes." Such interventions can be targeted toward the individual, organizational, and environmental level.

The SE model proposed can also help to reduce our feeling of being overwhelmed at the prospect of thinking about the socioecological context of HIV risk and prevention by reminding us that the key factors need to be identified only for the specific groups and locations under study. For this reason, all chapter authors in this book project have been asked to read this chapter and to locate their own research and thinking within or at least in relation to the SE model. One result of such a concerted effort is the overdue and urgently needed assessment and analysis of HIV risk in Latinos as not primarily a behavioral problem but as a multilevel problem that can include key elements of the historical and current experience of various Latino groups the United States, or marginalities, stigmas, and experiences of discrimination, as well as resilient responses, that need to be specified and utilized to facilitate HIV prevention more comprehensively. Furthermore, an SE approach to HIV risk and prevention can also provide a greater opportunity to facilitate the Latino community's ability to theorize local risk and prevention, by inviting members to share their relevant experiences, insights, and skills in order to advance the responsiveness and effectiveness of HIV prevention in Latino communities and beyond.

REFERENCES

Alaniz, M. L. (1994). Mexican farmworker women's perspectives on drinking in a migrant community. *The International Journal of the Addictions, 29*(9), 1173–1178.

Alderete, E., Vega, W. A., Kolody, B., & Aguilar-Gaxiola, S. (2000). Lifetime prevalence of and risk factors for psychiatric disorders among Mexican migrant farmworkers in California. *American Journal of Public Health, 90*(4), 608–614.

Bacon, D. (2008). *Illegal people: How globalization creates migration and criminalizes immigrants.* Boston: Beacon Press.

Blackmore, C. A., Limpakarnjanarat, K., Rigau-Perez, J. G., Albritton, W. L., & Greenwood, J. R. (1985). An outbreak of chancroid in Orange County, California: Descriptive epidemiology and disease-control measures. *Journal of Infectious Diseases, 151*(5), 840–844.

Blankenship, K. M., Bray, S. J., & Merson, M. H. (2000). Structural interventions in public health. *AIDS, 14,* S11–S21.

Borges, G., Medina-Mora, M. E., Orozco, R., Fleiz, C., Cherpitel, C., & Breslau, J. (2009). The Mexican migration to the United States and substance use in northern Mexico. *Addiction, 104*(4), 603–611.

Denner, J., Organista, K. C., Dupree, J. D., & Thrush, G. (2005). Predictors of HIV transmission among migrant and marginally housed Latinos. *AIDS and Behavior, 9*(2), 201–210.

Diaz, R. M., Ayala, G., & Bein, E. (2004). Sexual risk as an outcome of social oppression: Data from a probability sample of Latino gay men in three US cities. *Cultural Diversity & Ethnic Minority Psychology, 10*(3), 255–267.

Duke, M., & Gómez Carpinteiro, F. (2009). The effects of problem drinking and sexual risk among Mexican migrant workers on their community of origin. *Human Organization, 68*(3), 328–339.

Ehrlich, S. F., Organista, K. C., & Oman, D. (2007). Migrant Latino day laborers and intentions to test for HIV. *AIDS and Behavior, 11*(5), 743–752.

Finch, B. K., Catalano, R., Novaco, R., & Vega, W. A. (2003). Employment frustration and alcohol abuse/dependence among labor migrants in California. *Journal of Immigrant Health, 5*(4), 181–186.

Galvan, F. H., Ortiz, D. J., Martínez, V., & Bing, E. G. (2008). Sexual solicitation of Latino male day laborers by other men. *Salud Pública de México, 50,* 439–466.

García, V., & González, L. (2009). Juramentos and Mandas: Traditional Catholic practices and substance abuse in Mexican communities of Southeastern Pennsylvania. *NAPA Bulletin, 31*(1), 47–63.

Grzywacz, J. G., Quandt, S. A., Early, J., Tapia, J., Graham, C. N., & Arcury, T. A. (2006). Leaving family for work: Ambivalence and mental health among Mexican migrant farmworker men. *Journal of Immigrant and Minority Health, 8*(1), 85–97.

Hernández, M. T., Sanchez, M. A., Ayala, L., Magis-Rodríguez, C., Ruiz, J. D., Samuel, M. C., et al. (2009). Methamphetamine and cocaine use among Mexican migrants in

California: The California-Mexico epidemiological surveillance pilot. *AIDS Education and Prevention, 21*(5), 34–44.

Hovey, J. D., & Magaña, C. G. (2000). Acculturative stress, anxiety, and depression among Mexican immigrant farmworkers in the Midwest United States. *Journal of Immigrant Health, 2*(3), 119–131.

Hovey, J. D., & Magaña, C. G. (2003). Cognitive, affective, and physiological expressions of anxiety symptomatology among Mexican migrant farmworkers: Predictors and generational differences. *Violence & Abuse Abstracts, 9*(2), 87–166.

Kissinger, P., Liddon, N., Schmidt, N., Curtin, E., Salinas, O., & Narvaez, A. (2008). HIV/STI risk behaviors among Latino migrant workers in New Orleans post-hurricane Katrina disaster. *Sexually Transmitted Diseases, 35*(11), 924–929.

Magana, C. G., & Hovey, J. D. (2003). Psychosocial stressors associated with Mexican migrant farmworkers in the Midwest United States. *Journal of Immigrant Health, 5*(2), 12.

Martínez-Donate, A. P., Rangel, M. G., Hovell, M. F., Santibáñez, J., Sipan, C. L., & Izazola, J. A. (2005). HIV infection in mobile populations: The case of Mexican migrants to the United States. *Revista Panamericana de Salud Publica/Pan American Journal of Public Health, 17* (1 L2), 26(24).

Massey, D. S., Durand, J., & Malone, N. J. (2002). *Beyond smoke and mirrors: Mexican immigration in an era of economic integration.* New York: Russell Sage Foundation.

Mines, R., Mullenax, N., & Saca, L. (2001). *The binational farmworker health survey: An in-depth study of agricultural worker health in Mexico and the United States.* Davis, CA: California Institute for Rural Studies.

Munoz-Laboy, M., Hirsch, J. S., & Quispe-Lazaro, A. (2009). Loneliness as a sexual risk factor for male Mexican migrant workers. *American Journal of Public Health, 99*(5), 802–810.

Nandi, A., Galea, S., Lopez, G., Nandi, V., Strongarone, S., & Ompad, D. C. (2008). Determinants of access to and utilization of health services among undocumented Mexican immigrants in a US urban metropolitan area. *American Journal of Public Health, 98*, 2011–2020.

Ordonez, J. T. (2010). *Jornalero: The life and work of Latin American day laborers in Berkeley, California.* University of California, Berkeley.

Organista, K. C., Alvarado, N. J., Balblutin-Burnham, A., Worby, P., & Martinez, S. R. (2006). An exploratory study of HIV prevention with Mexican/Latino migrant day laborers. *Journal of HIV/AIDS & Social Services, 5*(2), 89–114.

Organista, K. C., & Balls Organista, P. (1997). Migrant laborers and AIDS in the United States: A review of the literature. *Aids Education and Prevention, 9*(1), 83–93.

Organista, K. C., Balls Organista, P., García de Alba, J. E., Castillo Morán, M. A., & Ureta Carrillo, L. E. (1997). Survey of condom-related beliefs, behaviors, and perceived social norms in Mexican migrant laborers. *Journal of Community Health, 22*(3), 185–198.

Organista, K. C., Carrillo, M., & Ayala, G. (2004). HIV prevention with Mexican migrants—Review, critique, and recommendations. *Journal of Acquired Immune Deficiency Syndromes, 37*(Suppl 4), S227–S239.

Organista, K. C., & Kubo, A. (2005). Pilot survey of HIV risk and contextual problems and issues in Mexican/Latino migrant day laborers. *Journal of Immigrant Health, 7*(4), 269–281.

Quesada, J. (1999). From Central American warriors to San Francisco day laborers: Suffering and exhaustion in a transnational context. *Transforming Anthropology, 8*(1&2), 162–185.

Rangel, M., Gudelia, Martinez-Donate, A. P., Hovell, M. F., Santibanez, J., Sipan, C. L., & Izazola, J. A. (2006). Prevalence of risk factors for HIV infection among Mexican migrants and immigrants: Probability survey in the North border of Mexico. *Salud Publica de México, 48*(1), 3–12.

Rhodes, S. D., Hergenrather, K. C., Griffith, D. M., Yee, L. J., Zometa, C. S., Montano, J., et al. (2009). Sexual and alcohol risk behaviors of immigrant Latino men in the south-eastern USA. *Culture Health & Sexuality, 11*(1), 17–34.

Shedlin, M., Decena, C. U., & Oliver-Velez, D. (2005). Initial acculturation and HIV risk among new Hispanic immigrants. *Journal of the National Medical Association, 97*(7 Suppl), 32S–27S.

Shedlin, M. G., Drucker, E., Decena, C. U., Hoffman, S., Bhattacharya, G., Beckford, S., et al. (2006). Immigration and HIV/AIDS in the New York Metropolitan Area. *Journal of Urban Health, 83*(1), 43–58.

Smedley, B. D., & Syme, S. L. (2000). *Promoting health intervention strategies from social and behavioral research.* Washington, DC: National Academy Press.

Sweat, M. D., & Denison, J. A. (1995). Reducing HIV incidence in developing countries with structural and environmental interventions. *AIDS, 9*(Suppl A), S251–S257.

Valenzuela, A., Jr. (2000). Working on the margins: Immigrant day labor characteristics and prospects for employment (Vol. Working Paper No. 22). La Jolla, California: The Center for Comparative Immigration Studies (CCIS).

Valenzuela, A., Jr. (2003). Day labor work. *Annual Review of Sociology, 29*, 303–333.

Valenzuela, A., Theodore, N., Meléndez, E., & Gonzalez, A. L. (2006). *On the corner: Day labor in the United States.* Los Angeles, CA: UCLA Center for the Study of Urban Poverty.

Vega, W. A., Kolody, B., Aguilar-Gaxiola, S., Alderete, E., Catalano, R., & Caraveo-Anduaga, J. (1998). Lifetime prevalence of DSM-III-R psychiatric disorders among urban and rural Mexican Americans in California. *Archives of General Psychiatry, 55*(9), 771–778.

Viadro, C. I., & Earp, J. L. (2000). The sexual behavior of married Mexican immigrant men in North Carolina. *Social Science & Medicine, 50*, 723–735.

Walter, N. (2000). *Structural violence and work injury: The experience of undocumented day laborers in San Francisco.* University of California UCB-UCSF Joint Medical Program, Masters Thesis.

Walter, N., Bourgois, P., & Loinaz, H. M. (2004). Masculinity and undocumented labor migration: Injured Latino day laborers in San Francisco. *Social Science & Medicine, 59*(6), 1159–1168.

Walter, N., Bourgois, P., Loinaz, H. M., & Schillinger, D. (2002). Social context of work injury among undocumented day laborers in San Francisco. *Journal of General Internal Medicine, 17*(3), 221–229.

Wong, W., Tambis, J. A., Hernandez, M. T., Chaw, J. K., & Klausner, J. D. (2003). Prevalence of sexually transmitted diseases among Latino immigrant day laborers in an urban setting—San Francisco. *Sexually Transmitted Diseases, 30*(8), 661–663.

Worby, P. (2007). *Accounting for context: Determinants of Mexican and Central American immigrant day laborer well-being and alcohol use.* Berkeley, CA: University of California, Berkeley [Doctoral Dissertation].

Worby, P., & Organista, K. C. (2007). Alcohol use and problem drinking among male Mexican and Central American immigrant laborers: A review of the literature. *Hispanic Journal of Behavioral Sciences, 29*, 413–455.

2 Enhancing Peer Norms, Self-Efficacy, Self-Esteem, and Social Support for Safe Sex in Naturalistic Environments

The Role of Community Involvement in Latino Gay, Bisexual, and Transgender Communities

Jesus Ramirez-Valles, Lisa M. Kuhns, and Haiyan Li

The purpose of this chapter is to explore the connection between community involvement and safe sex among gay and bisexual men and transgender individuals (GBT) of Latin American descent in the United States. Community involvement, especially in the form of activism and volunteerism, in lesbian, gay, bisexual, and transgender (LGBT) and HIV/AIDS-related issues is an environmental factor that may shape individuals' health behaviors. We propose that community involvement promotes safe sex practices through its influence on self-esteem, social support, peer norms, and safe sex self-efficacy. This proposition is consistent with the structural-environmental model presented in Chapter 1 because it envisions both HIV risk and prevention within a greater community context rather than overfocusing on risk behaviors.

It is well established that participation in groups and organizations promotes development of the self and improves well-being. This has been proposed by social integration and social movements theories (Bellah et al., 1996; Borgonovi, 2008; Durkheim, 1951; McAdam, 1989) and substantiated with solid empirical evidence (Puntnam, 2000; Piliavin & Siegl, 2007; Thoits & Hewitt, 2001; Musick & Wilson, 2008; Wilson & Musik, 1997). Many of the studies on community involvement and health outcomes (e.g., mental health, life satisfaction) have relied on sound and diverse methodology, such as longitudinal and qualitative approaches, including controlling for self-selection bias (Rietschlin, 1998; Thoits & Hewitt, 2001). Yet, data have come primarily from white, heterosexual, middle-class, and older populations in the United States.

Our knowledge of community involvement and its effects on Latino and GBT populations is limited. Until a few decades ago, GBT individuals had limited access to social spaces such as grassroots groups and community organizations addressing public affairs because of the prevailing homophobia. Many GBT would have been involved as activists and volunteers, but not always embracing an identity as gay, bisexual, or transgender individuals. With the rise of the gay movement, society's growing acceptance of homosexuality and gender nonconformity, and the AIDS epidemic, this has changed. Many GBT individuals are now involved in issues related to civil rights and HIV/AIDS and openly and proudly advance their identity as GBT (Omoto & Crain, 1995; Ramirez-Valles & Diaz, 2005).

The HIV/AIDS epidemic, in particular, generated a remarkable mobilization among gay men and their allies (Chambre, 2006; Ramirez-Valles, 2011; Stockdill, 2003). Still, most of them were white (Gould, 2009). The movement created by the epidemic aimed at making demands on state institutions, taking care of people living with HIV and AIDS, and developing prevention strategies. Later, the non-profit and governmental sector infusion of resources helped create a myriad of community-based organizations focused on HIV/AIDS. A large number of these organizations work with and for GBT. It is in this context that the contemporary Latino GBT community involvement has occurred (Cantu, 2000). Latino GBT have been involved in the gay and HIV/AIDS movement in fewer numbers than their white counterparts and such participation has been fostered mostly by HIV/AIDS organizations.

In what follows we discuss our conceptual framework to investigate the processes by which community involvement may shape safe sex practices among Latino GBT. Then, we test our hypotheses in a sample of Latino GBT from San Francisco and Chicago. After the discussion of our findings, we conclude by drawing implications for health-promoting interventions, especially among Latino GBT, in naturally occurring settings, such as community organizations.

CONCEPTUAL FRAMEWORK

Our theoretical model is based on a decade of work on community involvement and HIV/AIDS among GBT populations (Ramirez-Valles, 2002). But first, we clarify our use of the concept of community involvement, given its liberal use in the literature. Some of the terms used to describe individuals' involvement in community and societal affairs include volunteerism, activism, and civic involvement (Boehmer, 2000; Omoto & Snyder, 1995; Putnman, 2000). The terms may have ideological connotations. Volunteering, for example, may imply charity work performed by the middle classes (Taylor, 2005), whereas activism may denote the use of direct action in political issues.

Thus, to avoid ideological connotations and to be inclusive of work performed inside and outside of formal organizations, we use a definition of community involvement as individuals' unpaid work on behalf of others, or for a collective good, and in the context of a formal or semiformal organization and social networks, taking place outside the home and the family (Ramirez-Valles, 2002).

Elsewhere (Ramirez-Valles, 2002), we have proposed that community involvement works as a coping mechanism by moderating the negative effects that stress may cause on health outcomes. As in Chapters 7 (by Diaz et al.) and 8 (by Ayala), we refer to stress here as specifically derived from stigmatization based on racial categories, homosexuality (or gender nonconformity), and poverty. This role of community involvement, we offer, is due to four elements provided by involvement: self-esteem, social support, peer norms toward safe sex, and safe sex self-efficacy.

We have already found evidence of the moderating effects of community involvement among Latino GBT (Ramirez-Valles et al., 2010). In a prior analysis of these data, we compared two groups of Latino GBT: those involved in LGBT and HIV/AIDS organizations and causes in the previous year and those not involved in these organizations and causes. We evaluated the relationships between stigma based on race and homosexuality (or gender nonconformity) and two outcomes: sex under the influence of substances (i.e., alcohol and drugs) and unprotected sex. We presumed that the stress created by stigma would lead to unprotected sex through sex under the influence. What we found is that in the noninvolved group, experiences of stigma led to unprotected sex via the internalization of this stigma, which, in turn, was associated with sex under the influence. In the involved group, however, while experiences of stigma were related to internalization, this internalization was not associated with sex under the influence, and hence, with unprotected sex. Notably, general community involvement (e.g., helping the homeless, political parties) did not have any effect on sexual behavior. Likewise, the moderating effects of community involvement were attenuated when we considered lifetime involvement in LGBT and/or HIV organizations and causes (e.g., ever being involved vis-à-vis involvement in the previous year).

What remains to be explored, hence, is the processes by which involvement helps individuals deal with the stress created by stigma and prevents them from engaging in sexual risk behavior. In Figure 2.1, we identify the four elements hypothesized to mediate the association between community involvement and safe sex.

Self-Esteem

Community involvement is associated with psychological well-being among gay men (Bebbington & Gatter, 1994; Chambre, 1991; Omoto & Snyder, 2002; Ouellette et al., 1995; Schondel, Shields, & Orel, 1992; Stewart & Weinstein, 1997). Although most of these studies do not assess community involvement as we do here (in multiple formats, including level and frequency of involvement) and they rely on varied and questionable measures, their results are consistent.

The self-protective theory of stigma also provides support for the idea that community involvement may promote psychological well-being (Crocker & Major, 1989; Noh & Kaspar, 2003; Ramirez-Valles, 2011). When stigmatized individuals

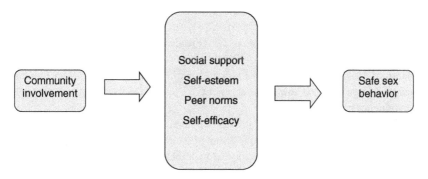

FIGURE 2.1 Conceptual model of the mechanisms of community involvement and safe sex among gay and bisexual men and transgender persons.

come together and mobilize, they see themselves as actors, not subjects or victims. They come to realize that their perceived shortcomings are actually perceptions created by the other, the larger society, rather than true characterizations of the self. This may promote self-esteem, which in turn leads to assertiveness in other realms, such as safe sex practices (Diaz, 1998).

Involvement fosters self-esteem by providing contact with peers, a sense of purpose in life, and a sense of competence (Allahyari, 2000; Frable et al., 1997; Moen & Fields, 1999; Ouellette et al., 1995; Wolfe, 1994). Individuals in social movements, for example, frequently experience a positive transformation of the self (McAdam, 1989; Snow et al., 1986). Latino GBT, thus, may become to see themselves not as victims, but as activists; and not as deviant and amoral subjects, but as proud and openly GBT (Kiecolt, 2000; Ramirez-Valles & Brown, 2003).

In one of our studies with Latino GBT (Ramirez-Valles & Diaz, 2003), we found a positive association between community involvement and self-esteem. The measure of involvement, while similar to the concept we use here, assessed it only in a dichotomous fashion (i.e., prior involvement versus no involvement). In an early study of AIDS volunteering, Schondel and colleagues (1992) found that AIDS volunteers reported higher personal satisfaction and self-esteem than nonvolunteers. Likewise, Wolfe (1994) argues that gay men who were members of ACT UP developed a strong sense of themselves as gay men through their involvement. Weitz (1991) makes a similar argument among people living with AIDS.

Social Support

This is the most common feature found in community involvement. People participate in groups and organizations looking for social connections and frequently they find them. Getting involved increases social support because it expands social networks, provides opportunity for face-to-face communication, and, as noted before, promotes a sense of belonging to a larger group or cause (Smith, 1994, 1997; Younis & Yates, 1997).

In Diaz's pioneer study on Latino gay men in New York City, Los Angeles, and Miami (Diaz et al., 2001; Ramirez-Valles & Diaz, 2005), community involvement (in Latino and LGBT organizations) was found to be associated with increased social support.

Self-Efficacy toward Safe Sex

Here we use the term self-efficacy as first defined by Bandura (1986): the extent to which one feels able to successfully perform a given behavior. Studies among volunteers have found increased general self-efficacy related to their participation as volunteers (Moen & Fields, 1999). As proposed by Social Cognitive Theory (Bandura, 1986), learning about safe sex and gaining confidence about practicing it may take place in social contexts, such as LGBT and AIDS organizations, through the influence of peers.

Community involvement may provide opportunities for vicarious learning and verbal persuasion. Participants may learn not only formally from the programs offered at organizations, but informally through their peers. They may share difficulties and encourage each other to practice safe sex. This sense of self-efficacy would theoretically be greater for individuals directly working within HIV/AIDS and LGBT organizations and if they feel a strong commitment toward the organizations.

We rely on social control theory to postulate that safe sex practices are partly shaped by peer norms. Peers within community organizations and social movements influence individuals' behaviors (Hirschi, 1969). Thus, if Latino GBT are involved in organizations promoting LGBT rights or HIV/AIDS prevention and care, they would likely acquire and follow the agenda of those organizations and the behaviors of their peers. Those not involved or who do not have a sense of bonding with those peers and their organizations would not feel compelled to act according to the organization's goals and norms.

In this chapter we advance our understanding of community involvement and its effects on health by looking at those four potential mediators: self-esteem, social support, peer norms toward safe sex, and safe sex self-efficacy. We already have good evidence that Latino GBT who are involved in AIDS and LGBT organizations are less likely to be affected by stigmatization and, therefore, less likely to engage in unprotected sex than those who are not involved. We are posing the following here: what are the factors by which community involvement helps Latino GBT practice safe sex?

METHODS
Sample

We collected data from 643 self-identified adult Latino gay/bisexual men and transgender individuals (male to female) living in Chicago ($n = 320$) and San Francisco ($n = 323$) in 2004. We chose these two cities to capture the experiences of Latinos from a variety of countries of origin in Latin America. In Chicago, the majority of the Latino population is of Mexican and Puerto Rican descent. In San Francisco, while Latinos of Mexican descent are the largest group, there is a sizable population from other Latin American regions (e.g., Central and South America). Also, the gay communities in these cities have experienced the HIV/AIDS epidemic and the AIDS and gay movements differently. San Francisco, in particular, has been an epicenter of both the epidemic and of the gay movement.

With the same objective of drawing a diverse and representative sample, we used an innovative sampling technique, respondent-driven sampling (RDS). It is close to impossible to obtain a random sample of Latino GBT because there is not a listing of the overall population (i.e., a sampling frame) and because those two social categories—Latino and GBT—are socially constructed. Moreover, GBT individuals are stigmatized, and therefore may not disclose their sexual orientation to others. RDS uses social networks as a means for sampling and therefore facilitates identification of eligible individuals through those networks. Peers recruit peers from inside their social network (Heckathorn, 1997, 2002). Thus, RDS derives generalizations not from individuals but from social networks to the entire population. Samples drawn using RDS are more representative of a hidden population than venue-based approaches (Ramirez-Valles et al., 2005). We provide details of our sample methodology elsewhere (Ramirez-Valles et al., 2005).

Measures

The entire questionnaire used in this study was developed by a team of seven bilingual researchers. We developed our measures using qualitative methods.

We collected life history data from Latino GBT in both cities. From these data and available measures in the literature, we composed measures (in both languages, English and Spanish). Then we pilot-tested the complete instrument in a sample of 200 Latino GBT in both cities. We used computer-assisted self-interviewing to collect data, which we believe helped promote reporting of sensitive information.

Sexual Risk

To measure sexual risk behavior, we used two sets of items: those reflecting sex under the influence of substances and those reflecting sex without the use of a condom or other barrier method. For the first one, participants reported how often they engaged in sexual activities (1) under the influence of alcohol and (2) under the influence of drugs in the previous 12 months. Response choices range from 1 = never to 4 = many times. Because the two variables were highly skewed (median = 1, mode = 1), we combined them to create one dichotomous variable (i.e., had sex under the influence of drugs or alcohol in the past 12 months, 1 = yes, 0 = no). Thirty-nine percent of the sample ($n = 249$) reported engaging in sex while under the influence of substances in the prior 12 months.

For unprotected sex, we relied on participants' reports of anal sex without a condom (either receptive or insertive) in the previous 12 months (1 = yes, 0 = no). Thirty-five percent of participants ($n = 224$) stated they engaged in unprotected sex in the prior 12 months.

Community Involvement

We measure involvement in general causes, as well as HIV/AIDS and LGBT-specific organizations and causes. Respondents were asked first to indicate whether they had ever done any volunteer work (defined as working in some way to help others without being paid, including activism and informal helping). Seventy-seven percent responded affirmatively, 71% in Chicago and 83% in San Francisco. Those who responded "yes" were then asked to indicate the causes or organizations for which they volunteered time (total of 20 causes listed). Participants who said "yes" to volunteering for either HIV/AIDS or LGBT causes were combined into one variable (1 = yes, 0 = no). Forty-eight percent of participants indicated that they had been involved in AIDS/GLBT organizations at some point in their lives. The percentage was higher in San Francisco (57%) than in Chicago (39%). In addition, we collected data on frequency and length of involvement (details are available from the authors).

Self-Esteem

For the measurement of self-esteem, we used the Rosenberg Self-Esteem Scale (Rosenberg, 1965), which includes 10 items answered on a four-point Likert-type scale (from strongly agree to strongly disagree). Statements included the following: I feel that I am a person of worth, at least on an equal basis with others; Overall, I am inclined to feel that I am a failure; I feel I have much to be proud of; and I am able to do things as well as most other people. We reverse-coded items as needed and computed an average for the self-esteem scale, with higher scores indicative of greater self-esteem. The Cronbach alpha for this variable in this sample is 0.82 (mean = 3.30, standard deviation = 0.47).

Social Support

General social support from friends and family was assessed via 10 items on a four-point frequency scale (i.e., always to never), except for two items rated on a seven-point frequency scale. Examples of these items include: How often do you talk to your friends? How often do you feel that there is no one to whom you can turn? How often do you have someone whose advice you really trust? An average of these items was computed to create the social support scale. The Cronbach alpha for the scale in this sample was 0.80 (mean = 3.42, standard deviation = 0.56).

Safe Sex Self-Efficacy

We operationalized this construct as safe sex self-efficacy and used nine items reflecting confidence in practicing safer sex techniques (e.g., I find it difficult to limit myself to safer sex all the time; If I want to, I can get a sexual partner to use condoms with me; and I can talk with my partners about things that I like to do to practice safer sex). Responses were rated on a four-point agreement scale, from strongly agree to strongly disagree. An average score was created from these nine items. The Cronbach alpha for this scale in this sample was 0.74 (mean = 3.10, standard deviation = 0.55).

Peer Norms toward Safe Sex

Similar to self-efficacy, we assessed this variable by means of the average response to seven items. Responses were coded in a four-point scale, from strongly agree to strongly disagree. Example items include the following: I believe that my friends always use condoms when having anal sex with new partners; I believe that many of my friends have unsafe sex; Most of my friends think that you should always use a condom when having anal sex; and my friends have talked to me about the importance of having safer sex. The Cronbach alpha for this scale in this sample was 0.77 (mean = 2.97, standard deviation = 0.49).

Sociodemographic Data

We also collected basic demographic data on all participants, including age, place of birth (U.S. born, non-U.S. born), education, city of residence (i.e., Chicago, San Francisco) and HIV status (HIV negative/untested, HIV positive). These data are presented in Table 2.1.

Analysis

We ran four different mediation analyses, one for each of our hypothesized mediators. A variable becomes a mediator between two correlated variables, if it is predicted by the primary independent variable (e.g., community involvement) and if it attenuates or eliminates the association between such variables (while being associated with the outcome). Following the traditional mediation analysis, we first assessed the association between community involvement and sexual risk behavior using logistic regression. Then we modeled the association between community involvement and the hypothesized mediators by means of multiple regression. Last, we ran logistic regression models regressing sexual risk on our main independent variable, community involvement and each of the four possible mediators.

Table 2.1 Demographic Characteristics of Latino GBT in San Francisco and Chicago, 2004 (N = 643)

	Chicago (n = 320) n (%)	San Francisco (n = 323) n (%)	Total (n = 643) n (%)
Age			
18–29	126 (39)	76 (23)	202 (31)
30–39	113 (35)	127 (39)	240 (37)
40–49	55 (17)	89 (28)	144 (23)
≥ 50	26 (8)	29 (10)	52 (9)
Gender			
Male	294 (92)	255 (79)	549 (85)
Transgender	26 (8)	68 (21)	94 (15)
Sexual orientation			
Homosexual/gay	264 (82.5)	275 (85)	539 (84)
Bisexual	56 (17.5)	48 (15)	104 (16)
Birthplace			
United States	99 (31)	46 (14)	145 (23)
Colombia	14 (4)	7 (2)	21 (3)
Cuba	8 (2.5)	15 (5)	23 (4)
El Salvador	0	26 (8)	26 (4)
Guatemala	8 (2.5)	11 (3)	19 (3)
Mexico	141 (44)	158 (49)	299 (47)
Nicaragua	0	15 (5)	15 (2)
Peru	4 (1)	17 (5)	21 (3)
Puerto Rico	27 (8)	7 (2)	34 (5)
Other	19 (6)	21 (6)	40 (5)
Education			
Less than High School	81 (25)	91 (28)	172 (27)
High School/GED	88 (28)	61 (19)	149 (23)
Technical/Vocational School	22 (7)	37 (11)	59 (9)
Some college	84 (26)	74 (23)	158 (25)
College degree	35 (11)	51 (16)	86 (13)
Graduate degree	10 (3)	9 (3)	19 (3)
Employment Status			
Full time	156 (49)	85 (26)	241 (37)
Part time	64 (20)	86 (27)	150 (23)
Unemployed	93 (29)	135 (42)	228 (35)
Other	7 (2)	15 (5)	22 (3)
Annual Income			
<10,000	95 (30)	165 (51)	260 (40)
10,000–19,999	108 (34)	64 (20)	172 (27)
20,000–29,999	70 (22)	50 (15)	120 (19)
30,000–39,999	34 (11)	28 (9)	62 (10)
≥40,000	13 (4)	16 (5)	29 (5)

	Chicago (n = 320) n (%)	San Francisco (n = 323) n (%)	Total (n = 643) n (%)
Relationship status			
Cohabitating, with partner	54 (17)	68 (21)	122 (19)
With partner but not cohabitating	108 (34)	89 (28)	197 (31)
Single/no primary partner	158 (49)	166 (51)	324 (50)
HIV tested			
Positive	57 (18)	113 (35)	170 (26)
Negative	208 (65)	184 (57)	392 (61)
Don't know	10 (3)	5 (1.5)	15 (2)
Not HIV tested	36 (11)	13 (4)	49 (8)
Refused to answer	9 (3)	8 (2.5)	17 (3)

In each instance, we evaluated the four indicators of community involvement (i.e., ever, AIDS/LGBT, and frequency of involvement and level of involvement in AIDS/LGBT). All the analyses were performed using unweighted data and controlling for age, education, place of birth, city, and HIV status. Elsewhere (Ramirez-Valles et al., 2008), we argue that as long as we control for those variables in our multivariable models, there is not need to weight observations (Winship and Radbill, 1994).

RESULTS

The sample included 643 self-identified Latinos between 18 and 73 years old (see Table 2.1). Thirty-one percent were between 18 and 29 years old, while 37% were between 30 and 39 and 23% between 40 and 49 years old. Only 9% of the sample was 50 years old or older. Regarding gender identity and sexual orientation, 85% identified as male and 15% transgender (most from San Francisco), and most identified as gay (84%); only 16% identified as bisexual.

The majority of the sample (77%) was born outside of the United States, mostly in Mexico (47%). The level of education achieved is relatively high, with 73% having completed at least high school. Yet only 37% of the sample was fully employed and 40% report less than $10,000 in annual income. The unemployment and poverty levels were especially high in San Francisco. This sample is not typical of the Latino population in the United States, where the level of educational achievement, for example, is much lower. We believe this reflects a particular immigration pattern of GBT. Many of them immigrate not in search of financial opportunities, but to avoid discrimination, either toward GBT or those living with HIV/AIDS.

Half of the sample was single or without a primary partner. This closely resembles the larger gay male population, where the majority is single. Last, 26% report being HIV positive.

Community Involvement and Sexual Risk

In logistic regression models we found no association between any of our measures of community involvement and sexual risk (see Table 2.2). In all these models, we

Table 2.2 Logistic Regression of Sexual Risk on Community Involvement among Latino GBT

Community Involvement Variable	Sex under Influence OR (95% CI)	Unprotected Sex OR (95% CI)
Ever community involved (general)	1.18 (0.79, 1.75)	1.16 (0.77, 1.75)
Ever AIDS/LGBT involved	1.24 (0.89, 1.74)	1.13 (0.80, 1.60)
Level of AIDS/LGBT involvement	1.02 (1.00, 1.07)	0.99 (0.97, 1.01)
Frequency of AIDS/LGBT involvement	0.93 (0.81, 1.07)	0.92 (0.80, 1.07)

All models controlled for age, education, place of birth, city, and HIV status.

controlled for age, education, place of birth, city, and HIV status. This confirms our previous finding using a different analytical approach (Ramirez-Valles et al., 2010). Being involved does not have a direct effect on sexual risk behavior. Based on these results, we were unable to test our main hypothesis, that self-esteem, social support, peer norms, and self-efficacy mediate the relationship between community involvement and sexual risk (i.e., because there is no significant relationship to be mediated). We, therefore, chose an alternative approach, to test indirect relationships between the intermediate psychosocial variables and our independent and dependent variables.

Community Involvement and Psychosocial Variables

In Table 2.3 we present the findings of the association between community involvement and our four psychosocial factors, controlling for age, education, place of birth, city, and HIV status. Ever being involved in any cause did not predict our four psychosocial variables. Yet, being involved in AIDS/LGBT organizations predicted peer norms ($b = 0.09$; $p < 0.05$), social support ($b = 0.13$; $p < 0.05$), and

Table 2.3 Linear Regression of Psychosocial Variables on Community Involvement among Latino GBT

Community Involvement Variable	Peer Norms B	Self-Esteem B	Social Support β	Safe Sex Self-Efficacy β
Ever community involved (general)	0.07	0.05	0.07	0.01
Ever AIDS/LGBT involved	0.09*	0.05	0.13*	0.11**
Level of AIDS/LGBT involvement	−0.01	0.00	0.00	0.00
Frequency of AIDS/LGBT involvement	0.01	0.01	0.05*	0.41*

All models controlled for age, education, place of birth, city, and HIV status.
*$p \leq 0.05$, **$p \leq 0.01$.

self-efficacy towards safe sex ($b = 0.11$; $p < 0.01$). The frequency of involvement in AIDS/LGBT organizations was also significantly associated with social support ($b = 0.05$; $p < 0.05$) and safe sex self-efficacy ($b = 0.41$; $p < 0.05$).

Psychosocial Variables and Sexual Risk

Table 2.4 presents the findings from the logistic regression models regressing sexual risk behavior on our four different psychosocial variables. As before, we controlled for sociodemographic factors in all the models. One psychosocial variable was significantly associated with sex under the influence: peer norms ($OR = 0.65$; $p < 0.05$).

For unprotected sex two variables were significantly associated: peer norms and safe sex self-efficacy. Peer norms were significantly associated with unprotected sex ($OR = 0.64$; $p < 0.05$) as was safe sex self-efficacy ($OR = 0.41$; $p < 0.01$). These results make sense, because self-efficacy and peer norms for safe sex are close to sexual risk while social support and self-esteem are distal in the casual sequence.

DISCUSSION

Our general goal in this chapter has been to explore how, if at all, naturally occurring environments, such as community involvement, foster preventive health behaviors among Latino GBT populations. Using the AIDS movement as an instance, we tested whether community involvement is associated with declines in sexual risk behavior and whether four potential psychosocial variables—self-esteem, social support, self-efficacy toward safe sex, and peer norms for safe sex—might mediate that association. Our results indicate that being involved in AIDS/LGBT organizations is only indirectly associated with sexual risk. Participation in these organizations seems to enhance social support, peer norms toward safe sex, and safe sex self-efficacy. In turn, peer norms and self-efficacy decrease the likelihood of engaging in sexual risk behavior. Involvement in other causes more generally does not

Table 2.4 Logistic Regression of Sexual Risk on Psychosocial Variables among Latino GBT

Psychosocial Variable	Sex under Influence OR (95% CI)	Unprotected Sex OR (95% CI)
Peer norms	0.65* (0.46, 0.92)	0.64* (0.45, 0.92)
Social support	0.90 (0.67, 1.21)	1.05 (0.77, 1.43)
Self-esteem	0.73 (0.51, 1.05)	1.01 (0.70, 1.46)
Safer sex self-efficacy	1.02 (1.00, 1.04)	0.41** (0.56, 0.99)

All models controlled for age, education, place of birth, city, and HIV status.

*$p \leq 0.05$, **$p \leq 0.01$.

make a difference. Thus, a socially natural setting and activity, such as community involvement in AIDS/LGBT organizations, may foster health prevention behaviors because this activity may provide exposure to safe sex peer norms and may promote safe sex self-efficacy (which may be promoted implicitly or explicitly by the organization's agenda).

These findings are consistent with the literature on volunteering and activism (Li & Ferraro, 2006). However, this is the first study, to our knowledge, showing evidence of the positive association between involvement and self-efficacy, peer norms, and social support among GBT populations. The results further our understanding of the processes by which community involvement affects health (Piliavin & Siegl, 2007; Ramirez-Valles, 2002).

Before elaborating on the implications of our research, we need to address the limitations of this study. This study is cross-sectional in design, thus, we cannot assume causal connections among our study variables. For example, it is quite possible that social support precedes community involvement, not the other way around. We rely on theory to make arguments about causation, but only longitudinal or experimental research designs may confirm them. We also need to note that self-esteem was not associated with either community involvement or sexual risk. This can be due to the fact that this variable was somewhat skewed toward higher scores. Alternatively, the concept (and its operationalization) may not accurate assess the self-concept among Latino GBT.

Participation in AIDS/LGBT organizations as a volunteer or activist develops peer norms and safe sex self-efficacy through several processes. As individuals get involved, they may embrace the agenda of the organization or movement (e.g., to prevent and fight HIV). A set of expectations, which directly shape peer norms, is created in the organization and among members regarding the practice of safe sex. These expectations become part of a social control process (Ramirez-Valles et al., 2010). That is, individuals act in accordance with social norms to avoid social exclusion and criticism. In addition, individuals have easy access to information about safe sex and may become comfortable talking about sexual practices and impediments and facilitators for safe sex. These features are rarely present in other organizations, such as political groups and those helping the homeless where Latino GBT may be involved.

This has implications for the way we, public health professionals and researchers, conduct HIV prevention programs for GBT and GBT of Latin American descent. Traditional pedagogical methods, referred to as "banking education" by Paulo Freire (1970), rely on transmitting information and practicing skills with a unidirectional and top-down approach (e.g., from an expert to the learner). These, according to Freire's pedagogy, may fail because they do not engage participants (e.g., learners) in the construction of their own knowledge and skills. This is particularly challenging with adult learners. Moreover, it is difficult to incorporate individuals' context and subjective knowledge using this approach. Interventions based solely on psychosocial or cultural factors, while showing some success, have similar limitations. They usually are individual-based, overlooking the social processes (e.g., the group) in which the self is embedded, and their effects may not be long lasting because these interventions are not built on existing resources and with the active participation of individuals themselves. Conversely, active participation in the solution of self and community's problems, such as the case of HIV/AIDS and discrimination against LGBT people, fosters ownership and critical understanding (Freire, 1970; Zimmerman et al., 1997). In this type of pedagogy, participants are not passive recipients of information, but colearners. Individuals learn as they collectively act. They learn from their actions and through their peers.

In practice, this means that we need to support and/or foster the above environments for Latino GBT. This is relevant not only because it may help HIV prevention activities, but because Latino GBT have very limited spaces in which to socialize as GBT people. Community organizations in which Latino GBT could get involved as volunteers or activists to help run programs and organize community groups are potential options. Internet-based social groups, for and by Latino GBT, may also work, but we have no evidence yet on their feasibility. School-based groups represent another option. We could tap on groups such as gay–straight alliances, that allow students to imagine and implement their own activities.

At the policy level, local, state, and federal agencies may want to emphasize community-based organizations in their allocation of resources and implementation of HIV prevention programs. Their policies need to advance the direct and active involvement of community members, that is, working with community members not as passive recipients of educational activities. They also need to further a bottom-up approach, in which programs are developed and implemented with community members and a reflective knowledge of the sociocultural context. Last, these policies ought to endorse the utilization of existing resources, such as naturally occurring environments and collaboration among organizations.

ACKNOWLEDGMENT

This research was supported by a grant from the National Institutes of Mental Health (R01MH62937-01) to Jesus Ramirez-Valles.

REFERENCES

Allahyari, R. A. (2000). *Visions of charity: Volunteer workers and moral community.* Berkeley, CA: University of California Press.

Bandura, A. (1986). *Social foundations of thought and action, a social cognitive theory.* Englewood Cliffs, NJ: Prentice-Hall.

Bebbington, A. C., & Gatter, P. N. (1994). Volunteers in an HIV social care organization. *AIDS Care, 6,* 571–585.

Bellah, R. N., Madsen, R., Sullivan, W. M., Swidler, A., & Tipton, S. M. (1996). *Habits of the heart: Individualism and commitment in American life.* Berkeley: University of California Press.

Boehmer, U. (2000). *The personal and the political: Women's activism in response to the breast cancer and AIDS epidemics.* Albany: State University of New York.

Borgonovi, F. (2008). Doing well by doing good. The relationship between formal volunteering and self-reported health and happiness. *Social Science & Medicine, 66*(11), 2321–2334.

Cantu, L. (2000). *Entre hombres/between men: Latino masculinities and homosexualities.* Thousand Oaks, CA: Sage.

Chambre, S. M. (1991). Volunteers as witness: The mobilization of AIDS volunteers in New York City, 1981–1988. *Social Services Review, 65,* 531–547.

Chambre, S. M. (2006). *Fighting for our lives: New York's AIDS community and the politics of disease.* New Brunswick, NJ: Rutgers University Press.

Crocker, J., & Major, B. (1989). Social stigma and self-esteem: The self-protective properties of stigma. *Psychological Review, 96*(4), 608–630.

Diaz, R. M. (1998). *Latino gay men and HIV: Culture, sexuality, and risk behavior.* New York: Routledge.

Diaz, R. M., Ayala, G., Bein, E., Henne, J., & Marin, B. V. (2001). The impact of homophobia, poverty, and racism on the mental health of gay and bisexual Latino men: Findings from 3 US cities. *American Journal of Public Health, 91*(6), 927–932.

Diaz, R. M., Morales, E. S., Bein, E., Dilan, E., & Rodriguez, R. A. (1999). Predictors of sexual risk in Latino gay/bisexual men: The role of demographic, developmental, social cognitive and behavioral variables. *Hispanic Journal of Behavioral Sciences, 21*(4), 480–501.

Durkheim, E. (1951). *Suicide.* New York: Free Press.

Frable, D. E., Wortman, C., & Joseph, J. (1997). Predicting self-esteem, well-being, and distress in a cohort of gay men: The importance of cultural stigma, personal visibility, community networks, and positive identity. *Journal of Personality, 65*(3), 599–624.

Freire, P. (1970). *Pedagogy of the oppressed.* New York: Seabury Press.

Gabard, D. L. (1995). Volunteers in AIDS service organizations: Motivations and values. *Journal of Health and Human Services Administration, 17,* 317–337.

Gould, D. (2009). *Moving politics: Emotion and ACT UP's fight against AIDS.* Chicago: University of Chicago Press.

Heckathorn, D. D. (1997). Respondent-driven sampling: A new approach to the study of hidden populations. *Social Problems, 44*(2), 174–199.

Heckathorn, D. D. (2002). Respondent-driven sampling II: Deriving valid population estimates from chain-referral samples of hidden populations. *Social Problems, 49*(1), 11–34.

Hirschi, T. (1969). *The causes of delinquency.* Berkeley: University of California Press.

Kiecolt, J. K. (2000). Self-change in social movements. In S. Stryker, T. J. Owen, & R. W. White (Eds.), *Self, identity, and social movements* (pp. 110–131). Minneapolis: University of Minnesota Press.

Li, Y., & Ferraro, K. F. (2006). Volunteering in middle life: Is health a benefit, barrier or both? *Social Forces, 85*(1), 497–519.

McAdam, D. (1989). The biographical consequences of activism. *American Sociological Review, 54*(5), 744–760.

Moen, P., & Fields, S. (1999). Retirement and well-being: Does community participation replace paid work? Paper presented at the American Sociological Association, Chicago, IL.

Musick, M. A., & Wilson, J. (2008). *Volunteers: A social profile.* Bloomington: Indiana University Press.

Noh, S., & Kaspar, V. (2003). Perceived discrimination and depression: Moderating effects of coping, acculturation, and ethnic support. *American Journal of Public Health, 93*(2), 232–238.

Omoto, A. M., & Crain, A. L. (1995). AIDS volunteerism: Lesbian and gay community-based responses to HIV. In G. M. Herek & B. Greene (Eds.), *AIDS, identity, and community: The HIV epidemic and lesbians and gay men* (pp. 187–209). Thousand Oaks, CA.: Sage Publications.

Omoto, A. M., & Snyder, M. (1995). Sustained helping without obligation: Motivation, longevity of service, and perceived attitude change among AIDS volunteers. *Journal of Personality & Social Psychology, 68*(4), 333–356.

Omoto, A. M., & Snyder, M. (2002). Considerations of community: The context and process of volunteerism. *American Behavioral Scientist, 45*(5), 846–867.

Ouellette, S. C., Cassel, B. J., Maslanka, H., & Wong, L. M. (1995). GMHC volunteers and the challenges and hopes for the second decade of AIDS. *AIDS Education and Prevention, 7*(5 Suppl), 64–79.

Pearlin, L. I., Menaghan, E. G., Lieberman, M. A., & Mullan, J. T. (1981). The stress process. *Journal of Health and Social Behavior, 22*(4), 337–356.

Piliavin, J. A., & Siegl, E. (2007). Health benefits of volunteering in the Wisconsin longitudinal study. *Journal of Health and Social Behavior, 48*(4), 450–464.

Putnam, R. D. (2000). *Bowling alone: The collapse and revival of American community.* New York: Simon & Schuster.

Ramirez-Valles, J. (2002). The protective effects of community involvement for HIV risk behavior: A conceptual framework. *Health Education Research, 17*(4), 389–403.

Ramirez-Valles, J. (2011). *Compañeros: Latino activists in the face of AIDS.* Chicago, IL: University of Illinois Press.

Ramirez-Valles, J., & Brown, A.U. (2003). Latino's community involvement in HIV/AIDS: Organizational and individual perspectives on volunteering. *AIDS Education and Prevention, 15*(1 Suppl A), 90–104.

Ramirez-Valles, J., & Diaz, R. M. (2005). Public health, race, and the AIDS movement: The profile and consequences of Latino gay men's community involvement. In A. M. Omoto (Ed.), *Processes of community change and social action* (pp. 51–66). Mahwah, NJ: Lawrence Erlbaum Associates.

Ramirez-Valles, J., Fergus, S., Reisen, C. A., Poppen, P. J., & Zea, M. C. (2005). Confronting stigma: Community involvement and psychological well-being among HIV-positive Latino gay men. *Hispanic Journal of Behavioral Sciences, 27*(1), 101–119.

Ramirez-Valles, J., Garcia, D., Campbell, R. T., Diaz, R. M., & Heckathorn, D. D. (2008). HIV Infection, sexual risk, and substance use among Latino gay and bisexual men and transgender persons. *American Journal of Public Health, 98*(6), 1036–1042.

Ramirez-Valles, J., Heckathorn, D. D., Vazquez, R., Diaz, R. M., & Campbell, R. (2005). From networks to populations: The development and application of respondent-driven sampling among IDUs and Latino gay men. *AIDS & Behavior, 9*(4), 387–402.

Ramirez-Valles, J., Kuhns, L., Diaz, R., & Campbell, D. (2010). The moderating effects of community involvement on health: Stigmatization and sexual risk among Latino sexual minorities. *Journal of Health & Social Behavior, 51*, 30–47.

Rietschlin, J. (1998). Voluntary association membership and psychological distress. *Journal of Health and Social Behavior, 39*, 348–355.

Rosenberg, M. (1965). *Society and the adolescent self-image.* Princeton, NJ: Princeton University Press.

Schondel, C., Shields, G., & Orel, N. (1992). Development of an instrument to measure volunteer's motivation in working with people with AIDS. *Social Work in Health Care, 17*(2), 53–71.

Smith, H. (1997). Grassroots associations are important: Some theory and a review of the impact literature. *Nonprofit and Voluntary Sector Quarterly, 26*, 269–306.

Smith, H. D. (1994). Determinants of voluntary association participation and volunteering: A literature review. *Nonprofit and Voluntary Sector Quarterly, 23*, 243–263.

Snow, D. A., Rochford, E. B., Worden, S. K., & Benford, R. D. (1986). Frame alignment processes, micromobilization, and movement participation. *American Sociological Review, 51*, 464–481.

Stewart, E., & Weinstein, R. S. (1997). Volunteer participation in context: Motivations and political efficacy within three AIDS organizations. *American Journal of Community Psychology, 25*(6), 809–837.

Stockdill, B. C. (2003). *Activism against AIDS: At the intersections of sexuality, race, gender, and class*. Boulder, CO: Lynne Rienner Publishers.

Taylor, R. F. (2005). Rethinking voluntary work. *The Sociological Review, 53,* 117–135.

Thoits, P. A., & Hewitt, L. N. (2001). Volunteer work and well being. *Journal of Health and Social Behavior, 42*(June), 115–131.

Weitz, R. (1991). *Life with AIDS*. New Brunswick, NJ: Rutgers University Press.

Wilson, J., & Musick, M. (1997). Who cares? Toward an integrated theory of volunteer work. *American Sociological Review, 62*(5), 694–713.

Winship, C., & Radbill, L. (1994). Sampling weights and regression analysis. *Sociological Methods and Research, 23*(2), 230–257.

Wolfe, M. (1994). The AIDS coalition to unleash power (ACT UP): A direct model of community research for AIDS prevention. In J. P. Van Vugt (Ed.), *AIDS prevention and services: community based research* (pp. 217–247). Westport, CT: Begin & Garvey.

Youniss, J., & Yates, M. (1997). *Community service and social responsibility in youth*. Chicago: University of Chicago Press.

Zimmerman, M., Ramirez-Valles, J., Suarez, E., De la Rosa, G., & Castro, M. (1997). An HIV/ AIDS prevention project for Mexican homosexual men: An empowerment approach. *Health Education & Behavior, 24,* 177–190.

3 Sexual Culture, Structure, and Change

A Transnational Framework for Studies of Latino/a Migration and HIV

Héctor Carrillo

INTRODUCTION

Over the past two decades, scholars increasingly have documented the role of population movement and international migration in the worldwide spread of HIV. The topic is enormously significant for Latinos/as in the United States because migrants constitute a considerable proportion of this population group. In 2007, the U.S. Census Bureau estimated that of 45.4 million people of Hispanic origin living in the United States, 18 million (40%) were foreign born (Grieco, 2009).[1] Among them, a majority were of Mexican origin (11.6 million). The literature on Latinos/as and HIV has provided a collective sense that migrant populations may be at increased risk for HIV due to cultural differences and the conditions of poverty, marginalization, and generalized social disadvantage that affect them in the United States. To date, however, knowledge of cultural differences between Latino/a migrants and the U.S.-born population remains somewhat limited.

This chapter discusses current depictions in the behavioral science literature of the relationship between Latino/a migrants' sexual cultures and HIV risk, and analyzes conceptual limitations that may hinder deeper understandings of how these two issues are interrelated. There is a tendency to draw conclusions about cultural differences between migrants and the U.S.-born population that are often unsubstantiated by empirical findings, primarily because behavioral studies typically are not designed to measure cultural factors. The result is a chain of assumptions and speculation about the sexual cultures of Latino/a subgroups that has ensued. The chapter also examines the limitations caused by a propensity to focus exclusively on the migrants' behaviors in the United States, without inquiring about their lives prior to migration or their continued contact with their home countries. Finally, the chapter analyzes the consequences of a widespread reliance on simple acculturation measures and on now problematic constructs such as *simpatía, familismo, machismo*, and *marianismo* (also discussed in this book's Latina-focused Chapters 4, 16, and 17). Such constructs were created to promote greater consideration of cultural issues in studies of HIV and other health issues affecting Latinos/as, but their use over the years has had the effect of representing so-called traditional Latino/a migrant culture as an unchanging, monolithic given.

Some of the current conceptual limitations in the behavioral study of HIV among Latino/a migrants may be addressed by the incorporation of a transnational framework, which may lead to a more accurate depiction of the factors influencing Latino/a migrants' sexual behaviors and sexual cultures and help develop a more comprehensive account of how the migrants' HIV risk is produced. HIV research with Latino/a migrants would benefit from giving greater consideration to the recent sociological and anthropological research on Latino/a migrants' sexualities. Not only has that research already incorporated a transnational framework, but it has also yielded a robust and nuanced body of knowledge on the effects of relocation on Latino/a migrants' sexual cultures and behaviors, including risk for HIV.

LATINO/A MIGRANTS IN THE HIV LITERATURE

Recent behavioral science articles on Latinos/as and HIV suggest the pervasiveness of a particular, shared understanding of Latino/a migrant sexual cultures. Typically, the literature has attempted to interpret HIV-related individual behaviors from a cultural perspective. In so doing, it has tended to replicate a generally untested perception of cultural difference between migrants and the U.S.-born population, where migrants are depicted as holding a constant set of "traditional" Latino/a values in relation to sexuality and gender, and U.S. society is assumed to be more sexually liberal by comparison.

The process seems to unfold as follows: Relying on the results yielded by simple acculturation measures, recent articles often cite older articles (which themselves may have cited even older articles going back to the late 1980s or early 1990s) in an attempt to provide a cultural explanation for differences detected among Latinos/as. They reproduce ideas about an essential and unchanging Latino/a sexual culture developed in the early days of the AIDS epidemic, and which often become encapsulated in a few simple (now reified) constructs, including *familismo, marianismo, machismo,* and *simpatía*.[2] Often those constructs are used without asking whether anything has changed in the past 20 years. The notion of a traditional Latino/a sexual culture is sometimes invoked even when actual study findings contradict it.[3]

The resulting profile of Latino/a migrant sexual culture that is repeatedly invoked is at best only partially accurate. At worst it becomes stereotypical and precludes consideration of important dimensions of sexual culture and the processes that shape it, including the diversity of lived experience among migrants and the dynamic sociocultural processes in the migrants' home countries. As we will see, the use of a limited, and static view of sexual culture creates conceptual problems for understanding: (1) how cultural and structural issues are interconnected; (2) the diversity that may exist among Latino/a migrants; and (3) how such diversity simultaneously reflects their experiences prior to migration, their continued interactions with their home countries, their interactions in the host country, and the processes of social and cultural change taking place in both the migrants' home countries and in the United States. This section summarizes some of the ways in which behavioral studies have typically addressed questions about culture and the conceptual problems that they seem to often contain.

HIV Information and Knowledge

Several studies have found that although many Latino/a migrants have accessed information about HIV and condom use, their knowledge about the disease and the proper use of condoms is low. In those studies Latinos/as often report misconceptions about HIV, even when many feel efficacious about preventing it (Apostolopoulos et al., 2006; Lopez-Quintero, Shtarkshall, & Newmark, 2005; Loue, Cooper, & Fiedler, 2003; Loue, Cooper, Traore, & Fiedler, 2004; Magis-Rodríguez et al., 2009; Organista & Kubo, 2005; Rhodes, Hergenrather, Wilkin, Alegria-Ortega, & Montano, 2006; Shedlin, Decena, & Oliver-Velez, 2005; Shedlin et al., 2006; Vissman et al., 2009).[4]

The literature has related little knowledge of HIV and condoms with generalized low education (Loue et al., 2003; Solorio & Galvan, 2009). Furthermore, based on a perceived need for more HIV information and education that specifically targets Latinos/as, the literature has often called for the production of culturally competent messages. It has proposed a range of strategies that emphasizes the creation of HIV educational materials and testing services in Spanish and prevention programs specific to Latinos/as; the use of Latino-specific media, including *novelas, telenovelas* (soap operas), and *fotonovelas* (comic-book like novelas as described by Painter et al. in Chapter 18); and the involvement of migrants as peer educators (Harper, Bangi, Sanchez, Doll, & Pedraza, 2009; Levy et al., 2005; Lopez-Quintero et al., 2005; Martínez-Donate et al., 2009; McQuiston & Uribe, 2001; Rhodes, Hergenrather, Bloom, Leichliter, & Montaño, 2009; Rhodes et al., 2006; Rios-Ellis et al., 2008; Solorio & Galvan, 2009; Vissman et al., 2009).

Unfortunately, the promotion of these well-intentioned strategies has sometimes further reified understandings of the nature of Latino/a migrant sexual cultures. Cultural competency is often conceived as requiring respect for a set of so-called traditional Latino/a sexual values, within which behavioral change then must be incorporated. In this view, the sexual culture of Latino/a migrants tends to be portrayed as homogeneous, unchanging, and untouchable, because stability seems necessary to make claims about cultural difference and to make culturally competent programs operationally feasible.

Traditional Latino/a Sexualities

Also in relation to cultural competency, the behavioral literature has assumed that general cultural differences exist with regard to sexuality between the United States and the Spanish-speaking countries of Latin America and the Caribbean (LAC). Although that may be the case, descriptions of what such cultural difference may consist of often are simplistic. Migrants from LAC are expected to hold so-called traditional Latino/a norms and values, including those related to gender and sexuality, which sometimes are represented with the shorthand constructs of *marianismo* and *machismo* (Apostolopoulos et al., 2006; Bourdeau, Thomas, & Long, 2008; Fernandez-Esquer et al., 2004; González-Guarda, Peragallo, Urrutia, Vasquez, & Mitrani, 2008; Jarama, Kennamer, Poppen, Hendricks, & Bradford, 2005; Lopez-Quintero et al., 2005; Loue et al., 2004; Magis-Rodríguez et al., 2009; Moreno, 2007; Olshefsky, Zive, Scolari, & Zuñiga, 2007; Rios-Ellis et al., 2008; Villarruel, Jemmott, Jemmott, & Ronis, 2007; Weidel, Provencio-Vasquez, Watson, & Gonzalez-Guarda, 2008). These Latino/a traditional sexual cultures are perceived as contrasting enormously with the more liberal sexual attitudes of the U.S. population. The picture, however, is more complicated if we take into account that LAC countries are changing rapidly in relation to gender and sexuality—sometimes faster than the United States—and also that the United States is by no means uniformly liberal.

Some isolated references to religiosity suggest that the conservative positions of the Catholic Church in relation to condom use, homosexuality, and sex outside of heterosexual marriage may function in the literature as an implicit marker of an imagined generalized sexual traditionalism ànd conservativeness among Latinos/as. However, the evidence of the influence of religiosity on Latino/a migrants sexual cultures is mixed (Villarruel et al., 2007). Indeed, many Latinos/as make pragmatic decisions that are different from what the Church says, and LAC societies have implemented policies that go against the Church's positions on sexual issues. Those policies include the legalization of abortion in Mexico City and of gay marriage in Argentina and Mexico City. Thus religiosity's influence may be less prominent than commonly assumed, and may be quite compartmentalized.

Perplexingly, conservative values informed by Catholicism would appear to be included in the package of traditional Latino/a values that culturally competent efforts are expected to protect and promote, in spite of the fact that some of those values can be extremely oppressive, in particular to Latino/a women and non-heterosexuals. Indeed, Marín (2003), a strong proponent of cultural analyses of Latino/a HIV risk, whose earlier work on the cultural constructs *familismo*, *machismo*, *marianismo*, and *simpatía* is widely cited, has noted that the gender disparities and homophobia that often accompany so-called traditional Latino/a sexualities can lead to a "cycle of disempowerment" (p. 188). By contrast, most of the literature overlooks the apparent tension between a proposed preservation of traditional Latino/a sexual culture and the potential benefits of cultural change. In a more dynamic view of sexual culture, where cultural change is allowed to play a role and sexual culture is no longer seen as static, cultural competency may take new meaning. It may be redefined to include the promotion of cultural change.

Sexual Communication

On a related topic, the literature also has reported patterns of sexual communication among Latino/a migrant populations that are different from those assumed to be more prevalent in the United States (Fernandez-Esquer et al., 2004; Loue et al., 2004; Weidel et al., 2008). A lack of open sexual communication—often labeled "sexual silence" (Carrillo, 2002; Díaz, 1998; Marín, 2003)—is perceived as prevalent (Fernandez-Esquer et al., 2004; Loue, 2006; Loue et al., 2004). Sexual silence is regarded as a barrier to HIV prevention because its strategies differ from the open negotiation and verbal communication that frequently are promoted within HIV prevention messages. (Chapter 16 features an intervention designed to "romper el silencio" [break the silence], but between mothers and daughters with regard to discussing sex and HIV, rather than between sexual partners as discussed below.)

Findings of sexual silence combine with notions of traditional sexual culture to create a sense that Latino/a migrants face greater cultural obstacles than the rest of the U.S. population in openly discussing sexuality and successfully adopting protective measures against HIV (Rojas-Guyler, Ellis, & Sanders, 2005). This assumption, however, fails to take into account that Latino/a migrants' sexual communication strategies may also have a productive side, particularly with regard to culturally based ideas about sexual passion (Carrillo, 2002).

Research conducted in Mexico found that expectations about strong bodily expression, not making everything verbally explicit, and a certain playfulness in talking about sex indirectly and with innuendo are often seen as contributing to a heightened sense of sexual pleasure and sexual intimacy, which people perceive as being weakened when a more "rational" way of negotiating sex is introduced (Carrillo, 2002). This view highlights the emphasis on a spontaneous flow of sex, and the sense that verbal sexual negotiation that focuses on health and hygiene, and that takes place during sex itself, may have the effect of "killing the moment." As one participant in Carrillo (2002) put it:

It's necessary to allow yourself to be taken by the moment, by the caresses, not think that you are in a relationship, not pressure yourself to think, because it all dies. My partner use to do something that totally turned me off. We would start touching and she would say, 'Did you wash your hands?' She killed me with that. (p. 198)

Although it might be tempting to assume that participants such as this one minimized the importance of HIV prevention, they did not. Indeed, many in this study saw safe sex as crucially important and were seeking alternative ways to enact it in a manner that was compatible with the kind of sexual flow that they favored. Generally they felt that open verbal communication about sex was necessary before and after sex, particularly in the context of ongoing (or stable) relationships. But during sex itself, words and sounds were perceived as playing two roles: (1) complementing bodily language through supportive moaning and other verbal expressions, and (2) acting as a recourse of last resort when the body failed to communicate refusal (Carrillo, 2002).

At issue here are the negative judgments that are often launched against forms of sexual communication such as the ones described above. This is a topic that has not been sufficiently researched with Latino/a migrants from a cultural perspective. Moreover, as the next subsection indicates, as Latino/a migrants become incorporated into U.S. life and society, and presumably become more exposed to the U.S. mainstream and adopt its forms of sexual communication, they do not seem to experience reductions in HIV risk but instead acquire new forms of risk.

Acculturation

Drawing on the extensive use of simple acculturation measures (most commonly based on language use or media preferences, although sometimes including variables such as length of residence in the United States or immigration status) the behavioral literature has divided the Latino/a population into acculturation subgroups (Ehrlich et al., 2007; Kinsler et al., 2009; Lopez-Quintero et al., 2005; Rojas-Guyler et al., 2005). In relation to HIV risk, the literature has reported conflicting findings about which subgroups of Latinos/as by acculturation are at higher risk for HIV, and whether less acculturated Latinos/as, the subgroup that is assumed to include a majority of recent Latino/a migrants, are at higher risk.

Over time, a sense has emerged that less acculturated Latinos/as face greater barriers to HIV prevention that are associated with traditional Latino/a sexual culture, but some studies also have highlighted negative effects of a loss of traditional Latino/a migrant sexual culture, including those associated with perceived forms of resilience such as the cultural emphasis on respect, collectivity, and family life (Lopez-Quintero et al., 2005; Loue et al., 2004; Marín, 2003; Rojas-Guyler et al., 2005). Highly acculturated Latino/a migrants, the argument goes, lose some of their original culture (and also the risks and resiliencies that accompany them) and acquire a more mainstream American sexual culture, which in turn leads to different risks and resiliencies.[5] The view is that acculturation leads to greater individuality (seen as positive from a decision making viewpoint, and negative from the loss of social supports associated with Latino/a collectivity), greater promiscuity among Latina women, sometimes less promiscuity among Latino men, possibly more egalitarian relationships, and greater exposure to racism and discrimination (due to greater contact with non-Latinos) (Rojas-Guyler et al., 2005). Confronted with the problem that acculturation seems to reduce some risks and increase others, some acculturation-based analyses have concluded that rather than assessing whether one subgroup of migrants is more at risk than the other, we must instead realize that different Latino/a groups face different challenges in terms of HIV; such analyses sometimes call for more research on acculturation (González-Guarda et al., 2008; Guilamo-Ramos, Bouris, Jaccard, Lesesne, & Ballan, 2009; Loue, 2006; Loue et al., 2004; Moreno, 2007; Organista, Carrillo, & Ayala, 2004; Rojas-Guyler et al., 2005).[6]

Although the concept of acculturation has become extremely popular for explaining cultural differences among Latino/a subgroups, a strong critique has also been launched that points to its conceptual limitations (Abraído-Lanza, Armbrister, Flórez, & Aguirre, 2006; Hunt, Schneider, & Comer, 2004). Concern exists about the oversimplifications that result from the use of acculturation measures that rely on language (or other indirect and simple factors) as proxies for complex cultural phenomena (Cabassa, 2003; Hunt et al., 2004). In fact, although the concept of acculturation was first developed within anthropology and sociology in the early part of the twentieth century, it has been long abandoned by those disciplines because of its limitations in accounting for complex cultural processes (Hunt et al., 2004). Recent critiques of the use of acculturation measures in public health and the behavioral sciences have noted that it tends to lead to sweeping statements about Latino/a culture—statements that do not do justice to the complexity of culture, and in particular sexual culture (Abraído-Lanza et al., 2006; Cabassa, 2003; Deren et al., 2005; Hunt et al., 2004).

Furthermore, the concept of acculturation often is also used alongside the aforementioned Latino/a cultural constructs, and the combined effect is a tendency to reify Latino/a sexual culture and to conceive it as static. In this sense, when the literature discusses the sexual cultural practices of less acculturated Latinos/as (often meaning migrants) the view of their sexual culture that emerges fails to take into account the diverse cultural experiences that migrants have within the complex societies from which they came, as well as how sexuality is changing there.

Structural Explanations

The literature has associated the marginalized position of many Latino/a migrants within U.S. society, and the many factors that cause it, with an increase in vulnerability toward HIV. The migrants' frequent undocumented status, low English skills, poverty and economic instability, as well the negative effects of racism, homophobia, violence, and social discrimination all emerge as potential structural barriers to HIV prevention (Apostolopoulos et al., 2006; Díaz, 1998; Díaz, Ayala, Bein, Henne, & Marín, 2001; Loue, 2006; Magis-Rodríguez et al., 2009; Marín, 2003; Moreno, 2007; Organista & Kubo, 2005; Parrado, Flippen, & Uribe, 2010; Rhodes et al., 2006; Solorio & Galvan, 2009; Weidel et al., 2008). The effects of the lack of access to adequate educational and health services, which may also limit exposure to appropriate HIV education and testing, condoms, and counseling, have also been noted. And scholars have also associated these structural issues with some of the negative psychosocial consequences of migration, including social isolation, loneliness, depression, and increased alcohol and substance use (Apostolopoulos et al., 2006; Díaz et al., 2001; Ehrlich et al., 2007; Magis-Rodríguez et al., 2009; Marín, 2003; Organista & Kubo, 2005; Parrado et al., 2010; Solorio & Galvan, 2009; Vissman et al., 2009).[7] Several of these factors are noted as producing the environmental conditions for HIV risk. For example, male migrants' involvement in sex with sex workers may follow from loneliness or prolonged separations from wives or steady partners, and may sometimes be structurally facilitated by the migrants' employers (Apostolopoulos et al., 2006; Painter, 2008; Parrado et al., 2010; Shedlin et al., 2005).

The behavioral literature, however, has had some difficulties relating these various structural factors to processes of cultural formation, and thus the relationship between individuals, culture, and structure in the production of HIV risk remains obscured. This difficulty may be connected to overreliance on the concept of acculturation and the view of sexual culture that results, which cannot account for the dynamic nature of sexual culture and its connections to structural changes in both the Latino/a migrants' sending countries and the United States (Deren et al., 2005). With such an absence, it is hard to envision how and whether broader structural issues can be addressed as part of culturally based HIV prevention programs (i.e., how a structural level of analysis can be best conceived and linked to other sociocultural issues affecting individual and relationship-based HIV risk). In Chapter 6, Hirsch and Vasquez offer a multisectorial approach to help us envision needed structural directions in HIV prevention.

More generally, the potential for structural approaches that could address Latino/a migrants' HIV might not be feasible without first adopting a transnational perspective. It seems necessary to take into account the structural inequalities produced in the relationship between host and home countries and the conditions that lead to the migration flows in the first place. It also seems necessary to consider the migrants' transnational connections with their home countries, and whether psychosocial issues such as isolation and loneliness may be somewhat mitigated by those connections. Little is known, for instance, about the effects of the availability of cheap and accessible technologies—from phone cards, cell phones, and texting, to Skype—and the role that those technologies may play in facilitating the receipt of social support from abroad.

In summary, the various issues discussed in this section suggest that the behavioral research on HIV among Latino/a migrants has developed an overly narrow and potentially inaccurate understanding of their sexual cultures, which limits the potential to consider processes of sexuality-related cultural change and possible connections with programs oriented toward addressing broader structural issues. Although the literature has made some inroads into exploring the associations between Latino/a migration and HIV, for the field to move forward and achieve greater nuance and a deeper understanding of how those associations operate, current conceptual limitations such as the ones noted in this section must be addressed. The sections that follow propose two possible expansions that may help in this regard, namely the inclusion of a transnational framework of analysis and the greater incorporation of the approaches and findings of the recent sociological and anthropological literatures on sexuality, gender, and migration.

A TRANSNATIONAL FRAMEWORK

The integration of a transnational perspective requires a shift in the overall strategies of design and measurement in studies of HIV risk in Latino/a migrant populations. Although several, overlapping definitions of transnationalism are in circulation, a common denominator among them is the notion that international migrants often maintain strong affective, social, cultural, economic, and political ties with their places of origin, even many years after relocation (Faist, 2001; Levitt, 2001; Levitt & Jaworsky, 2007; Vertovec, 2009). Increasingly facilitated by the availability of fast communication technologies, those links can remain as strong as (or stronger than) those that migrants develop and establish within host societies, and they do not necessarily decline after migrants become fully and formally incorporated into the host country through stable employment, marriage, permanent residency, or citizenship.

In relation to various Latino/a migrant national subgroups in the United States—Mexicans, Dominicans, Puerto Ricans—there is now a substantial social scientific literature that has demonstrated these groups' strong transnational ties (Itzigsohn, Dore Cabral, Hernández Medina, & Vázquez, 1999; Levitt, 2001; Smith, 2006). For instance, Smith (2006) described how transnational linkages have influenced the sense of identity and community among Mexicans living in New York who came from a particular small town in southern Mexico. Those migrants have established formal migrant associations that significantly shape the economic, social, and political life of their home town.

In addition, they use their transnational connections as a primary point of reference that informs their cultural understandings and also helps them shape those of their children (the so-called 1.5 and second generations, who have been socialized in the United States). In this regard, Smith (2006) found that when migrant parents saw their children setting out on a path that they found troubling—such as showing signs that they were joining a gang—they sometimes sent the children for extended visits to Mexico. This strategy was meant to instill values that migrant parents felt would help their children stay away from trouble, as part of what Smith calls "redefining their Mexicanness" (p. 169). Sometimes the strategy worked, as in the case of Toño, who had joined a gang in New York. Upon returning from Mexico, "Toño left his old friends and began cultivating friendships with more upwardly mobile Mexicans in college. His social life centered on his family and steady girlfriend. He graduated from college in 2002. His return to Ticuani helped change his life in enduring, positive ways" (p. 170).[8]

In response to the limitations of Mexican local governments, the migrant associations fund public works, which give the migrants local stature and a level of political power that they do not enjoy in the United States. Their transnational ties also compel them to deeply assess the cultures that exist in their home towns and compare them with those that they perceive as prevailing in New York City. The result is the construction of largely hybrid cultures that draw from both. Those cultures end up simultaneously affecting and being affected by the cultures at both ends of the transnational circuit. In this sense, Latino/a migrants and their children change as a result of migration, but they also keep a strong connection to their cultures of origin. They contribute to cultural changes in both locations, via what migration scholars have called "social remittances" (Levitt, 2001).

Rather than depicting migrants as passive recipients of culture (as is often implied in behavioral analyses of acculturation and HIV), transnational studies have recognized the role of Latino/a migrants as agents of change in their own right. As we will see below, this and other features of transnationalism have multiple implications for HIV prevention studies among Latino/a migrants. A transnational perspective questions many of the assumptions noted in the previous section, and also makes evident the limitations of analytical frameworks that pay no attention to the migrants' lives in their home countries, the cultural and social changes taking place there, or the continued relationship that they retain with their places of origin. Such a perspective also provides analytical tools for understanding Latino/a migrant cultures—not as static, but in motion, both spatially and across time—and lends additional support for views of culture that are prevalent among sociologists and anthropologists who study migrant sexuality. Those views are discussed in the following section.

Furthermore, the concept of transnationalism raises important questions about the adequacy of the concept of acculturation as a framework to understand migrants' sexual lives and HIV risk (Santelli, Abraido-Lanza, & Melnikas, 2009). The notion that migrants abandon their own sexuality-related understandings and simply adopt those imagined to be prevalent among the U.S. mainstream inadequately represents transnational practices. Some acculturation models have tried to solve this limitation by measuring biculturalism, but this adjustment, although helpful, cannot fully capture the dynamic ways in which migrants make compatible contradictory understandings that stem from different cultural systems, as well as how they use different understandings selectively and pragmatically depending on the interactions taking place in specific sexual contexts and situations. (For example, the cultural logic informing a Latina migrant's sexual behavior with a non-Latino partner may differ from that which may inform the same woman's behavior should the partner be Latino/a or someone from her home country.) It also cannot account for the specific cultural paths that migrants follow in the United States, which appear to greatly depend on their starting points in their home country.

My work in progress on sexuality and HIV with Mexican gay migrants in San Diego, for instance, shows that if we consider more closely their various patterns of experience in Mexico, depending on their social class position and their rural or urban origin, among other variables, the diversity of their patterns of sexual behavior and HIV risk in the United States becomes much clearer. My participants' experiences in Mexico influenced to whom they were sexually attracted upon arrival, how easy it was for them to access the mainstream gay community in San Diego, how familiar they were with the concept of a steady gay relationship, their attitudes about casual sex, and ultimately what kinds of HIV risks they incurred during sexual encounters with U.S. partners. In this sense, the shift from acculturation to a transnational framework also shifts the analysis from a linear process of incorporation into U.S. society to one in which HIV outcomes in the United States can be linked to the migrants' experiences before migration (Carrillo, 2010; Carrillo & Fontdevila, 2011; Carrillo, Fontdevila, Brown, & Gómez, 2008).

This kind of analysis, however, requires consideration of the migrants' lived experiences and trajectories in their countries of origin, prior to migration. This means breaking open the black box in which the HIV behavioral literature has tended to place the lives and experiences that migrants had (or continue to have) in their home country. Furthermore, a transnational perspective requires paying close attention to developments in the migrants' home countries that may noticeably signify shifts in the sexual cultures there—shifts that may also influence the migrants (Carrillo, 2007). Examples are the public debates about issues such as women's rights, LGBT (lesbian, gay, bisexual, transgender) rights, abortion, sex education, and HIV itself that routinely take place throughout the LAC region.

Obviously, not all sexuality-related changes in the LAC region are liberal or progressive, and the effects of conservative efforts to prevent progressive change must also be considered. But the implementation of progressive changes in the LAC region forces us to question the assumption that the sexual cultures and existing policies in the United States are by definition more liberal, particularly since LAC countries have put in place several policies that surpass in scope those available in the United States. In fact, Latin Americans are regularly exposed to a variety of sexuality-related opinions and ideologies—more than the behavioral literature has been inclined to recognize—and the Latin American media allows broadcasts that are not possible in the open-access U.S. networks. For instance, compared to the United States, in several LAC countries there are fewer limitations on condom and HIV prevention advertising. Also, the federal governments of several LAC countries have implemented national antihomophobia campaigns, which in addition to emphasizing the right for all people to not suffer from discrimination, have linked homophobia structurally to HIV risk (Carrillo, 2007; Donohoe, Reyes, Armas, & Mandel, 2008). Although discussions about conducting similar campaigns have taken place among activists in the United States, it remains unlikely that a federally funded antihomophobia campaign could be implemented.

This last example also raises questions about the examination of the potential for binational structural approaches in HIV work with Latino/a migrants. A transnational framework invites questions about what kinds of international collaborations could help address the structural factors that have been identified as promoting HIV risk.[9] It also suggests the importance of analyses that address potential linkages between migration policy—both in the United States in the migrants' home countries—and health and HIV-related policies.

LATINO/A TRANSNATIONAL SEXUAL CULTURES AND CHANGE

Recent sociological and anthropological studies of gender and sexuality among Latino/a migrants have incorporated a transnational framework in their design. Drawing on studies conducted with Mexican migrants, this section discusses conceptual and methodological innovations that may be particularly helpful for HIV research. These examples also illustrate well the extent to which sociological and anthropological studies of migrant gender and sexuality have departed from acculturation-based accounts in favor of more nuanced analyses of Latino/a sexual cultures.

Shifts in Sexual Culture

The theme of change in sexual and gender cultures is common in the recent sociological and anthropological literature on gender and sexuality among Mexican migrants. It has also demonstrated that the cultural changes that migrants experience cannot be interpreted as resulting exclusively from exposure to new sexual cultures in the United States. Instead, they relate to (1) broader cultural changes happening in the migrants' home countries, (2) generational differences, and (3) a resulting desire among migrants to live their sexuality and gender relations differently in a new location. In one example, Hirsch (2003), who studied Mexican heterosexual migrant couples in the United States and Mexico, reported a shift from an emphasis on *respeto* (respect) to an emphasis on *confianza* (trust) as a main feature of marriage. This shift signals a redefinition of patriarchal marriage and its transformation into what Hirsch and other scholars call "companionate marriage" (p. 2). Hirsch (2003) also found that the shift toward companionate marriage had been facilitated by relocation, not just because of new cultural possibilities within the United States, but also due to the distance that migrants placed between themselves and their home town in Mexico.

The important role of distance from familiar places emerges also in studies of Mexican gay male migrants (Cantú, 2009; Carrillo, 2010). As evidenced by these studies, distance becomes an important facilitator to implement changes that may seem daunting when gay men are surrounded by family, and in this sense these men tend to interpret migration to the United States retrospectively as leading to sexual liberalization.

In this literature, heterosexual men and women, as well as gay men, have reported dissatisfaction with machista attitudes. Gay male migrants also reported dissatisfaction with homophobia. And both gay and heterosexual migrants often expressed a desire to live their relationships differently from their parents and saw this desire as consistent with broader cultural changes taking place throughout Mexico. Their assessments suggest that although these migrants may appear "traditional" upon arrival in the United States, they also carry with them a desire for sexual and gender-related change, which in itself may constitute a motivation to migrate. The changes that they experience thus cannot be interpreted solely as a result of exposure to the sexual cultures that they encounter in the United States. Moreover, as indicated by Deren et al. (2005), sometimes the changes are produced by new necessities that emerge after migration, such as when single men are put in the position of having to do housework (because they migrated alone, or because their female partners, who now work full-time, demand it).

This literature has provided evidence that some Mexican migrants undergo considerable sexuality- and gender-related changes sometimes without much direct or substantial contact with people who are part of the so-called U.S. mainstream (although some do have considerable social and sexual contact with non-Latinos in the United States). Hirsch (2003), for instance, commented that she often was the only non-Latina with whom some of her participants discussed personal issues, and most did not watch English TV or movies. This suggests that direct contact with non-Latinos is not necessary for exposure to a variety of sexuality-related cultural interpretations—including those deemed American—that appear regularly on Mexican television and also on Spanish U.S. television (which in itself is considerably transnational). In this sense, migration to the United States is not a prerequisite for migrants to have considered alternative ways of living their sexual lives after migrating.

In spite of the limitations that migrants encounter in the United States, they often experience some upward mobility—at least in comparison to their previous situations in their home country—and also shifts in family life that facilitate sexuality-related change and a reformulation of gender relations. For instance, González-López (2005), who studied Mexican migrants in Los Angeles, reported that the conditions of employment and family life in the United States provided women greater sexual autonomy and independence, which in turn helped them reconstitute their relations with male partners. In this study, both men and women alike also articulated a desire to provide more open sex education to their children, in a manner that would help the younger generation protect themselves against harm and live better sexual lives. The argument here is that new structural conditions, life in a new environment, and distance from the conditions that surrounded migrants in their home country influence the transformations in their sexual culture, and this puts into question the idea that cultural change results solely from acculturation. The usefulness of a transnational cultural/structural framework—one that pays close attention to the migrants' points of reference in both their home country and the United States—for understanding how sexual cultures change should be evident.

The various findings from this literature have direct implications in terms of HIV prevention. Instead of being trapped in a traditional Mexican sexual culture, migrants may be seeking new spaces where they can make effective changes that they perhaps have envisioned even before leaving Mexico. Such a desire for change may provide important opportunities for HIV prevention. For instance, Latino gay migrants in San Francisco participating in *Hermanos de Luna y Sol,* an HIV prevention program specially designed for them, use their desires for change to engage in considerable self- and group-reflection about how to implement HIV prevention, while addressing the social forces that oppress them and the broader changes in their sexualities that they seek (Díaz, 1998). This program examines the gay immigrants' experiences of rejection and abuse "to promote participants' awareness about the difficulties involved in their dual-minority status" as gay/bisexual in a homophobic society and as belonging to an ethnic minority in a racist society (p. 164). The program also seeks to create a strong bond among participants based on their shared experiences, and to link it to reflection about their HIV risk in the context of an emerging strong sense of mutual social support. The activities also include an emphasis on "contextual or person-situation factors that either compete with or facilitate the enactment of safer sex intentions" (p. 168). Progressive change, and the role of individuals and social groups in producing it, seems to permeate the program.

The desire for change is also evident in Hirsch's (2003) findings about how Mexican migrant couples are reconstituting the concept of heterosexual marriage. The enactment of companionate marriage opens up possibilities for the promotion of HIV prevention that cannot be envisioned if Latino/a heterosexual marriage is conceived as a traditional, stable, and unchanging institution, but it also points toward potential new challenges. The emphasis on trust that Hirsch noted is important for two contrasting reasons. On the one hand, trust has been linked to greater HIV risk within steady relationships, particularly when it is accompanied by HIV risk denial caused by a perceived need to avoid information that can lead to mistrusting a sexual partner (Carrillo, 2002; Hirsch, Higgins, Bentley, & Nathanson, 2002). On the other hand, trust has been found to provide opportunities for sexual communication within relationships (specifically for women to confront male infidelity), which may provide a possible path for promoting HIV prevention (Hirsch et al., 2002). These implications, however, cannot be considered if Latino/a migrant culture is conceived only as traditional.

Cultural Hybridity

These studies have also demonstrated that enacting cultural change does not simply involve discarding one set of Latino traditional cultural interpretations and straight-forwardly adopting a new "Americanized" set, as some of the acculturation models seem to presuppose. Indeed, the shifts in sexual cultures that Latino/a migrants experience appear far from linear. They include instead the construction of hybrid cultural interpretations. Such construction, which Carrillo (2002) labeled "sexual hybridity" (following from García Canclini's (1995) broader concept of cultural hybridity), involves the strategic, combined use of interpretations taken from different sets of sexual scripts (Gagnon & Simon, 1973) and sexual categories— interpretations that on the surface may appear contradictory or incompatible, but that make sense within a more flexible logic and can be adapted as needed for specific contexts and situations.

In the study by Hirsh (2003), for instance, young heterosexual migrant couples incorporated perceptions that are consistent with an idealized, trust-based, egalitarian U.S. version of marriage, while also retaining cultural interpretations that circulate in Mexico, such as the notion of a separation between the worlds of the street (as the space of men) and the home (as the space of women). In Atlanta, the streets became a more comfortable space for women and a less comfortable one for men, although both experienced the pleasures of lowered social vigilance and greater anonymity. But back in Degollado, Mexico, where women often asked permission from their husbands to go out by themselves, migrant women chose to not just enact the patterns of greater freedom to which they had become accustomed in Atlanta; they instead renegotiated their own freedom of movement by strategically managing their husband "por las buenas" (by getting on their good side), "by attending to the chores about which her husband cares most" (p. 119). They thus combined, in a hybrid fashion the scripts of interaction acquired in Atlanta with strategies that they felt were more consistent with the social conditions in their small town in Mexico.

Their hybrid practices and interpretations represented a kind of Mexican modernity that differed from that thought to be prevalent in the U.S. mainstream, but also from the more traditional (or stereotypical) views of Mexican sexual culture. The migrants managed to consolidate these hybrid interpretations while living in the United States, but they also took them back with them when they returned to Mexico and adapted them to the local customs. Through their strategic adaptations, their now hybrid interpretations made sense and appeared local and not foreign, because they were compatible with a cultural logic that was recognizable to those around them, even when they also included changes motivated by exposure to a different way of viewing marriage that had been facilitated by travel to the United States.

The process of cultural hybridization involves multiple influences that originate both in the migrants' home and host countries and, in this case, one could say that this version of companionate marriage crafted by migrants is then exported back to Mexico. Companionate marriage, as understood by Hirsch's informants, constituted a kind of social remittance, because it sent the message to people in Degollado that change is possible regarding the dynamics of marriage. And it would be consistent with, and strengthen, changes in marriage also taking place within Mexico, as evidenced by Hirsch's interpretation that the migrants did not want to be seen at home as "left behind" (p. 165), meaning that they perceived that people in Mexico were also changing rapidly while they were absent. This also suggests that in enacting this change, although being in the United States helped, the migrants' cultural points of reference were largely in Mexico and to a lesser degree in the United States.

Cultural hybridity, the back and forth movement of cultural practices between Mexico and the United States, and the existence of transnational cultural points of reference have implications for how HIV prevention programs ought to be conceptualized. They demonstrate that by solely conceiving of change as related to Latino/a migrants' acculturation to an imagined core, mainstream U.S. culture may miss important features of the processes of personal and cultural change. Instead, they point toward the importance of developing measures that can take into account the migrants' lives in both their home countries and the United States. They also suggest the need to consider deeply the social and cultural changes that are taking place in the migrants' home countries, and comparing them to those occurring in the United States. And finally, they highlight the relevance of adaptations that migrants may implement in order to function in different social contexts, as well as to interact with different kinds of partners.

Rather than seeing culture as stable, and acculturation (or even biculturality) as a linear and permanent process of change, cultural hybridity challenges us to think of culture as specific to context, and of migrants as having the ability to get the most out of their participation in different social and sexual contexts. This way of thinking of Latino/a migrant sexual culture is consistent with the sociological view of culture as a toolkit (Swidler, 2003), where migrants may gain simultaneous access to more than one cultural toolkit and may draw from each as needed depending on the context or situation.

Culture and Structure

Finally, another important feature of these studies is the inclusion of a transnational political economic perspective that seeks to situate the individual changes that migrants experience within a larger set of structural forces that foster or limit such changes. Sexual culture then is seen not as a characteristic of individuals, but rather as shaped by a combination of social and structural forces, emphasizing the idea that sexuality contains a dimension of power (Cantú, 2009; Deren et al., 2005). Furthermore, as Hirsch is careful to remind us, personal change must be seen through the lens of a (transnational) social theory of sexuality. It then would be a mistake to interpret changes in sexual culture as related exclusively to individual choice and individual ideological change, as is common in individually-oriented studies of sexual behavior and HIV risk.

In relation to this topic, Cantú (2009) explained that heteronormativity is a force behind the marginalization and stigmatization of gay people (in both Mexico and the United States, I would add), which influences the desire of a subgroup of gay Mexicans to seek sexuality-related change through migration. But instead of relying on a sense of Mexican traditional culture, Cantú emphasized the need to consider oppressive structural factors similar to those addressed by the *Hermanos de Luna y Sol* program described earlier (namely homophobia, racism, and poverty). He also noted the importance of considering how these structural factors link sexuality to migration in order to imagine producing the kinds of cultural change sought by gay migrants. His concern was that stereotypical views of culture can become in themselves a reflection of (and support for) structural factors of oppression, in this case via the creation of a cultural deficit model that perpetuates the exoticization and othering of Latino/a migrants. Cantú (2009) concluded that:

While culture is important analytically, its importance is not necessarily greater for nonhegemonic groups. When 'culture' is used as a factor of analysis only of U.S. minorities or non-Western peoples, there is a tendency to either directly of indirectly imply that their 'culture,' which is a 'backwards' culture, is to 'blame' for what are represented as pathological traits or what may be called 'cultural pathologization.' (p. 79)

As also noted in the discussion of the *Hermanos de Luna y Sol* program, gay migrants, however, sometimes find that in the United States other structural forces can limit them, including the fact that they often join economically disadvantaged communities within U.S. society or become subjected to racial discrimination. As these examples suggest, structure is thus implicated in propelling sexual migration, as well as shaping the processes of cultural change that migrants collectively undergo during and after migration. An understanding of the reciprocal relationship between culture and structure—in terms of how cultural practices may be the product of the social structure, and also how culture may reproduce or question structural forces—is essential to analyzing how HIV risk is produced.

CONCLUSIONS

In a 2004 review article on HIV prevention among Mexican migrants (Organista et al., 2004) my colleagues Kurt Organista, George Ayala, and I noted that we

may be witnessing diminishing returns on the behavioral science approach, with respect to infection rates and levels of safer sex as well as its limitations in conducting cross-cultural research. Thus, a continued sole reliance on an overly individualistic cognitive approach is likely to result in a reproduction of limited past findings. (p. S228)

We proposed that a new approach was needed—one that paid close attention to the social and cultural contexts in which individual behaviors are enacted. We felt then, as I do now, that a contextual approach would allow us to better conceptualize the relationship between culture and structure in HIV risk, as well as how social change can be incorporated in analyses of how HIV risk is produced and can be mitigated.

It is encouraging that over the course of this decade, some behavioral scientists and HIV researchers working with Latino/a migrants have in fact conducted analyses that pay close attention to the shifts in contexts that migrants experience, and also to the sociocultural and political changes taking place in the migrants' home and host countries. One interesting example is provided by Parrado, Flippen, and McQuiston (2005), who in conducting a quantitative study with Mexican migrants in North Carolina used the sociological and anthropological literature on migration and gender to analyze the relationship between women's power and HIV risk. These authors generated a nuanced analysis that "challenges the common assumption of a positive association between women's power and migration" (p. 366), but also concluded that these women's

elevated risk of HIV is not merely reducible to cultural traits that dictate low interpersonal power. Rather, the experience of migration, which is associated with scarce social resources and informal marriage, and the precarious position of migrant women in the United States are integral contributing factors. Considerable variation in power among Mexican women in both Mexico and the United States according to education and other resources also challenges the idea that culture, rather than poverty or limited opportunities, is the root of powerlessness for these women. (p. 368)

As suggested by this quotation, this study incorporated several welcome conceptual shifts. It offered an explanation that helps us understand how the contextual and environmental challenges created by migration may trump the cultural changes that Latina migrant women may experience as a result of migration. It considered the diversity of experience among migrants, and the sociodemographic factors that may be behind it. And it avoided pointing it to a reified traditional Latino/a culture as the main force behind migrant women's HIV risk, and instead recognized the role of poverty and other structural factors. This analytical approach, which is consistent with the framework proposed in this chapter, opens up the possibility of investigating the relative effects that cultural and social changes may have in comparison with broader contextual and structural factors that limit or enable those changes.

The recent literature on HIV and Latino/a migrants contains other similarly promising examples (Díaz et al., 2004; Harvey, Beckman, Browner, & Sherman, 2002; Miguel Muñoz-Laboy, Hirsch, & Quispe-Lazaro, 2009). But there remain many recently published articles that fully rely on simple measures of acculturation and make sweeping claims about traditional Latino/a sexual and gender culture. This makes ever more important the implementation of studies with Latino/a migrants that explicitly incorporate a transnational perspective, seek to develop a nuanced understanding of sexual culture, and pursue a better understanding of the mutually constitutive manner in which culture and structure seem to operate in the production of HIV risk.

NOTES

1. These estimates classify the more than 4 million individuals who were born in Puerto Rico and who currently live in the 50 states and the District of Columbia as natives of the United States, and not as immigrants (Grieco, 2009). The criterion used by the U.S. Census Bureau is that Puerto Ricans have the right to U.S. citizenship at birth, even if they were born in Puerto Rico. If Puerto Ricans born on the island but living in the United States were reclassified as "foreign born," the proportion of immigrants within the U.S. Hispanic population would increase to 53%.

2. Exceptions are studies concerned exclusively with migrant populations or Latino gay men, which have tended to focus less on acculturation. Some of these studies are also reflective about the need to consider cultural diversity within Latino/a populations. Examples include the articles by Carballo-Diéguez et al. (2005), Díaz, Ayala, and Bein (2004), Ehrlich, Organista, and Oman (2007), Muñoz-Laboy and Dodge (2007), Organista and Kubo (2005), Ramirez-Valles, Garcia, Campbell, Diaz, and Heckathorn (2008), Solorio and Galvan (2009), and Zea, Reisen, and Díaz (2003).

3. Interesting examples of the struggle to interpret findings that contradict conventional understandings of Latino/a sexual culture are provided by Fernandez-Esquer, Atkinson, Diamond, Useche, and Mendiola (2004) and Fernández et al. (2004).

4. One interesting exception is Fitzgerald, Chakraborty, Shah, Khuder, and Duggan (2003), who found that women "did surprisingly well when compared to other surveys of HIV knowledge in Latino migrant farm worker groups" (p. 34).

5. In some analyses, a perceived loss of "Hispanidad"—and not necessarily acculturation per se—is seen as leading to increased HIV risk (Fernández, Jacobs, Warren, Sanchez, & Bowen, 2009; Hernández et al., 2009).

6. See Deren, Shedlin, Decena and Mino (2005) for an interesting account that sought a broader approach in analyses of HIV risk among Latino/a migrants—one that would not

discard a focus on acculturation, but would combine it with a focus on the cultures that the migrants bring with them and the conditions in their home countries.

7. To be sure, the literature has also reported resiliencies that mitigate some of the negative effects of these structural factors among some Latino/a migrants. See, for instance, Organista and Kubo (2005).

8. Ironically, Smith also found that this strategy has resulted in the exportation of gangs to Mexico, as some of the returnees ended up replicating in Mexico the patterns that they learned in New York.

9. An important example is provided by the Health Initiative of the Americans at the University of California, Berkeley (http://hia.berkeley.edu/).

REFERENCES

Abraído-Lanza, A. F., Armbrister, A. N., Flórez, K. R., & Aguirre, A. N. (2006). Toward a theory-driven model of acculturation in public health research. *American Journal of Public Health, 96*(8), 1342–1346.

Apostolopoulos, Y., Sonmez, S., Kronenfeld, J., Castillo, E., McLendon, L., & Smith, D. (2006). STI/HIV risks for Mexican migrant laborers: Exploratory ethnographies. *Journal of Immigrant and Minority Health, 8*(3), 289–300.

Bourdeau, B., Thomas, V. K., & Long, J. K. (2008). Latino sexual styles: Developing a nuanced understanding of risk. *Journal of Sex Research, 45*(1), 71–81.

Cabassa, L. J. (2003). Measuring acculturation: Where we are and where we need to go. *Hispanic Journal of Behavioral Sciences, 25*(2), 127–146.

Cantú, L. (2009). *The sexuality of migration: Border crossing and Mexican immigrant men.* New York: New York University Press.

Carballo-Diéguez, A., Dolezal, C., Leu, C.-S., Nieves, F., Decena, C., & Balan, I. (2005). A randomized controlled trial to test an HIV-prevention intervention for Latino gay and bisexual men: Lessons learned. *AIDS Care, 17*(3), 314–328.

Carrillo, H. (2002). *The night is young: Sexuality in Mexico in the time of AIDS.* Chicago: University of Chicago Press.

Carrillo, H. (2007). Imagining modernity: Sexuality, policy, and social change in Mexico. *Sexuality Research & Social Policy, 4*, 74–91.

Carrillo, H. (2010). Leaving loved ones behind: Mexican gay men's migration to the USA. In F. Thomas, M. Haour-Knipe, & P. Aggleton (Eds.), *Mobility, sexuality and HIV* (pp. 24–39). London: Routledge.

Carrillo, H., & Fontdevila, J. (2011). Rethinking sexual initiation: Pathways to identity formation among gay and bisexual Mexican male youth. *Archives of Sexual Behavior, 40*, 1241–1254.

Carrillo, H., Fontdevila, J., Brown, J., & Gómez, W. (2008). Risk across borders: Sexual contexts and HIV prevention challenges among Mexican gay and bisexual immigrant men—Findings and recommendations from the Trayectos Study, Available from http://www.caps.ucsf.edu/projects/Trayectos/monograph/EnglishFinal.pdf.

Deren, S., Shedlin, M., Decena, C. U., & Mino, M. (2005). Research challenges to the study of HIV/AIDS among migrant and immigrant Hispanic populations in the United States. *Journal of Urban Health: Bulletin of the New York Academy of Medicine, 83*(2, Suppl 3), iii13–iii25.

Díaz, R. M. (1998). *Latino gay men and HIV.* New York: Routledge.

Díaz, R. M., Ayala, G., & Bein, E. (2004). Sexual risk as an outcome of social oppression: Data from a probability sample of Latino gay men in three U.S. Cities. *Cultural Diversity and Ethnic Minority Psychology, 10*(3), 255–267.

Díaz, R. M., Ayala, G., Bein, E., Henne, J., & Marín, B. V. (2001). The impact of homophobia, poverty, and racism on the mental health of gay and bisexual latino men: Findings from 3 US cities. *American Journal of Public Health, 91*(6), 927–932.

Donohoe, T., Reyes, M., Armas, L., & Mandel, N. (2008). Continuum of care for HIV patients returning to Mexico. *Journal of the Association of Nurses in AIDS Care, 19*(5), 335–337.

Ehrlich, S. F., Organista, K. C., & Oman, D. (2007). Migrant Latino day laborers and intentions to test for HIV. *AIDS Behavior, 11*, 743–752.

Faist, T. (2001). Beyond national and post-national models: Transnational spaces and immigrant integration. In L. Tomasi (Ed.), *New horizons in sociological theory and research: The frontiers of sociology at the beginning of the twenty-first century* (pp. 277–312). Burlington, VT: Ashgate Publishing Co.

Fernandez-Esquer, M. E., Atkinson, J., Diamond, P., Useche, B., & Mendiola, R. (2004). Condom use self-efficacy among U.S.—and foreign-born Latinos in Texas. *Journal of Sex Research, 41*(4), 390–399.

Fernández, M. I., Collazo, J. B., Hernández, N., Bowen, G. S., Varga, L. M., Vila, C. K., et al. (2004). Predictors of HIV risk among Hispanic farmworkers in south Florida: Women are at higher risk than men. *AIDS and Behavior, 8*(2), 165–174.

Fernández, M. I., Jacobs, R. J., Warren, J. C., Sanchez, J., & Bowen, G. S. (2009). Drug use and Hispanic men who have sex with men in south Florida: Implications for intervention development. *AIDS Education and Prevention, 21*(Suppl B), 45–60.

Fitzgerald, K., Chakraborty, J., Shah, T., Khuder, S., & Duggan, J. (2003). HIV/AIDS knowledge among female migrant farm workers in the Midwest. *Journal of Immigrant Health, 5*(1), 29–36.

Gagnon, J. H., & Simon, W. (1973). *Sexual conduct: The social sources of human sexuality* (Vol. 15). Chicago: Aldine Publishing Co.

García Canclini, N. (1995). *Hybrid cultures: Strategies for entering and leaving modernity.* Minneapolis: University of Minnesota Press.

González-Guarda, R. M., Peragallo, N., Urrutia, M. T., Vasquez, E. P., & Mitrani, V. B. (2008). HIV risks, substance abuse, and intimate partner violence among Hispanic women and their intimate partners. *Journal of the Association of Nurses in AIDS Care, 19*(4), 252–266.

González-López, G. (2005). *Erotic journeys: Mexican immigrants and their sex lives.* Berkeley: University of California Press.

Grieco, E. M. (2009). *Race and Hispanic origin of the foreign-born population in the United States: 2007.* Washington, DC: U.S. Census Bureau.

Guilamo-Ramos, V., Bouris, A., Jaccard, J., Lesesne, C., & Ballan, M. (2009). Familial and cultural influences on sexual risk behaviors among Mexican, Puerto Rican, and Dominican Youth. *AIDS Education and Prevention, 21*(Suppl B), 61–79.

Harper, G. W., Bangi, A. K., Sanchez, B., Doll, M., & Pedraza, A. (2009). A quasi-experimental evaluation of a community-based HIV prevention intervention for Mexican American female adolescents: The SHERO's Program. *AIDS Education and Prevention, 21*(Suppl B), 109–123.

Harvey, S. M., Beckman, L. J., Browner, C. H., & Sherman, C. A. (2002). Relationship power, decision making, and sexual relations: An exploratory study with couples of Mexican origin. *Journal of Sex Research, 39*(4), 282–291.

Hernández, M. T., Sanchez, M. A., Ayala, L., Magis-Rodríguez, C., Ruiz, J. D., Samuel, M. C., et al. (2009). Methamphetamine and cocaine use among Mexican migrants in California: The California–Mexico epidemiological surveillance pilot. *AIDS Education and Prevention, 21*(Suppl B), 34–44.

Hirsch, J. S. (2003). *A courtship after marriage: Sexuality and love in Mexican transnational families*. Berkeley: University of California Press.

Hirsch, J. S., Higgins, J., Bentley, M. E., & Nathanson, C. A. (2002). The social constructions of sexuality: Marital infidelity and sexually transmitted disease: HIV risk in a Mexican migrant community. *American Journal of Public Health, 92*(8), 1227–1237.

Hunt, L. M., Schneider, S., & Comer, B. (2004). Should "acculturation" be a variable in health research? A critical review of research on US Hispanics. *Social Science and Medicine, 59*, 973–986.

Itzigsohn, J., Dore Cabral, C., Hernández Medina, E., & Vázquez, O. (1999). Mapping Dominican transnationalism: Narrow and broad transnational practices. *Ethnic and Racial Studies, 22*(2), 316–337.

Jarama, S. L., Kennamer, J. D., Poppen, P. J., Hendricks, M., & Bradford, J. (2005). Psychosocial, behavioral, and cultural predictors of sexual risk for HIV infection among Latino men who have sex with men. *AIDS and Behavior, 9*(4), 513–523.

Kinsler, J. J., Lee, S.-J., Sayles, J. N., Newman, P. A., Diamant, A., & Cunningham, W. (2009). The impact of acculturation on utilization of HIV prevention services and access to care among an at-risk Hispanic population. *Journal of Health Care for the Poor and Underserved, 20*(4), 996–1011.

Levitt, P. (2001). *The transnational villagers*. Berkeley: University of California Press.

Levitt, P., & Jaworsky, B. N. (2007). Transnational migration studies: Past developments and future trends. *Annual Review of Sociology, 33*, 129–156.

Levy, V., Page-Shafer, K., Evans, J., Ruiz, J., Morrow, S., Reardon, J., et al. (2005). HIV-related risk behavior among Hispanic immigrant men in a population-based household survey in low-income neighborhoods of Northern California. *Sexually Transmitted Diseases, 32*(8), 487–490.

Lopez-Quintero, C., Shtarkshall, R., & Newmark, Y. D. (2005). Barriers to HIV-testing among Hispanics in the United States: Analysis of the national health interview survey, 2000. *AIDS Patient Care and STDs, 19*(10), 672–683.

Loue, S. (2006). Preventing HIV, eliminating disparities among Hispanics in the United States. *Journal of Immigrant Health, 8*, 313–318.

Loue, S., Cooper, M., & Fiedler, J. (2003). HIV knowledge among a sample of Puerto Rican and Mexican men and women. *Journal of Immigrant Health, 5*(2), 59–65.

Loue, S., Cooper, M., Traore, F., & Fiedler, J. (2004). Locus of control and HIV risk among a sample of Mexican and Puerto Rican women. *Journal of Immigrant Health, 6*(4), 155–165.

Magis-Rodríguez, C., Lemp, G., Hernandez, M. T., Sanchez, M. A., Estrada, F., & Bravo-García, E. (2009). Going north: Mexican migrants and their vulnerability to HIV. *Journal of Acquired Immune Deficiency Syndromes, 51*(Suppl 1), S21–S25.

Marín, B. V. (2003). HIV prevention in the Hispanic community: Sex, culture, and empowerment. *Journal of Transcultural Nursing, 14*(3), 186–192.

Martínez-Donate, A. P., Zellner, J. A., Fernández-Cerdeño, A., Sañudo, F., Hovell, M. F., Sipan, C. L., et al. (2009). Hombres sanos: Exposure and response to a social marketing HIV prevention campaign targeting heterosexually identified Latino men who have sex with men and women. *AIDS Education and Prevention, 21*(Suppl B), 124–136.

McQuiston, C., & Uribe, L. (2001). Latino recruitment and retention strategies: Community-based HIV prevention. *Journal of Immigrant Health, 3*(2), 97–105.

Moreno, C. (2007). The relationship between culture, gender, structural factors, abuse, trauma, and HIV/AIDS for Latinas. *Qualitative Health Research, 17* (3), 340–352.

Muñoz-Laboy, M., & Dodge, B. (2007). Bisexual Latino men and HIV and sexually transmitted infections risk: An exploratory analysis. *American Journal of Public Health, 97*(6), 1102–1106.

Muñoz-Laboy, M., Hirsch, J. S., & Quispe-Lazaro, A. (2009). Loneliness as a sexual risk factor for male Mexican migrant workers. *American Journal of Public Health, 99*(5), 802–810.

Olshefsky, A. M., Zive, M. M., Scolari, R., & Zuñiga, M. (2007). Promoting HIV risk awareness and testing in Latinos living on the U.S.–Mexico border: The Tú No Me Conoces social marketing campaign. *AIDS Education and Prevention, 19*(5), 422–435.

Organista, K. C., Carrillo, H., & Ayala, G. (2004). HIV prevention with Mexican migrants: Review, critique, and recommendations. *Journal of Acquired Immune Deficiency Syndromes, 37*(4), S227–S239.

Organista, K. C., & Kubo, A. (2005). Pilot survey of HIV risk and contextual problems and issues in Mexican/Latino migrant day laborers. *Journal of Immigrant Health, 7*(4), 269–281.

Painter, T. M. (2008). Connecting the dots: When the risks of HIV/STD infection appear high but the burden of infection is not known—The case of male Latino migrants in the southern United States. *AIDS Behavior, 12,* 213–226.

Parrado, E. A., Flippen, C. A., & McQuiston, C. (2005). Migration and relationship power among Mexican women. *Demography, 42*(2), 347–372.

Parrado, E. A., Flippen, C. A., & Uribe, L. (2010). Concentrated disadvantages: Neighbourhood context as structural risk for Latino immigrants in the USA. In F. Thomas, M. Haour-Knipe, & P. Aggleton (Eds.), *Mobility, sexuality and AIDS* (pp. 40–54). London: Routledge.

Ramirez-Valles, J., Garcia, D., Campbell, R. T., Diaz, R. M., & Heckathorn, D. D. (2008). HIV infection, sexual risk behavior, and substance use among Latino gay and bisexual men and transgender persons. *American Journal of Public Health, 98*(6), 1036–1042.

Rhodes, S. D., Hergenrather, K. C., Bloom, F. R., Leichliter, J. S., & Montaño, J. (2009). Outcomes from a community-based, participatory lay health adviser HIV/STD prevention intervention for recently arrived immigrant Latino men in rural North Carolina. *AIDS Education and Prevention, 21*(Suppl B), 103–108.

Rhodes, S. D., Hergenrather, K. C., Wilkin, A., Alegria-Ortega, J., & Montano, J. (2006). Preventing HIV infection among young immigrant Latino men: Results from focus groups using community-based participatory research. *Journal of the National Medican Association, 98*(4), 564–573.

Rios-Ellis, B., Frates, J., D'Anna, L. H., Dwyer, M., Lopez-Zetina, J., & Ugarte, C. (2008). Addressing the need for access to culturally and linguistically appropriate HIV/AIDS prevention for Latinos. *Journal of Immigrant and Minority Health, 10*(5), 445–460.

Rojas-Guyler, L., Ellis, N., & Sanders, S. (2005). Acculturation, health protective sexual communication, and HIV/AIDS risk behavior among Hispanic women in a large Midwestern city. *Health Education & Behavior, 32*(6), 767–779.

Santelli, J. S., Abraido-Lanza, A. F., & Melnikas, A. J. (2009). Migration, acculturation, and sexual and reproductive health of Latino adolescents. [Editorial]. *Journal of Adolescent Health, 44,* 3–4.

Shedlin, M. G., Decena, C. U., & Oliver-Velez, D. (2005). Initial acculturation and HIV risk among new Hispanic immigrants. *Journal of the National Medican Association, 97*(7), 32S–37S.

Shedlin, M. G., Drucker, E., Decena, C. U., Hoffman, S., Bhattacharya, G., Beckford, S., et al. (2006). Immigration and HIV/AIDS in the New York Metropolitan Area. *Journal of Urban Health: Bulletin of the New York Academy of Medicine, 83*(1), 43–58.

Smith, R. C. (2006). *Mexican New York: Transnational lives of new immigrants.* Berkeley: University of California Press.

Solorio, M. R., & Galvan, F. H. (2009). Self-reported HIV antibody testing among Latino urban day laborers. *Journal of the National Medican Association, 101*(12), 1214–1220.

Swidler, A. (2003). *Talk of love: How culture matters*. Chicago: University of Chicago Press.

Vertovec, S. (2009). *Transnationalism*. New York: Routledge.

Villarruel, A. M., Jemmott III, J. B., Jemmott, L. S., & Ronis, D. L. (2007). Predicting condom use among sexually experienced Latino adolescents. *Western Journal of Nursing Research*, 29(6), 724–738.

Vissman, A. T., Eng, E., Aronson, R. E., Bloom, E. R., Leichliter, J. S., Montano, J., et al. (2009). What do men who serve as lay health advisers really do?: Immigrant Latinos share their experiences as Navegantes to prevent HIV. *AIDS Education and Prevention*, 21(3), 220–232.

Weidel, J. J., Provencio-Vasquez, E., Watson, S. D., & Gonzalez-Guarda, R. (2008). Cultural considerations for intimate partner violence and HIV risk in Hispanics. *Journal of the Association of Nurses in AIDS Care*, 19(4), 247–251.

Zea, M. C., Reisen, C. A., & Díaz, R. M. (2003). Methodological issues in research on sexual behavior with Latino gay and bisexual men. *American Journal of Community Psychology*, 31(3/4), 281–291.

4 Love, Sex, and Power Revisited

The Integration of a Gendered Context in HIV Prevention among Latinas

Monica D. Ulibarri, Anita Raj, and
Hortensia Amaro

INTRODUCTION

This chapter provides a review of the conceptual and empirical work on HIV prevention specific to Latinas that has developed since Amaro's (1995) "Love, Sex, and Power" article was published in *The American Psychologist*. By 1995, it had become evident that HIV and AIDS were serious epidemics disproportionately affecting Latina women in the United States (Centers for Disease Control and Prevention, 1995b). The "Love, Sex, and Power" article has been highly cited (462 citations) and has influenced a generation of HIV activists and researchers seeking to provide better guidance and insight into the unique vulnerabilities that women, particularly poor and minority women, face in the context of HIV prevention. Although the Amaro (1995) study addressed the status of HIV/AIDS research among U.S. women in general, many of the author's suggestions have been applicable to HIV/AIDS prevention research with Latina women specifically (e.g., see Chapter 17) and have provided important conceptual guidelines for future theoretically based work.

We begin this chapter with an overview of HIV/AIDS epidemiology and risk factors among Latinas in the United States. We then highlight existing HIV prevention interventions for Latina women with a special emphasis on programs that have taken a gendered context approach or included aspects of the structural-environmental (SE) model by addressing gender-based violence, relationship power, history of childhood abuse, and alcohol and drug use. Lastly, we provide a summary of advances in HIV prevention among Latinas in the past 15 years and propose what the next generation of HIV prevention efforts for Latinas should include.

It is important to note that this chapter focuses primarily on Latina women in the United States because the nature of Latina women's HIV risk in other countries involves socioeconomic and political considerations beyond the scope of this chapter. It is also important not to assume homogeneity among Latina women as a group. Latinas are composed of various races; they come from various regions in the United States and Latin America, and they represent all levels of socioeconomic status and acculturation (Peragallo et al., 2005). Nonetheless, many experiences, cultural values, and beliefs are common to Latinas as a whole (Arredondo, 2002).

BRIEF HISTORY OF WOMEN, LATINAS, AND HIV IN THE UNITED STATES, 1970s TO 1995

Recognition of HIV/AIDS in the United States began in the 1970s, when a growing number of severe and fatal medical cases developed among mostly gay men; during this period it was in fact assumed to be a disease exclusively of men. By the 1980s, HIV/AIDS was named and identified as a deadly infectious disease disproportionately affecting gay men, people with hemophilia, and injection drug users (IDUs), populations exclusively or predominantly male, though female infections began to be identified in the United States as early as 1982 (Centers for Disease Control and Prevention, 1989; Corea, 1992).

Women were largely invisible in discussions of HIV prevention, diagnosis, and treatment throughout the 1980s (Corea, 1992). Nonetheless, during this same period, service providers and activists working with vulnerable populations of women (e.g., illicit drug-using women, women in prison) were seeing increasing numbers of their patients and clients with indications of HIV infection, but diagnoses were difficult because diagnostic criteria at that time were largely based on how the condition manifested in males (Corea, 1992). Thus, by the late 1980s, a movement began to increase awareness of HIV among women and redefine diagnostic criteria and service provision to be more inclusive of HIV-infected women (Corea, 1992).

By 1992, women, particularly black women and Latinas, were identified as one of the fastest rising populations in the United States in terms of HIV acquisition (Centers for Disease Control and Prevention, 1992). In 1993, AIDS became the fourth leading cause of death among U.S. women aged 25–44 years (Centers for Disease Control and Prevention, 1994). By 1994, there was a more than 3-fold increase in the proportion of female to male HIV cases in the United States over the previous decade (Centers for Disease Control and Prevention, 1995b). This same period also saw a dramatic increase in AIDS cases among Latinos (see Figure 4.1). By 1995, Latinas accounted for one in five female AIDS cases in the United States. HIV/AIDS among women could no longer be ignored; unfortunately, much of the discussion of women and HIV/AIDS focused on women as vectors and vessels of infection for men and children (Corea, 1992; O'Leary & Jemmott, 1996).

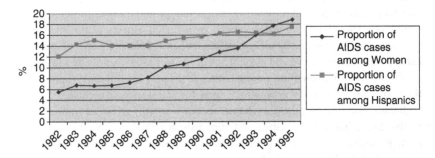

FIGURE 4.1 Proportion of cumulative female and Hispanic AIDS cases from 1982 to 1995. Data from CDC HIV surveillance reports 1982 to 1995 (Centers for Disease Control and Prevention, 2011).

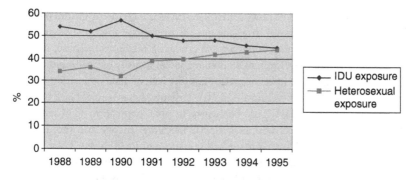

FIGURE 4.2 Proportion of Hispanic women with AIDS by exposure category from 1988 to 1995. Data from HIV/AIDS Surveillance Reports 1988 to 1995 (Centers for Disease Control and Prevention, 2011).

During the mid-1990s, epidemiologic data in the United States were documenting a shift in the primary means of HIV exposure among women: HIV was now more likely to be acquired from heterosexual sex than from injection drug use (Centers for Disease Control and Prevention, 1995b) (see Figure 4.2). The issue of HIV/AIDS and women was at a crisis point and appeared to be a more generalized epidemic for Latina and black women (Centers for Disease Control and Prevention, 1995b). Among Latinas, those born outside of the United States (inclusive of Puerto Rico) were particularly affected by heterosexual HIV transmission (Centers for Disease Control and Prevention, 1995a). In 1995, more than half of AIDS cases among non-U.S.-born Latinas involved heterosexual exposure as compared to only 39% and 16% of U.S.- and Puerto Rican-born Latinas with AIDS, respectively (Centers for Disease Control and Prevention, 1995a). Concerns were raised regarding the impact that growing rates of HIV/AIDS among Latina and black women would have on the health and stability of communities and families (Centers for Disease Control and Prevention, 1995b, 1996). Women, again particularly Latinas and blacks, required greater prioritization for prevention programming. It was in the above context that Amaro's (1995) "Love, Sex and Power" was written.

Context and Impact of "Love, Sex, and Power"

By 1995, a number of HIV prevention efforts had been published and had demonstrated a significant impact on reducing HIV risk behaviors (e.g., unprotected sex, multiple sex partners) among gay men, injection drug users (active or in recovery), and non-IDU substance-using populations (Card, Benner, Shields, & Feinstein, 2001). These efforts were individually based and cognitively focused, utilizing social and behavioral theories such as Social Cognitive Theory (Bandura, 1986), Theory of Reasoned Action (Ajzen & Fishbein, 1977, 1980; Fishbein & Ajzen, 2010), and Diffusion of Innovation Theory (Kelly et al., 1992; Kelly, St. Lawrence, Brasfield, & Hood, 1989; Kelly, St. Lawrence, Diaz, & Stevenson, 1991). As highlighted in "Love, Sex and Power," these theories were likely of limited utility for women at risk for HIV in heterosexual relationships because all of these theories were premised on individual control over sexual behavior and failed to recognize the powerful role of gender norms in sexual behavior. Such perspectives negated the reality of women's lives and heterosexual dyadic relationships, which are entrenched in power inequities advantaging men.

Amaro (1995) asked us how women's desire to use condoms in sexual relationships with men could result in actual use of condoms if men, the likely wearers of the condom, refuse. If women are experiencing relationship abuse, economic dependence, or are simply reliant on men for social security or positioning, how do they safely engage in condom negotiation in the face of male opposition? In 1995, only one U.S.-based intervention—SISTA, targeting heterosexual black women—significantly reduced HIV risk behaviors in this population (DiClemente & Wingood, 1995). SISTA, based on Social Learning Theory and the Theory of Gender and Power, addressed many of the issues put forth in the "Love, Sex, and Power" article by emphasizing ethnic and gender pride and condom-use communication, negotiation, and norms within heterosexual relationships.

EPIDEMIOLOGY OF HIV/AIDS AMONG LATINAS IN THE UNITED STATES TODAY

The disproportionate impact of HIV on the Latino community relative to white communities continues. Although Latinos currently represent 15% of the U.S. population, they account for 16% of new HIV diagnoses among U.S. women (Centers for Disease Control and Prevention, 2008; Hall et al., 2008). Recent evidence documents that the estimated lifetime risk (ELR) for contracting HIV among U.S. Latinas is 0.94% (i.e., a 1 in 106 chance); this is almost five times the ELR for white females in the United States (Centers for Disease Control and Prevention, 2010a).

For women generally, and Latinas specifically, heterosexual sex remains the predominant means of exposure. Among Latinas, 84% of newly diagnosed HIV cases were acquired via heterosexual sex; 16% were acquired via injection drug use (Centers for Disease Control and Prevention, 2008). As described previously, among Latina women, IDU-related infections were more likely among U.S.-born women (inclusive of Puerto Rico) than among immigrant women (Centers for Disease Control and Prevention, 2008). However, whereas in 1995, the major mode of transmission among women in the United States and Puerto Rico was associated with IDU, today the major single category of risk for women is heterosexual transmission (Centers for Disease Control and Prevention, 2008). This shift to heterosexual transmission suggests that we may be moving toward a more generalized epidemic in Latino communities, as indicated by recent data from the CDC (Denning & DiNenno, 2010).

UNAIDS defines a generalized epidemic as one in which the HIV rate among the general population is greater than 1% (UNAIDS, 2010). Although the United States maintains an HIV rate of less than 1%, recent research from the CDC documents that in impoverished urban areas in the United States (typically those with greater numbers of black and Hispanic residents), the HIV prevalence rate is 2.1%, demonstrating a generalized epidemic for these populations (Denning & DiNenno, 2010). Additionally, these data demonstrate that although Latinos in the United States generally fare better than blacks in terms of likelihood of HIV infection (Centers for Disease Control and Prevention, 2008), in these poor urban environments, likelihood of HIV infection does not vary between these racial/ethnic groups (Denning & DiNenno, 2010).

Overall, this review of existing national surveillance efforts indicates an ongoing need for HIV interventions tailored to Latinas at risk for HIV via heterosexual sex. Such at-risk women may not easily be identified via their own sexual risk practices, in the context of a growing generalized HIV epidemic in poor urban areas. But rather these interventions may better be targeted to these geographic areas themselves, because residence within such areas confers risk for HIV beyond that solely explained by women's or their partners' sex practices. Such findings corroborate the relationally focused "Love, Sex and Power" approach by adding neighborhood context and poverty as contributors to the HIV epidemic among Latinas, and as potential intervention targets of employment, housing, and microfinance supports as a means of reducing HIV risk in these communities.

HIV RISK AMONG LATINAS

As highlighted in the previous section on the epidemiology of HIV among women, the primary mode of HIV risk for Latinas is through heterosexual contact followed by injection drug use. However, there are several gendered factors (e.g., traditional gender norms, intimate partner violence, and relationship power) as well as structural-environmental factors (migration and acculturation issues, poverty, and access to health care) that impact individual level factors such as lack of accurate HIV/AIDS knowledge, self-efficacy, substance use and abuse, and psychological distress, further exacerbating Latinas' behavioral risks for HIV (Herbst et al., 2007; Marín, 2003; Newcomb & Carmona, 2004; Peragallo et al., 2005; Simoni et al., 2010; Weeks, Schensul, Williams, & Singer, 1995). In this section, we focus on relationship power, intimate partner violence, psychological distress, substance abuse, and HIV risk, which are most relevant to Amaro's (1995) gendered context model and the SE model, with consideration of how cultural constructs may influence Latinas' HIV risk behavior.

Relationship Power and Intimate Partner Violence

There are two predominant definitions of relationship power in women's HIV prevention literature: one emphasizes women's economic status (e.g., higher education and income level) (Babcock, Waltz, Jacobson, & Gottman, 1993) and the other emphasizes control and decision making in sexual relationships (Billy, Grady, & Sill, 2009; Pulerwitz, Gortmaker, & DeJong, 2000). Both play a key role in women's HIV risk by impeding a woman's ability to initiate or negotiate condom use (Amaro et al., 2007; Pulerwitz, Amaro, De Jong, Gortmaker, & Rudd, 2002; Pulerwitz et al., 2000; Raj, Silverman, & Amaro, 2004; Simoni et al., 2010; Suarez-Al-Adam, Raffaelli, & O'Leary, 2000; Ulibarri, Sumner, Cyriac, & Amaro, 2010). In addition, unequal economic status in heterosexual relationships may further disempower Latinas by making them more dependent on men for economic and social stability (Simoni et al., 2010). Latinas' recognition of this and interest in inclusion of economic supports as a means of HIV prevention were documented in a needs assessment study conducted by the National Council of La Raza (2006).

HIV risk through heterosexual contact among Latinas may be further complicated by the presence of intimate partner violence (IPV) in the relationship (El-Bassel et al., 2007; Wu, El-Bassel, Witte, Gilbert, & Chang, 2003). For example, in clinic and emergency department-based studies with predominantly minority women (inclusive of Latinas) in New York, IPV was associated with increased likelihood of engaging in unprotected sex and having multiple sex partners, a history of sexually transmitted infection (STI), and/or a high-risk male partner (e.g., injection drug using or HIV-infected male partner) (El-Bassel et al., 2007; Wu et al., 2003).

Although these studies did not conduct separate analyses by ethnic group, they were some of the first empirical studies to document the relationship between IPV and HIV risk among ethnic minority women and acknowledge the importance that violence plays in the gendered context of Latina and African American women's heterosexual relationships.

More recently, in a study of HIV risk and IPV among a community sample of Latinas and their intimate partners in South Florida, Gonzalez-Guarda and colleagues (2008) did not find a direct relationship between IPV and condom use, but IPV was associated with the women's history of STIs and male partners' HIV risk behaviors (e.g., history of STIs, ever injected drugs, sex with other men, being a sex worker, or an IDU). Gonzalez-Guarda and colleagues suggested that these findings indicate that Latinas' risk for HIV may be more influenced by their partners' behaviors than their own. The implications of these studies are that Latinas may be at risk for HIV not only through their own behavior, but through the risk behaviors of their abusive male partners, and that the power structure and dynamics in intimate relationships may shape the choices Latinas have or do not have with respect to their own risk behaviors.

Further research is needed to fully understand the influence of relationship power and intimate partner violence on Latina women's HIV risk behaviors. Subsequent research should consider including male partners and utilizing dyad-based methodology and analyses to obtain better information about the context of the relationship in which many risk behaviors occur. Research with a predominantly Latino sample of men documents that those reporting IPV perpetration and traditional gender role ideologies are significantly more likely to report risky sex practices including unprotected sex and multiple partnering (Raj et al., 2006; Santana, Raj, Decker, La Marche, & Silverman, 2006), suggesting the utility of assessing men for IPV perpetration. However, the safety of women in dyadic interventions must be taken into consideration because research including male partners may be contraindicated in cases where extreme IPV is present (Witte et al., 2004).

Substance Abuse and Cooccurring Psychological Disorders

Research consistently documents high rates of HIV risk among women with serious mental illnesses [e.g., depression, bipolar disorder, posttraumatic stress disorder (PTSD)], cooccurring substance abuse, and a history of gender-based violence such as childhood sexual abuse, rape, and IPV (Friedman & Loue, 2007; Ulibarri, Sumner, et al., 2010). However, there is relatively little research in the area of HIV risk, substance abuse, and cooccurring psychological disorders among Latinas. Psychological disorders may increase HIV risk through participation in self-destructive behaviors (e.g., sexual promiscuity and unprotected sex with high-risk partners), increased drug use to self-medicate psychiatric symptoms, and drug-related risk behaviors (e.g., sharing needles, trading sex for drugs) (Devieux et al., 2007; Parillo, Freeman, Collier, & Young, 2001). For example, a recent study of HIV sexual risk behavior among Puerto Rican women with severe mental illness (i.e., depression, bipolar disorder, schizophrenia) found that women suffering from increased severity of psychiatric symptoms were more likely to report sex with an injection drug user, sex while high on drugs or alcohol, and trading sex for money or drugs (Heaphy, Loue, Sajatovic, & Tisch, 2010). Likewise, an empirical study of PTSD and HIV risk among African American and Latina women accessing emergency room services showed an association between having PTSD symptoms and sex with multiple sexual partners, sex with a male risky partner (e.g., injection drug using), and having experienced partner violence related to condom use compared to women who did not exhibit PTSD symptoms (El-Bassel, Gilbert, Vinocur, Chang, & Wu, 2011). These studies provide evidence for the importance of considering psychological distress and substance use when assessing HIV risk among Latinas, and the need for HIV prevention interventions that address multiple factors associated with HIV risk.

Latino Cultural Constructs

Latino cultural constructs, such as *machismo* and *marianismo* (male and female gender role ideology, respectively), likely serve as facilitators or inhibitors of HIV risk. Unfortunately, there is a paucity of empirical research that measures these cultural constructs specifically and their relation to HIV risk behaviors among Latinas (see Carillo's critique of these constructs in Chapter 3).

Many theorize that the traditional gender role of *machismo*, which accepts male dominance as a proper form of male conduct (Castro & Hernandez, 2004), may encourage risky sexual behaviors such as having multiple sex partners, engaging in unprotected sex, and dominance over women (Alvarez et al., 2009; Marín, 2003; Pérez-Jiménez, Seal, & Serrano-García, 2009; Weidel, Provencio-Vasquez, Watson, & Gonzalez-Guarda, 2008). Goodyear, Newcomb, and Allison (2000) found that Latino young men with more traditional gender role ideologies had greater pregnancy involvement and endorsement of coercive sex. Conversely, it is proposed that the more positive aspects of *machismo*, such as protecting and honoring the welfare of the family (Galanti, 2003), may motivate Latino men to reduce their risk behaviors to protect their family's well-being (Alvarez et al., 2009). However, there are still very few empirical studies with males or females that measure *machismo*, or even traditional gender roles more broadly, and its relation to HIV risk in the Latino community.

Marianismo is the female traditional gender role counterpart to *machismo*. The word is derived from the Virgin Mary and refers to the belief that women should be saintly, pure, self-sacrificing, and deferent to men (Arredondo, 2002; Simoni et al., 2010). As with *machismo*, empirical research documenting and measuring *marianismo* is still evolving and is yet to be incorporated into HIV research with Latinas. However, it is theorized that adherence to *marianismo* may affect Latinas' sexual decision-making control, placing them at greater risk for HIV (Marín, 2003; Simoni et al., 2010).

There are several other Latino cultural constructs that are purported to influence HIV risk behaviors among Latinas. For example, it is thought that *familismo*, the importance of family, including a strong emphasis on placing family needs before one's own gratification (Clauss-Ehlers & Levi, 2002; Raffaelli & Ontai, 2004), may be used as a motivating factor for Latinas to engage in safer sex practices to ensure their healthy longevity and ability to care for their families. In addition, *simpatía,* maintaining harmonious and nonconfrontational interpersonal relationships, and *respeto,* respect and attention to issues of social position in interpersonal relationships, may have important implications for Latina women's condom negotiation. Latinas, especially those who fear IPV, may wish to avoid confrontation with male sex partner, and consequently avoid being more assertive and asking partners about their sexual histories and condom use.

Latino cultural constructs that dictate traditional gender roles and gender stereotypes, as well as script what is considered to be acceptable communication and behavior surrounding sex, may be important influences on relationship power and HIV risk prevention among Latina women and their male sexual partners. However, further research is needed to determine the actual effect of these gender role beliefs and scripts among Latinos/as. Latinas of different generations, levels of acculturation, and socioeconomic levels may or may not conform to these beliefs, or if they do, may do so to varying degrees (Arredondo, 2002). In addition, further examination of the relationship among power, social status, and cultural constructs in the context of HIV research is needed. It is not known whether they may operate as direct-effect causal factors of HIV risk behavior or as moderators or mediators of the direct influence of other causal variables of risk behavior (Castro & Hernandez, 2004; Ulibarri et al., 2010). However, once known, this information may have important implications for the design of effective HIV prevention education for Latina women. Interestingly, Rios-Ellis in Chapter 16 of this book reports on an intervention designed to facilitate communication about sex and HIV between mothers and daughters.

HIV PREVENTION INTERVENTIONS WITH LATINAS

Since the publication of "Love, Sex, and Power," there have been a few interventions with demonstrated effectiveness that were designed to address issues such as relationship power, gender-based violence, substance abuse, or cooccurring mental health problems for Latina women. Most of these are listed among the CDC's Best Evidence or Promising Evidence Interventions (Centers for Disease Control and Prevention, 2009a, 2009c); however, there remain no studies developed specifically for adult Latinas on the CDC's Diffusion of Effective Behavioral Interventions (DEBI) list (CDC and AED, 2009).

In this section we highlight a few of the Best Evidence and Promising Evidence interventions for Latinas that we felt were good examples of work with a gendered contextual approach. This list is not intended to be a comprehensive review of the literature regarding HIV prevention with Latinas, which is outside the scope of this chapter; rather it is a selection of successful interventions that we believe illustrate the necessary components of a gendered context approach. For a more in-depth review of the adaptation and dissemination of DEBI interventions in Hispanic/Latino populations see Stallworth and colleagues (2009).

The Women's Health Promotion (WHP) program (Amaro, Raj, Reed, & Cranston, 2002; Centers for Disease Control and Prevention, 2007; Raj et al., 2001), tailored for Spanish-speaking, heterosexual, HIV-negative Latina women, utilized tenets of Social Cognitive Theory, the Theory of Reasoned Action, and the Health Belief Model to reduce risky sexual behavior among a community sample of Latinas in Boston. In addition to HIV/AIDS and STI education, condom practice, and negotiation skills, WHP also included participant-suggested sessions that addressed the women's larger structural environment or gendered context such as general mental health, depression, cervical cancer, diabetes, nutrition, non-HIV-related partner communication, partner violence, oppression, and social justice. Gender-specific programming elements included emphasis on female physiology, the effect of partner violence on sexual risk, and sexual negotiation with consideration of relationship power dynamics (Massachusetts Department of Public Health, 1998). Women in the specialized WHP intervention group demonstrated a substantial increase in condom use at the 3-month follow-up evaluation as compared to women in the wait-list control group who received only HIV prevention material and referrals (Raj et al., 2001). This Latina-focused evaluation study was a direct result of the "Love, Sex, and Power" article, building on the framework presented in that work. To date, the WHP is still the only program on the CDC Best Evidence list that is solely for adult Latinas and is gender, culturally, and linguistically tailored to their needs. These findings clearly highlight the need for increased attention to the creation of effective HIV prevention models for Latinas, with consideration of the diverse cultures and regional variations of this population.

Project SEPA [Salud, Educación, Prevención y Autocuidado (Health, Education, Prevention and Self-Care)] (Peragallo et al., 2005) is a culturally sensitive intervention designed to reduce high-risk HIV sexual behaviors among low-income Mexican American and Puerto Rican women (also reviewed in Chapter 17). One of the CDC's Promising Evidence Interventions (as opposed to Best Evidence) (Centers for Disease Control and Prevention, 2009c), it is noteworthy because of the input researchers obtained during its design from the Latina community. They incorporated important themes, such as interpersonal violence, identified through focus groups with their target population and were sensitive to cultural issues surrounding the delivery of the intervention (Peragallo et al., 2005). An essential element in their intervention was the use of Latina bilingual and bicultural facilitators who understood the perspective of the participants and tailored the sessions to their specific needs. However, these specific elements were not assessed in the evaluation of the intervention. Project SEPA was efficacious in decreasing perceived barriers to condom use and increasing HIV knowledge, partner communication, and risk-behavior intentions. It did not, however, change perceived safer-sex peer norms. Compared to the control group, a greater proportion of the intervention group reported increased condom use at 3-month follow-up; however, their sample size lacked statistical power to detect a difference between the groups at the $p = 0.05$ level. Nonetheless, Project SEPA illustrates the importance of involving Latinas in developing the content of interventions and utilizing facilitators who have the necessary expertise and experiences to gain the trust of the Latina women who they serve.

Although not Latina-specific, Project Connect (Centers for Disease Control and Prevention, 2009b; El-Bassel et al., 2001, 2003, 2005) is a DEBI-listed, six-session HIV/STD relationship-based intervention to increase condom use, decrease STD transmission, and reduce the number of sexual partners. It was originally tested among both African American and Latino heterosexual couples (54.3% African American, 38.3% Latino). Although it did not draw from any gender-specific theoretical framework, Project Connect's strengths are that it recognized the importance of relationship dynamics and focused on couple communication to empower women to initiate and sustain condom use with their long-term intimate partners. This intervention is also significant in that it demonstrates the feasibility of couples-based HIV interventions among ethnic minority heterosexual couples (El-Bassel et al., 2001). However, it is important to note that the intervention outcome data were not analyzed separately for each ethnic group.

Another example of a more gender and structural environmental approach to HIV prevention is the Boston Consortium Model (Amaro et al., 2004), which was part of the SAMHSA-funded Women, Co-Occurring Disorders and Violence Study (WCDVS) and is listed in the National Registry of Evidence-Based Programs and Practices (NREPP, 2011). The Boston Consortium Model (BCM) of integrated trauma, mental health, and substance abuse treatment was implemented in substance abuse treatment sites in Boston. The study assessed HIV risk behaviors, mental health, trauma, and substance abuse outcomes among women receiving the BCM and those receiving substance abuse services as usual. Although not Latina specific (the sample was close to evenly divided among Latina, African American, and non-Latina white women), this study illustrates the importance of comprehensive and integrated care in the context of HIV prevention among low-income women with cooccurring psychiatric and substance use disorders and a history of sexual or physical abuse.

The intervention focused on the system of care as well as the individual client levels. At the system of care level, the intervention integrated a trauma-informed approach (Amaro et al., 2004) through comprehensive staff training on trauma and its link to mental health and addiction disorders, integrated assessment and treatment planning for trauma and addiction disorders, and connections between the mental health and addictions treatment systems of care. At the individual client level, the intervention provided a series of manualized skills-based interventions (i.e., economic, family reunification, and leadership skills) and a trauma-specific intervention group. The intervention contained group sessions addressing trauma, coping skills, empowerment, safety, and increasing awareness of the association between substance abuse, mental health problems, and trauma; the control group received standard treatment for substance abuse. Women who received the integrated trauma treatment intervention were more likely to demonstrate reduced sexual risk behaviors relative to the control group at 6 and 12 month follow-up (Amaro et al., 2007). Additionally, results indicated that women in the intervention had higher relationship power at 6 and 12 months and that those with higher relationship power scores were less likely to engage in unprotected sex than women with lower scores. The intervention also produced significantly greater reductions in trauma and mental health symptomatology and drug abstinence.

The BCM results illustrate the value of comprehensive interventions that address multiple gender- and structural-level issues in the context of HIV prevention research. As a whole, these studies provide evidence that incorporating concepts of gender empowerment, mental health, substance abuse, and trauma treatment are important to consider when designing future HIV behavioral risk-reduction interventions for high-risk women.

RECOMMENDATIONS FOR THE NEXT GENERATION OF HIV PREVENTION INTERVENTIONS FOR LATINAS

Since the publication of "Love, Sex, and Power," there have been several advances in HIV prevention and treatment in the United States. There are now several efficacious behavioral HIV prevention interventions available for women (CDC and AED, 2009). However, very few address issues of gender and power or are culturally specific to Latinas. There have also been significant advances in the prevention of perinatal HIV transmission, resulting in a near elimination of HIV in infants and children in the United States (De Cock, Jaffe, & Curran, 2011; Dieffenbach & Fauci, 2011). However, the rate of HIV/AIDS perinatal transmission in Latino children remains four times greater than among white children (Centers for Disease Control and Prevention, 2010b). Likewise, there have been advances in the treatment of HIV and AIDS through antiretroviral therapy (ART). Yet Latina and black women with HIV and AIDS are at greater risk for death compared to white women. Further, recent findings demonstrate that antiretroviral treatment of infected individuals leads to significant reduced risk of transmission of the virus to their sexual partners (National Institute of Allergy and Infectious Diseases, 2011) and postexposure prophylaxis against HIV by using ART (Barber & Benn, 2010) provides an important prevention tool that has high relevance for women, including women rape survivors. However, it is yet to be seen whether Latinas will benefit from these biomedical advances in HIV prevention. Access to and widespread implementation of the advances in the use of antiretroviral and postexposure treatment as tools for prevention of HIV among Latinas will require significant effort and research to identify the most efficacious methods for dissemination.

Reducing these health disparities should be the focus of the next generation of HIV/AIDS prevention and treatment research for Latina women. In addition, despite many of the advances in interventions for Latina women over the past 15 years, important gaps continue to exist in our understanding of the relationships among power, socioeconomic status, Latino cultural values, gender-based violence, and HIV risk and infection. There are several areas in which the next generation of HIV prevention interventions for Latina women must be improved.

First, we must include the end users, in this case, Latinas, in the development, implementation, and evaluation of HIV/AIDS outreach, education, and intervention programs. We must also identify critical elements of culturally specific interventions in order to understand what works best for Latina women. Methods such as community-based participatory research may be especially helpful in the development of original and adaptation of existing evidence-based prevention interventions (Alvarez et al., 2009; Castro, Barrera, & Martinez, 2004). Obtaining the input of the Latina community throughout the entire process will ensure cultural appropriateness and promote ownership and further dissemination of the resulting intervention.

The use of *promotoras*, Latina community members who disseminate health messages (Ramos, Hernandez, Ferreira-Pinto, Ortiz, & Somerville, 2006), may serve as a cost-effective method for HIV prevention and education. Although research on HIV prevention programs for Latinas using *promotoras* is sparse, there are a few promising studies that have demonstrated success in increasing HIV knowledge and testing among Latina women along the United States–Mexico border (Ramos, Ferreira-Pinto, Rusch, & Ramos, 2010; Ramos, Green, & Shulman, 2009). *Promotora*-based models may be especially helpful in reaching less acculturated Latinas who are otherwise unlikely to access HIV prevention services (Gonzalez, Hendriksen, Collins, Durán, & Safren, 2009). However, further investigation on the utility and cost-effectiveness of the use of *promotoras* relative to other methods is needed.

Second, further research on Latino cultural constructs and how they contribute relationship power dynamics and HIV risk is needed. Many of the proposed relationships between Latino cultural values such as *machismo* and *marianismo* and HIV risk remain theoretical and have not been empirically demonstrated. However, as advancements in the measurement of these constructs are made, more research including these constructs should be possible.

Third, cultural adaptations of existing interventions for women should be developed and tested, especially in resource-poor settings in which time and monetary resources may not be available for more extensive culturally specific development. There is a strong body of literature providing guidelines for the cultural adaptation of evidence-based interventions (Barrera & Castro, 2006; Bernal, 2006; Castro et al., 2004). In addition, the CDC's Division of HIV/AIDS Prevention (DHAP)

Capacity Building and Prevention Program Branches have made significant efforts to adapt existing DEBI interventions for the Latino community (Stallworth et al., 2009). There have been several successful adaptations of DEBI interventions for use among Latinas (Stallworth et al., 2009). For example, Sisters Informing Sisters on Topics About AIDS (SISTA), originally designed for African American women, has been adapted for Latinas by the American Psychological Association (APA) Behavioral and Social Science Volunteer (BSSV) Program in collaboration with the CDC (American Psychological Association, 2011). However, publication of outcome results from the actual implementation of SISTA with Latinas is still needed. It is likely that we will continue to see more adaptations of existing DEBI interventions for Latinas in the future, and we look forward to the documentation of this process and results in the literature.

Fourth, embedding HIV prevention into the context of other services that Latina women are likely to use such as health care settings, prenatal care, family planning and reproductive health clinics, community-based organizations, substance abuse and mental health treatment, domestic violence services, and schools may improve access for Latina women. In addition, it may reduce the stigma associated with seeking HIV-specific services (Alvarez et al., 2009). El-Bassel and colleagues (El-Bassel et al., 2007, 2011; Sormanti, Wu, & El-Bassel, 2004) have demonstrated effective screening for HIV risk behaviors, intimate partner violence, substance use, and posttraumatic stress disorder among African American and Latina women in outpatient clinics and emergency medical care settings. HIV prevention interventions that utilize existing services may prove cost-effective and improve outreach to Latinas.

Lastly, interventions should routinely screen for gender-based violence and incorporate treatment for trauma (Ulibarri, Sumner, et al., 2010). In the past 15 years, increased attention to gender issues in HIV prevention has yielded research documenting gender-based violence as a factor that contributes to Latina women's risk of HIV infection (El-Bassel et al., 2007, 2011; Gonzalez-Guarda et al., 2008; Gonzalez-Guarda, Vasquez, Urrutia, Villarruel, & Peragallo, 2011; Raj et al., 2004). HIV intervention approaches need to address issues of gender-based violence and relationship power as risk factors that can directly affect women's ability to negotiate condom use and engage in sexually protective behaviors with their male partners (Amaro et al., 2007; El-Bassel et al., 2001, 2003, 2005). Interventions that address these issues show great promise (El-Bassel et al., 2005; Peragallo et al., 2005; Raj et al., 2001) and should be disseminated and adapted to other high-risk Latina populations.

CONCLUSIONS

In the past 15 years, Latinas have become one of the fastest growing populations at risk for HIV. A history of abuse, such as intimate partner violence, substance abuse, and cooccurring mental disorders, is a structural environmental and gender-based issue that further complicates their risk. Whereas integrated intervention efforts for gender-based violence, trauma, and substance abuse are necessary to address HIV risk among women generally and Latinas specifically, consideration must also be given to structural issues related to women's and girls' capacity to protect themselves from HIV. Though effective HIV interventions in the United States are largely focused on individual or dyadic sexual risk reduction efforts (Centers for Disease Control and Prevention, 2009a), growing international work documents the importance of improving gender-equity ideologies among men (Jewkes et al., 2006, 2008; RISHTA, 2007; Schensul et al., 2009) and increasing economic autonomy of women (Kim et al., 2007; Pronyk et al., 2006) as a means of reducing women's risk and vulnerability to HIV in their sexual relationships with men. These more recent works document the importance of addressing social and structural risk factors (e.g., gender inequities, poverty) that reinforce sexual risk for HIV, as a means of reducing HIV risks. There is documentation of greater structural risks for Latinos relative to non-Latino populations in the United States, in terms of education, employment, and income (Pew Hispanic Center, 2011), and certainly gender inequities exist within the culture as described previously. Hence, these types of social-structural interventions targeting men as well as women may prove very useful in reducing HIV/AIDS in Latino communities.

Since the publication of "Love, Sex, and Power," the recognition of the gender-specific nature of women's HIV risk has gained attention, with some DEBI programs having a sound conceptual framing of these issues; however, the advances in HIV prevention interventions for Latinas specifically have been quite limited. In fact, still applicable today are many of the issues originally discussed by Amaro in 1988 (Amaro, 1988) regarding the need for specific HIV prevention interventions for Latinas and the examination of structural, cultural, and gender-based factors impacting Latina's HIV risk. Because Latinos are the largest minority group and are projected to constitute 29% of the population by the year 2050 (Pew Hispanic Center, 2008), the continued lack of progress in HIV prevention for Latinas represents a serious scientific gap that will contribute to the rising rates of HIV among Latina women. The advancement of research in the area of Latino cultural constructs and their relation to HIV risk is central to the development of improved HIV prevention methods. Currently, research on Latino cultural constructs is still speculative. Cultural adaptations for Latinas of existing evidence-based interventions are viable, but documentation of the efficacy and outcomes of these adaptations remains sparse.

There is great need for a sustained program of research and efficacy studies at the National Institutes of Health and the Centers for Disease Control and Prevention to create a knowledge base that will inform the development of HIV prevention strategies among Latinas. We look forward to the next generation of HIV prevention research among Latina women and hope that it yields answers to many of our remaining questions and produces efficacious prevention interventions that can stop the current trend of increasing HIV infection in Latinas.

ACKNOWLEDGMENTS

Monica Ulibarri was supported in part by a grant from the National Institute on Drug Abuse (K01 DA026307).

REFERENCES

Ajzen, I., & Fishbein, M. (1977). Attitude-behavior relations: A theoretical analysis and review of empirical research. *Psychological Bulletin, 84*(5), 888–918. doi: 10.1037/0033-2909.84.5.888.

Ajzen, I., & Fishbein, M. (1980). *Understanding attitudes and predicting social behavior.* Englewood Cliffs, NJ: Prentice-Hall.

Alvarez, M. E., Jakhmola, P., Painter, T. M., Taillepierre, J. D., Romaguera, R. A., Herbst, J. H., & Wolitski, R. J. (2009). Summary of comments and recommendations from the CDC consultation on the HIV/AIDS epidemic and prevention in the Hispanic/Latino community. *AIDS Education and Prevention, 21*(5), 7–18. doi: 10.1521/aeap.2009.21.5_supp.7.

Amaro, H. (1988). Considerations for prevention of HIV infection among Hispanic women. *Psychology of Women Quarterly, 12*(4), 429–443. doi: 10.1111/j.1471-6402.1988.tb00976.x.

Amaro, H. (1995). Love, sex, and power: Considering women's realities in HIV prevention. *American Psychologist, 50*(6), 437–447.

Amaro, H., Larson, M. J., Zhang, A., Acevedo, A., Dai, J., & Matsumoto, A. (2007). Effects of trauma intervention on HIV sexual risk behaviors among women with co-occurring disorders in substance abuse treatment. *Journal of Community Psychology, 35*(7), 895–908.

Amaro, H., McGraw, S., Larson, M. J., Lopez, L., Nieves, R., & Marshall, B. (2004). Boston consortium of services for families in recovery: A trauma-informed intervention model for women's alcohol and drug addiction treatment. *Alcoholism Treatment Quarterly, 22*(3–4), 95–119. doi: 10.1300/J020v22n03_06.

Amaro, H., Raj, A., Reed, E., & Cranston, K. (2002). Implementation and long-term outcomes of two HIV intervention programs for Latinas. *Health Promotion Practice, 3,* 245–254.

American Psychological Association. (2011). Resource guide for adapting SISTA for Latinas. Retrieved February 16, 2011, from http://www.apa.org/pi/aids/programs/bssv/sista.pdf.

Arredondo, P. (2002). Mujeres latinas—Santas y marquesas. *Cultural Diversity and Ethnic Minority Psychology, 8*(4), 308–319. doi: 10.1037/1099-9809.8.4.308.

Babcock, J. C., Waltz, J., Jacobson, N. S., & Gottman, J. M. (1993). Power and violence: The relation between communication patterns, power discrepancies, and domestic violence. *Journal of Consulting and Clinical Psychology, 61*(1), 40–50.

Bandura, A. (1986). *Social foundations of thought and action: A social cognitive theory.* Englewood Cliffs, NJ: Prentice-Hall, Inc.

Barber, T. J., & Benn, P. D. (2010). Postexposure prophylaxis for HIV following sexual exposure. *Current Opinion in HIV and AIDS, 5,* 322–326. doi: 10.1097/COH. 0b013e32833a5e6c.

Barrera, M., Jr., & Castro, F. G. (2006). A heuristic framework for the cultural adaptation of interventions. *Clinical Psychology: Science and Practice, 13*(4), 311–316. doi: 10.1111/j.1468-2850.2006.00043.x.

Bernal, G. (2006). Intervention development and cultural adaptation research with diverse families. *Family Process, 45*(2), 143–151. doi: 10.1111/j.1545-5300.2006.00087.x.

Billy, J. O., Grady, W. R., & Sill, M. E. (2009). Sexual risk-taking among adult dating couples in the United States. *Perspectives on Sexual and Reproductive Health, 41*(2), 74–83.

Card, J. J., Benner, T., Shields, J. P., & Feinstein, N. (2001). The HIV/AIDS prevention program archive (HAPPA): A collection of promising prevention programs in a box. *AIDS Education and Prevention: Official Publication of the International Society for AIDS Education, 13*(1), 1–28.

Castro, F. G., Barrera, M., Jr., & Martinez, C. R., Jr. (2004). The cultural adaptation of prevention interventions: Resolving tensions between fidelity and fit. *Prevention Science, 5*(1), 41–45. doi: 10.1023/B:PREV.0000013980.12412.cd.

Castro, F. G., & Hernandez, N. T. (2004). A cultural perspective on prevention interventions. In R. J. Velasquez, L. M. Arellano, & B. W. McNeill (Eds.), *The handbook of Chicana/o psychology and mental health* (pp. 371–397). Mahwah, NJ: Lawrence Erlbaum Associates.

CDC and AED. (2009). The diffusion of effective behavioral interventions (DEBI) project retrieved 02/16/2011, 2011, from http://www.effectiveinterventions.org/.

Centers for Disease Control and Prevention. (1989). Current trends first 100,000 cases of acquired immunodeficiency syndrome. *Morbidity and Mortality Weekly Report, 38*(32), 561–563.

Centers for Disease Control and Prevention. (1992). Update: Acquired immunodeficiency syndrome—United States, 1991. *Morbidity and Mortality Weekly Report, 41*(26), 463–468.

Centers for Disease Control and Prevention. (1994). Annual summary of births, marriages, divorces, and deaths; United States, 1993. *Monthly Vital Statistics Report* (Vol. 42, pp. 18–20). Hyattsville, MD: U.S. Department of Health and Human Services, Public Health Service.

Centers for Disease Control and Prevention. (1995a). HIV/AIDS surveillance report year-end. 7(2).

Centers for Disease Control and Prevention. (1995b). Update: AIDS among women—United States, 1994. *Morbidity and Mortality Weekly, 40*(5), 81–84.

Centers for Disease Control and Prevention. (1996). AIDS among children—United States, 1996. *Morbidity and Mortality Weekly, 45*(46), 1005–1010.

Centers for Disease Control and Prevention. (2007). Best-evidence: Women's health promotion (WHP). Retrieved March 3, from http://www.cdc.gov/hiv/topics/research/prs/resources/factsheets/WHP.htm.

Centers for Disease Control and Prevention. (2008). HIV surveillance report, Volume 20. Retrieved February 18, 2011, from http://www.cdc.gov/hiv/topics/surveillance/resources/reports/.

Centers for Disease Control and Prevention. (2009a). Best-evidence interventions. Retrieved February 16, 2011, from http://www.cdc.gov/hiv/topics/research/prs/best-evidence-intervention.htm.

Centers for Disease Control and Prevention. (2009b). Best-evidence: Connect (couple or woman-alone). Retrieved March 1, 2011, from http://www.cdc.gov/hiv/topics/research/prs/resources/factsheets/Connect.htm.

Centers for Disease Control and Prevention. (2009c). Promising-evidence. Retrieved February 16, 2011, from http://www.cdc.gov/HIV/topics/research/prs/resources/factsheets/SEPA.htm.

Centers for Disease Control and Prevention. (2010a). Estimated lifetime risk for diagnosis of HIV infection among Hispanics/Latinos—37 states and Puerto Rico, 2007. *Morbidity and Mortality Weekly Report, 59*(40), 1297–1300.

Centers for Disease Control and Prevention. (2010b). Racial/ethnic disparities among children with diagnoses of perinatal HIV infection—34 states, 2004–2007. *Morbidity and Mortality Weekly Report, 59*(4), 97–101.

Centers for Disease Control and Prevention. (2011). Reports: Past issues. Retrieved March 22, 2011, from http://www.cdc.gov/hiv/topics/surveillance/resources/reports/past.htm#surveillance.

Clauss-Ehlers, C. S., & Levi, L. L. (2002). Violence and community, terms in conflict: An ecological approach to resilience. *Journal of Social Distress & the Homeless, 11*(4), 265–278. doi: 10.1023/a:1016804930977.

Corea, G. (1992). *The invisible epidemic: The story of women and AIDS.* New York: HarperCollins.

DiClemente, R. J., & Wingood, G. M. (1995). A randomized controlled trial of an HIV sexual risk-reduction intervention for young African-American women. *JAMA: The Journal of the American Medical Association, 274*(16), 1271–1276. doi: 10.1001/jama.274.16.1271.

De Cock, K. M., Jaffe, H. W., & Curran, J. W. (2011). Reflections on 30 years of AIDS. *Emerging Infectious Diseases, 17*(6), 1044–1048.

Denning, P., & DiNenno, E. (2010). Communities in crisis: Is there a generalized HIV epidemic in impoverished urban areas of the United States? Retrieved September 13, 2010, from http://www.cdc.gov/hiv/topics/surveillance/resources/other/poverty.htm.

Devieux, J. G., Malow, R., Lerner, B. G., Dyer, J. G., Baptista, L., Lucenko, B., & Kalichman, S. (2007). Triple jeopardy for HIV: Substance using severely mentally ill adults. *Journal of Prevention & Intervention in the Community, 33*(1–2), 5–18.

Dieffenbach, C. W., & Fauci, A. S. (2011). Thirty years of HIV and AIDS: Future challenges and opportunities. *Annals of Internal Medicine, 154*(11), 766–771.

El-Bassel, N., Gilbert, L., Vinocur, D., Chang, M., & Wu, E. (2011). Posttraumatic stress disorder and HIV risk among poor, inner-city women receiving care in an emergency department. *American Journal of Public Health, 101*(1), 120–127.

El-Bassel, N., Gilbert, L., Wu, E., Chang, M., Gomes, C., Vinocur, D., & Spevack, T. (2007). Intimate partner violence prevalence and HIV risks among women receiving care in emergency departments: Implications for IPV and HIV screening. *Emergency Medicine Journal, 24*(4), 255–259.

El-Bassel, N., Witte, S. S., Gilbert, L., Sormanti, M., Moreno, C., Pereira, L., & Steinglass, P. (2001). HIV prevention for intimate couples: A relationship-based model. *Families, Systems & Health, 19*(4), 379–395.

El-Bassel, N., Witte, S. S., Gilbert, L., Wu, E., Chang, M., Hill, J., & Steinglass, P. (2003). The efficacy of a relationship-based HIV/STD prevention program for heterosexual couples. *American Journal of Public Health, 93*(6), 963–969.

El-Bassel, N., Witte, S. S., Gilbert, L., Wu, E., Chang, M., Hill, J., & Steinglass, P. (2005). Long-term effects of an HIV/STI sexual risk reduction intervention for heterosexual couples. *AIDS and Behavior, 9*(1), 1–13.

Fishbein, M., & Ajzen, I. (2010). *Predicting and changing behavior: The reasoned action approach.* New York: Psychology Press.

Friedman, S. H., & Loue, S. (2007). Incidence and prevalence of intimate partner violence by and against women with severe mental illness. *Journal of Women's Health (2002), 16*(4), 471–480.

Galanti, G.-A. (2003). The Hispanic family and male-female relationships: An overview. *Journal of Transcultural Nursing, 14*(3), 180–185. doi: 10.1177/1043659603014003004.

Gonzalez, J. S., Hendriksen, E. S., Collins, E. M., Durán, R. E., & Safren, S. A. (2009). Latinos and HIV/AIDS: Examining factors related to disparity and identifying opportunities for psychosocial intervention research. *AIDS and Behavior, 13*(3), 582–602. doi: 10.1007/s10461-008-9402-4.

Gonzalez-Guarda, R. M., Peragallo, N., Urrutia, M. T., Vasquez, E. P., & Mitrani, V. B. (2008). HIV risks, substance abuse, and intimate partner violence among Hispanic women and their intimate partners. *The Journal of the Association of Nurses in AIDS Care, 19*(4), 252–266.

Gonzalez-Guarda, R. M., Vasquez, E. P., Urrutia, M. T., Villarruel, A. M., & Peragallo, N. (2011). Hispanic women's experiences with substance abuse, intimate partner violence, and risk for HIV. *Journal of Transcultural Nursing: Official Journal of the Transcultural Nursing Society/Transcultural Nursing Society, 22*(1), 46–54.

Goodyear, R. K., Newcomb, M. D., & Allison, R. D. (2000). Predictors of Latino men's paternity in teen pregnancy: Test of a mediational model of childhood experiences, gender role attitudes, and behaviors. *Journal of Counseling Psychology, 47*(1), 116–128. doi: 10.1037/0022-0167.47.1.116.

Hall, H. I., Song, R., Rhodes, P., Prejean, J., An, Q., Lee, L. M., & Janssen, R. S. (2008). Estimation of HIV incidence in the United States. *Journal of the American Medical Association, 300*(5), 520–529. doi: 10.1001/jama.300.5.520.

Heaphy, E. L. G., Loue, S., Sajatovic, M., & Tisch, D. J. (2010). Impact of psychiatric and social characteristics on HIV sexual risk behavior in Puerto Rican women with severe mental illness. *Social Psychiatry and Psychiatric Epidemiology, 45*(11), 1043–1054.

Herbst, J. H., Kay, L. S., Passin, W. F., Lyles, C. M., Crepaz, N., & Marín, B. V. (2007). A systematic review and meta-analysis of behavioral interventions to reduce HIV risk behaviors of Hispanics in the United States and Puerto Rico. *AIDS and Behavior, 11*(1), 25–47.

Jewkes, R., Nduna, M., Levin, J., Jama, N., Dunkle, K., Khuzwayo, N., & Duvvury, N. (2006). A cluster randomized-controlled trial to determine the effectiveness of stepping stones in preventing HIV infections and promoting safer sexual behaviour amongst youth in the rural Eastern Cape, South Africa: Trial design, methods and baseline findings. *Tropical Medicine & International Health, 11*(1), 3–16.

Jewkes, R., Nduna, M., Levin, J., Jama, N., Dunkle, K., Puren, A., & Duvvury, N. (2008). Impact of stepping stones on incidence of HIV and HSV-2 and sexual behaviour in rural South Africa: Cluster randomised controlled trial. *British Medical Journal, 337*(a506). doi: 10.1136/bmj.a506.

Kelly, J. A., St. Lawrence, J. S., Brasfield, T. L., & Hood, H. V. (1989). Group intervention to reduce AIDS risk behaviors in gay men: Applications of behavioral principles. In V. M. Mays, G. W. Albee, & S. F. Schneider (Eds.), *Primary prevention of AIDS: Psychological approaches.* (pp. 225–241). Thousand Oaks, CA: Sage Publications, Inc.

Kelly, J. A., St. Lawrence, J. S., Diaz, Y. E., & Stevenson, L. Y. (1991). HIV risk behavior reduction following intervention with key opinion leaders of population: An experimental analysis. *American Journal of Public Health, 81*(2), 168–171. doi: 10.2105/ajph.81.2.168.

Kelly, J. A., St Lawrence, J. S., Stevenson, L. Y., Hauth, A. C., Kalichman, S. C., Diaz, Y. E., & Morgan, M. G. (1992). Community AIDS/HIV risk reduction: The effects of endorsements by popular people in three cities. *American Journal of Public Health, 82*(11), 1483–1489.

Kim, J. C., Watts, C. H., Hargreaves, J. R., Ndhlovu, L. X., Phetla, G., Morison, L. A., &. Pronyk, P. (2007). Understanding the impact of a microfinance-based intervention on women's empowerment and the reduction of intimate partner violence in South Africa. *American Journal of Public Health, 97*(10), 1794–1802.

Marín, B. V. (2003). HIV prevention in the Hispanic community: Sex, culture, and empowerment. *Journal of Transcultural Nursing: Official Journal of the Transcultural Nursing Society/ Transcultural Nursing Society, 14*(3), 186–192.

Massachusetts Department of Public Health. (1998). Women's health promotion program.

National Council of La Raza. (2006). Redefining HIV/AIDS for Latinos: A promising new paradigm for addressing HIV/AIDS in the Hispanic community. Washington, DC.

National Institute of Allergy and Infectious Diseases. (2011). Treating HIV-infected people with antiretrovirals protects partners from infections: Findings result from NIH-funded international study. Retrieved May 12, 2011, from http://www.niaid.nih.gov/news/newsreleases/2011/pages/hptn052.aspx.

Newcomb, M. D., & Carmona, J. V. (2004). Adult trauma and HIV status among Latinas: Effects upon psychological adjustment and substance use. *AIDS and Behavior, 8*(4), 417–428.

NREPP. (2011). SAMHSA's national registry of evidence-based programs and practices. Retrieved March 15, 2011, from http://www.nrepp.samhsa.gov/.

O'Leary, A., & Jemmott, L. S. (Eds.). (1996). *Women and AIDS: Coping and caring.* New York: Plenum.

Parillo, K. M., Freeman, R. C., Collier, K., & Young, P. (2001). Association between early sexual abuse and adult HIV-risky sexual behaviors among community-recruited women. *Child Abuse & Neglect, 25*(3), 335–346.

Peragallo, N., Deforge, B., O'Campo, P., Lee, S. M., Kim, Y. J., Cianelli, R., & Ferrer, L. (2005). A randomized clinical trial of an HIV-risk-reduction intervention among low-income Latina women. *Nursing Research, 54*(2), 108–118.

Pérez-Jiménez, D., Seal, D. W., & Serrano-García, I. (2009). Barriers and facilitators of HIV prevention with heterosexual Latino couples: Beliefs of four stakeholder groups. *Cultural Diversity and Ethnic Minority Psychology, 15*(1), 11–17. doi: 10.1037/a0013872.

Pew Hispanic Center. (2008). U.S. population projections 2005–2050. Retrieved March 21, 2011, from http://pewhispanic.org/reports/report.php?ReportID=85.

Pew Hispanic Center. (2011). Statistical portrait of Hispanics in the United States, 2009. Retrieved March 21, 2011, from http://pewhispanic.org/factsheets/factsheet.php?FactsheetID=70.

Pronyk, P. M., Hargreaves, J. R., Kim, J. C., Morison, L. A., Phetla, G., Watts, C., & Porter, J. D. (2006). Effect of a structural intervention for the prevention of intimate-partner violence and HIV in rural South Africa: A cluster randomised trial. *Lancet, 368*(9551), 1973–1983.

Pulerwitz, J., Amaro, H., De Jong, W., Gortmaker, S. L., & Rudd, R. (2002). Relationship power, condom use and HIV risk among women in the USA. *AIDS Care, 14*(6), 789–800.

Pulerwitz, J., Gortmaker, S. L., & DeJong, W. (2000). Measuring sexual relationship power in HIV/STD research. *Sex Roles, 42*(7), 637–660.

Raffaelli, M., & Ontai, L. L. (2004). Gender socialization in Latino/a families: Results from two retrospective studies. *Sex Roles, 50*(5–6), 287–299. doi: 10.1023/b:sers.0000018886.58945.06.

Raj, A., Amaro, H., Cranston, K., Martin, B., Cabral, H., Navarro, A., & Conron, K. (2001). Is a general women's health promotion program as effective as an HIV-intensive prevention program in reducing HIV risk among Hispanic women? *Public Health Reports (Washington, DC: 1974), 116*(6), 599–607.

Raj, A., Santana, C., La Marche, A., Amaro, H., Cranston, K., & Silverman, J. G. (2006). Perpetration of intimate partner violence associated with sexual risk behaviors among young adult men. *American Journal of Public Health, 96*(10), 1873–1878.

Raj, A., Silverman, J. G., & Amaro, H. (2004). Abused women report greater male partner risk and gender-based risk for HIV: Findings from a community-based study with Hispanic women. *AIDS Care, 16*(4), 519–529.

Ramos, R. L., Ferreira-Pinto, J. B., Rusch, M. L. A., & Ramos, M. E. (2010). Pasa la voz (spread the word): Using women's social networks for HIV education and testing. *Public Health Reports (Washington, DC: 1974), 125*(4), 528–533.

Ramos, R. L., Green, N. L., & Shulman, L. C. (2009). Pasa la Voz: Using peer driven interventions to increase Latinas' access to and utilization of HIV prevention and testing services. *Journal of Health Care for the Poor and Underserved, 20*(1), 29–35.

Ramos, R. L., Hernandez, A., Ferreira-Pinto, J. B., Ortiz, M., & Somerville, G. G. (2006). Promovisión: Designing a capacity-building program to strengthen and expand the role of promotores in HIV prevention. *Health Promotion Practice, 7*(4), 444–449. doi: 10.1177/1524839905278868.

RISHTA. (2007). Addressing gupt rog: Narrative prevention counseling for STI/HIV prevention—A guide to AYUSH and allopathic practitioners., from http://www.popcouncil.org/pdfs/NPC_manual.pdf.

Santana, M. C., Raj, A., Decker, M. R., La Marche, A., & Silverman, J. G. (2006). Masculine gender roles associated with increased sexual risk and intimate partner violence perpetration among young adult men. *Journal of Urban Health, 83*(4), 575–585.

Schensul, S. L., Saggurti, N., Singh, R., Verma, R. K., Nastasi, B. K., & Mazumder, P. G. (2009). Multilevel perspectives on community intervention: An example from an Indo-US HIV prevention project in Mumbai, India. *American Journal of Community Psychology, 43* (3–4), 277–291. doi: 10.1007/s10464-009-9241-0.

Simoni, J. M., Evans-Campbell, T., Andrasik, M. P., Lehavot, K., Valencia-Garcia, D., & Walters, K. L. (2010). HIV/AIDS among women of color and sexual minority women. In H. Landrine & N. F. Russo (Eds.), *Handbook of diversity in feminist psychology,* (pp. 335–365). New York: Springer Publishing Co.

Sormanti, M., Wu, E., & El-Bassel, N. (2004). Considering HIV risk and intimate partner violence among older women of color: A descriptive analysis. *Women & Health, 39*(1), 45–63.

Stallworth, J. M., Andía, J. F., Burgess, R., Alvarez, M. E., & Collins, C. (2009). Diffusion of effective behavioral interventions and Hispanic/Latino populations. *AIDS Education and Prevention, 21*(5), 152–163. doi: 10.1521/aeap.2009.21.5_supp.152.

Suarez-Al-Adam, M., Raffaelli, M., & O'Leary, A. (2000). Influence of abuse and partner hypermasculinity on the sexual behavior of Latinas. *AIDS Education and Prevention, 12*(3), 263–274.

Ulibarri, M. D., Strathdee, S. A., Lozada, R., Magis-Rodriguez, C., Amaro, H., O'Campo, P., & Patterson, T. L. (2010). Intimate partner violence among female sex workers in two Mexico–U.S. Border cities: Partner characteristics and HIV risk behaviors as correlates of abuse. *Psychological Trauma: Theory, Research, Practice, and Policy, 2*(4), 318–325. doi: 10.1037/a0017500.

Ulibarri, M. D., Sumner, L. A., Cyriac, A., & Amaro, H. (2010). Power, violence, and HIV risk in women. In M. Paludi & F. L. Denmark (Eds.), *Victims of sexual assault and abuse: Resources and responses for individuals and families: Vol. 1. Incidence and psychological dimensions* (Vol. 1, pp. 211–236). Santa Barbara, CA: Praeger.

UNAIDS. (2010). UNAIDS report on the global AIDS epidemic. Retrieved February 18, 2011, from http://www.unaids.org/globalreport/Global_report.htm.

Weeks, M. R., Schensul, J. J., Williams, S. S., & Singer, M. (1995). AIDS prevention for African-American and Latina women: Building culturally and gender-appropriate intervention. *AIDS Education and Prevention, 7*(3), 251–264.

Weidel, J. J., Provencio-Vasquez, E., Watson, S. D., & Gonzalez-Guarda, R. (2008). Cultural considerations for intimate partner violence and HIV risk in Hispanics. *The Journal of the Association of Nurses in AIDS Care, 19*(4), 247–251.

Witte, S. S., El-Bassel, N., Gilbert, L., Wu, E., Chang, M., & Steinglass, P. (2004). Recruitment of minority women and their main sexual partners in an HIV/STI prevention trial. *Journal of Women's Health (2002), 13*(10), 1137–1147.

Wu, E., El-Bassel, N., Witte, S. S., Gilbert, L., & Chang, M. (2003). Intimate partner violence and HIV risk among urban minority women in primary health care settings. *AIDS and Behavior, 7*(3), 291–301.

5 Demonstrated Effectiveness and Potential of Community-Based Participatory Research for Preventing HIV in Latino Populations

Scott D. Rhodes

INTRODUCTION

Having one of the most rapidly growing Latino populations in the United States, North Carolina reflects current trends in Latino immigration to the United States (U.S. Census Bureau, 2009). Much of the growth of the Latino population has occurred in rural communities (Southern State Directors Work Group, 2008). Jobs in farm work, construction, and factories, coupled with dissatisfaction with the quality of life in traditional U.S. destinations, have led many immigrants to leave higher-density regions of the United States and relocate to the Southeast (Kasarda & Johnson, 2006; Rhodes, Eng, et al., 2007). Increasingly, however, immigrants are bypassing typical U.S. destinations and coming to the Southeast directly. Their demographics differ from Latinos who traditionally immigrated to Arizona, California, New York, and Texas; for example, they tend to come from rural communities in southern Mexico and Central America, report lower educational backgrounds, have arrived more recently, and arrive in communities in the United States without histories of immigration. These communities also lack developed infrastructures to meet their needs (Asamoa et al., 2004; Harari, Davis, & Heisler, 2008; Hayes-Bautista, 2004; Kasarda & Johnson, 2006; North Carolina Institute of Medicine, 2003; Rhodes, Eng, et al., 2007; Rhodes, Hergenrather, Griffith, et al., 2009; U.S. Census Bureau, 2009). Chapter 14 offers New Orleans as an example of such a new destination for predominantly Honduran migrant day laborers.

Furthermore, immigrant Latinos in the southeastern United States are arriving and settling in communities in which antiimmigration sentiment often is high. There is a general fear among immigrant Latinos, documented and undocumented, of racial profiling and detention and deportation. Publicity over partnerships between local law enforcement and U.S. Immigration and Customs Enforcement and recent allegations that public health department records have been used in deportation proceedings have further made the environment difficult for immigrant

Latinos (Rhodes, Eng, et al., 2007; Rhodes, Hergenrather, Griffith, et al., 2009; Rhodes, Hergenrather, et al., 2010; Vissman et al., 2011).

Within this context, our community-based participatory research (CBPR) partnership comprised of community members; representatives from community-based organizations (CBOs), including Latino-serving organizations; and academic researchers has been engaged in nontoken, collaborative research to explore HIV risk and a broad range of intervention approaches to meet the priorities and needs, and build on the assets, of recently arrived immigrant Latinos in the Southeast. This partnership evolved from a local initiative that had a history of success designing and implementing interventions and programs originally focused on diabetes within African American faith communities in rural North Carolina. We initially focused on adult heterosexually active Latino men; however, based on the partnerships established, the trust gained, and the expansion of diverse voices within the partnership, our research has expanded to identify and address the priorities of Latino men who have sex with men (MSM) and Latina women. Simply, this research is conducted in partnership with the affected community and follows a systematic process that begins with formative research and moves toward action, including intervention development, implementation, and evaluation.

This chapter outlines some of the community-based research that our partnership has conducted in the southeastern United States. Although I am not Latino and I lack a personal immigration experience, I report how our research, which is designed to explore and reduce the burden of HIV among immigrant Latinos who are politically, socially, and economically disenfranchised, has unfolded. I present the systematic process of how we have applied CBPR, including its values and principles and the processes that are aligned with CBPR, to identify community priorities and needs—and assets on which to build—and to support and contribute to the potential impact of community-driven solutions to reduce HIV exposure and transmission of immigrant Latinos in the United States.

I describe how our partnership built on early successes developing, implementing, and evaluating HIV prevention interventions designed by, and for, heterosexually active Latino men to expand our HIV prevention research in partnership with Latino MSM and Latina women during the past 10 years. I also outline factors that contribute to our CBPR partnership's successes. These factors may serve to help others to develop authentic and successful CBPR projects.

THE RATIONALE FOR COMMUNITY-BASED PARTICIPATORY RESEARCH (CBPR)

We know that understanding and intervening on the complex behavioral, situational, and environmental factors that influence HIV risk benefit from the multiple perspectives, experiences, and expertise of community members, organizational representatives, and academic researchers (Cashman et al., 2008; Hergenrather & Rhodes, 2008; Institute of Medicine, 2000; Israel, Schulz, Parker, & Becker, 1998; Minkler & Wallerstein, 2002; Rhodes, Malow, & Jolly, 2010). Blending the real lived experiences of Latino community members, the insights of organizational representatives based in service provision, and sound science has the potential to develop deeper and more informed understandings of phenomena, and, thus, produce more likely impactful interventions. An ideal approach to blending the perspectives of community members, organizational representatives, and academic researchers is CBPR.

CBPR lends itself to identifying the factors delineated in the structural-environmental (SE) model of HIV risk and prevention presented in Chapter 1. CBPR can help to illustrate the progression or how the SE model can be a framework for moving from individual-level influences to the more complex environmental and situational factors that influence HIV risk behavior among immigrant Latinos. It is through iterative processes that a more informed understanding of HIV risk can be outlined and subsequently tested and intervened upon. The Latino-focused partnership that I have been working with for the past decade in North Carolina has been exploring these broader contextual influences, but the development of interventions to address these influences has been slow. This is in part because of the community's expressed sense of urgency in terms of the HIV epidemic and the ability to more easily address individual-level variables. It has made sense for our partnership to move to focusing on SE and system changes after establishing a well functioning partnership, a shared understanding of research, and trust with health department leaders, for example. However, it must be acknowledged that the types of interventions that research mechanisms fund tend to be short-term individual-level interventions, interventions that focus on the individual Latino and his or her behavior and not SE factors such as poor living and working conditions, immigration and documentation status, fair living wages, discrimination, etc. (see Chapter 6 in which Hirsch and Vasquez describe such multisectorial contextual factors for Mexican migrants). Thus, our partnership is slowly developing evidence in order to infuse these broader contextual factors into its research without reaching too far from the expected. Of course, the challenges facing community members would best be served by highly innovative interventions, but given the funding process and the politicization and stigmatization of vulnerable populations including Latinos, we have far to go.

COMMUNITY-BASED PARTICIPATORY RESEARCH (CBPR) DEFINED

CBPR is an approach to research designed to ensure authentic, full, and equal participation of community members (including those most affected by the issue being studied), organizational representatives, and academic researchers throughout the entire research process. CBPR moves from individuals within a community being objects or "targets" of research to fully involved research partners. CBPR emphasizes colearning, reciprocal transfer of expertise and sharing of decision-making power among partners. CBPR is democratic and acknowledges and emphasizes that community members, organizational representatives, and academic researchers are equal as they strive for knowledge generation for health promotion and disease prevention. By inclusion of the various perspectives, knowledge generated and thus the understanding of phenomena are more informed and improved than less collaborative approaches. Community members provide perspectives on the lived experiences from within the community itself. They often know what is important and meaningful for themselves in particular and the community in general and have local theories on association and causation. Moreover, because community members do not speak in one voice, the diversity of community perspectives can capture the multidimensionality of experiences. Similarly, organizational representatives have invaluable insights based on their ongoing work "in the field" and "on the street." They have perspectives on what is happening in aggregate terms and often can identify "exceptions to the rule." Finally, academic researchers bring scientific expertise and an understanding of research that can inform community priorities and intervention development, and help communities build evidence for resources and advocacy.

Within our HIV prevention research, for example, Latino community members and representatives from CBOs provide particular insights into the priorities and needs of Latino communities as well guidance into research question formulation, research design, instrumentation and data collection, intervention development and content, and report preparation and dissemination. Their role is not limited to establishing priorities, providing the formative data that guide intervention content, or serving on community advisory boards (CABs); rather, they have an active role throughout the entire research endeavor.

Simply, community members, organizational representatives, and academic researchers participate in and share control over all phases of the research process, e.g., assessment; problem definition; methodology selection; data collection, analysis, and interpretation; dissemination of findings; and application of the results (action). A distinctive feature of CBPR is that research should move toward action through translation of findings into their application in the community (Cornwall & Jewkes, 1995; Israel, Eng, Schulz, & Parker, 2005; Minkler, 2005; Rhodes, Eng, et al., 2007; Rhodes, Hergenrather, Montano, et al., 2006; Rhodes, Hergenrather, et al., 2007; Rhodes, Malow, et al., 2010). Such action may include further research to better understand phenomena to intervene more effectively; or intervention development, pilot or full implementation, and/or evaluation. Action may include multilevel action, including individual, group, community, policy, and social change as advocated in chapters throughout this book.

Thus, CBPR is inherently translational. It ensures that basic, more formative research is conducted with an eye on its potential and practical use to improve community health. Research may begin with an assessment of needs, and to understand phenomena, based in community perceptions and epidemiologic data, but a hallmark of CBPR is the translation of research findings into action and community change, precisely what is needed to confront HIV in Latino communities.

PARTNERSHIP DEVELOPMENT WITH IMMIGRANT LATINOS

Our CBPR partnership is based on a firm foundation lain by the North Carolina Community-Based Public Health Initiative (CBPHI). Members of a North Carolina CBPHI-organized CBPR partnership that had a history of successfully implementing community-based diabetes interventions within African American faith communities in rural North Carolina (Margolis et al., 2000; Parker et al., 1998) wanted to explore the health priorities and needs of the growing Latino community (Rhodes, Eng, et al., 2007). They were concerned that in their community in which a former Grand Wizard of the Ku Klux Klan, David Duke, led a well-publicized anti-Latino immigration rally on the steps of the town hall, the priorities and needs of their immigrant Latino neighbors were being neglected (Cuadros, 2006; Rhodes, Eng, et al., 2007).

Because Latino community members were not sufficiently represented within the CBPR partnership, local Latino community members were recruited to join the partnership. Much effort went into the process of building trust with and recruiting community members because the existing CBPR partners knew the importance of, and were committed to, working shoulder to shoulder with community members for improved community health. Partners met informally with Latino community members to discuss the partnership.

Although building trust to expand involvement can challenge any collaborative process, within this community, building trust was complicated by local and national debates about immigration that fueled rallies and crimes against Latinos and Latino-serving organizations (Cuadros, 2006; Rhodes, Eng, et al., 2007; Rhodes, Hergenrather, Griffith, et al., 2009; Rhodes, Hergenrather, et al., 2009; Streng et al., 2004; Vissman et al., 2011). Many members and leaders of the local Latino community, documented and undocumented, were hesitant to participate in a process that they initially did not understand. They did not trust partnership members including those who were Latino, and worried whether they would be safe to participate in or collaborate with the partnership. Much effort went into trust building through informal networking and dialogue.

The president of a large multicounty soccer league of more than 1800 adult Latino men in rural North Carolina was identified as a leader potentially willing to serve on the CBPR partnership. Representatives of our partnership approached the league president and began a dialogue about the partnership and its mission, his potential involvement (and the potential involvement of his soccer league), and the potential to explore and address the priorities and needs of the Latino community over time. Partners met with the league president every 2 weeks over dinner, explaining his potential role on the partnership and asking for referrals and recommendations about others who might be key to recruit to the CBPR partnership. After each dinner, he requested time to think about his involvement and the involvement of his league and scheduled a subsequent dinner meeting. After 8 months of having dinner every 2 weeks with CBPR partnership representatives, the president brought his wife to dinner. She humorously asked, "Why do you continue to take my husband to dinner?" Hearing the partners discuss his role and the importance of his involvement in the third person resonated with him. His wife also approved of his involvement, and he was ready to move forward rapidly.

The league president and a small representation from the soccer league began to attend meetings of the partnership. At this point the partnership also included new members, including representatives from a local *tienda* (small Latino grocery store), two Spanish-language churches, and a statewide farmworker advocacy group that was working in the area with the North Carolina Migrant Education Program; and the director of a statewide coalition to promote Mexican leadership. Because the partnership wanted to ensure that all members were committed to a participatory approach to research, the partnership principles, which continue to guide the partnership, were refined (Rhodes, Hergenrather, et al., 2011; Rhodes, Malow, et al., 2010). These partnership principles are outlined in Table 5.1.

These partnership principles establish a common foundation and shared expectations among partners, guide how partners relate to one another, and help to ensure the highest level of engaged and equitable participation possible. Partnership principles also establish a foundation for partners to build on each other's strengths and develop their roles as change agents working together to improve the overall health of communities.

PRIORITIZING MEN'S HEALTH

The partners quickly decided to explore Latino men's health given that at that point the majority of immigrant Latinos in the southeastern United States were male.

Table 5.1 Principles Guiding Our CBPR Partnership in North Carolina

To improve community health, we strive to build and maintain trust among each of us—community members, organizational and agency representatives, academic researchers, and clinicians—through:

Mutual respect and genuineness;

Establishing and utilizing formal and informal partnership networks and structures;

Committing to transparent processes and clear and open communication;

Roles, norms, and processes evolving from the input and agreement of all partners;

Agreeing on the values, goals, and objectives of research and practice;

Building upon each partner's strengths and assets;

Offering continual feedback among members;

Balancing power and sharing resources;

Sharing credit for the accomplishments of the partnership;

Facing challenges together;

Developing and using relationships and networks outside of the partnership;

Incorporating existing environmental structures to address partnership focuses;

Taking responsibility for the partnership and its actions; and

Disseminating conclusions and findings to research and clinical audiences, community members, and policy makers.

In general, these immigrant Latino men were healthy and had few health concerns. However, the soccer league president and members of the soccer league were certain that sexual health would be a priority given that Latino men had reported having been infected by a sexually transmitted disease (STD), worrying about infection, and/or hearing about someone they knew being infected (Rhodes, Eng, et al., 2007; Rhodes, Hergenrather, Wilkin, Alegria-Ortega, & Montaño, 2006).

INITIAL QUALITATIVE DATA COLLECTION, ANALYSIS, AND INTERPRETATION

Partners elected to begin their CBPR process by collecting formative data on Latino men's health priorities. Partners were clear to stay focused on action, and although the academic researcher partners had a variety of research questions, partners maintained a focus on knowledge necessary for community-level action. This process involved the partners answering two important questions: "*What* do we want to know?" and "*Why* do we want to know it?" This discussion was important because partners recognized that knowledge for knowledge sake (i.e., the accumulation of scientific knowledge) can be important, but the application of knowledge to improve the health and wellbeing of the local Latino community was more important. Partners chose to explore health priorities and sexual health using focus groups. Although partners wondered whether Latino men would discuss sexual health in a focus group setting, with other Latino men, they recognized that assumptions about immigrant Latino men living within a new context with little support needed to be tested.

Partners came to agreement on the research and recruitment design and the roles and contributions of the partners. A subgroup of the partnership created, reviewed, revised, and approved a focus group moderator's guide. Recruitment of participants for each focus group was coordinated by the league president at the

89

Demonstrated Effectiveness and Potential of Community-Based Participatory Research for Preventing HIV in Latino Populations

tienda where representatives from the league met for their weekly Saturday morning planning meetings. Two partnership members served as the focus group moderator and the note taker, who documented nonverbal reactions of the participants and tracking participant dialogue. The note taker was an academic researcher proficient in Spanish. A Latino-serving CBO hosted the focus groups. Seven focus groups were completed. Each focus group was audiotaped with the signed consent of each participant.

The focus group transcripts were analyzed by the analysis team, another subgroup of the partnership; each transcript was coded by both native Spanish and English speakers. Research suggests that collaborative analysis of qualitative data by speakers of different languages simultaneously and with iterative discussion, reflection, and negotiation of codes and themes yields higher quality and more accurate findings (MacQueen, McLellan, Kay, & Milstein, 1998; Shibusawa & Lukens, 2004).

To minimize bias, the analysis team completed a multistage inductive interpretative thematic process by separately reading and rereading the transcripts to identify potential codes, coming together to create a common coding system and data dictionary, and then separately assigning agreed-upon codes to relevant text. Subsequently, the analysis team convened to compare broad content categories and begin the process of developing and interpreting themes. They compared and revised themes, and these themes were presented to the entire partnership for further refinement and interpretation through four iterative discussions. During these discussions, preliminary themes were written on flip charts in both Spanish and English, but the process included much dialogue to overcome literacy challenges. The partners discussed and revised the themes and their interpretation. All partners were equitably involved in each phase of the research process, including data analysis and interpretation. The scientific advantage included increasing the quality and accuracy of findings and their interpretation (Altman, 1995; Cashman et al., 2008; Israel et al., 1998; Streng et al., 2004).

USE OF THE DATA AND INTERVENTION DEVELOPMENT

Findings were disseminated through community and national presentations, reports, and peer-reviewed papers. Because action is a key characteristic of CBPR, the findings also were used for funding proposals and intervention design. All partners had equal access to the findings; for example, representatives from a Latino-serving CBO used findings for grant preparation, and community members used the findings to advocate for Latino men's health.

A finding from the initial focus groups was the potential of harnessing the naturally existing social network of the soccer league to reduce HIV sexual risk among heterosexually active Latino men by selecting natural leaders from various soccer teams to be trained to serve as lay health advisors for their teams. Thus, the partnership wrote a funded proposal to develop, implement, and evaluate an intervention entitled: *HoMBReS: Hombres Manteniendo Bienestar y Relaciones Saludables* (Men: Men Maintaining Wellbeing and Healthy Relationships) (Rhodes, Hergenrather, Montano, et al., 2006). Further details about the development, implementation, and evaluation of the *HoMBReS* intervention are available in Chapter 18 (by Painter, Organista, Rhodes, & Sañudo). Briefly, the HoMBReS intervention included the training of lay health advisors, known as "Navegantes" (Navigators). Navegantes were trained to serve as health advisors to provide information and resources, opinion leaders to change expectations and norms about sexual health and what it means to be a Latino man, and community advocates to bring the voices of the community to the agencies that offer health services. The *Navegantes* worked formally and informally with their teammates for 18 months. At postintervention assessment, the intervention was found to have increased condom use and HIV testing among teammates in the intervention compared to their peers in the comparison control group (Rhodes, Hergenrather, Bloom, Leichliter, & Montaño, 2009). The *HoMBReS* intervention has since been included in the CDC *Compendium of Evidence-Based HIV Behavioral Interventions* (http://www.cdc.gov/hiv/topics/research/prs/resources/factsheets/hombres.htm) as the first best evidence *community-level* intervention.

During implementation of HoMBReS, and before postintervention assessment data had been collected and analyzed, the state of North Carolina Department of Health and Human Services published a request for applications (RFA) to fund HIV prevention interventions within North Carolina. However, the RFA required CBOs and AIDS service organizations (ASOs) to implement interventions that had evidence of effectiveness with an emphasis on interventions that were part of the Dissemination of Effective Behavioral Intervention (DEBI) Project of the CDC. Although Latinos were clearly disproportionately affected by HIV, only two Latino-focused interventions with evidence of effectiveness existed within the DEBI Project. One focused on reducing drug use and injection-related HIV risk behaviors in Puerto Ricans (Robles et al., 2004); the other focused on urban Hispanic men and women (predominantly from Puerto Rico) and African American men and women within STD clinics (O'Donnell, O'Donnell, San Doval, Duran, & Labes, 1998). Partners felt that although these interventions offered insights into HIV prevention within the Latino community, they were less relevant to meet the sexual prevention needs of Latino men in the southeastern United States where injecting drug use among Latinos was low. Partners also wanted to meet the prevention needs of men *before* they had reason to go to an STD clinic. Thus, because the partners were beginning to understand the power of evidence, together they developed a study to test a small-group intervention for heterosexually active Latino men.

The intervention was known as HoMBReS-2. The HoMBReS-2 intervention was not a lay health advisor intervention; rather, it was a multisession small-group intervention designed to increase condom use and HIV testing among Latino men. HoMBReS-2 included rapport and trusting-building activities; didactic teaching; DVD segments that served as triggers for discussion and role modeling; role plays; group discussion; and skills building, practice, and feedback. It was based on social cognitive theory (Bandura, 1986) and empowerment education (Freire, 1973) and blended locally collected data on risk among heterosexually active Latino men (Rhodes, 2009; Rhodes, Eng, et al., 2007; Rhodes & Hergenrather, 2007; Rhodes, Hergenrather, Bloom, et al., 2009; Rhodes, Hergenrather, Griffith, et al., 2009; Rhodes, Hergenrather, Montano, et al., 2006; Rhodes, Hergenrather, Wilkin, et al., 2006). The intervention was designed to address the priorities established by the CBPR partnership, including (1) increasing awareness of the magnitude of HIV and STD infection among Latinos in the United States and North Carolina; (2) providing information on types of infections, modes of transmission, signs and symptoms, and local counseling, testing, care, and treatment options; (3) increasing condom use; (4) bolstering the positive and reframing the negative aspects of what it means to be a man, a Latino man, and an immigrant Latino man; and (5) increasing the use of health care within an environment that lacks bilingual and bicultural services and

91

Demonstrated Effectiveness and Potential of Community-Based Participatory Research for Preventing HIV in Latino Populations

within communities in which antiimmigration sentiment is high (Rhodes, Eng, et al., 2007).

One DVD segment that was produced for the *HoMBReS-2* intervention was designed to demystify the process of accessing health department HIV testing services. The segment followed a Spanish-speaking Latino man as he went through the actual testing process at a local health department. It showed the difficulties of getting an interpreter, the embarrassment of having a female interpreter and nurse, and types of questions that one is asked and the rationale behind the data that the health department or other testing sites collect. A facilitated discussion subsequently allowed participants to discuss what they learned from the DVD segment and get their follow-up questions answered.

Three peer leaders known as "compañeros de salud" (peer health partners) from the community were trained to cofacilitate the intervention during implementation. The *compañeros de salud* received training in the epidemiology of HIV and health disparities, HIV transmission, risk behavior, cultural and social influences on sexual health, access to health care services, and predictors of behavior change. Role-playing exercises provided opportunities to practice skills and receive feedback to enhance their communication skills. One session also reviewed the study design and basic research concepts, including fidelity, bias, and evaluation, and human subjects protection. Through their involvement in intervention pretesting, didactic instruction, and interactive exercises, the *compañeros de salud* became familiar with the theories and partnership-informed logic underlying the intervention, effective implementation strategies, and behavioral change methods. *Compañeros de salud* were evaluated pre- and posttraining, and the results of these evaluations were used to tailor the training to their needs. The project coordinator and an observer were present during all intervention sessions to assess and ensure fidelity.

The HoMBReS-2 intervention was pilot tested comparing immigrant Latino men randomized to the HIV prevention intervention group to those randomized to the one-session comparison cancer education group. The mean age of participants ($n = 142$) was 31.6 years and 60% reported being from Mexico. Adjusting for baseline behaviors, relative to their peers in the cancer education comparison, participants in the HIV prevention intervention were more likely to report consistent condom use [adjusted odds ratio (AOR) = 3.52; 95% confidence interval (CI) = 1.29–9.63] and receiving an HIV test (AOR = 5.18; 95% CI = 2.26–11.9) at 3-month follow-up (Rhodes, McCoy, Vissman et al., 2011).

FURTHER DEVELOPMENTS RESULTING FROM INITIAL RESEARCH WITH LATINO MEN
Latino MSM

Since the implementation and evaluation of the *HoMBReS* and *HoMBReS-2* interventions, two groups of immigrant Latinos emerged and requested HIV prevention programming. First, a group of five Latino MSM, who were not part of the *HoMBReS* intervention but where aware of the intervention, given that they were living in the same communities in which implementation was occurring, met with the Latino-serving CBO that had hosted the focus groups. They asked about HIV prevention resources that were available for Latino MSM. Partners realized that they did not know much about Latino MSM and their priorities and needs in rural North Carolina.

A subgroup of the partnership met with the original five Latino MSM informally to get a sense of their perceptions of the community, their experiences, and potential needs. Included in this discussion was a discussion of the oftentimes protracted timeline associated with research. Partners wanted to be realistic with the MSM that while movement can occur, often the research endeavor is slow. Based on recruitment of Latino MSM to the partnership and ongoing dialogue, the partnership began a series of studies to explore HIV prevention and begin a systematic intervention development process. The research began with community assessments to understand some of the environmental and situational factors facing Latino MSM that influence risk. These assessments included interviews with Latino-serving providers and Latino MSM, and a respondent-driven sampling (RDS) study (Rhodes, Fernandez, et al., 2011; Rhodes, Hergenrather, et al., 2010, 2011; Rhodes, Malow, et al., 2010; Rhodes, McCoy, et al., 2011; Rhodes, Yee, & Hergenrather, 2006).

RDS, which is an extension of chain-referral methods but provides a basis to calculate unbiased estimates of population parameters, relies on respondents to recruit a limited number of subsequent respondents who are part of their social networks (Heckathorn, 1997, 2002). Among 190 Latino MSM RDS study participants, the average age was 25.5 years old (±5.4; range: 18–48). The average number of years living in the United States was about 10 years with a range from a few months to 25 years, and over two-thirds of participants lived in the United States fewer than 10 years. Over 75% reported Mexico as their country of origin. The prevalence estimates of HIV risk behaviors among MSM populations were limited, and this study provided the first estimates available for Latino MSM coming to the Southeast. The RDS-weighted prevalence estimate of sex with at least one woman was 21.2% [95% confidence interval (CI): 11.1, 28.4]; sex with multiple male partners was 88.9% (95% CI: 88.3, 98.3); and inconsistent condom use during anal sex was 54.1% (95% CI: 43.4, 60.8), during the past 3 months.

RDS was particularly successful because Latino MSM were accustomed to referring one another to local resources. For example, Latino MSM have reported that they commonly provide guidance to social network members about job and housing opportunities, buying a car, and getting other needs met. Harnessing these naturally existing networks for recruitment was easily understood and implemented by respondents (Rhodes, Hergenrather, et al., 2011; Rhodes, McCoy, et al., 2011).

Blending the various locally collected data led the partnership to develop two interventions for Latino MSM. These interventions are currently being implemented by our partnership. The first intervention is a lay health advisor intervention entitled *HOLA: Hombres Ofreciendo Liderazgo y Apoyo (Hello: Men Offering Leadership and Help)*. This intervention is based on the *HoMBReS* intervention; however, rather than utilizing the social structure of the soccer league, it harnesses informal social networks of Latino MSM in rural communities. Lay health advisors or Navegantes, are trained to work with their friends to increase condom use and HIV testing.

The *HOLA* intervention is designed to meet the priorities established by the partnership, including (1) increasing awareness of the magnitude of HIV and STD infection; (2) providing information on types of infections, modes of transmission, and signs and symptoms; (3) offering guidance on local counseling, testing, care, and treatment services, eligibility requirements, and "what to expect" in health care encounters; (4) building condom use skills (e.g., how to communicate effectively, how to properly select, use, and dispose of condoms); (5) changing health-compromising norms of what it means to be an immigrant, a Latino man, a gay man, and an MSM; (6) building supportive relationships and sense of community; and (7) providing skills building to successfully help others.

Latino gay men have reported that sometimes they may take risks because they do not feel as if they are meeting the sociocultural expectations of what it means to be a man. They are gay, which can be taboo within some Latino communities, and some Latino MSM have reported that MSM are not perceived as "real" men by others, as noted by Diaz et al. in Chapter 7. They also may feel that their masculinity is further negated by the challenges they face in the United States (e.g., discrimination, harsh living and working conditions); they may feel that they are unable to meet their responsibilities as men (Rhodes, Hergenrather, Griffith, et al., 2009). Thus, for some men, having multiple partners and engaging in other risk behaviors may "affirm" their manhood. The HOLA intervention includes activities to deconstruct these sociocultural norms and expectations and learn strategies to cope with these pressures, reframe them, and support one another as a community of men who have power over how they view themselves and each other. They are taught how behaviors, the environment, and individuals influence one another, using constructs from social cognitive theory (Bandura, 1986) and empowerment education (Freire, 1973), specifically consciousness raising, critical reflection, and reciprocal determinism.

The second intervention that emerged is entitled HOLA en Grupos, a small-group intervention for Latino MSM, also designed to increase condom use and HIV testing. This intervention was "homegrown," based on the immediate needs of Latino MSM, prior to the collection and analysis of locally collected formative data. The process of developing the intervention was iterative with CBPR partners, specifically staff from a CBO and Latino MSM from the community, developing and revising the intervention based on (1) review of other interventions that target Latinos in general and MSM, including Hermanos de Luna y Sol (http://www.caps.ucsf.edu/projects/HLS/and http://cci.sfsu.edu/taxonomy/term/37), (2) learning from ongoing implementation of the evolving intervention, and (3) the experiences with other interventions that the partners and CBO staff had developed for the Latino community including HoMBReS and HoMBReS-2 (Rhodes, Eng, et al., 2007; Rhodes, Hergenrather, Bloom, et al., 2009; Rhodes, Hergenrather, Montano, et al., 2006); Promotoras Unidas Educando de la Sexualidad (PUEdeS), a reproductive health and HIV/STD prevention intervention for Latina women; and Wise Decisions, a teen pregnancy prevention intervention for adolescents.

The CBPR partnership was able to secure funding for the further refinement, implementation, and rigorous evaluation of the HOLA and HOLA en Grupos interventions.

Latina Women

Since the partners began their intervention research with immigrant Latino men, Latinas (e.g., girlfriends, wives, partners, sisters, and cousins of male participants) stepped forward and asked for HIV prevention programming tailored to their needs and priorities. For example, during implementation of the HoMBReS-2 intervention, it was common for Latina women to request to attend. Study staff explained to these Latinas that the intervention was designed for men and reported back to the partnership that Latinas wanted some type of programming.

After ongoing discussions, the partners initiated focus groups with adult Latinas and in-depth interviews with local service providers in central North Carolina. Partners leveraged the interest of a core group of Latina partners, who either were current or recently recruited members of the CBPR partnership, and two female Spanish-speaking graduate students. This formative research explored health priorities, sociocultural determinants of sexual risk, and potentially effective intervention approaches (Cashman, Eng, Simán, & Rhodes, 2011).

A total of 42 sexually active Latinas participated in one of four focus groups. Over half reported Mexico as their country of origin; other participants reported being from El Salvador, Guatemala, and Honduras. Approximately 75% reported completing middle school or less. About two-thirds reported speaking and understanding only Spanish, while another 35% reported speaking "more Spanish than English." Participants reported working in factories and restaurants, and as house cleaners, childcare providers, and housewives. Half of the participants reported living with a male partner, about one-third reported being single, and approximately one-fifth reported either living alone but having a partner in their country of origin or having an "other" type of living situation. Participants reported no illicit drug use but about 20% reported ever having injected vitamins.

After a systematic process of qualitative data analysis, priorities for HIV prevention interventions among immigrant Latinas were identified. These priorities included (1) clarifying misunderstandings about anatomy and increasing knowledge about sexual and reproductive organs and their functions, including information on HIV and STD transmission and prevention; (2) building skills for condom use and to negotiate condom use; (3) providing guidance on how to access available resources and what to expect during HIV testing visits; (4) building skills to effectively and safely communicate with partners, peers, adult family members, and health care providers; (5) harnessing natural helpers within informal social networks of Latinas; (6) leveraging Latino cultural values, specifically collectivism and familismo; and (7) utilizing a variety of teaching strategies (see Latina focused Chapters 4 and 17 in this book for more on Latina-focused HIV prevention priorities).

Based on this formative research, partners developed a culturally congruent intervention entitled *Mujeres Juntas Estableciendo Relaciones Saludables* (*MuJEReS*). The intervention, which is designed to reduce the disproportionate HIV burden borne among Latinas in the United States, trains Latina lay health advisors, known as "Comadres" from the community, to work within their existing informal social networks. Lay community Latinas chose the term "Comadre" because of its common use to mean a trusted friend or neighbor who can be relied upon for advice and assistance. In addition to the formal and informal health advising in which Comadres engage, partners determined that each Comadre also holds six 60- to 90-minute group sessions during intervention implementation with their social network members. These group sessions include (1) hosting a fiesta to inaugurate the Comadre's role as a resource within her social network; (2) learning and practicing correct condom use skills; (3) brainstorming and discussing ways to overcome communication barriers with sex partners; (4) brainstorming and discussing ways to overcome communication barriers with providers; (5) demystifying the HIV testing process through describing available testing options, delineating the process (eligibility, etc.), and illustrating challenges that will be faced and how they can be surmounted; and (6) exploring what it is like to be an immigrant Latina

95

Demonstrated Effectiveness and Potential of Community-Based Participatory Research for Preventing HIV in Latino Populations

through facilitated dialogue designed to build positive self images and supportive relationships.

FACILITATORS OF SUCCESSFUL CBPR

Our community-based HIV prevention research with Latinos has been particularly successful based on seven factors. These factors are presented in Table 5.2.

Building Trust

Initially there was little Latino representation in the partnership; however, through networking and building trust, the partnership was able (and continues) to expand. Currently, there are over 50 partnership members most of whom are located in northwest and central North Carolina. Although each partner may not prioritize HIV in its own organizational mission, each partner is committed to the health and wellbeing of immigrant Latinos in North Carolina, and has contributed to exploring HIV prevention, care and support, and treatment needs for several years.

Trust, however, requires ongoing maintenance. Facilitators of trust for academic researchers include being visible and in the community during events such as festivals; doing volunteer work such as serving on organizational boards and participating in health fairs; and soliciting, and remaining open to, new ideas and perspectives from community members and organizational representatives.

Power Sharing among Partners

Partners have continued to share power. Early on, the expanded partnership made decisions using the 70% consensus rule. This decision-making process encourages consensus by asking whether each partner can support a given decision by at least 70% . This operating norm was found effective within other CBPR partnerships (Israel et al., 2001). Our partnership has also found that this process functions well; however, after a decision has been made, community members may take the decision back to their constituents, other community members, and get their perspectives and feedback. In our partnership with the soccer league, for example, decisions were reworked if the broader soccer league did not agree with what the partnership decided. This occurred despite a decision reflecting what their own representatives

Table 5.2 Factors Contributing to Successful Community-Based Research with Latinos

Building trust
Power sharing among partners
Building on existing community knowledge
Harnessing community creativity
Testing assumptions
Focusing on action
Taking incremental research steps

to the partnership wanted. Of course, this type of shared decision making and power over the decision-making process requires partners to continually communicate to ensure a thorough understanding of partner perspectives. This process may take time but is worth the investment.

A proxy for power sharing may be shared control over financial resources. Our partnership has allocated 40–50% of the direct federally funded cost of HIV-related research projects to organizations within our CBPR partnership. Staff from CBOs serve as official coinvestigators or coprincipal investigators, and supervise intervention development, implementation, and evaluation of staff. This also ensures that community capacity continues to be developed.

Building on Existing Community Knowledge

Our partnership has built on what community members and organizational representatives already know. We have worked to ensure that research is not a barrier to community progress but rather is a complement to meeting the priorities and needs of communities. Rather than assuming that knowledge must be collected and assembled in certain formats by trained researchers, our partnership has recognized the foundation of knowledge existing within communities. In addition to the collaborative processes of building on partner perspectives, community forums and town hall meetings have supplemental formats to gauge what is known and unknown within the community and help identify and/or validate priorities. These types of events allow for broad perspectives that reach beyond existing partners. Furthermore, well facilitated forums, which include key community members, organizational representatives, and academic researchers, can explore what should and can happen in terms of next steps. Our approach used triggers based in empowerment education to lead an action-oriented discussion (Rhodes, Hergenrather, et al., 2011; Rhodes, Hergenrather, Wilkin, & Jolly, 2008). For example, we held a community forum to explore how to meet the prevention needs of MSM that led to multiple action steps designed to support the health and wellbeing of Latino MSM (Rhodes, Hergenrather, et al., 2011). Specifically, the North Carolina Department of Health and Human Services allocated funds to create safe spaces and Spanish-language programming for Latino MSM throughout North Carolina, a CBO increased offsite after-hour HIV testing in Spanish-speaking communities in rural North Carolina, and grant writing teams convened to apply for both programmatic and research funding to meet the HIV prevention needs of Latino MSM.

These discussions move beyond presentation of findings or the current situation to what can be done (action) based on a process in which participants evaluate (1) what is important and (2) what is changeable. This process also includes the identification of partners who are going to lead each component of action.

Harnessing Community Creativity

We do not merely blend community, organizational, and academic perspectives of partnership members for more informed understanding of phenomena; rather, we rely on the creativity of community members to ensure that study designs and data collection procedures have the highest potential to succeed. Furthermore, intervention approaches, content, and activities are developed in partnership with community members. We also work with community members who are not part of the partnership to ensure that the drafted content and activities are meaningful.

We revise the intervention based on the feedback. This iterative process is completed several times prior to pretesting.

To illustrate the process, a subgroup of our partnership developed the *HoMBReS-2* intervention. This subgroup contained community members, including heterosexually active Latino men; representatives from CBOs, including an ASO, a Latino-serving political advocacy group, and public health departments; and academic researchers from three universities. The intervention included an activity that allowed Latino men to practice reframing the types of health-compromising statements that they may hear within the Latino community, such as "Why worry about AIDS, I will die from something any way," "What doesn't kill me, makes me stronger," "AIDS only affects gays," "I am a man, I can take anything," and "The health department is only for pregnant women." These statements were developed by community members who brainstormed and discussed these statements.

As the intervention further developed, meetings with diverse community members were held to review the intervention to ensure that activities were relevant and engaging and content was received as it was intended. Partnership members made revisions based on these meetings. These revisions were then reviewed again by community members. This process continued until the intervention was deemed ready for pretesting by partners and other community members.

This review by community members who are not part of the partnership is vital because community members who join the partnership are at least slightly different from those who do not join. Furthermore, over time, they may lose some of their community insights as they become more invested in the partnership. Review by community members who are not part of the partnership also builds further buy-in among community members. This buy-in may yield increased community acceptability of and participation in CBPR studies.

Testing Assumptions

Our partnership also questions and tests assumptions. For example, during our initial exploration of the health priorities of immigrant Latino men, partners were not certain that Latino men, who were part of a multicounty soccer league, would discuss sexual health within a focus group. However, participants engaged in animated discussions about sexual behavior, including perspectives on and personal experiences with condom use. Thus, although the use of focus groups was not without weaknesses (e.g., discussions of same-sex sexual behavior were absent), the focus group format was more successful than some of the partners presumed.

Focusing on Action

Partners are clear that our research must lead to improving the health and wellbeing of immigrant Latinos within our communities; thus, we maintain a focus on collecting only necessary data that can be readily used to inform action. Action may include multilevel action, including individual, group, community, policy, and social change. For example, after our partnership conducted the initial focus groups with the soccer league, we used these findings to write a proposal that was funded to develop, implement, and evaluate the *HoMBReS* intervention. Organizational representatives also used preliminary findings to apply for funding to produce and air Spanish-language radio commercials to increase HIV knowledge within their catchment communities.

Using an Incremental Approach to Research

Our partnership has used an incremental process to research that builds understanding of health phenomena. We begin the research process based on what the partners collectively know, compare this knowledge to what is available in the literature, and build sequential research questions. We tend to start small to build evidence. This approach helps communities understand how evidence is accumulated and builds their capacity to identify and answer questions.

The incremental approach also helps our partnership build a history of success. Because the research process can be lengthy, our partnership celebrates successes and highlights process-related findings. For example, we celebrated high retention rates in both our studies to evaluate the *HoMBReS* and *HoMBReS-2* interventions prior to knowing whether the interventions were effective. These types of incremental successes are important for all partners, particularly given the protracted time systematic research takes.

Furthermore, our partnership has only begun to address larger change. The success of these efforts is based in part on our step-by-step approach. We began by being more focused on individual change; however, we are progressing to focusing on structural environmental and system changes now that we established a well functioning partnership, a shared understanding of research, and trust with health department leaders, for example.

CONCLUSIONS

Our partnership is strong and well established. We have established partnership principles to which partners adhere. We work together, recognizing that no one person or type of person—community member, organizational representative, academic researcher—has the answer or can identify and meet the priorities and needs of communities alone. Because we want to make a difference in the HIV epidemic within the local Latino community, our partnership is committed to working together to blend perspectives and expertise.

Of course, our work as a partnership has not been without challenges. Community members and organizational representatives face the realities of HIV infection every day and know that something must be done for the communities of which they are part. The slow pace of securing research funding is a continual frustration and challenge.

Furthermore, communities themselves are not infallible; community members and members of community-based partnerships may have strongly held prejudices about one another. For example, some members who were part of the original CBPR partnership advocated against prioritizing Latino health. They had negative feelings about Latinos whom they perceived as undocumented and unwelcome. In addition, when Latino MSM stepped forward to advocate for HIV prevention programming, some partners had initial misconceptions about MSM. Facilitating a partnership around sensitive issues that include race and sexuality has required ongoing support.

Our partnership has multiple projects that have grown and developed synergistically. Although this growth has seemed slow, the products of our research have been profound. We now have two HIV prevention interventions designed for heterosexually active Latino men that have evidence of effectiveness. These interventions have a high level of cultural congruence given the iterative process of community participation in their development. CBPR has also contributed to strong study designs; we have had high retention rates. In the *HoMBReS* intervention study, 81% of participants were retained 18 months after initiation of the intervention. In the *HoMBReS-2* intervention study, 98% of participants were retained at 3-month postintervention follow-up.

Our partnership has since developed three other interventions—two for Latino MSM and one for Latina women—that are currently being tested. During intervention development, partners continued to use an approach that ensured that the developed interventions built on the lived experiences of community members, the perspectives of organizational representatives based in service provision, and the scientific expertise of academic researchers.

We have had great success using systematic CBPR processes to meet the priorities and needs of immigrant Latinos in this part of the country. We are committed to CBPR because it maximizes the probability that what we do together is based on what the community itself prioritizes, is more informed due to the sharing of broad perspectives and ideas, and builds the capacity of all partners to solve community problems and build on community assets, and conduct meaningful research.

REFERENCES

Altman, D. G. (1995). Sustaining interventions in community systems: On the relationship between researchers and communities. *Health Psychology, 14*(6), 526–536.

Asamoa, K., Rodriguez, M., Gines, V., Varela, R., Dominguez, K., Mills, C. G., et al. (2004). Report from the CDC. Use of preventive health services by Hispanic/Latino women in two urban communities: Atlanta, Georgia, and Miami, Florida, 2000 and 2001. *Journal of Women's Health, 13*(6), 654–661.

Bandura, A. (1986). *Social foundations of thought and action: A social cognitive theory.* Englewood Cliffs, NJ: Prentice-Hall.

Cashman, R., Eng, E., Simán, F., & Rhodes, S. D. (2011). Exploring the sexual health priorities and needs of immigrant Latinas in the southeastern US: A community-based research approach. *AIDS Education and Prevention, 23*(3), 236–248.

Cashman, S. B., Adeky, S., Allen, A. J., Corburn, J., Israel, B. A., Montano, J., et al. (2008). The power and the promise: Working with communities to analyze data, interpret findings, and get to outcomes. *American Journal of Public Health, 98*(8), 1407–1417.

Cornwall, A., & Jewkes, R. (1995). What is participatory research? *Social Science & Medicine, 41*(12), 1667–1676.

Cuadros, P. (2006). *A home on the field: How one championship team inspires hope for the revival of small town America.* New York: Harpercollins.

Freire, P. (1973). *Education for critical consciousness.* New York: Seabury Press.

Harari, N., Davis, M., & Heisler, M. (2008). Strangers in a strange land: Health care experiences for recent Latino immigrants in Midwest communities. *Journal of Health Care for the Poor and Underserved, 19*(4), 1350–1367.

Hayes-Bautista, D. (2004). *La Nueva California: Latinos in the Golden State.* Berkeley, CA: University of California.

Heckathorn, D. D. (1997). Respondent-driven sampling: A new approach to the study of hidden populations. *Social Problems, 44*(2), 174–199.

Heckathorn, D. D. (2002). Respondent-driven sampling II: Deriving valid population estimates from chain-referral samples. *Social Problems, 49*(1), 11–34.

Hergenrather, K. C., & Rhodes, S. D. (2008). Community-based participatory research: Applications for research in health and disability. In T. Knoll (Ed.), *Focus on disability: Trends in research and application* (Vol. 2, pp. 59–87). New York: Nova Science.

Institute of Medicine. (2000). *Promoting health: Intervention strategies from social and behavioral research.* Washington, DC: National Academy Press.

Israel, B. A., Eng, E., Schulz, A. J., & Parker, E. A. (2005). Introduction to methods in community-based participatory research for health. In B. A. Israel, E. Eng, A. J. Schulz, & E. A. Parker (Eds.), *Methods in community-based participatory research* (pp. 3–26). San Francisco, CA: Jossey-Bass.

Israel, B. A., Lichtenstein, R., Lantz, P., McGranaghan, R., Allen, A., Guzman, J. R., et al. (2001). The Detroit community-academic urban research center: Development, implementation, and evaluation. *Journal of Public Health Management and Practice, 7*(5), 1–19.

Israel, B. A., Schulz, A. J., Parker, E. A., & Becker, A. B. (1998). Review of community-based research: Assessing partnership approaches to improve public health. *Annual Review of Public Health, 19,* 173–202.

Kasarda, J. D., & Johnson, J. H. (2006). *The economic impact of the Hispanic population on the state of North Carolina.* Chapel Hill, NC: Frank Hawkins Kenan Institute of Private Enterprise.

MacQueen, K. M., McLellan, E., Kay, K., & Milstein, B. (1998). Codebook development for a team-based qualitative analysis. *Cultural Anthropology Methods, 10*(2), 31–36.

Margolis, L. H., Stevens, R., Laraia, B., Ammerman, A., Harlan, C., Dodds, J., et al. (2000). Educating students for community-based partnerships. *Journal of Community Practice, 7*(4), 21–34.

Minkler, M. (2005). Community-based research partnerships: Challenges and opportunities. *Journal of Urban Health, 82*(2 Suppl 2), ii3–ii12.

Minkler, M., & Wallerstein, N. (2002). Improving health education through community building organization and community building: A health education perspective. In M. Minkler (Ed.), *Community organizing and community building for health* (pp. 30–52). New Brunswick, NJ: Rutgers University Press.

North Carolina Institute of Medicine. (2003). *NC Latino health 2003.* Durham: North Carolina Institute of Medicine.

O'Donnell, C. R., O'Donnell, L., San Doval, A., Duran, R., & Labes, K. (1998). Reductions in STD infections subsequent to an STD clinic visit. Using video-based patient education to supplement provider interactions. *Sexually Transmitted Diseases, 25*(3), 161–168.

Parker, E. A., Eng, E., Laraia, B., Ammerman, A., Dodds, J., Margolis, L., et al. (1998). Coalition building for prevention: Lessons learned from the North Carolina community-based public health initiative. *Journal of Public Health Management and Practice, 4*(2), 25–36.

Rhodes, S. D. (2009). Tuberculosis, sexually transmitted diseases, HIV, and other infections among farmworkers in the eastern United States. In T. A. Arcury & S. A. Quandt (Eds.), *Latino farmworkers in the Eastern United States: Health, safety and justice* (pp. 131–152). New York: Springer.

Rhodes, S. D., Eng, E., Hergenrather, K. C., Remnitz, I. M., Arceo, R., Montano, J., et al. (2007). Exploring Latino men's HIV risk using community-based participatory research. *American Journal of Health Behavior, 31*(2), 146–158.

Rhodes, S. D., Fernandez, F. M., Leichliter, J. S., Vissman, A. T., Duck, S., O'Brien, M. C., et al. (in press). Medications for sexual health available from non-medical sources: A need for increased access to healthcare and education among immigrant Latinos in the rural southeastern USA. *Journal of Immigrant and Minority Health, 13*(6), 1183–1186.

Rhodes, S. D., & Hergenrather, K. C. (2007). Recently arrived immigrant Latino men identify community approaches to promote HIV prevention. *American Journal of Public Health, 97*(6), 984–985.

Rhodes, S. D., Hergenrather, K. C., Aronson, R. E., Bloom, F. R., Felizzola, J., Wolfson, M., et al. (2010). Latino men who have sex with men and HIV in the rural south-eastern USA: Findings from ethnographic in-depth interviews. *Culture, Health & Sexuality, 12*(7), 797–812.

Rhodes, S. D., Hergenrather, K. C., Bloom, F. R., Leichliter, J. S., & Montaño, J. (2009). Outcomes from a community-based, participatory lay health advisor HIV/STD prevention intervention for recently arrived immigrant Latino men in rural North Carolina, USA. *AIDS Education and Prevention, 21*(Suppl 1), 104–109.

Rhodes, S. D., Hergenrather, K. C., Griffith, D., Yee, L. J., Zometa, C. S., Montaño, J., et al. (2009). Sexual and alcohol use behaviours of Latino men in the south-eastern USA. *Culture, Health & Sexuality, 11*(1), 17–34.

Rhodes, S. D., Hergenrather, K. C., Montano, J., Remnitz, I. M., Arceo, R., Bloom, F. R., et al. (2006). Using community-based participatory research to develop an intervention to reduce HIV and STD infections among Latino men. *AIDS Education and Prevention, 18*(5), 375–389.

Rhodes, S. D., Hergenrather, K. C., Vissman, A. T., Stowers, J., Davis, A. B., Hannah, A., et al. (2011). Boys must be men, and men must have sex with women: A qualitative CBPR study to explore sexual risk among African American, Latino, and white gay men and MSM. *American Journal of Men's Health, 5*(2), 140–151.

Rhodes, S. D., Hergenrather, K. C., Wilkin, A., Alegria-Ortega, J., & Montaño, J. (2006). Preventing HIV infection among young immigrant Latino men: Results from focus groups using community-based participatory research. *Journal of the National Medical Association, 98*(4), 564–573.

Rhodes, S. D., Hergenrather, K. C., Wilkin, A. M., & Jolly, C. (2008). Visions and voices: Indigent persons living with HIV in the southern United States use photovoice to create knowledge, develop partnerships, and take action. *Health Promotion Practice, 9*(2), 159–169.

Rhodes, S. D., Hergenrather, K. C., Yee, L. J., Wilkin, A. M., Clarke, T. L., Wooldredge, R., et al. (2007). Condom acquisition and preferences within a sample of sexually active gay and bisexual men in the Southern USA. *AIDS Patient Care & STDS, 21*(11), 861–870.

Rhodes, S. D., Malow, R. M., & Jolly, C. (2010). Community-based participatory research: A new and not-so-new approach to HIV/AIDS prevention, care, and treatment. *AIDS Education and Prevention, 22*(3), 173–183.

Rhodes, S. D., McCoy, T. P., Hergenrather, K. C., Vissman, A. T., Wolfson, M., Alonzo, J., et al. (2011). Prevalence estimates of health risk behaviors of immigrant Latino men who have sex with men in rural North Carolina. *Journal of Rural Health, 27*(16), 361–373.

Rhodes, S. D., McCoy, T. P., Vissman, A. T., DiClemente, R. J., Duck, S., Hergenrather, K. C., et al. (2011). A randomized controlled trial of a culturally congruent intervention to increase condom use and HIV testing among heterosexually active immigrant Latino men. *AIDS and Behavior, 15*(8), 1764–1775.

Rhodes, S. D., Yee, L. J., & Hergenrather, K. C. (2006). A community-based rapid assessment of HIV behavioural risk disparities within a large sample of gay men in south-eastern USA: A comparison of African American, Latino and white men. *AIDS Care, 18*(8), 1018–1024.

Robles, R. R., Reyes, J. C., Colon, H. M., Sahai, H., Marrero, C. A., Matos, T. D., et al. (2004). Effects of combined counseling and case management to reduce HIV risk behaviors among Hispanic drug injectors in Puerto Rico: A randomized controlled study. *Journal of Substance Abuse Treatment, 27*(2), 145–152.

Shibusawa, T., & Lukens, E. (2004). Analyzing qualitative data in a cross-language context: A collaborative model. In D. K. Padgett (Ed.), *The qualitative research experience* (pp. 175–186). Belmont, CA: Wadsworth/Thompson Learning.

Southern State Directors Work Group. (2008). *Southern states manifesto: Update 2008. HIV/ AIDS and sexually transmitted diseases in the south.* Birmingham, AL: Southern AIDS Coalition.

Streng, J. M., Rhodes, S. D., Ayala, G. X., Eng, E., Arceo, R., & Phipps, S. (2004). Realidad Latina: Latino adolescents, their school, and a university use photovoice to examine and address the influence of immigration. *Journal of Interprofessional Care, 18*(4), 403–415.

U.S. Census Bureau. (2009). *2008 American community survey data profile highlights: North Carolina fact sheet* (Vol. 2009). Washington, DC: United States Department of Commerce.

Vissman, A. T., Bloom, F. R., Leichliter, J. S., Bachmann, L. H., Montaño, J., Topmiller, M., et al. (2011). Exploring the use of non-medical sources of prescription drugs among immigrant Latinos in the rural southeastern USA. *Journal of Rural Health, 27*(2), 159–167.

6 Mexico–U.S. Migration, Social Exclusion, and HIV Risk

Multisectoral Approaches to Understanding and Preventing Infection

Jennifer S. Hirsch and Emily Vasquez

INTRODUCTION

The risk of HIV infection ranks relatively low in the day-to-day concerns of many Mexican migrants. Before coming to the United States, many worry about dying in transit from dehydration, snakes in the desert, or the rapaciousness of their fellow humans (Archibold, 2007; Jimenez, 2009; Cleaveland, 2011). Once here, they worry about how to work in places in which there is limited public transportation and in which they are unable to secure a driver's license or car insurance (Bazar, 2008; Preston & Gebeloff, 2010). At work, they worry about discrimination (Marin, Grzywacz, et al., 2009), exposure to toxic levels of pesticides (Villarejo, 2003), fatal construction accidents (Cierpich, Styles, et al., 2008; Cunningham, Ruben, et al., 2008; Gany, Dobslaw, et al., 2011), about being kept late to care for others' children so that they cannot care for their own (Ehrenreich & Hochschild, 2002; Hondagneu-Sotelo, 2007), and that they might be robbed of their cash wages on their way home (Londoño & Vargas, 2007; Abel & Amrhein, 2009). During moments of rest at the end of 6-day weeks, they worry about the physical and economic well-being of loved ones back home (Hovey & Magana, 2002; Sullivan & Rehm, 2005; Grzywacz, Quandt, et al., 2006; Snipes, Thompson, et al., 2007; Cervantes, Mejia, et al., 2010; Familiar, Borges, et al., 2011; Negi, 2011). Given the limited recreational options and unbalanced sex ratios in the communities in which they frequently reside, they may drown those worries in alcohol (Loury, Jesse, et al., 2011) or seek solace with a commercial sex worker (Parrado, Flippen, et al., 2004; Hirsch, Munoz-Laboy, et al., 2009; Munoz-Laboy, Hirsch, et al., 2009).

The fact that a variety of threats and concerns might seem more pressing for vulnerable migrant populations, however, does not mean that their risk of HIV infection is low. Latino migrants, including Mexicans, increasingly settle in areas with relatively high prevalence (Painter, 2008). Recent data show that some of the metropolitan areas that have experienced the largest percent increase in foreign-born population between 2000 and 2009, including Jackson, Charlotte, Jacksonville, and Atlanta, also had some of the highest rates in the nation of diagnosis of new infections by 2009 (Centers for Disease Control and Prevention, 2011; The Brookings Institution, 2011).[1] This is not to say that there is a causal relation between one and the other, or even to make claims about possible prevalence rates among Mexican migrants, but rather to point out that migration itself often puts Mexicans in a setting in which prospective sexual partners are more likely to be HIV positive than they would be in Mexican sending communities. Moreover, life in the United States frequently involves engagement in practices and exposure to contexts that put Mexican migrants at risk of infection (Apostolopoulos, Sonmez, et al., 2006; Kissinger, Liddon, et al., 2008; Painter, 2008; Parrado & Flippen, 2010; Rhodes, Bischoff, et al., 2010; Wilson, Eggleston, et al., 2010; Albarrán & Nyamathi, 2011), and their generally limited access to health care is reflected in the disproportionate numbers of Mexican-origin individuals in the United States presenting late or with "dual diagnoses." That is, by the time they receive a diagnosis of HIV, they have reduced CD4 cell counts or are already sick with AIDS (Levy, Prentiss, et al., 2007; Espinoza, Hall, et al., 2008; Dennis, Napravnik, et al., 2011). This late presentation is associated with an increased likelihood of passing the virus on to others and with poorer therapeutic outcomes for those who receive antiretroviral therapy (ART) (Battegay, Fluckiger, et al., 2007).

As discussed in the introduction to this volume, a *Structural Environmental* framework enables us to consider how HIV risk is produced by the broader social context in which Mexican migrants live (Sweat, Denison, et al., 1995; Parrado & Flippen, 2010; Ward, 2010; Albarrán & Nyamathi, 2011; Winett, Harvey, et al., 2011). In this chapter, we explore sources of HIV risk at the structural level, looking at the influence of policies across multiple sectors. We connect this point about the multisectoral determinants of risk to the robust critique that has emerged of individual-level behavioral interventions, arguing that a structural approach to HIV prevention should encompass policy reform relevant to housing, transportation, urban development, occupational safety, health insurance, and immigration, all of which shape the broader context of HIV risk for Mexican migrants.[2]

Additionally, we draw on a systems perspective (Leischow, Best, et al., 2008), as well as our own ethnographic encounters with Mexican migrants, to think about the research, advocacy, and policy implications of HIV being only one of many threats to the health and well-being of Mexican migrants in the United States. Instead of responding to this issue as one of competing priorities (i.e., should advocates be fighting for more attention to diabetes and other chronic diseases, which take such a heavy toll, or to HIV prevention, where the disparities are also quite clear?) we underline the common structural causes of HIV and other urgent health risks. We thus note that intervention at the structural level could impact both HIV risk and other health outcomes that are of considerable importance in relation to population health. Not secondarily, those outcomes may also be experienced by migrant communities as more pressing priorities. As such, we urge HIV researchers, many of whom already work from a multilevel perspective, to make common cause with researchers focused on other health outcomes.

It may be obvious to those of us who have devoted our careers to research on HIV or Latino health that HIV is a pressing issue, and this single-disease focus is reinforced by disease-specific funding streams. It is possible, however, that researchers could build a more effective platform to shape policy by demonstrating the multiple outcomes that could be improved by structural interventions. Furthermore, this "multiple-exposure, multiple outcome" perspective is relevant to advocates in strengthening the health justification for policy reform and in building broad coalitions that would include both those interested in other health disparities relevant to the Latino community and those working outside the health sector. As the saying goes, *Unidos, si se puede!*

MEXICAN MIGRANTS, HIV RISK, AND AIDS CARE

To understand the risks facing Mexican migrants, it is important first to understand who those migrants are, and how the demography of labor migration between Mexico and the United States has changed over recent decades. Early settlement patterns of Mexican migrants in the United States were shaped by the demand for (and recruitment of) labor by agricultural growers, the U.S. rail industry and mining companies, who together represented a significant force by the start of the twentieth century (Massey, Durand, et al., 2002). By 1942, this migrant flow was institutionalized under the auspices of the Bracero Program, which formalized U.S. dependence on Mexican labor (Durand, Massey, et al., 2000; Massey, Durand, et al., 2002). At that time, the principally male migrant circuits had clear nodes of concentration in California, Texas, and Illinois, with more minor migrant streams up and down the East and West coasts and through Midwestern states, which followed the harvests (Durand, Massey, et al., 2000). After the termination of the Bracero Program in 1964, when a series of increasingly stringent caps were first imposed on Mexican immigration, it remained principally young men—especially bachelors or those in the early stages of family formation intent on a short-term stay—who continued to follow these well-established migrant paths. They did so illegally, in response to persistent demand, engaging in a sort of cat-and-mouse routine with the Immigration and Naturalization Service (INS) in which they risked what amounted to an essentially symbolic arrest and a short-lived deportation, a risk they could stand to face again should the need arise for a return migration (Massey, Durand, et al., 2002).

The dynamics of Mexican migration to the United States changed drastically, however, with the 1986 Immigration Reform and Control Act (IRCA). This legislation channeled significant funding to U.S. border control, which served to militarize traditional crossing-points and, importantly, complicated old patterns of return migrations (Massey, Durand, et al., 2002). Settlement became increasingly permanent, as a result, and more frequently included wives and children (Massey, Durand, et al., 2002). Simultaneously, IRCA authorized a massive legalization of migrants who could prove their residency in the United States since 1982 and provided for the legal immigration of the families of those who qualified. Reflecting settlement trends up to that point, 54% (2.3 million) of those who applied for this asylum were living in California. But, as Massey and Capoferro (2008) explain, given the economic decline and rising antiimmigrant sentiment in that state, as well as the ongoing restructuring of U.S. industry nationwide, their new legal status enabled millions to respond to labor demands in new destinations. Hence, the path was hewn for new immigrant communities in states including Nevada, Colorado, Utah, Georgia, North Carolina, and Kansas, and in cities such as New York City, Phoenix, Las Vegas, Denver, Charlotte, Atlanta, and Raleigh-Durham (Durand, Massey, et al., 2000; Card & Lewis, 2007; Leach & Bean, 2008). The typical Mexican migrant, once a young, single man working in agriculture, increasingly moved to urban destinations where he began working in the service sector and where he was joined by growing numbers of women (Durand, Massey, et al., 1999).

According to the American Community Survey, Mexican immigrants in the United States totaled nearly 11.5 million in 2009 and accounted for 29.9% of the foreign born (Pew Hispanic Center, 2011). Half were undocumented (Pew Hispanic Center, 2011). Their geographic distribution across the country reflected this trend toward increasingly diverse settlement patterns—though 37.5% of Mexican migrants were residing in California, 20.9% in Texas, and 6% in Illinois, steadily growing communities had developed elsewhere with 5.1% in Arizona, 2.4% in Florida and Georgia, another 2.1% in North Carolina (as described in Chapter 5 by Scott Rhodes) and Colorado, and 2.0% in New York (Pew Hispanic Center, 2011). While the Mexican-born population in the United States grew by another 25% between 2000 and 2010 (Pew Hispanic Center, 2011), during that period births in the United States of Mexican-American babies surpassed immigration as the primary driver of growth in the Mexican-origin population, reflecting not only the fertility of Mexican-born individuals in the United States, but also a significant decline in the rate of Mexican immigration, which, likely a reflection of economic conditions in the United States, fell from more than one million in 2006 to just 404,000 in 2010 (a 60% reduction) (Passel & Cohn, 2009). Interestingly, the slowing pace of immigration was also accompanied by a slowing pace in return migration—about 450,000 Mexicans returned to Mexico annually in 2006 and 2007, compared to 319,000 in 2010 (Pew Hispanic Center, 2011).

The American Community Survey also provides evidence that about a third of Mexican migrants in the United States worked in service occupations in 2009, whereas only about 5% worked in the agricultural industry. Among those over 25 years old 61.2% had achieved less than a high school diploma (U.S. Census Bureau, 2009). More than 25% lived in poverty and 57% had no health insurance coverage (U.S. Census Bureau, 2009). Importantly, men significantly outnumbered women, comprising nearly 60% of those aged 18 to 34 years (U.S. Census Bureau, 2009). Finally, the majority of Mexican migrants (58.2% of men and 57.9% of women) were married, though not necessarily cohabiting with their spouses, while 33.3% of men and 25% of women had never been married (U.S. Census Bureau, 2009).

Despite the feminization of the Mexican migrant flows to the United States over time, unattached men (which includes both single men and men who migrate without their wives) have continued to represent a significant proportion of the Mexican immigrant population—indeed, there were at least a million more Mexican-born men than women in the United States in 2009, equivalent to the population of the entire state of Rhode Island—and there is substantial evidence to suggest that widespread sexual risk practices exist among these men. This does not necessarily imply that they are more or less sexually active than other groups, only that evidence exists that migrant men do, not surprisingly, have sex while they are in the United States, and that, like most other people, they do not always use condoms when they do so.

Research suggests that Mexican men living in the United States engage in several HIV risk behaviors, including sex with commercial sex workers, selling sex themselves, sex between men, low rates of condom use, and substance use. For example, in a sample of 442 randomly selected migrant men in North Carolina (71% Mexican), Parrado et al. (2004) found that rates of engaging with a sex worker were as high as 40% among married men unaccompanied by their wives and 46% among unmarried men. Parrado et al. also found that although HIV knowledge and reported condom use were quite high, the men surveyed reported being less likely to use condoms as they grew more familiar with a particular sex worker (Parrado, 2004). In a study of 450 Latino day laborers in Los Angeles (nearly half of whom were of Mexican origin), Galvan (2008) found that 37% of the sample reported being solicited for sex by another man while seeking work and 9.4% reported having had sex with their solicitors, that drug dependence was associated with doing so, and that most did not use condoms during anal sex with their solicitors. As we argue in the sections that follow, the social isolation, loneliness, boredom, and limited access to health services that research has shown to be linked to sexual risk taking are socially produced characteristics of the migration experience rather than inevitable aspects of life as a migrant (see also Viadro & Earp, 2000; Apostolopoulos, Sonmez, et al., 2006; Rhodes, 2006; Munoz-Laboy, Hirsch, et al., 2009; Seña, 2010; Wilson, Eggleston, et al., 2010).

Despite evidence of these high-risk behaviors among Mexican migrants, surveillance-based information regarding HIV infection in this group is limited, especially among those who return periodically to their sending communities (Painter, 2008). We do know, however, that in general Hispanics in the United States are disproportionately affected. Indeed, Hispanics were diagnosed with HIV in 2009 at a rate of more than three times that of whites (22.8 vs. 7.2 per 100,000), a rate second in the nation only to that of blacks (Centers for Disease Control and Prevention, 2011). Reflecting a pattern evident across all race/ethnicities in the United States, Hispanic men were diagnosed with HIV at a higher rate than Hispanic women (48.3 vs. 11.9 per 100,000) (Centers for Disease Control and Prevention, 2011). Additional subgroup differences have also been reported between the rates of infection depending on U.S. and foreign-born status, as well as national origin. Assessing data from 33 states and 5 independent areas, Espinoza et al. (2008) found that between 2003 and 2006 the annual number of diagnoses was stable for Hispanics overall, but the number of diagnoses increased among Hispanic males born in Mexico by approximately 8.8% each year and among males and females from Central America by 18.6% and 24.6% each year, respectively. Importantly, Painter (2008) has suggested that the prevalence of HIV infection among Mexican migrants is also likely to vary by state. In states in which settlement began more recently—with the dramatic shift in settlement patterns in the wake of IRCA—he suggests that migrants may be at increased risk for HIV infection due to less stable social support systems and sexual networks, which would be more readily available in traditional settlement areas (Painter, 2008).

Overall, HIV prevalence among adults in the United States is twice that in Mexico (UNAIDS, 2010) and Mexican HIV surveillance data offer some evidence of the connection between migration and HIV risk in Mexico, especially in rural sectors (although the collection of data related to migration history has not been consistent) (Magis-Rodriguez, Gayet, et al., 2004). Mexican HIV surveillance data show, for example, that approximately 33% of AIDS cases in Mexico have occured in those states that export the highest number of number of migrants to the United States (Magis-Rodriguez, Gayet, et al., 2004). A study in the Mexican states of Michoacán and Jalisco revealed that by the end of 2000, more than one in five people living with HIV/AIDS there had previously resided in the United States (Magis-Rodriguez, Gayet, et al., 2004), and there is evidence that migrants who have been to the United States within a year report more sexual partners and noninjecting drug use than nonmigrant Mexicans (Magis-Rodriguez, Lemp, et al., 2009).

The bodily exclusion of Mexican migrants in the United States further manifests itself in health inequalities among those diagnosed with HIV. Although the focus of this chapter is the contextual organization of risk, questions of access to care and clinical outcomes are relevant because they emphasize the acute nature of this health inequality; in addition, new evidence about infectiousness and disease stage makes it clear that enhancing access to care is of signal importance for the broader dynamics of the epidemic. Hispanics born in Mexico and Central America are almost twice as likely to be diagnosed with AIDS within 12 months of receiving an HIV diagnosis, in comparison with Hispanics born in the United States (Schwarcz, Hsu, et al., 2006; Levy, Prentiss, et al., 2007; Espinoza, Hall, et al., 2008; see also Dennis, Napravnik, et al., 2011). Late disease-stage presentation is also particularly common in men, who rarely utilize health services, as compared to women, who frequently engage with the health care system due to reproductive health needs (Espinoza, Hall, et al., 2008).

Once infected, access to care varies considerably depending on geographic location. In every state, an HIV diagnosis and sufficiently advanced disease stage are the only eligibility criteria for receiving ART through the AIDS Drug Assistance Program (ADAP)—but because ADAP is funded at the state level, qualifying for coverage is not synonymous with receiving care (Sack, 2010). Here, curiously, is a case in which the lack of a policy seems to be beneficial for Mexican migrants who engage with available services. If states were forced to legally specify whether residency status should make one eligible for financial assistance in paying for medications, it is unlikely that there would be widespread support for treating HIV-positive Mexicans—an outcry for deportation is more likely.

Linked to this apparent loophole, there is evidence of a surprising paradox in regards to Hispanic survival after diagnosis with AIDS—both U.S. born and foreign-born Hispanics appear to fare as well as whites in terms of survival 12 and 36 months after diagnosis with AIDS (Espinoza, Hall, et al., 2008). However, it is not clear whether these findings may be due to inconsistencies in the data or, perhaps, to the return of immigrants with advanced disease to their country of origin (Espinoza, Hall, et al., 2008).

THE LESSONS OF 30 YEARS OF HIV INTERVENTIONS

At the start of the fourth decade of the global HIV pandemic, more than 5 million people worldwide are benefiting from antiretroviral therapy, representing a 13-fold increase in global coverage since 2004 alone, though 10 million more are eligible but are not receiving treatment. As Gupta et al. (2008) have argued, given that the rate of infection still far exceeds the rate of treatment initiation, it is clear that "we cannot treat our way out of this epidemic" (p. 485). Prevention remains key to the global fight against HIV and an emerging paradigm in prevention strategy, addressing the structural factors that drive the unequal distribution of risk at the population level, is gaining ground. This new paradigm of "combination prevention" strives for synergy among "behavioral, biomedical and structural approaches based on scientifically derived evidence with the wisdom and ownership of communities" (Merson, O'Malley, et al., 2008, p. 475). Finally, it seems, structural interventions are gaining ground not just as "a nice accompaniment to 'the real stuff' of HIV prevention strategies" but as absolutely central to them (Hankins & de Zalduondo, 2010, p. S72).

The shift away from programs focused on behavioral change alone comes in the wake of broad recognition that although behavioral change strategies—which typically attempt to delay onset of first intercourse, decrease the number of sexual partners, increase condom use, encourage testing, and decrease sharing of needles and substance use—have often had demonstrable short-term success in the modification of specific behaviors, under rigorous evaluation they have not proven sustainable or efficacious in regards to reduction of the incidence of HIV infection (Coates 2008; Hankins & de Zalduondo, 2010; Ross, 2010; de Wit, Aggleton, et al., 2011). Individual-level behavioral interventions, it is now understood, were doomed from the start given their failure to consider societal conditions, such as gender inequality, sexual culture, poverty, and access to HIV services (Hankins & de Zalduondo, 2010). These were lessons decades (and millions of dollars) in coming, and our delay is difficult to justify. After all, the most significant strategies through which public health practice has lengthened and improved people's lives are those that change the context in which individuals live, rather than those which exhort people to choose healthier behaviors. For example, 25 of the 30 years by which life expectancy in the United States has increased from the beginning to the end of the twentieth century is attributable to structural interventions ranging from vaccination to safer and healthier food to fluoridation of drinking water (Centers for Disease Control and Prevention, 1999). Government regulation, collective action, and the transformation of institutions and systems played key roles in those gains.

In the United States, the trajectory of HIV prevention among Mexican migrants has reflected this long-standing global emphasis on individual-level intervention. In their 2004 review of available research outcome literature on HIV prevention with Mexican migrants, Organista, Carrillo, et al. (2004) reported that prevention efforts to that point consisted primarily of HIV/AIDS education, condom promotion and distribution, HIV testing and counseling, and support groups for people living with HIV and AIDS. The structural factors that create risky environments for Mexican migrants, they argued, were underresearched and efforts to address them, with few exceptions, were consequently stalled (Organista, Carrillo, et al., 2004). It is our perspective that although the call to integrate a structural approach into the response to HIV risk among Mexican migrants in the United States has since been widely echoed by advocates and academics, as we shall detail below, little headway has been made in terms of effecting real change at the structural level to reduce Mexican migrant HIV risk. Below, we outline the landscape of contextual risk that persists today.

Of course, with great concern, we recognize that the structural level interventions we identify will confront an ugly, xenophobic reality: The Joe Wilson "you lie!" moment during President Obama's speech on health insurance reform emphasized the exclusion of Mexican migrants from the American social body, and the socially constituted lack of value placed on the health of their individual bodies (see Scherer, 2009). This xenophobic reaction was evidence of a long-running and heated opposition to the provision of health care to Mexican migrants—a sentiment previously embodied perhaps most palpably in California's Proposition 187, which in 1994 denied the provision of health care in that state to the foreign born, including pregnant women. That measure was deemed unconstitutional in Federal court and eventually repealed, but the sentiment that produced that legislation, and that was reproduced by it, is alive and well today, if not even more powerful.

LANDSCAPES OF RISK AND SUFFERING: THE DAILY LIVES OF MEXICAN MIGRANTS
Housing

A drive past the apple farms in Western New York State, the peach farms of Georgia and South Carolina, the tomato and strawberry fields in Florida, or the vast agricultural lands in the Salinas Valley provides a graphic reminder of the dismal living conditions of migrant agricultural laborers, most of whom are of Mexican origin (Early, Davis, et al., 2006; Vallejos, Quandt, et al., 2009, 2011). This is hardly, however, a purely rural phenomenon; their economic and legal vulnerability means that in suburban and urban contexts as well, Mexican immigrants are likely to face overcrowding and poorly maintained housing (Pader, 1994; Krivo, 1995; Schill, Friedman, et al., 1998; Rosenbaum & Schill, 1999; Clark, Deurloo, et al., 2000). Landlords may be less assiduous about maintaining properties in which tenants are most unlikely to complain to municipal authorities, and low wages may make trailers and apartments in aging complexes that have fallen into disrepair the only housing that is affordable to migrants. Limited access to the banking system can concentrate migrants in low-quality housing by making it impossible for them to secure a mortgage or even establish the credit rating necessary to rent in many places.

An emerging literature has documented the relationship between unstable housing and both increased HIV risk and poorer clinical outcomes for individuals living with AIDS (Wolitski, Kidder, et al., 2010; Aidala, Cross, et al., 2005; Aidala, Lee, et al., 2007; Aidala & Sumartojo, 2007; Holtgrave, Briddell, et al., 2007; Kidder, Wolitski, et al., 2007; Friedman, Marshal, et al., 2009; Royal, Kidder, et al., 2009). Other work has looked quite specifically at how housing conditions shape HIV risk among various Latino groups or in some cases among Mexican migrants (Parrado & Flippen, 2010). In that work, Parrado found that neighborhood-level gender imbalances and external social organization (i.e., "broken windows") were related to exposure to sexual risk. Another path through which residential patterns can shape sexual risk is via the recreational options available in the places in which people live. When the first author was living in Atlanta, migrant workers were concentrated in neighborhoods in which leisure-time spaces consisted primarily of places to play pool, play soccer, pray, or drink—and that was the more urbanized areas (Hirsch, Munoz-Laboy, et al., 2009). In migrant camps found in rural areas, buying sex may be one of very few opportunities for diversion (Magis-Rodriguez, Lemp, et al., 2009).

Transportation

Both directly and indirectly, transportation infrastructure and policies are part of the context of HIV risk. Acknowledging the challenges posed by what might seem a relatively quotidian part of the day—the morning commute—serves to highlight both the basic indignities of social exclusion and the ways in which this particular element of context might exacerbate HIV risk. Many of the new migrant-receiving destinations to which Mexicans have flocked over the past two decades lack adequate public transportation infrastructure, and some of those same states also have legislation that makes it hard if not impossible for undocumented immigrants to acquire a driver's license. The number of states with this type of legislation has actually increased over the past decade, coincident with (and perhaps in part due to) both the post 9/11 political climate and the contracting economy which has made immigrants the targets for political ill-will (Bazar, 2008; Lacey, 2011). Even in relatively immigrant-friendly states such as New York, it proved impossible for a popular governor with substantial political capital to use a public-safety argument (making driver's licenses accessible enables all drivers to buy auto insurance and enables the state to have better information about its residents) to expand access to driver's licenses (Hakim, 2007).

The challenges posed by driver's license laws are characteristic of the social exclusion faced by undocumented Mexican migrants; that alone should be understood as part of the context of HIV risk (Hirsch, Munoz-Laboy, et al., 2009). But constrained access to transportation also intertwines with the issues related to housing described above. The combined difficulty of getting around and the limited options for recreation in the neighborhoods in which Mexican migrants can afford to live mean that for many migrant men, spending a portion of their earnings to buy sex is one of the few forms of gratification and entertainment available to them.

Occupational Safety and Health

There are two ways in which occupational safety is relevant to thinking about HIV risk. In the broadest sense, due to the relatively higher prevalence of HIV in the United States, men's risk of HIV infection is enhanced by the mere fact of being here at all, and they are here as workers—mowing lawns, butchering hogs, hanging sheetrock, or delivering Chinese food—because the global organization of labor and capital has made it hard for them to earn a living in their communities of origin. In other words, it is not the jobs per se that put them at risk of HIV infection—the low-wage, physically demanding jobs filled by migrant workers may not even offer indoor plumbing or a place to wash their hands, much less opportunities for on-the-job sex—but rather these men's location in the global economic order that put them physically in places in which there is an increased risk of sex with an HIV-positive individual. Mexican men certainly engage in multiple partnerships and extramarital liaisons while at home (Pulerwitz, Izazola-Licea, et al., 2001; Parrado, Flippen, et al., 2004; Hirsch, Smith, et al., 2009), but being far from home—understood as including the watching eyes of one's neighbors, the comforts of family and kin, and access to a stable sexual partner such as one's wife or fiancée—does increase the likelihood of engaging in extramarital or casual partnerships. For those immigrants who engage in sex work as part of a strategy for economic survival, of course, HIV is a much more direct part of on-the-job risk (Galvan, Ortiz, et al., 2008).

Of course, the distal connection between economic organization and HIV risk is complemented by much more direct occupational health concerns faced by Mexican migrant workers. The rate of work-related deaths in the United States has dropped by 15% in the past 15 years, but the rate of workplace fatalities is consistently higher among Hispanics as compared to the rate for all U.S. workers, with the majority (70%) of deaths among Hispanic workers occurring among those who are Mexican born (Cierpich, Styles, et al., 2008). Why do these deaths (which foreground thousands of injuries each year) occur disproportionately among Mexican migrants? Here we suspect that it is not necessarily a lack of policy relevant to occupational safety, but an insufficient and unequal enforcement of existing policy, which is reflected in these statistics. Furthermore, that Mexican migrant bodies are ignored, while Mexican migrant labor is readily exploited in the United States, is a reality for which government, business, and *consumers* must take responsibility. The lust of the American consumer for cheap protein, housing, and berries, for manicured hands and just as neatly manicured lawns, contributes to the maintenance of a migration regime dependent upon low-cost (and therefore necessarily undocumented) migrant labor.

Just as we have become increasingly socially responsible regarding the environmental impact of our consumption, we believe that consumers' recognition of their impact on the health of workers may foster demand for change. The link between occupational injuries and mortality, the increased risk of HIV encountered by Mexican migrant laborers in the United States, even the limits on access to health care imposed by jobs (as discussed below), are all externalities associated with commodities we use everyday. Whether it is takeout pizza or a steak in a fine restaurant, most meals in America are served with a side of HIV risk, and so one step toward expanding how we think of the structural interventions that might mitigate HIV risk would be to begin a more honest conversation about the ways in which American consumers benefit from and contribute to the conditions of vulnerability in which many Mexican migrants live.

Access to Health Care

Mexican migrants face significant challenges in terms of access to health care in the United States. They are concentrated in economic sectors that do not provide employer based health insurance (Cunningham, Ruben, et al., 2008), which limits opportunities for clinic-based primary prevention, and long work hours and low wages further complicate access to available services. Undocumented Mexican-origin individuals represent a significant portion of the 50 million people living in the United States who do not have access to health insurance; it is estimated that about 20% of the uninsured are foreign born, noncitizens, who were specifically excluded from the major reforms in health care advanced during the first years of the Obama administration (Kaiser Commission on Medicaid and the Uninsured, 2010). Language can be an issue as well—as migrants have moved beyond traditional migrant receiving locations such as Chicago and California to settle in almost every state in the union, many of these newer migrant communities are entirely without bilingual service providers—not to mention interpreters who speak Purepécha (Nandi, Galea, et al., 2008).

Primary care provides opportunities for sexual risk reduction messaging, STD testing, HIV testing and counseling, and for linkages to ART and AIDS care for those who are HIV positive. Beyond the relevance to thinking about opportunities for HIV prevention or to link migrants with care, understanding the ways that Mexican migrants do (or do not) engage with the U.S. health care system is part of acknowledging the many other health inequalities faced by this population. Despite a substantial literature on the Hispanic birth outcome "paradox," there are health outcomes in which clear disparities emerge, related both to contextual factors and to the above-mentioned limited access to primary health care. These include oral health (Horton & Barker, 2010) and obesity (Kaplan, Huguet, et al., 2004). Analysis from the Mexican Migration Project of premigration and postmigration health also found a higher prevalence of heart disease, mental health disorders, and smoking among nonmigrants. The noxious intersection between undocumented status and the organization of health care in the United States is emphasized by a recent extreme case in which an individual who had been receiving dialysis at a public hospital in Atlanta, Georgia, was told that the only way she could continue to do so was to be sick enough that she had to go to an emergency room, which as a provider of last resort would, unlike the clinic she had been attending, be legally required to provide her with care, but even then only on a temporary basis (Sack, 2011). HIV researchers may be singularly concerned with the penises of Mexican migrants, but it should be remembered that those migrants themselves may be more concerned with health issues related to their kidneys, backs, or teeth.

Migration Policy

It is not surprising that men who are far away from their spouses for extended periods of time are more likely to have a nonmarital partner (Parrado & Flippen, 2010).

Before "Operation Hold the Line" in El Paso, Texas, and similar initiatives that went into effect along the southern border (Lowell & Perderzini, 2006), greatly increasing the danger and expense of crossing the border, it was not uncommon for migrant men to return home annually for an extended visit. Some Mexican migrants, both men and women, continue with this old pattern of annual circular migration, but changes in border management have resulted in many migrant men spending years away from their families. Migration policy's influence on sexual risk practices is hardly the primary reason for a critique of the current policy regime among those who are opposed to it, nor are the policy's noxious health consequences likely to hold much sway among proponents of even more restrictive policies. Nevertheless, a more contextual approach to thinking about the social factors that facilitate HIV risk practices makes it relevant to consider policies that restrict the ability of migrants to travel home to see their families and that severely limit the circumstances under which migrants can legally arrange for their families to join them in the United States.

A Risk-Producing Context

A host of other factors have been shown to contribute to HIV risk for Mexican migrants. These include isolation, anxiety, and loss of familial and social support networks, a situation associated with seeking multiple casual sex partners, engaging in sex with commercial sex workers, and using illicit drugs and alcohol abuse (Munoz-Laboy, Hirsch, et al., 2009), as well as exposure to a social culture that is often more open and permissive with regard to sexual and drug-using behaviors (Magis-Rodriguez, Gayet, et al., 2004). Migrants have also been shown to adopt new sexual practices such as oral and anal sex and same-gender partners (Magis-Rodriguez, Lemp, et al., 2009).

These experiences of invisibility, vulnerability, and alienation can make the migrant sojourn an intensely alienating experience. As one migrant man said in Atlanta, "You get used to the idea that you are alone here. You have to understand that, that it is you against the world: to face whatever comes, whether it is good or bad. You live together with other people but as much for them as for you they are beating this pressure alone, to try to make life lighter." Another man emphasized the relation between consumption of commercial sex and the alienation of migrant life, noting that when he had sex with a sex worker it was "the only time I felt like a human being" (Hirsch, Munoz-Laboy, et al., 2009).

In addition to those aspects of social inequality that broadly shape the social organization of HIV risk (sexual inequality/heteronormativity, racial inequality, gender inequality, stigma and discrimination against drug users), we have tried to show here that social, economic, and health policies exacerbate vulnerability to HIV for Mexican migrant workers. They are not HIV policies, and indeed they are not all even health policies, but they influence the conditions in which migrants live, and the circumstances under which their sexual practices take shape, in ways that have clear implications for the risk of sexual transmission of HIV.

CONCLUSIONS

In sum, Mexican migrants face many other pressing health inequalities; behavioral interventions for HIV prevention have largely proven to be ineffective, unsustainable, or not scalable, and for both political and epidemiological reasons, Mexican migrants are unlikely to be high on the priority list even if effective interventions were developed. Moreover, sexual relations are a social behavior, not simply a health behavior, and thus the sexual risk practices produced by a complicated web of social factors are unlikely to be amenable to any sort of single intervention.

Although we might appear to be building toward an argument against any public health action related to HIV prevention among Mexican migrants as both unjustified and unlikely to be effective, that is not in fact our point. Our point, rather, is that the combination of these insights makes it necessary to think in an entirely different way about public health approaches to HIV prevention for these vulnerable individuals. All of this should make clear that there is no "clean-water" equivalent of sexual risk reduction—that is, no one population-level intervention that it could reasonably be argued would by itself be likely to significantly reduce the risk that a Mexican migrant in the United States would become infected with HIV. Rather, we argue that advocates and researchers should consider this as justification for more multisectoral approaches—indeed, for making common cause with initiatives that are either relevant to many other sectors of the population, or that address health issues of particular concern to the Mexican immigrant population other than HIV.

Specifically, we are making a case for three kinds of research. First, there is a need for multisited research to assess the relation between HIV risk practices and aspects of social context such as housing availability and conditions, publicly funded recreational options, transportation infrastructure, and local labor markets. Migrants who arrive in cities with established Spanish-speaking populations and good public transportation lead vastly different lives than they would if they were living in isolated trailer parks in rural areas, and the impact of variation in these aspects of social context can be most convincingly studied through comparison. Cities may offer both greater risks—more sexual partners, populations with very high rates of HIV infection, easy access to injection drugs—but may also provide more salutary forms of recreation. The point is not to build an evidence base that would lead to changing housing, transportation, or labor policy as an HIV prevention intervention. Rather, the goal would be to develop an expanded sense of what it could mean to talk about structural interventions by tracing out the processes through which specific configurations of social institutions affect HIV-relevant practices. We wonder, for example, how DREAM Act legislation (now passed in 12 states) might influence the life projects and therefore potentially impact the sexual risk-taking of Mexican immigrant youth who benefit from it? There is a great deal of enthusiasm for "combined prevention," but it would still be useful to develop more possibilities for the macrolevel and mesolevel interventions.

Second, we are trying to make a case for multioutcome research that looks at the broad impact of these state and local-level policy changes. It certainly seems logical that limiting access to drivers licenses would have a clear and immediate impact on the mental health of undocumented populations; any traffic stop becomes a possible route to deportation. We are reminded of a young woman living in a trailer park outside of Atlanta who assessed her time in the United States succinctly: "me siento en la carcel." But what is the impact of these policies on HIV risk? On nutrition and obesity? School performance and high-school drop-out rates? Much is made of developing culturally appropriate interventions for various ethnic populations, and in a sense our argument here takes us in the other direction, suggesting instead that researchers explore the health implications of changes in social institutions that affect many populations. The goal would be to build an evidence base that could be used for making common cause across racial and ethnic lines—in essence, to use health research as a tool for transcending identity politics to work collectively toward the broader social good. Although we are not so naive as to believe in a direct causal link between research and policy, evidence can be useful to advocates pressing for policy change and can provide useful cover to policymakers seeking to make change.

Running through this chapter has been a more general argument about the relation between social exclusion and HIV risk, and this leads us to the third recommendation, which is to look specifically at the multiple health impacts of various migration regimes. Despite severe (and growing) threats to the stability of their social safety nets, a number of EU countries have managed to explicitly define health as a human right and ensure access to care to migrants regardless of their immigration status. The United States appears for the moment to be headed in the opposite direction, with migrant workers treated as cannon fodder in the global wars of capitalism—with an unquenchable desire for the inexpensive "mano de obra," with no responsibility taken for the bodies to which those arms are attached. How is living in fear bad for people? Conversely, how does engagement in mobilization to protect and promote immigrants' rights—the Immokalee workers, the college students' advocacy for passage of the federal DREAM act—affect various health outcomes? If HIV risk practices are in part a product of social exclusion and alienation, it is not inconceivable that these claims to citizenship would be relevant for practices of self-care (although anyone who has ever worked on a political campaign or as a community organizer knows that doing so greatly increases one's risk for late-night pizza consumption). In Chapter 2, Ramirez-Valles et al. provided empirical evidence that AIDS activism and community involvement decrease HIV risk in LGBT Latinos.

These suggestions regarding a research agenda to learn about how social context shapes HIV risk for one of the most vulnerable sectors of the Latino community are driven by a commitment to public health as social justice. Our goal is not only to produce information that could be used to reduce HIV risk among a population whose lives are otherwise unchanged, but also to inspire the production of knowledge that could contribute in some small way to more fundamental improvements in the lives of the disenfranchised—a category that, in the United States, most certainly includes many Mexican migrants.

NOTES

1. The foreign-born population in Jackson, Mississippi, grew by 104.5% between 2000 and 2009—growth surpassed in the nation only in Cape Coral, Florida. Jackson ranked third in the nation for its rate of new HIV infections in 2009 (39.2 cases per 100,000). The metropolitan area Charlotte–Gastonia–Concord in North and South Carolina likewise saw a 90% increase in its foreign-born population during this time and ranked tenth in the nation in 2009 for new HIV cases (30.2 cases per 100,000). Jacksonville, Florida, saw an increase of 77.2% in foreign-born residents and was ranked seventh in the nation for its rate of diagnosis of HIV infection in 2009 (36.4 cases per 100,000). Atlanta, Georgia, is ranked fifth in the nation for its rate of diagnosis of HIV infection (37.7 cases per 100,000), an area that saw an increase of 68% in its foreign-born population between 2000 and 2010.

2. Given the relatively large proportion of the Mexican-origin population in the United States that is undocumented, these socially produced vulnerabilities are of variable relevance in understanding the challenges faced by other sectors of the Latino population; the structural exclusions created by the legal challenges of navigating daily life as an

undocumented person are shared by a great many Central-American and some Dominican immigrants, but are of much less relevance to Latinos whose roots lie in Cuba or Puerto Rico. Furthermore, our focus in this chapter is not the Mexican-origin population as a whole, but rather those Mexican-born individuals who have migrated to the United States as workers. This excludes those "1.5" generation individuals, who face other challenges specific to growing up in a society in which they may lack legal citizenship but which may be the only home they know, and it also excludes the risks facing second and subsequent generation Mexican-origin individuals.

REFERENCES

Abel, J., & Amrhein, S. (2009, January 4). Easy targets. *St. Petersburg Times*, p. 3A.

Aidala, A., Cross, J. E., et al. (2005). Housing status and HIV risk behaviors: Implications for prevention and policy. *Aids and Behavior, 9*(3), 251–265.

Aidala, A. A., Lee, G., et al. (2007). Housing need, housing assistance, and connection to HIV medical care. *Aids and Behavior, 9*(6), S101–S115.

Aidala, A. A., & Sumartojo, E. (2007). Why housing? *Aids and Behavior, 11*(6), S1–S6.

Albarrán, C. R., & Nyamathi, A. (2011). HIV and Mexican migrant workers in the United States: A review applying the vulnerable populations conceptual model. *The Journal of the Association of Nurses in AIDS Care, 22*(3), 173–185.

Apostolopoulos, Y., Sonmez, S., et al. (2006). STI/HIV risks for Mexican migrant laborers: Exploratory ethnographies. *Journal of Immigration & Minority Health, 8*(3), 291–302.

Archibold, R. C. (2007, September 15). At U.S. border, desert takes a rising toll. *The New York Times*, p. A1.

Battegay, M., Fluckiger, U., et al. (2007). Late presentation of HIV-infected individuals. *Antiviral Therapy, 12*(6), 841–851.

Bazar, E. (2008, January 30). Fewer licenses for illegal migrants; More states require legal status to drive. *USA Today*, p. 3A.

Card, D., & Lewis, E. G. (2007). The diffusion of Mexican immigrants during the 1990s: Explanations and impacts. In G. J. Borjes (Ed.), *Mexican immigration to the United States* (pp. 193–228), Chicago, IL: University of Chicago Press.

Centers for Disease Control and Prevention. (1999). *Ten great public health achievements— United States, 1990–1999* (pp. 241–243). Atlanta, GA.

Centers for Disease Control and Prevention. (2011). HIV surveillance report 2009. 12.

Cervantes, J. M., Mejia, O. L., et al. (2010). serial migration and the assessment of extreme and unusual psychological hardship with undocumented Latina/o families. *Hispanic Journal of Behavioral Sciences, 32*(2), 275–291.

Cierpich, H., Styles, L., et al. (2008). Work-related injury deaths among Hispanics—United States, 1992-2006. *Morbidity and Mortality Weekly Report, 57*(22), 597–600.

Clark, W. A. V., Deurloo, M. C., et al. (2000). Housing consumption and residential crowding in U.S. housing markets. *Journal of Urban Affairs, 22*(1), 49–63.

Cleaveland, C. (2011). 'In this country, you suffer a lot': Undocumented Mexican immigrant experiences. *Qualitative Social Work*, August 9, 2011, 1–21. Retrieved from http://qsw. sagepub.com/content/early/2011/06/25/1473325011409475.

Coates, T. J. (2008). Behavioural strategies to reduce HIV transmission: How to make them work better. *The Lancet, 372*(9639), 669–684.

Cunningham, A. S., Ruben, J. D., et al. (2008). Health of foreign-born people in the United States: A review. *Health Place, 14*(4), 623–635.

de Wit, J. B., Aggleton, P., et al. (2011). The rapidly changing paradigm of HIV prevention: Time to strengthen social and behavioural approaches. *Health Education Research, 26*(3), 381–392.

Dennis, A. M., Napravnik, S., et al. (2011). Late entry to HIV care among Latinos compared with non-Latinos in a southeastern US cohort. *Clinical Infectious Diseases, 53*(5), 480–487.

Durand, J., Massey, D. S., et al., (1999). The new era of Mexican migration to the United States. *The Journal of American History, 86*(2), 518–536.

Durand, J., Massey, D. S., et al. (2000). The changing geography of Mexican immigration to the United States: 1910–1996. *Social Science Quarterly, 81*(1), 1–15.

Early, J., Davis, S., et al. (2006). Housing characteristics of farmworker families in North Carolina. *Journal of Immigrant and Minority Health, 8*(2), 173–184.

Ehrenreich, B., & Hochschild, A. (Eds.) (2002). *Global woman: nannies, maids and sex workers in the new economy.* New York: Metropolitan Press.

Espinoza, L., Hall, H. I., et al. (2008). Characteristics of HIV infection among Hispanics, United States 2003–2006. *Journal of Acquired Immune Deficiency Syndrome, 49*(1), 94–101.

Familiar, I., Borges, G., et al. (2011). Mexican migration experiences to the US and risk for anxiety and depressive symptoms. *Journal of Affective Disorders, 130*(1–2), 83–91.

Friedman, M. S., Marshal, M. P., et al. (2009). Associations between substance use, sexual risk taking and HIV treatment adherence among homeless people living with HIV. *AIDS Care-Psychological and Socio-Medical Aspects of AIDS/HIV, 21*(6), 692–700.

Galvan, F. H., Ortiz, D. J., et al. (2008). Sexual solicitation of Latino male day laborers by other men. *Salud Publica De Mexico, 50*(6), 439–446.

Gany, F., Dobslaw, R., et al. (2011). Mexican urban occupational health in the US: A population at risk. *Journal of Community Health, 36*(2), 175–179.

Grzywacz, J. G., Quandt, S. A., et al. (2006). Leaving family for work: Ambivalence and mental health among Mexican migrant farmworker men. *Journal of Immigrant and Minority Health, 8*(1), 85–97.

Gupta, G. R., Parkhurst, J. O., et al. (2008). Structural approaches to HIV prevention. *The Lancet, 372*(9640), 764–775.

Hakim, D. (2007, November 14). Spitzer dropping his driver's license plan. *The New York Times,* p. A1.

Hankins, C. A., & de Zalduondo, B. O. (2010). Combination prevention: A deeper understanding of effective HIV prevention. *AIDS, 24*(Suppl 4), S70–S80.

Hirsch, J. S., Munoz-Laboy, M., et al. (2009). They miss more than anything their normal life back home: Masculinity and extramarital sex among Mexican migrants in Atlanta. *Perspectives on Sexual and Reproductive Health, 41*(1), 23–32.

Hirsch, J. S., Smith, D. J., et al. (2009). *The secret: Love, marriage, and HIV.* Nashville, TN: Vanderbilt University Press.

Holtgrave, D. R., Briddell, K., et al. (2007). Cost and threshold analysis of housing as an HIV prevention intervention. *AIDS and Behavior, 11*(6), S162–S166.

Hondagneu-Sotelo, P. (2007). *Domestica: Immigrant workers cleaning and caring in the shadows of affluence.* Berkeley, CA: University of California Press.

Horton, S., & Barker, J. C. (2010). Stigmatized biologies: Examining the cumulative effects of oral health disparities for Mexican American farmworker children. *Medical Anthropology Quarterly, 24*(2), 199–219.

Hovey, J. D., & Magana, C. G. (2002). Exploring the mental health of Mexican migrant farm workers in the midwest: Psychosocial predictors of psychological distress and suggestions for prevention and treatment. *Journal of Psychology, 136*(5), 493–513.

Jimenez, M. (2009). Humanitarian crisis: Migrant deaths at the U.S.-Mexico border. American Civil Liberties Union of San Diego & Imperial Counties.

Kaiser Commission on Medicaid and the Uninsured. (2010). The uninsured: A primer.

Kaplan, M. S., Huguet, N., et al. (2004). The, association between length of residence and obesity among Hispanic immigrants. *American Journal of Preventive Medicine, 27*(4), 323–326.

Kidder, D. P., Wolitski, R. J., et al. (2007). Access to housing as a structural intervention for homeless and unstably housed people living with HIV: Rationale, methods, and implementation of the housing and health study. *AIDS and Behavior, 11*(6), S149–S161.

Kissinger, P., Liddon, N., et al. (2008). HIV/STI risk behaviors among Latino migrant workers in New Orleans post-hurricane Katrina disaster. *Sexually Transmitted Diseases, 35*(11), 924–929.

Krivo, L. (1995). Immigrant characteristics and Hispanic-Anglo housing inequality. *Demography, 32*(4), 599–615.

Lacey, M. (2011, August 24). License access in New Mexico is heated issue. *The New York Times*, p. A1.

Leach, M. A., & Bean, F. D. (2008). The structure and dynamics of Mexican migration to new destinations in the United States. In D.S. Massey (Ed.), *New faces in new places: The changing geography of American immigration* (pp. 51–74). New York: Russell Sage Foundation.

Leischow, S. J., Best, A., et al. (2008). Systems thinking to improve the public's health. *American Journal of Preventive Medicine, 35*(2S), S196–S203.

Levy, V., Prentiss, D., et al. (2007). Factors in the delayed HIV presentation of immigrants in Northern California: Implications for voluntary counseling and testing programs. *Journal of Immigrant and Minority Health, 9*(1), 49–54.

Londoño, E., & Vargas, T. (2007, October 26). Robbers stalk Hispanic immigrants, seeing ideal prey. *Washington Post*, p. A01.

Loury, S., Jesse, E., et al. (2011). Binge drinking among male Mexican immigrants in rural North Carolina. *Journal of Immigrant and Minority Health, 13*(4), 664–670.

Lowell, B. L., Perderzini, C. P., et al. (2006). The demography of Mexico/U.S. migration. In A. E. Latapi & S. F. Martin (Eds.), *Mexico-U.S. migration management: A binational approach* (pp. 1–32). Lantham, MD: Lexington Books.

Magis-Rodriguez, C., Gayet, C., et al. (2004). Migration and AIDS in Mexico: An overview based on recent evidence. *Journal of Acquired Immune Deficiency Syndrome, 37*(Suppl 4), S215–S226.

Magis-Rodriguez, C., Lemp, G., et al. (2009). Going north: Mexican migrants and their vulnerability to HIV. *Journal of Acquired Immune Deficiency Syndrome, 51*(Suppl 1), S21–S25.

Marin, A. J., Grzywacz, J. G., et al. (2009). Evidence of organizational injustice in poultry processing plants: Possible effects on occupational health and safety among Latino workers in North Carolina. *American Journal of Industrial Medicine, 52*(1), 37–48.

Massey, D. S., & Capoferro, C. (2008). The geographic diversification of American immigration. In D. S. Massey (Ed.), *New faces in new places: The changing geography of American immigration* (pp. 25–50). New York: Russell Sage Foundation.

Massey, D. S., Durand, J., et al. (2002). *Beyond smoke and mirrors: Mexican immigration in an era of economic integration.* New York: Russell Sage Foundation.

Merson, M. H., O'Malley, J., et al. (2008). The history and challenge of HIV prevention. *Lancet, 372*(9637), 475–488.

Munoz-Laboy, M., Hirsch, J. S., et al. (2009). Loneliness as a sexual risk factor for male Mexican migrant workers. *American Journal of Public Health, 99*(5), 802–810.

Nandi, A., Galea, S., et al. (2008). Access to and use of health services among undocumented Mexican immigrants in a US urban area. *American Journal of Public Health, 98*(11), 2011–2020.

Negi, N. J. (2011). Identifying psychosocial stressors of well-being and factors related to substance use among Latino day laborers. *Journal of Immigrant and Minority Health, 13*(4), 748–755.

Organista, K. C., Carrillo, H., et al. (2004). HIV prevention with Mexican migrants: Review, critique, and recommendations. *JAIDS Journal of Acquired Immune Deficiency Syndromes, 37*, S227–S239.

Pader, E. J. (1994). Spatial relations and housing policy: Regulations that discriminate against Mexican-origin households. *Journal of Planning Education and Research, 13*(2), 119–135.

Painter, T. M. (2008). Connecting the dots: When the risks of HIV/STD infection appear high but the burden of infection is not known—the case of male Latino migrants in the southern United States. *AIDS Behavior, 12*(2), 213–226.

Parrado, E. A. (2004). Use of commercial sex workers among Hispanic migrants in North Carolina: Implications for the spread of HIV. *Perspectives on Sexual and Reproductive Health, 36*(4), 150–156.

Parrado, E. A., & Flippen, C. (2010a). Community attachment, neighborhood context, and sex worker use among Hispanic migrants in Durham, North Carolina, USA. *Social Science & Medicine, 70*(7), 1059–1069.

Parrado, E. A., & Flippen, C. A. (2010b). Migration and sexuality: A comparison of Mexicans in sending and receiving communities. *Journal of Social Issues, 66*(1), 175–195.

Parrado, E. A., Flippen, C. A., et al. (2004). Use of commercial sex workers among Hispanic migrants in North Carolina: Implications for the spread of HIV. *Perspectives on Sexual and Reproductive Health, 36*(4), 150–156.

Passel, J. S., & Cohn, D. V. (2009). *Mexican immigrants: How many come? How many leave?* Washington, DC: Pew Hispanic Center.

Pew Hispanic Center. (2011) Statistical portrait of the foreign-born population in the United States, 2009. Washington, DC.

Preston, J. & Gebeloff, R. (2010, December 10). Some unlicensed drivers risk more than a fine. *The New York Times*, p. A1.

Pulerwitz, J., Izazola-Licea, J.-A., et al. (2001). Extrarelational sex among Mexican men and their partners' risk of HIV and other sexually transmitted diseases. *American Journal of Public Health, 91*(10), 1650.

Rhodes, S. D. (2006). Preventing HIV infection among young immigrant Latino men: Results from focus groups using community-based participatory research. *Journal of the National Medical Association, 98*(4), 564–573.

Rhodes, S. D., Bischoff, W. E., et al., (2010). HIV and sexually transmitted disease risk among male Hispanic/Latino migrant farmworkers in the Southeast: Findings from a pilot CBPR study. *American Journal of Industrial Medicine, 53*(10), 976–983.

Rosenbaum, E., & Schill, M. H. (1999). Housing and neighborhood turnover among immigrant and native-born households in New York City, 1991 to 1996. *Journal of Housing Research 10*(2), 209–233.

Ross, D. A. (2010). Behavioural interventions to reduce HIV risk: What works? *AIDS, 24*(Suppl 4), S4–14.

Royal, S. W., Kidder, D. P., et al. (2009). Factors associated with adherence to highly active antiretroviral therapy in homeless or unstably housed adults living with HIV. *AIDS Care-Psychological and Socio-Medical Aspects of AIDS/HIV, 21*(4), 448–455.

Sack, K. (2010, July 1). Slump cripples aid for drugs to treat H.I.V. *New York: The New York Times*, p. A1.

Sack, K. (2011, September 2). Clinic rejects immigrants after impasse with hospital. New York: *The New York Times*, p. A12.

Scherer, M. (2009, September 10) 'You Lie!': Representative Wilson's outburst. *Time*. Retreived from http://www.time.com/time/politics/article/0,8599,1921455,00.html.

Schill, M. H., Friedman, S., et al., (1998). The housing conditions of immigrants in New York City. *Journal of Housing Research 9*(2), 201–235.

Schwarcz, S., Hsu, L., et al. (2006). Late diagnosis of HIV infection: Trends, prevalence, and characteristics of persons whose HIV diagnosis occurred within 12 months of developing AIDS. *Journal of Acquired Immune Deficiency Syndrome, 43*(4), 491–494.

Seña, A. C. (2010). Feasibility and acceptability of door-to-door rapid HIV testing among Latino immigrants and their HIV risk factors in North Carolina. *AIDS Patient Care and STDs, 24*(3), 165–173.

Snipes, S. A., Thompson, B., et al. (2007). Anthropological and psychological merge: Design of a stress measure for Mexican farmworkers. *Culture Medicine and Psychiatry 31*(3), 359–388.

Sullivan, M. M., & Rehm, R. (2005). Mental health of undocumented Mexican immigrants— A review of the literature. *Advances in Nursing Science, 28*(3), 240–251.

Sweat, M. D., Denison, J. A., et al. (1995). Reducing HIV incidence in developing countries with structural and environmental interventions. *AIDS 9*(Suppl A), S251–S257.

The Brookings Institution. (2011). Change in foreign-born population since 2000. from http://soma.brookings.edu/DownloadHandler.axd?mode=indicator&ind=55.

UNAIDS. (2010). UNAIDS Report on the Global AIDS Epidemic, 2010.

U.S. Census Bureau (2009). 2009 American Community Survey.

Vallejos, Q. M., Quandt, S. A., et al. (2009). *The condition of farmworker housing in the eastern United States Latino farmworkers in the eastern United States* (pp. 37–67). New York: Springer.

Vallejos, Q. M., Quandt, S. A., et al. (2011). Migrant farmworkers' housing conditions across an agricultural season in North Carolina. *American Journal of Industrial Medicine, 54*(7), 533–544.

Viadro, C. I., & Earp, J. A. (2000). The sexual behavior of married Mexican immigrant men in North Carolina. *Social Science and Medicine, 50*(5), 723–735.

Villarejo, D. (2003). The health of U.S. hired farm workers. *Annual Review of Public Health, 24*, 175–193.

Ward, L. S. (2010). Farmworkers at risk: The costs of family separation. *Journal of Immigrant and Minority Health, 12*(5), 672–677.

Wilson, K. S., Eggleston, E., et al. (2010). HIV/STI risk among male Mexican immigrants in Dallas, Texas: Findings from a pilot study. *Journal of Immigrant and Minority Health, 12*(6), 947–951.

Winett, L., Harvey, S. M., et al. (2011). Immigrant Latino men in rural communities in the Northwest: Social environment and HIV/STI risk. *Culture, Health and Sexuality, 13*(6), 643–656.

Wolitski, R. J., Kidder, V., et al. (2010). Randomized trial of the effects of housing assistance on the health and risk behaviors of homeless and unstably housed people living with HIV. *Aids and Behavior, 14*(3), 493–503.

Section II
Illuminating Complex Dimensions of HIV Risk in Diverse Latino Populations, Environments, and Situations

7 Inequality, Discrimination, and HIV Risk

A Review of Research on Latino Gay Men

Rafael M. Díaz, Jorge Sánchez, and Kurt Schroeder

INTRODUCTION

A recent Centers for Disease Control and Prevention (CDC) report on the prevalence of HIV infection among men who have sex with men (MSM) reminds us that gay men—and in particular gay men of color—continue to carry the major burden of the HIV epidemic in the United States (Centers for Disease Control and Prevention, 2010). The surveillance study found that one in five gay men in the United States are infected with HIV, in sharp contrast to a prevalence rate of less than 1% in the U.S. general population. The study also showed that HIV prevalence was unevenly distributed among ethnoracial groups: 28% of Black gay men and 18% of Latino gay men, in comparison to 16% of white gay men, are infected with HIV. Similarly among those HIV infected, lack of awareness of own HIV status in disproportionately higher in Black (59%) and Latino (46%) gay men, in comparison to white gay men (26%). Above all, the CDC statistics emphasize the fact that the HIV epidemic is not just a serious and damaging disease, but also a marker of larger structural-environmental, social, and cultural forces of discrimination and inequality on the basis of sexual orientation, race, ethnicity, and even immigration status. That is, HIV/AIDS data reveal patterns that are not random but that mirror many ingrained patterns of racism, stigma, and discrimination that create multiple marginalities and vulnerabilities to morbidity and mortality related to larger psychosocial and health problems.

Within the Latino U.S. community, gay men also carry the brunt of the epidemic. Latino gay men account for over half of all AIDS cases among Latino males in the United States (Centers for Disease Control and Prevention, 2008). This percentage is much higher in the Western United States, where Latino gay men represent 80–90% of all AIDS cases among Latino males. It is clear that no sound policy or effective programs that address HIV/AIDS in Latino communities could be developed without taking into account the particular social and structural factors that place Latino gay men at risk. In this spirit, we offer a critical review of the research literature from the perspective of social, structural, and environmental forces that explain the disproportionate burden of HIV in this most affected subgroup of Latinos.

DEFINING THE POPULATION OF LATINO GAY MEN

We use the term "Latino gay men" to broadly define the population of Latino men who have sex with men (MSM), but more precisely those men whose same-sex sexual activity expresses an underlying homosexual or homoerotic sexual orientation. These men typically self-identify with a variety of words and categories that indicate a nonheterosexual orientation, such as gay, homosexual, bisexual, or queer. These words describe not only their erotic interests and behavior, but also a deeply felt personal identity based on their sexual, emotional, and romantic involvement with other men. In fact, for the majority of these men, their sexual orientation and identity organize a large portion of their lives; important life choices—separation from families of origin, migration to the United States, moving to gay-friendly cities such as San Francisco, career trajectories, and choices of friendship networks—are made to facilitate and support the lived expression of their homosexual orientation (Diaz, 1998; Carrillo et al., 2008).

The specific definition of Latino gay men, and this review, exclude two important categories of persons that often interact and participate in different aspects of this community, namely, Latino MSM who identify as heterosexual, sometimes referred to as MSMW, and male-to-female (MTF) transgender individuals. We believe that this (temporary and functional) exclusion is justified because the substantial differences and circumstances of the excluded groups merit their own assessments, analyses, and conclusions. Our omission of data on transgender persons and heterosexual MSM is done respectfully in order to avoid gross generalizations, and also as an admission of our limited knowledge.

PREVALENCE OF HIV AND RISK BEHAVIOR

Two national studies that involve probability samples suggest that—consistent with recent CDC statistics—approximately 20% of Latino gay men of all ages in large U.S. urban centers are infected with HIV. In a household probability sample (Urban Men Health Study; $N = 2,881$) of geographic areas with a high concentration of MSM in four major U.S. cities (San Francisco, Los Angeles, Chicago, and New York), a substantial number of Latinos ($N = 246$, or 10% of the sample) were included. In this study, 19% of the Latino sample reported an HIV-positive status (Catania et al., 2001). In a second study, a probability sample ($N = 912$) of Latino gay/bisexual men who attend Latino gay venues in the cities of Los Angeles, Miami, and New York yielded a somewhat similar, though slightly higher prevalence of 22% (Diaz & Ayala, 2001). From these two studies, and taking into account the limitations of self-reporting a stigmatized status, it can be said with some confidence and conservatively that about one out of five Latino gay and bisexual men in large U.S. urban centers are infected with HIV (Diaz, Peterson, & Choi, 2007).

In the three-city study, involving a venue-based probability sample of Latino gay men in three U.S. cities, rates of unprotected anal intercourse were 28% (estimated by sexual activity in the past 2 months) and 37% (estimated by sexual activity with the last two sexual partners within a 12-month period). However, the data from the last two partners suggest that only about half of the 37% of men who report unprotected anal intercourse (or 18% of the sample) do so with a nonmonogamous partner. Thus, it must be noted that a large majority of Latino gay men are genuinely attempting to be safe in their sexual activity, by either condom use and/or monogamy practices (Diaz, Ayala, & Bein, 2004).

A more recent study (Ramirez-Valles et al., 2008) drew a representative sample of Latino gay men in San Francisco (N = 323) and Chicago (N = 320) using respondent-driven sampling (RDS). The study estimated the prevalence of HIV at 35% among Latino gay men in San Francisco, much higher than the national estimates in earlier studies, and higher than the prevalence for Chicago of 21.5%. About 21% of the sample in San Francisco reported engaging in unprotected anal intercourse (7% did so with known serodiscordant partners). Notably, although the prevalence of HIV is much higher in San Francisco than Chicago, no differences were found in the rates of unprotected anal sex between the two cities. This latter finding suggests that given the higher background prevalence of HIV in San Francisco, a single act of unprotected anal intercourse in this city carries a higher risk of infection than in communities with lower HIV prevalence.

HOMOSEXUAL IDENTITY AND DISCLOSURE IN LATINO CULTURE

For Latino men who have sex with other men, homosexual identification is impacted by multiple cultural meanings, particularly gender ideologies and family values (Carrier, 1995; Carrillo, 2002; Diaz, 1998). Traditional masculine ideologies define homosexuality as a gender deviation and, consequently, male homosexuals as not "real men" as noted by Rhodes in Chapter 5. Because families are highly valued as the most important agent of gender role socialization, homosexuality is perceived to be a disappointment and dishonor to families. In the context of gender norms and the strong values placed on lifelong family cohesion (*Familismo*), Latino gay men face enormous challenges in adopting and disclosing a homosexual or gay identity. Although research suggests that gender ideologies do change with increasing acculturation to mainstream U.S. culture, it is also clear that the value of familism, where families are seen as the main source of emotional and social support throughout the lifespan, resists acculturation and remains a central defining characteristic of Latino culture and identity (Vega, 1995). See Chapters 16 and 17 for more discussion on familism.

It is thus not surprising that the processes of homosexual identification and disclosure ("outness") are impacted by cultural norms of sexual silence and existing sexual prejudice (homophobia) within Latino families. For example, many Latino gay men choose to come out openly only to friends, but not to their families, with the perception that openly disclosed homosexuality is a terrible burden to their families. Many immigrant Latino gay men choose to migrate and come out far away from their families, as a way to negotiate the tensions between *familismo* and the adoption of a homosexual identity and social life. The often-heard phrase *"everybody knows, but we do not talk about it"* illustrates how some Latino families negotiate the tension between the love for their sons and the heteronormative aspects of their culture (Diaz, 1998). On the other hand, there is increasing evidence that Latino families do change and grow, and younger men seem more able to come out in the context of a supportive family. Nonetheless, studies to date show that family acceptance of Latino gay males, particularly those who are effeminate and gender nonconforming, is relatively low (Ryan et al., 2009).

For those who identify as homosexual, a variety of terms exist including gay, homosexual, bisexual, or queer. Some men may use culturally nuanced terms such as *loca, joto, pato,* or *maricón* (equivalents of *queen, fairy, sissy,* or *faggot*) to self identify and to refer to one another warmly, even though these terms have often been used against them as a derogatory expression of sexual discrimination. The majority of Latino gay men feel they belong to a diverse and inclusive gay world or community sometimes referred to as *de ambiente*, of the ambiance, or *entendido*, those who understand; the two concepts illustrate the adaptive cultural capacity of this community to privately acknowledge what is not publicly disclosed, a capacity that is not quite appropriately described by the term "sexual silence" (Carrillo, 2002).

Of central importance to the purpose of this review is the fact that cultural dimensions of homosexual identity and disclosure may impact Latino gay men's integration to the mainstream gay culture in the United States—a culture that often demands uncompromised "outness" and public openness about homosexuality—as well as their sensitivity to messages about HIV/AIDS, including access to HIV treatment and prevention services. These cultural factors are therefore of crucial importance when designing programs and services that target this population.

LATINO BISEXUALITIES

Bisexuality refers to a person's concurrent sexual attraction and/or behavior toward both male and female individuals. Experts agree that the phenomenon of bisexuality within Latino communities takes multiple forms and behavioral expressions, hence the notion of bisexualities. For some Latino MSM, the label "bisexual" may serve as a transitional identification that facilitates the development of a gay identity, that is, a stage in the coming out process. But for many others, bisexuality may be a genuine sexual orientation, where the person—regardless of behavioral expression—experiences sexual attraction and desire for members of both genders (Muñoz-Laboy & Dodge, 2005). For those who have a bisexual orientation, substantial variation exists in the predominance of attraction to either gender, with some individuals being attracted *mostly* to women or *mostly* to men (Chapter 10 presents an interesting chapter on bisexual Latino male sex markets in New York City by Muñoz-Laboy and colleagues). For some, equal bisexuality happens when the gender of the person is not a major factor in the attraction or selection of sexual partners. For some men, whose sexual orientation and identification are heterosexual, bisexual behavior can be an expression of temporary necessity or circumstances rather than sexual attraction, as in the case of individuals who are sex workers or those who are incarcerated (see Chapter 12 for a description of HIV risk and Latinos in the criminal justice system).

Regardless of a bisexual or homosexual orientation, the fact is that a substantial number of Latino MSM also have sex with women for a variety of reasons, ranging from genuine sexual attraction to the internal experience of social pressure; at times, Latino gay men may have sex with women out of a desire to be more "normal" and fit with cultural expectations of masculine behavior. Latino values of familism lead some men to opt for bisexual life choices—such as getting married to a woman at the same time that a male lover is maintained at the margins of family life—in order to live and express their homosexual desire at the same time that they minimize potential cultural conflicts (Muñoz-Laboy et al., 2009). Some men who have a homosexual orientation may want to have a family and children of their own, and do get married as a way to enact such a family desire. Also, having their own heterosexual family allows men for a fuller participation in extended families, religious institutions, and other organizations in a mostly heteronormative Latino civil society (Muñoz-Laboy, 2008).

There are important reasons why different Latino bisexualities must be taken into account when designing HIV prevention programs for MSM. The first reason is that in many circumstances, sex with men may happen in secret, in silence, and at the margin of family life and/or gay community. "Closet" issues may accompany bisexual life choices, and the marginality and silence of sexual behavior may be conducive to risk for HIV. For example, given the close relation between HIV and homosexuality in the Latino community, the use of condoms or discussions about safer sex with steady female partners may be avoided, given that it could be interpreted as a disclosure of extramarital affairs including homosexual encounters outside the relationship (Muñoz-Laboy & Dodge, 2005). Latino MSM who do not participate in organized groups or gay community may be less responsive to prevention campaigns or be less willing to participate in prevention programs because those programs may be viewed as a potential "outing." Second, the majority of HIV prevention programs that target MSM rely on images, language, and assumptions of a mainstream gay culture that frowns upon bisexuality as a denial of a gay identity. Such programs may lack cultural sensitivity to the particular needs of Latino men who have sex with both men and woman for the different reasons mentioned above.

EXPERIENCES OF DISCRIMINATION AND OPPRESSION

The most comprehensive data on experiences of homophobia and racism among Latino gay and bisexual men come from the time/location probability sample of 912 men drawn from Latino gay social venues in the cities of Miami, Los Angeles, and New York; the three cities were chosen not only because of their obvious regional diversity, but also because they represent the three largest Latino ethnic subgroups in the United States, namely, Cubans in Miami, Puerto Ricans in New York, and Mexicans in Los Angeles. The survey was preceded by a qualitative focus group study ($N = 298$) and, based on the qualitative data, survey items were created that quantitatively measured past experiences of social discrimination on account of race, class, and sexual orientation. The main focus of the study was to document experiences of social discrimination and oppression, and test their impact on the health and wellbeing of Latino gay and bisexual men in the United States, particularly their HIV risk (Diaz & Ayala, 2001). In Chapter 8, Ayala provides an empirical test of the relation between HIV risk and social discrimination and oppression in Latino and African American MSM.

In the focus group meetings, men spoke about experiencing both verbal and physical abuse, police harassment, and decreased economic opportunities on account of their being gay and/or perceived as effeminate. They spoke about powerful messages—both explicit and covert—in their communities, telling them that their homosexuality made them "not normal" and not truly men; that they would grow up alone without children or families; and that ultimately their homosexuality is dirty, sinful, and shameful to many of their families and loved ones. Some men mentioned having to opt for exile and migration in order to live their homosexual life away from their loved ones, whom they worried would be hurt if they opted to express their homosexual desires openly. And many others admitted they had to live double lives and pretend to be straight in order to maintain social connections and employment opportunities.

Similarly, men reported multiple instances of discrimination, verbal and physical violence, police harassment, and decreased sexual and social opportunities on account of their being Latino, immigrant, Spanish-speaking, and/or of a darker skin color. A great deal of racism was experienced in the context of gay community and gay venues, where men reported not feeling at ease, not feeling welcomed, and some even reported being "escorted out" of venues on account of their different looks, color, or accent. Some men felt sexually objectified by white boyfriends and lovers, who stereotypically paid more attention to their skin color or Spanish accents than to their personal selves. Many of these men felt invisible, believing that they were just being used as fantasy material, rather than being part of a more authentic and equitable relationship. Many others encountered overt racist rejection in the context of sexual and lover relations.

Many focus group participants also reported experiencing poverty both while growing up and in the present. Men talked about difficulties meeting their day-to-day living expenses and often struggled with inconsistent employment and sources of income. Many reported not having health insurance or access to decent health care. Others reported they did not have their own place to live, and had to rely on friends or relatives for temporary housing. Anger often surfaced among those who were children of Mexican migrant farmworkers when remembering the poor conditions of their families of origin, in the face of obvious social inequality. Others had to face the harsh reality of extreme poverty and misery in the inner city, with a deep sense of lack of control and unsettled resignation. Voices from the South Bronx, one of the poorest and more devastated areas in the country, often made an implicit connection between the poverty of the neighborhood and the seemingly inevitability of HIV infection.

The subsequent quantitative survey confirmed that the overwhelming majority of Latino gay men have experienced homophobia personally and quite intensely: approximately two-thirds of the men (64%) were verbally insulted as children for being gay or effeminate, 70% felt that their homosexuality hurt and embarrassed their family, 64% had to pretend to be straight in order to be accepted, 71% heard as a child that gays would grow old alone, 29% had to move away from their family on account of their homosexuality, and 20% reported instances of police harassment on account of their homosexuality. Similarly, the data showed that about one-third of Latino gay men have experienced racism in the form of verbal harassment as children (31%) and by being treated rudely as adults on account of their race or ethnicity (35%). One out of four men (26%) have experienced discomfort in white gay spaces because of their ethnicity, and more than one out of five (22%) have experienced racially related police harassment. Interestingly, the majority (62%) reported experiencing racism in the form of sexual objectification from other gay men. The quantitative data also revealed that within a 1-year period, more than half of the sample ran out of money for basic necessities (61%) and had to borrow money to get by (54%). With unemployment rates around 30%, close to one-half of the men (45%) had to look for work in the past year.

HIV STIGMA AND DISCLOSURE

In the three-city study, analysis of the data for HIV-negative men revealed a high prevalence of stigmatizing attitudes toward people infected with HIV (Diaz, 2006). More than half of the sample (57%) believed that HIV-positive individuals are responsible for getting infected, and close to half (46%) of the sample believed that HIV-positive persons are to blame for the spread of AIDS. In addition, 52% of the sample saw HIV-positive men as more sexually promiscuous, and 18% believed that they are people who cannot be trusted. In the realm of sexual interactions and romantic relationships, the overwhelming majority (82%) of HIV-negative men felt that sex with HIV-positive men is dangerous, with 57% saying that they are not willing to have sex with an HIV-positive person, even if condoms were available. Close to two-thirds (57%) of HIV-negative men reported that they are not willing to have an HIV-positive person as a boyfriend or girlfriend.

Not surprisingly, a large proportion of HIV-positive men in the sample reported that being HIV positive has negatively impacted their social and sexual lives, beyond the physical/medical challenges posed by their HIV infection. For example, about half of the sample (46%) felt that HIV has made it more difficult for them to find sex and an even lager proportion (58%) felt that HIV made it more difficult to find lover relationships. Two-thirds (66%) of the sample reported that HIV has made it harder for them to enjoy sex. Nearly half (46%) of all HIV-positive participants reported having been treated unfairly because of their serostatus and 45% believed that they had to hide their status to find acceptance from their families and friends. The overwhelming majority (82%) of HIV-positive men thought sexual partners might reject them if they knew their HIV serostatus, a finding that not surprisingly exactly mirrors the fact (reported above) that 82% of HIV-negative men believed that sex with HIV-positive men is dangerous.

More recently, Zea and her colleagues studied the relationship between HIV disclosure and mental health outcomes in a sample of 301 HIV-positive Latino gay and bisexual men in the Northeastern United States (Zea et al., 2005, 2006; Zea, 2008). Very appropriately, the researchers measured HIV disclosure separately to specific targets (mother, father, closest friend, and main male partner) and to target groupings (family members and close friends). According to Zea's research, Latino MSM who are HIV positive are less likely to disclose their HIV status to their families than their white MSM counterparts possibly because many Latino MSM want to protect their families from the suffering that such disclosure may engender. In addition, fear of stigmatizing attitudes that are highly prevalent in many Latino communities engender expectations of social and sexual rejection that discourage disclosure. Zea's research also found lower rates of HIV disclosure among more recent immigrants because many fear that they may not stay legally in this country as HIV-positive persons or because their perceived (or real) lack of access to care.

Although rates of HIV disclosure to main male partner and closest friend were relatively high (78% and 85%, respectively), disclosure rates to mother (37%) and to father (23%) were very low, controlling for having parents alive after diagnosis. Because HIV status is associated with homosexuality in Latino as well as other communities, the investigators commented that the low level of family disclosure is also likely related to homophobia experienced in the context of the immediate family. Not surprisingly, the researchers found that HIV disclosure was strongly related to greater quality of social support, higher self-esteem, and lower levels of depression. Because nondisclosure is strongly related to a sense of isolation (47% of the sample reported that after disclosing they felt "less lonely than before"), nondisclosure to family members can have a very negative consequence for Latino men who strongly value family ties and family support. Further multivariate analyses confirmed that the quality of social support mediates the effect of HIV disclosure on both depression and self-esteem. The researchers also showed that Latino MSM living with HIV who do not disclose their serostatus to someone during a sexual encounter are more depressed. Depression itself can increase HIV risk as Latino MSM may unwittingly attempt to gain some relief or distraction from their painful mental state by engaging in unprotected sex.

CONTEXTS OF HIV RISK AS AN OUTCOME OF SOCIAL OPPRESSION

In Latino gay men, high-risk sexual practices occur in the presence of substantial knowledge about HIV/AIDS and in the presence of relatively strong personal intentions and skills to practice safer sex. HIV risk behavior tends to occur within particular contexts and situations—such as sexual activity aimed to alleviate exhaustion and depression, sexual activity within relationships of unequal power, or sexual activity under the influence of drugs and/or alcohol—in which it is subjectively difficult to act according to personal intentions for health and sexual safety. Men who are knowledgeable, capable of, and skillful at safer sex practices confess a certain helplessness and inability to be safe in those situations researchers such as Organista et al. in Chapter 1 have labeled "risky." Because the same individual can act safely in some situations and unsafe in another, Díaz and his collaborators have conceptualized "risk" as a property of contexts and situations, rather than as an intraindividual characteristic.

Studies show that the strongest predictor of unprotected anal intercourse among Latino gay men is participation in high-risk situations, particularly situations that involve the use of alcohol and drugs. More importantly, participation in those difficult and risky situations are strongly predicted by individual and group histories of social discrimination and financial hardship, and to the negative impact of such discrimination and hardships on men's social connectedness and sense of self-worth (Diaz et al., 2004). Recent multivariate analysis (structural equation modeling) of data from the San Francisco-Chicago RDS study suggests that experiences of both homosexual and racial stigma are strong predictors of the use of alcohol and drugs in sexual situations, which in turn is a strong predictor of unprotected anal intercourse (Ramirez-Valles et al., 2010). Interestingly, although the relation between racial stigma and sex under the influence of alcohol and drugs was direct, the relation between experiences of homosexual stigma and those situations of risk were mediated by *internalized* homophobia. Findings to date emphasize the need to understand sexual and racial oppression, as well as its social, sexual, and psychological impact in the lives of Latino gay men, in order to address the increased risk for HIV in this population. It is clear that prevention services must address not only Latino cultural factors but also the social and structural factors of oppression and discrimination that impact the social and sexual lives of Latino gay men.

THE IMPACT OF IMMIGRATION AND ENCULTURATION

A substantive number of Latino gay men in the United States are immigrants whose life trajectories, social contexts, and sexual lives have been deeply impacted and transformed by the migration experience. For many of these men, their reasons for migration into the United States are strongly related to their homosexuality—a desire for a fuller expression of homoerotic desire and relationships—as well as to economic factors. For some Latino gay men, migration to the United States is pressured by difficult circumstances related to family and social rejection of homosexuality; some come to the United States seeking asylum on account of severe histories of threats and abuse, police harassment, and discrimination on the basis of both their homosexuality and HIV-positive status. For many of these men, life as open gay men in their own towns and cities of origin is simply out of the question; the motivation to migrate is thus a combination of personal safety and protection of family and loved ones who would be hurt and embarrassed by openly lived homosexuality.

The most recent and comprehensive study on the impact of immigration on sexuality and health among Latino gay and bisexual men was conducted in the San Diego/Tijuana area by Hector Carrillo and colleagues (Carrillo, Fontdevila, Brown, & Gomez, 2008). The ethnographic study, named *"Trayectos"* ("Pathways"), wisely included not only Mexican immigrant gay men but also two important groups that would bring a larger perspective to the study of immigration effects: gay men of Mexican descent born in the United States and non-Latino gay men who had been recently involved—romantically and/or sexually—with Mexican immigrant gay men. The rest of this section reports *Trayecto's* major findings to date. (See Chapter 3 by Carrillo whose theorizing about HIV risk and migration is partly informed by *Trayecto's* project.)

The researchers found that Trayecto immigrant participants are in general willing to protect themselves and their sexual partners from transmission of HIV—about half of the immigrant men in Trayectos were using condoms consistently for anal sex. However, safer sex behavior was challenging for many others, particularly when they encountered sexual contexts and situations that were unfamiliar to them given the new cultural context. Specifically, immigrant men are more prone to engage in HIV risk behavior when they enter into sexual contexts—casual or romantic—in which they do not know "the rules of the game," that is, when they apply assumptions about sexual behavior that may have been true in Mexico but do not apply in the new U.S. context. Consider, for example, an encounter between an HIV-negative immigrant man and an HIV positive U.S.-born man, where the U.S.-born man will take the active penetrating position. Based on prior experience in Mexico, the immigrant man may assume that sexual partners always act with the intention of protecting others (a rule of mutual, *collective responsibility*), such that the active partner's neglect or refusal to use condoms might be interpreted as a sign that the partner is not infected and thus not likely to transmit HIV. On the other hand, in that same situation, the penetrating sexual partner might be assuming that each person is responsible for themselves (a rule of *personal responsibility*) and thus assume that the immigrant man's lack of insistence on using condoms is an indication that he is already HIV infected and is not concerned about issues of reinfection. This case demonstrates a situation in which immigrants' different set of rules, assumptions, and expectations clash with those of the new sexual contexts they encounter, thus increasing the risk of HIV transmission.

Beyond differences in rules, expectations, and assumptions, immigrant gay men also encounter novel and highly charged sexual contexts, such as gay bathhouses in the United States, where limited English language skills and lack of clarity about venue etiquette may inhibit requests for condom use. The situation is further complicated by the high sexual arousal and intensity of pleasure some men may experience in the presence of those who look and feel different or foreign, and whom they find irresistibly attractive and powerful. Immigrant men may also be at increased risk for HIV in romantic involvements in which cultural expectations of trust, intimacy, fidelity, and love interfere with condom use, as when condom use is construed as a sign of mistrust or infidelity. The study authors note that participation in these contexts of increased HIV risk vary according to the sexual cultures and contexts immigrant men participate in *before* migration as well as the sexual cultures and contexts they find ("the landing pad") *after* their arrival. In addition, motives for migration can influence the level of risk as when strong needs for self-expression after years of imposed restraint lead these men to find, shortly after migration, a set of sexual contexts that is difficult to negotiate competently to reduce risk, such as Internet-mediated sexual encounters where drugs are involved.

The investigators of the Trayecto's study encourage public health officials and HIV prevention workers to take into account the wide diversity that exists in the migration experience for Latino gay men and avoid careless and trite generalizations. They argue for the need to take into account immigrants' participation in sexual cultures before migration as well as the reasons for migration, given that these interact with new and challenging contexts in ways that may lead to the increased risk for HIV. Specifically, the sexual histories prior to migration, and the specific reasons that motivate migration, shape the sexual assumptions and expectations as well as the different sexual contexts in which immigrant men will more likely participate. Above all, similar to other researchers who have studied HIV risk among Latino gay men in the United States, Trayecto's researchers argue for the need to understand social contexts, rather than simply individual psychological and cognitive factors, as the main source of HIV risk, encouraging prevention workers and policy makers to take into account both cultural assets and vulnerabilities.

MENTAL HEALTH

In the study of 912 Latino gay men in three U.S. cities, the investigators measured the frequency of five symptoms of psychological distress, including symptoms related to anxiety and depression, experienced during the 6 months prior to the survey (Diaz et al., 2001; Diaz, Bein, & Ayala, 2006). The most frequently reported symptoms were depressed mood and sleep difficulties. During the past 6 months, an estimated 80% of Latino gay men experienced feelings of sadness and depression at least once or twice during the time period, with 22% experiencing a depressed mood at a relatively high ("many times") frequency. Close to two-thirds of the sample (61%) suffered sleep problems at least once or twice during the previous 6 months, with 20% experiencing sleep problems many times. Feelings of anxiety (i.e., experiences of fear and/or panic with no apparent reason) and a general feeling of being sick or not well were experienced by about half of the sample, at least once or twice during a 6-month period. The most serious symptom of psychological distress—thoughts of taking one's own life—was experienced by 17% at least once or twice during a 6-month period, with 6% having suicidal ideation a few times or more. On all measures of psychological distress, men who are HIV positive reported more frequent symptoms; for example, 25% of HIV-positive men reported they had contemplated suicide in the previous 6 months.

More importantly, the above study showed that psychological symptoms among Latino gay men were strongly predicted by experiences of homophobia, racism, and financial distress. The authors reported strong associations between specific experiences of homophobia, racism, and financial hardship, and suicidal ideation within the past 6 months. Of the 24 Chi-square analyses conducted to test the bivariate association between specific items of social discrimination and suicidal thoughts, 18 (or 75%) were statistically significant; of the remaining six tests, three had marginally significant probabilities between 0.06 and 0.10. The multivariate analysis showed that homophobia, racism, and poverty had independent and cumulative effects on symptoms of psychological distress, and that those effects were partially mediated by their negative impact on self-esteem and social support (Diaz et al., 2001).

In a recent study of lesbian, gay, and bisexual young adults in San Francisco (with half of the sample being Latino), Ryan and colleagues found that family rejection of their child's homosexuality during adolescence was a strong predictor of mental health outcomes in young adulthood. Those who had experienced higher rates of family rejection during adolescence on account of their homosexuality or gender nonconformity were 5.9 times more likely to show signs of depression and 5.6 more likely to have suicidal thoughts in young adulthood. Those who were highly rejected were and 8.4 times more likely to have attempted suicide during their lifetime. Very important for the purpose of this review is the fact that rates of family rejection were highest for Latino gay males (Ryan et al., 2009).

SUBSTANCE USE

Studies that involved venue-based probability samples of Latino gay men in large U.S. urban centers estimate the prevalence of illicit substance use at approximately 50%, with over one-third of men reporting regular marijuana use and 15–20% reporting recent use of stimulants, including cocaine, methamphetamine, ecstasy, and amyl nitrate inhalants/poppers. The prevalence data from San Francisco show that rates of substance use in the past 6 months, particularly stimulants and other so-called "party" or "club" drugs, vary significantly according to the type of venues in which men were recruited. Those recruited in mainstream (mostly white) gay venues show higher rates of drug use than those recruited in Latino-identified gay venues (50% vs. 37%), suggesting increased use of drugs as a function of increased acculturation and participation in mainstream gay culture (Diaz, Heckert, & Sanchez, 2004).

By far, the highest rates of drug use, particularly stimulants, within Latino MSM in San Francisco were found among men who were recruited from Internet sex chat rooms and sex phone lines; of these, 62% reported recent methamphetamine use, 53% recent use of poppers, and 39% recent use of ecstasy. The high prevalence of drug use among Internet users was also reported by Fernández et al. (2005) in a study of club drug use and risky sex among Latino MSM recruited on Internet chat rooms in Miami. The researchers reported that close to half (48.5%) of those recruited in the Internet study used "club drugs," defined as cocaine (15.8%), crystal meth (11.7%), poppers (31.6%), ecstasy (14%), gamma-hydroxybutyrate (GHB, 3.5%), ketamine (3.5%), and Viagra (19.3%). The lower rates of stimulant use found among Miami users in comparison to San Francisco users must be interpreted with caution, given the different recruitment procedures and aims of the two studies, the different Internet sites sampled, and possible cultural differences between East and West coast drug users. The most recent and reliable comparison of two RDS samples of Latino gay men in Chicago and San Francisco show similar rates in the general use of stimulants, but differences in the types of stimulants used. For example Latino gay men in San Francisco were more likely to use methamphetamine (19% versus 9%), but the pattern was reversed in Chicago, where they were more likely to use cocaine (19% versus 9%).

In a recent study of 300 Latino stimulant-using gay men, randomly selected from social and sexual venues in San Francisco, 51% reported methamphetamine, 44% reported cocaine, and 5% reported crack as their most frequently used stimulant. The investigators assessed the reasons for use for the participant's specific most frequently used stimulant. Reasons for stimulant use clustered by five main factors including, in order of reported frequency, energy, sexual enhancement, social connection, coping with stressors, and focused work productivity (Diaz, Heckert, & Sanchez, 2005). Methamphetamine users gave reasons more frequently related to sexual enhancement (to have better sex, more sex, and more anal sex) whereas cocaine users gave reasons more often related to social connections (to be more sociable and to fit in with other gay men). The findings suggest that Latino gay men use stimulants for reasons that are important in their social, emotional, work, and sexual lives. However, there is no empirical evidence to suggest that reasons or motivations for stimulant use among Latino gay men are qualitatively or quantitatively different from reasons reported by men from other ethnic groups. In fact, similar to studies of non-Latino whites, Latino gay men were found to rely on methamphetamine for reasons related to sexual enhancement, possibly to meet cultural expectations and norms of sexual prowess and sexual success in the gay community.

It is important to note that the most important and most frequently cited reason reported for stimulant use is "energy." Qualitative data from the same study suggest that many Latino gay men rely on stimulants to meet the demand of heavy work schedules and to deal with the exhaustion of highly stressed out lives. Stimulant use, particularly the use of methamphetamine and cocaine, plays an important and "functional" role for men who, exhausted by work demands, use the drug in order to participate in the joys of social and sexual life in the context of the gay community (Diaz, 2007). Unfortunately, particularly in the case of highly addictive substances such as methamphetamine, the "functional" use often becomes "dysfunctional," resulting in a host of negative consequence including loss of employment, estrangement from partners and friends, physical depletion, and psychological symptoms such as severe depression and paranoia. Although increased frequency of use is related to increased acculturation and participation in the mainstream gay community, it is not clear at this time how experiences of social discrimination (both inside and outside the gay community) may play a role in the frequency and patterns of substance use or abuse among Latino gay men.

In all studies that have measured both drug use and HIV risk among Latino gay men, the two variables have been strongly correlated. In multivariate analyses of the Miami study, the use of club drugs was associated with higher number of partners, unprotected receptive anal intercourse, and social isolation. In the San Francisco study, methamphetamine users had the highest rates (72%) of unprotected anal intercourse ever reported for any subsample of Latino MSM.

Rates of unprotected intercourse with multiple and casual partners were much higher among methamphetamine than cocaine users. Within-user comparisons showed that users were more likely to be at situations of sexual risk when they are under the influence of a stimulant than a nonstimulant (e.g., marijuana). Methamphetamine use had stronger relations than cocaine use to negative life consequences such as interpersonal conflicts with families, friends, and at work, as well as physical, emotional, and sexual problems (Diaz, 2007).

To date, no study has exclusively focused on Latino gay men's use of alcohol, even though both qualitative and quantitative studies of HIV risk show a strong correlation between alcohol use and unprotected anal intercourse. Nonpublished data from the three-city study of 912 Latino gay men, reported only in the context of a presentation, suggest a linear association between increased frequency and amount of alcohol use and the risk of HIV (Diaz, Ayala, & Bein, 1999). Published data from the same study also show a strong correlation between sexual episodes under the influence of alcohol and reported unprotected anal intercourse with nonmonogamous partners (Diaz et al., 2004). Interestingly, rates of heavy alcohol use and sex under the influence of alcohol tend to be much lower in San Francisco than in Chicago. In the two-city RDS study, only 15% of the men in San Francisco reported heavy alcohol use in comparison to 37% of men in Chicago (Ramirez-Valles et al., 2008). Similarly, only 27% of the men reported having sex under the influence of alcohol in San Francisco, while 41% reported so in Chicago. Sex under the influence of drugs was similar in Chicago than in San Francisco (20% vs. 19%). Thus, it is not clear what variables may explain the relatively lower alcohol use found among Latino gay men in San Francisco. It is important to recognize, however, that even though at lower levels, the use of alcohol during sex is strongly correlated with unprotected sex in San Francisco as well as in other places were the two variables have been assessed.

TWO SOURCES OF VULNERABILITY: CHILDHOOD SEXUAL ABUSE AND INTIMATE PARTNER VIOLENCE

The prevalence of two important markers of mental health problems—childhood sexual abuse (CSA) and intimate partner violence (IPV)—are disproportionately high among Latino gay men in comparison to men from other ethnicities. Furthermore, the two variables—CSA and IPV—have been shown to be strong predictors of HIV risk among Latino gay men, including sex under the influence of drugs and alcohol. Latino gay/bisexual men with a history of CSA are significantly more likely to engage in unprotected anal intercourse with a nonprimary partner or a partner with a different HIV status than those who had not been sexually abused as children; the higher the level of coercion during CSA, the greater the risk of HIV infection. Similarly, Latino gay men with a history of IPV are more likely to participate in sexual situations, such as peer pressure to discard condoms and situations of unequal power, that are shown to increase the likelihood of unprotected anal intercourse.

Data for the Urban Men's Health Study, a random-digit telephone probability survey of 2881 adult men who have sex with men (MSM) residing in four U.S. cities show that Latino MSM are twice as likely (22% vs.11%) to report sexual abuse before age 13 than non-Latino MSM (Arreola et al., 2005). Other qualitative work by Arreola and colleagues suggests that those who experienced CSA were targeted for that abuse mostly because of their nonconforming gender attitudes and behavior. Thus, the high prevalence of CSA is strongly correlated with experiences of homophobia and masculinity ideologies that see homosexuality as a gender deviation and homosexuals as not truly men.

Similarly, the three city study of 912 Latino gay men showed that rates for different types of IPV are consistently higher than the reported IPV rates (across all ethnic groups) for the Urban Men's Health Study. Specifically, Greenwood et al. (2002) reported rates of intimate partner "battering" as 34% for psychological/symbolic, 22% for physical, and 5% for sexual battering among all 2881 MSM studied in the Urban Men's Health Study. In the three-city sample of 912 Latino gay men, Feldman et al. (2008) reported rates of intimate partner victimization of 45% for psychological, 33% for physical, and 9.5% for sexual victimization. Although neither the IPV survey items nor the studies' sampling strategies are exactly comparable, the data from these two probability studies suggest that Latino MSM have much higher rates of different types of IPV, a finding that parallels findings about CSA.

Because histories of both CSA and IPV are strongly correlated with anxiety, depression, substance-related problems, and HIV risk, these data suggest the need to take into account these two variables when planning HIV prevention programs.

The importance of CSA in HIV prevention is underscored by a recent analysis of data from 4295 MSM who participated in the EXPLORE intervention. The intervention involved individual intensive counseling sessions in which participants were asked to consider their own sexual choices and reflect on situations that trigger them to be more or less safe. The intervention study showed not only that CSA is strongly related to HIV risk behavior and seroconversion but that for those MSM with histories of CSA the EXPLORE program had no effects in lowering their risk for HIV infection (Mimiaga et al., 2009).

SOURCES OF RESILIENCY AND STRENGTH

When Latino gay men are asked to describe what in their lives has helped them deal and cope with difficulties, their responses can be categorized into six different factors: family acceptance, social connectedness, sexual satisfaction, community involvement, social activism, and the presence of gay role models while growing up. All these factors serve to alleviate feelings of social isolation and increase self-esteem, which in turn reduce their risk for HIV. In other words, men who can speak openly to their families, who have satisfactory relationships with friends and lovers, who are involved with other men like themselves to create a more just society, and who have witnessed the possibility of a satisfying and productive life as a gay man are less likely to have problems related to mental health, substance abuse, or the risk for HIV. It is clear that all six factors point to social contexts and situations in which men are accepted and feel socially connected. Studies of family acceptance (Ryan et al., 2009) and community involvement (Ramirez-Valles, 2010) show that these two variables serve as strong protective factors against mental health problems, substance abuse, and the risk for HIV. In the study by Ramirez-Valles, the expected negative relation between social discrimination (homophobic and racial) and negative health outcomes did not show for men who had been involved in social activism for gay and HIV-related causes.

SUMMARY AND IMPLICATIONS FOR HIV PREVENTION WITH LATINO GAY MEN

In conclusion, we offer a set of statements that we believe captures the most important findings of the literature on Latino gay men to date:

- HIV risk is the property of contexts shaped by experiences of discrimination and oppression—homophobia, racism, poverty, HIV stigma, and forced migration.
- The subjective experience of oppression is a deep sense of loneliness/isolation, a lowered sense of self-esteem/self-worth, and a reduced sense of personal agency.
- Sexual identities, life choices, and sexual behavior are shaped by two important cultural factors: masculinity ideologies and loyalty to families of origin.
- Two sources of psychosocial vulnerability—childhood sexual abuse and intimate partner violence—are highly correlated with HIV risk.
- Substances, in particular alcohol and stimulants, are used functionally to meet economic, social, and sexual demands. However, functional use easily turns into dysfunctional abuse, increasing the risk for HIV transmission.
- Two sources of resiliency and strength—family/social support and community involvement/social activism—can be promoted to reduce the vulnerability to HIV among Latino gay men.

The findings from this literature review suggest that HIV prevention programs for Latino gay men must address, first and foremost, the fact that their higher risk for HIV is strongly related to their own histories of inequality and discrimination. Promoting critical awareness of these discriminatory forces, and channeling the consequent outrage into constructive community involvement and social activism, can become the major motivating force to help men to take care of their own health and one another's. The awareness of a shared history of oppression can serve as an important bond of solidarity and help men reframe safer sex practices as acts of social responsibility and mutual care. Of crucial importance is the need to address the fact that histories of childhood sexual abuse and intimate partner violence, highly prevalent in this population, are important mediators of the effects of discrimination on HIV risk. Programs can help men explore situations of sexual risk that undermine their ability to protect themselves, including sex under the influence of alcohol and drugs, and offer alternative strategies for men to maximize sexual pleasure and intimacy while minimizing the risk of HIV transmission.

Experiences of homophobia, poverty, racism, and forced migration are internalized and subjectively experienced as a deep sense of social alienation and diminished self-worth. The sense of isolation is deepened for those who feel rejected by their families and those who are forced to sexual silence in order to maintain meaningful social connections and participate in family life. Needless to say, deep feelings of loneliness and low self-esteem undermine Latino gay men's desire and effort to protect themselves against the transmission of HIV. It is thus paramount that beyond a critical awareness of the effects of discrimination on men's social and sexual lives, programs must foster a sense of family solidarity and communality. As men become aware that others genuinely care for their lives, and that they can access social support when needed, they will be more likely to undertake the enormous effort needed to sustain safer sex practices over time during this too long and too tragic epidemic.

REFERENCES

Arreola, S. G., Neilands, T. B., Pollack, L. M., Paul, J. P., & Catania, J. A. (2005). Higher prevalence of childhood sexual abuse among Latino men who have sex with men than non-Latino men who have sex with men: Data from the Urban Men's Health Study. *Child Abuse and Neglect, 29*(3), 285–290.

Carrier, J. (1995). *De Los Otros: Intimacy and homosexuality among Mexican men.* New York: Columbia University Press.

Carrillo, H. (2002). *The night is young: Sexuality in Mexico in the times of AIDS.* Chicago: University of Chicago Press.

Carrillo, H., Fontdevvila, J., Brown, J., & Gomez, W. (2008). *Risk across borders; Sexual contexts and HIV prevention challenges among Mexican gay and bisexual immigrant men.* Trayectos Study, San Francisco State University and the Center for Research on Gender and Sexuality.

Catania, J. A., Binson, D., Dolcini, M., et al. (2001). The continuing HIV epidemic among men who have sex with men. *American Journal of Public Health, 91,* 907–914.

Centers for Disease Control and Prevention. (2008). HIV prevalence and awareness of HIV infection among MSM—21 cities, United States, 2008. *Morbidity and Mortality Weekly Report, 59*(37), 1201–1207.

Centers for Disease Control and Prevention. (2010). HIV prevalence estimates—United States, 2006. *Morbidity and Mortality Weekly Report, 57*(39), 1073–1076.

Diaz, R. M. (1998) *Latino gay men and HIV: Culture, sexuality and risk behavior.* New York: Routledge.

Díaz, R. M. (2006). In our own backyard: HIV stigmatization in the Latino gay community. In N. Teunis (Ed.), *Sexual inequalities* (pp. 50–65). Berkeley: University of California Press.

Díaz, R. M. (2007). Methamphetamine use and its relation to HIV risk: Data from Latino gay men. In I. Meyer & M. Northridge, (Eds.), *The health of sexual minorities: Public health perspectives on lesbian, gay, bisexual and transgender populations* (pp. 584–603). New York: Springer.

Diaz, R. M., & Ayala, G. (2001). *Social discrimination and health: The case of Latino gay men and HIV risk.* New York: The Policy Institute of the National Gay and Lesbian Task Force.

Diaz, R. M., Ayala, G., & Bein, E. (1999). *Substance use and sexual risk: Findings from the national latino gay men's study.* Invited presentation at the HIV Center for Clinical and Behavioral Studies. New York: Columbia University.

Díaz, R. M., Ayala, G., & Bein, E. (2004). Sexual risk as an outcome of social oppression: Data from a probability sample of Latino gay men in three US cities. *Cultural Diversity and Ethnic Minority Psychology, 10*(3), 255–267.

Díaz, R. M., Ayala, G., Bein, E., Henne, J., & Marin, B. V. (2001). The impact of homophobia, poverty and racism on the mental health of gay and bisexual Latino men: Findings from 3 U.S. cities. *American Journal of Public Health, 91*(6), 927–932.

Díaz, R. M., Bein, E., & Ayala, G. (2006). Homophobia, poverty and racism: Triple oppression and mental health outcomes in Latino gay men. In A. Omoto & H. Kurtzman (Eds.), *Research on sexual orientation, mental health: Examining identity and development in lesbian, gay, and bisexual people.* (pp. 207–224). Washington, DC: APA Books.

Díaz, R. M., Heckert, A, L., & Sánchez, J. (2004). *Fabulous effects, disastrous consequences: Stimulant use among Latino gay men in San Francisco.* Presentation at the National Institute on Drug Abuse, Washington, DC.

Diaz, R. M., Heckert, A. H., & Sanchez, J. (2005). Reasons for stimulant use among Latino gay men in San Francisco: A comparison between methamphetamine and cocaine users. *Journal of Urban Health, 82*(1), 71–78.

Díaz, R. M., Peterson, R. M., & Choi, K. H. (2007). Social discrimination and health outcomes in African-American, Latino and Asian/Pacific Islander gay men. In R. Wolitski, R. Stall, & R. Valdisseri (Eds.), *Unequal opportunity: Health disparities among gay and bisexual men in the United States* (pp. 327–354). New York: Oxford University Press.

Feldman, M., Díaz, R.M., Ream, G., & El-Bassel, N. (2008). Intimate partner violence and HIV sexual risk among Latino gay men. *Journal of LGBT Health Research; 3*(2), 9–19.

Fernández, M. I., Perrino, T., Collazo, J. B., et al. (2005). Surfing new territory: Club-drug use and risky sex among Hispanic men who have sex with men recruited on the Internet. *Journal of Urban Health, 82*(1), i79–i88.

Greenwood, G. L., Relf, M. V., Huang, B, et al. (2002). Battering victimization among a probability sample of men who have sex with men. *American Journal of Public Health, 92,* 1964–1969.

Mimiaga, M. J., Noonan, E., Donnell, D., Safren, S. A., Koenen, K. C., Gortmaker, S., O'Cleirigh, C., Chesney, M. A., Coates, T. J., Koblin, B. A., & Mayer, K. H. (2009). Childhood sexual abuse is highly associated with HIV risk-taking behavior and infection among MSM in the EXPLORE study. *Journal of Acquired Immune Deficiency Syndrome, 51,* 340–348.

Muñoz-Laboy, M. (2008). Familism and sexual regulation among bisexual Latino men. *Archives of Sexual Behavior.* 37(5), 773–782.

Muñoz-Laboy, M., & Dodge, B. (2005). Bi-sexual practices: Patterns, meanings, and implications for HIV/STI prevention among bisexually active Latino men and their partners. *Journal of Bisexuality;* 5(1), 81–100.

Muñoz-Laboy; M., Yon Leau, C., Sriram, V., Weinstein, H., Vasquez del Aquila, E., & Parker, R. (2009). Bisexual desire and familism: Latino/a bisexual young men and women in New York City. *Culture, Health & Sexuality,* 11(3), 331–344.

Ramirez-Valles, J., Garcia, D., Campbell, R, T., Diaz, R. M., & Heckathorn, D. D. (2008). HIV infection, sexual risk, and substance use among Latino gay and bisexual men and transgender persons. *American Journal of Public Health,* 98, 1028–1035.

Ramirez-Valles, J., Kuhns,M., Campbell, R. T., & Diaz, R. M. (2010). Social integration and health: community involvement, stigmatized identities, and sexual risk in Latino sexual minorities. *Journal of Health and Social Behavior,* 51(1), 30–47.

Ryan, C. C., Huebner, D., Díaz, R. M., and Sanchez, J. (2009). Family rejection as a predictor of negative health outcomes in white and Latino lesbian, gay, and bisexual young adults. *Pediatrics,* 123(1), 346–352.

Valleroy, L., MacKellar, D., Karon, J., et al. (2000). HIV prevalence and associated risks in young men who have sex with men. *JAMA, 284,* 198–204.

Vega, W. (1995). The study of Latino families: A point of departure. In E. Zambrana (Ed.), *Understanding Latino families: Scholarship, policy, and practice* (pp. 3–17). Thousand Oaks, CA: Sage Publications.

Zea, M. C. (2008). Disclosure of HIV status and mental health among Latino men who have sex with men. In S. Loue (Ed.), *Health issues confronting minority men who have sex with men* (pp. 217–228). New York: Springer.

Zea, M. C., Reisen, C. A., Poppen, P. J., Bianchi, F. T., & Echeverry, J. J (2005). Disclosure of HIV status and psychological well-being among Latino gay and bisexual men. *AIDS and Behavior,* 9, 15–26.

Zea, M. C., Reisen, C. A., Poppen, P. J., Echeverry, J. J., & Bianchi, F. T (2004). Disclosure of HIV-positive status to Latino gay men's social networks. *American Journal of Community Psychology,* 33, 107–116.

8 Homophobia, Racism, Financial Hardship, and AIDS

Unpacking the Effects of Social Discrimination on the Sexual Risk for HIV among Latino Gay Men

George Ayala

INTRODUCTION

Gay men and other men who have sex with men (MSM) continue to account for the majority of new HIV cases in the United States (CDC, 2008a, 2008b). Racial/ethnic disparities in HIV prevalence and incidence persist within this group with black and Latino MSM particularly hard hit (CDC, 2005; Diaz & Ayala, 2001; Valleroy et al., 2000). For example, the estimated AIDS incidence rate among Latino/Hispanic men was 31.0 per 100,000 compared with 10.6 per 100,000 among white men, a 3-fold difference (CDC, 2008b). Among Latino/Hispanic men, male-to-male sexual contact is the most commonly reported mode of HIV transmission; about one-half of estimated AIDS cases among Latino men reported in 2007 was due to male-to-male sexual contact (CDC, 2009). The disproportionate impact HIV is having on Latino gay men and other MSM suggests an underlying structural basis for the apparent social shape of the AIDS epidemic. See Chapter 7 by Diaz, Sánchez, and Schroeder for an updated review of the literature on this topic.

Researchers have increasingly looked to the compounding effects of social discrimination to explain persistent racial/ethnic disparities across a range of health issues (Krieger, 1993, 2003). For example, racial prejudice can affect health outcomes in at least two ways (Cain & Kingston, 2003). First, racial discrimination and ethnic discrimination usually result in social practices and economic policy that restrict employment, housing education, and health care opportunities, which in turn can produce negative health outcomes. Second, racism can produce negative emotional and stress responses in those experiencing discrimination (Williams, Neighbors, & Jackson, 2003).

In the HIV field, there have been various studies that have examined the potential effects of homophobia, racism, and financial hardship on the sexual health of Latino gay men and other MSM. These studies show that experiences of social discrimination are associated with: poor mental health (Diaz et al., 2001; Williams, Neighbors, & Jackson, 2003), participation in difficult sexual situations that may lead to heightened behavioral risk for HIV (Diaz, Ayala, & Bein, 2004), and increased substance use and unprotected receptive anal intercourse (Bruce, Ramirez-Valles, & Campbell, 2008; Nakamura & Zea, 2010). Our own past qualitative research suggests that Latino gay men experience racial stereotyping, segregation, and social exclusion, even from mainstream gay communities (Ayala & Diaz, 2001). Racial segregation and stereotyping have the potential to influence sexual partner selection, shape sexual expectations, and determine the characteristics of sexual networks in ways that might heighten the risk for HIV transmission (Wilson et al., 2009; Laumann & Youm, 1999). For example, race-based sexual stereotyping may result in segregation of sexual networks that in turn creates a heightened risk for HIV transmission because of elevated background HIV seroprevalence among racial/ethnic minority MSM. More specifically, if overall HIV prevalence is higher among Latino MSM and sexual partnering choices that Latino MSM make are influenced by segregation—limiting their choices of sexual partners to other Latino MSM—their risk for HIV exposure is potentially greater than that of men whose sexual partnering choices are not constrained by racial segregation.

Although experiences of discrimination might help explain why Latino gay men and other MSM continue to be disproportionately affected by the AIDS epidemic, there is still a need to better understand (1) the specific sources and types of social discrimination experienced by Latino MSM, (2) the additive effects of experiencing two or more forms of discrimination, and (3) the specific mechanisms through which these experiences influence disparities in HIV/AIDS. In an effort to begin filling these knowledge gaps, this chapter reviews the findings of recent research focused on the impact of social discrimination on HIV risk among Latino gay men and other MSM and discusses their implications for intervention development and research. As of the writing of this chapter, two of these studies were in review for publication. Separately, they each offer important insights about how social discrimination operates to heighten the risk for HIV transmission among Latino gay men. Together, these studies begin to make the case for a social and structural approach to addressing HIV in this group.

SOURCES AND TYPES OF RACISM AND HOMOPHOBIA EXPERIENCED BY LATINO MSM
Summary of Study Procedures

Focusing on the sources and types of social discrimination Latino gay men are experiencing is important for at least two reasons: (1) it helps to "unpack" or "distill" the constellation of interrelated factors at the structural, social, and interpersonal levels that constitute discrimination; and (2) it identifies possible loci for prevention intervention.

Ayala, Paul, and Choi (2010) conducted a qualitative study that describes (1) how African American, Asian, or Pacific Islander (API) and Latino MSM experience racism and homophobia; (2) the sources and types of these experiences as described by study participants; and (3) the ways these experiences vary across race/ethnicity. An underlying impetus for their paper was to deepen our understanding of the persistent HIV-related disease burden shouldered by MSM of color.

In July and August 2005, the research team convened six focus groups with respondents who met the following inclusion criteria: men who (1) were between 18 and 50 years old, (2) reported having sex with other men within the past

6 months, (3) reported having had a new male sexual partner in the past 12 months, (4) were African American, API, or Latino, and (5) resided in Los Angeles County. A stratified purposive sampling method was utilized to ensure age and racial/ethnic balance among focus group respondents (Kuzel, 1999). In other words, focus groups were stratified by age (18–29 years, 30–50 years) and race/ethnicity (one ethnic group per age group). The focus group sample ranged in age from 21 to 49 years, and consisted of 17 African Americans, 16 APIs, and 17 Latinos. The mean age was 30.7 years.

In addition, between December 2005 and August 2006, Ayala, Paul, and Choi conducted 35 individual in-depth interviews with men who reported having had sex with other men in the prior 6 months, lived in Los Angeles County, and were either African American, API, or Latino. Inclusion criteria were based upon purposive sampling, with cells stratified once again by age and race/ethnicity. A total of 12 African American, 12 API, and 11 Latino men were interviewed. Sixteen men were 18 to 29 years old; 19 men were 30 years or older. The age range was 20 to 60 years, with a mean age of 33.2 years and a median age of 31 years.

The team began with the focus groups (two for each ethnic group) using a semistructured interview guide to elicit information on three broad topic areas: (1) experiences of social discrimination and coping with ethnic and sexual minority status; (2) descriptions of social networks and their perceived role in respondents' lives; and (3) experiences of meeting sexual partners. Next, the team conducted individual in-depth interviews with a separately and conveniently recruited sample of participants using a semistructured open-ended interview guide that followed and expanded upon the topics examined in the focus groups by eliciting the personal narratives of study participants related to these areas of concern. This mode of data collection allowed for in-depth discussion of experiences with meeting sexual and dating partners, general partner selection preferences, the influence of one's social network, experiences of and the impact of discrimination and racism, personal coping strategies, and sexual risk practices. For the purposes of this chapter, presented below are the results from the focus group and in-depth interviews conducted with Latino MSM research participants.

THREE LEVELS OF SOCIAL DISCRIMINATION
Racism and Homophobia in Mainstream Los Angeles

The study found that experiences of racism and homophobia were commonly reported among both focus group and in-depth interview study participants. Latino respondents all reported experiencing racism in Los Angeles from mainstream society (including at work and from police) and the mainstream gay community. Men interviewed reported feeling excluded or believing they had been denied opportunities afforded to others. Respondents also expressed concern about negative race-based stereotyping of ethnic minorities by mainstream society. For example, Latino MSM reported being ethnically and economically homogenized, assumed to be from a lower socioeconomic status (e.g., Mexican gardeners or janitors).

Latino men participating in this study also reported experiencing homophobia from mainstream society in their day-to-day lives in Los Angeles (e.g., at work, on the street). For example, respondents commonly described being called names, made fun of, judged and treated differently for being gay.

Homophobia at Home

While many respondents in this study reported strong ties to their respective communities of color and families, these were also environments in which study participants commonly reported experiencing homophobic reactions and a sense of being unwelcome due to their sexual orientation. Many Latino MSM described cultural pressures to be macho or manly, and that being identified as gay meant being perceived as feminine or less than a man. Some participants expressed concern about what others thought and about the level of discomfort others felt being around gay people. Most felt frustrated by the constraints these pressures imposed on being able to live their lives in an authentic manner. Homophobia seemed especially troubling to respondents when evident within their families of origin. Many study participants felt uncomfortable at family functions, due to ongoing pressure from the family to marry and to have children, and fear of disgracing or being rejected by their families. The following are excerpts from interviews conducted with Latino MSM:

I mean I know—I know people and over the years people that have been beaten by their fathers and their families and thrown out of their houses you know and have to go live on the streets. As a matter of fact, the first gay pride we ever went to—um, in 1989, was in Long Beach. And one of the guys with us, his family happened to be watching TV and saw him on the news. When he got home his shit was outside on the porch—"We don't want to know anything about you. We don't want to have anything to do with you." That could have been any one of us . . . [33-year-old Latino in-depth interview participant]

Yeah . . . first of all—my mom's religious—she's Catholic—and growing up she'd say, 'If you ever turned gay I'd cut off your dick.' Like she would always like—bring that up—like in high school. [24-year-old Latino focus group member]

. . . my mom [thought] . . . of all the kids she thought I'd be the first to give her a grandson. [25-year-old Latino focus group member]

Respondents also commonly described feeling unwelcome and unvalued in the mainstream gay community as experienced during visits to West Hollywood, Los Angeles' most identifiable mainstream gay enclave. Specifically, Latino respondents reported feeling invisible, being patronized, sexually objectified, and/or rejected for sex, having difficulty finding love relationships, and being self-conscious about their body types or physical appearance. And for some Latino participants, sexual objectification often meant being reduced to a piece of "Latin meat."

. . .when you're in. . .a city where. . .there's predominantly White people and you go in a store. . .you can tell their eyes light up like, 'Oh, you're Latino meat'. . . [25-year-old Latino in-depth interview participant]

In summary, Latino gay men in this study reported experiencing racism from mainstream gay communities in the form of race-based sexual objectification and rejection and homophobia from their racial/ethnic communities of origin and families from which they felt unwelcomed and pressured to conform to strict masculine gender roles. This was in addition to their day-to-day experiences of discrimination from mainstream society in Los Angeles. These findings raise the following questions in relation to the heightened risk for HIV among Latino gay men: (1) *Do source and type of discrimination matter;* and (2) *Is there an additive effect from experiencing multiple types of discrimination from multiple sources?*

143

Homophobia, Racism, Financial Hardship, and AIDS

THE ADDITIVE EFFECTS OF RACISM, HOMOPHOBIA, AND FINANCIAL HARDSHIP

Summary of Study Procedures

For Latino gay men who are poor or working class, marginalization and/or discrimination can be experienced on the basis of race/ethnicity, sexual orientation, and/or class status. The differential and additive effects of multiple forms of social discrimination are still poorly understood yet must have the potential to exact some kind of cumulative toll at times.

Using cross-sectional quantitative survey data collected in 2006 from 1081 Latino MSM, recruited with respondent-driven sampling (RDS) techniques, from Los Angeles and New York, Mizuno et al. (2011) examined the extent to which Latino gay men and other MSM reported exposure to social discrimination (i.e., experienced both homophobia and racism, homophobia only, racism only, or neither homophobia nor racism), and explored how such exposure is associated with HIV risk behaviors, after controlling for potential confounders. Eligible participants had to identify as male, be 18 years of age or older, report sex (oral sex, anal sex, or mutual masturbation) with a man in the past 12 months, and be a resident of the area in which they were recruited. Participation was open to men who were HIV positive, HIV negative, or of unknown serostatus.

Experiences of homophobia in the past 12 months were assessed using five items: In the past 12 months, how often have you (1) been hit or beaten up; (2) been treated rudely or unfairly; (3) been made fun of or called names; (4) had to act more manly than usual to be accepted; and (5) felt uncomfortable in a crowd of straight Latinos in your city because people thought you were homosexual or not manly enough?

Experiences of racism in the past 12 months were assessed using the following five items: In the past 12 months, how often have you (1) been hit or beaten up; (2) been treated rudely or unfairly; (3) felt uncomfortable in a crowd of white gay men; (4) had trouble finding a male lover or boy friend; and (5) been turned down for sex because of your race or ethnicity?

Following Mays and Cochran's (2001) approach, the research team created a homophobia index indicating whether a participant reported experiencing any of the five homophobic items in the past 12 months (yes/no). A comparable index was also created for racism. An index of discrimination measure was also created, indicating whether a participant reported any homophobic or racist experience in the past 12 months (yes/no).

The team examined demographic and socioeconomic factors (i.e., age, income, education) and sociocultural factors (i.e., place of birth). In addition, the team collected results of HIV tests conducted as part of the study. These data are summarized in Table 8.1.

It is important to note that the majority (57%) of this sample of Latino MSM reported being born outside of the United States. In addition, the sample was undereducated and underemployed with 73% reporting an annual income of less than $20,000 a year. Last, more than a third of the men who participated in the study (39%) were HIV positive. These background variables may be the function of the

Table 8.1 Demographic Characteristics of the Latino MSM Sample
(N = 1081), 2005–2006

Characteristics	Latino MSM n (%)
Age (years)	
18–29	432 (40)
30–39	339 (31)
40 and older	307 (29)
Highest education completed	
Less than high school graduate	243 (22)
High school graduate or GED	461 (43)
Technical school graduate or A.A. degree	204 (19)
Four-year college degree or higher	170 (16)
Employment	
Full time	328 (30)
Part time	298 (28)
Unemployed	268 (25)
Unable to work (disabled)	172 (16)
Retired	13 (1)
Annual income before taxes	
Less than $5,000	317 (30)
$5,000–$9,999	232 (22)
$10,000–$19,999	218 (21)
$20,000–$29,999	128 (12)
$30,00 and above	152 (15)
Born in United States	
Yes	460 (43)
No	620 (57)
HIV Status (based on testing done in study)	
HIV positive	416 (39)
HIV negative	661 (61)
Length of time known HIV positive (among HIV-positive/aware men)	
Up to 5 years	103 (28)
6–10 years	109 (29)
Over 10 years	158 (43)

recruiting methods utilized for the study—RDS, which can at times tap networks that are poorer and more hidden than other sampling strategies. The demographic characteristics of the sample are important in relation to interpreting the study findings discussed below. For example, immigration status may exacerbate financial hardship and amplify the subjective experiences of racism and homophobia in ways that are unique to Latino gay men.

To determine the sexual risk for HIV, the study assessed whether participants had engaged in unprotected insertive or receptive anal intercourse with main or casual male partners in the past 3 months. Other risk behaviors used in this analysis were two substance use variables, binge drinking in the past 3 months, and drug use in the past 3 months.

Summary of Main Findings

Mizuno found more than 40% of respondents experienced both homophobia and racism in the past 12 months. Factors associated with exposure to social discrimination were study site, income, education, marital status, and self-reported HIV status. Overall, men with lower income and education and those who reported being HIV positive were more likely to report experiencing both types of social discrimination. Adjusting for potential confounders, men exposed to both homophobia and racism were more likely to report unprotected receptive anal intercourse with a casual sex partner (AOR = 1.92, 95% CI, 1.18–3.24) and binge drinking (AOR = 1.42, 95% CI, 1.02–1.98) as compared to men exposed to neither form of discrimination during the past year.

These findings are important for showing the detrimental and additive effects of social discrimination on the sexual risk for HIV among Latino MSM. *How* racism and homophobia operate to elevate risk is still an open question, especially when taking into account other background or demographic variables such as immigration, socioeconomic status, and HIV serostatus.

MECHANISM THROUGH WHICH SOCIAL DISCRIMINATION INFLUENCES HIV RISK FOR LATINO MSM
Summary of Study Procedures

In another recent analysis, Ayala, Bingham, Millet, Kim, and Millet (2011) modeled the impact of social discrimination and financial hardship on the sexual risk for HIV among Latino ($n = 1081$) and black MSM ($n = 1154$) recruited using respondent-driven sampling (RDS) techniques using data taken from the same CDC-funded, three-city study—Brothers y Hermanos—referenced above in the Mizuno analysis. In this instance, the research team examined the correlations between experiences of social discrimination, financial hardship, and the sexual risk for HIV among Latino and black MSM living in Los Angeles County, New York City, and Philadelphia. They combined a traditional mediation analysis with the results of a path analysis to examine simultaneously the direct, indirect, and total effects of explanatory variables on men's participation in unprotected anal intercourse (UAI) with casual male partners in the past 3 months. The team hypothesized that the following:

1. Experiences of social discrimination (defined as racism and homophobia, e.g., being made fun of, called names, treated unfairly in the last 12 months), financial hardship (e.g., running out of money for basic necessities in the last 12 months), and lack of social support (e.g., feeling isolated and alone, no one to talk with) would each be positively associated with UAI with casual male partners.
2. Experiences of social discrimination and financial hardship would be positively associated with lack of social support.
3. Experiences of social discrimination, financial hardship, and lack of social support would each be associated with reports of being in situations that make safer sex more difficult such as sex in exchange for drugs, money, or a place to sleep, using drugs before or during sex, having a partner who is perceived to be more masculine than one's self, and having sex in a causal partner's home.

4. Participation in riskier sexual situations would mediate the associations between social discrimination, financial hardship, and lack of social support on UAI with casual male partners.

Testing the Hypothesized Links between Discrimination and HIV Risk

To test the first hypothesis, the research team entered experiences of homophobia, racism, and financial hardship as predictors of lack of social support in a multiple linear regression equation. The results supported Hypothesis 1 with experiences of discrimination and financial hardship predicting lack of social support (homophobia—β = 0.50, p < 0.0001; racism—β = 0.51, p = 0.0003; and financial hardship—β = 0.75 p < 0.0001). To test the second hypothesis, the team then entered experiences of social discrimination, financial hardship, and lack of social support as predictors of participation in potentially risky sexual situations. Lack of social support (β = 0.03, p < 0.0001), together with experiences of homophobia (β = 0.12, p = 0.0001), racism (β = 0.11, p = 0.006), and financial hardship (β = 0.14, p < 0.0001), were associated with participation in potentially risky sexual situations.

Risky Sexual Situations as Mediators

Finally, to test whether risky sexual situations mediate the associations between social discrimination, financial hardship, and lack of social support on the risk for HIV, the research team entered all variables into a logistic regression equation as predictors of risk. As illustrated in Table 8.2, the addition of the hypothesized mediation variable (participation in potentially risky sexual situations) to the full model reduced the direct associations of almost all of the explanatory variables, meeting Baron and Kenny's (1986) criteria for partial mediation. Complete mediation would have been achieved had there not been a significant effect of racism on UAI. Experiences of racism retained a small direct effect on UAI with a casual partner (OR = 1.2, p = 0.03).

Table 8.2 Logistic Regression Equation with Homophobia, Racism, Financial Hardship, Lack of Social Support, and Difficult Sexual Situations as Predictors of UAI among Latino and black MSM

Predictor	OR	95% CI	p-value
Homophobia	1.0	0.88–1.1	0.94
Racism	1.2	1.0–1.4	0.03
Financial hardship	1.1	0.91–1.4	0.25
Lack of social support	1.0	0.99–1.0	0.07
Riskier sexual situations (ref = none)*	1.0	—	—
One	2.6	2.0–3.4	<0.0001
Two	7.3	5.5–9.7	<0.0001
Three to five	13	10–18	<0.0001

*The dependent variable for difficult sexual situations is modeled as a four-level continuous variable: the experience of none, one, two, or three to five difficult situations.

Social Discrimination and Sexual Risk: Race/Ethnicity Differences

Building on the results of the meditational analysis, the research team then began building a model of sexual risk among Latino and black MSM using path analysis. They found that the direct and indirect effects between experiences of social discrimination, financial hardship, lack of social support, participation in risky sexual situations, and UAI with a casual partner were similar for both Latino and black MSM. Path coefficients are presented in Figure 8.1 and are reported along with path analysis procedures in an article by Ayala and colleagues (2011).

As illustrated in Figure 8.1, the research team found a statistically significant direct path between experiences of racism and UAI with a casual partner among black MSM. Interestingly, this path was not statistically significant for Latino MSM. On the other hand, the path between racism and lack of social support was statistically significant only for Latino MSM. Furthermore, the path between lack of social support and UAI with a casual partner was statistically significant among Latino MSM but not among black MSM. Finally, the path between financial hardship and UAI with a casual partner was statistically significant among Latino MSM but not among black MSM. In other words, mediating factors that could explain *how* racism and financial hardship might influence the risk for HIV for Latino and black gay men differed in some important ways. The team speculated that skin color and immigration status may play a role in the differential experiences of racism and financial hardship for black and Latino MSM, respectively, factors that were not examined in their study but that merit future in-depth investigation.

Racism and financial hardship may be instigated and influenced by skin color and immigration status among other factors, which together represent a complicated constellation of factors that shapes how and who experiences these particular forms of social discrimination. It is important to highlight here, as noted above, the majority of the study participants were poor, underemployed, and undereducated immigrants living with HIV. How racism is enacted and experienced among Latino

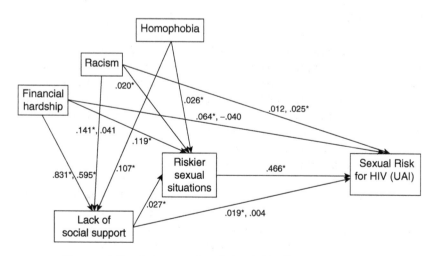

FIGURE 8.1 The associations between racism, homophobia, financial hardship, and unprotected anal intercourse with casual male partners among Latino and black MSM. *p-value < 0.05. [Partially restricted model; path coefficients are listed for both Latinos (*listed first*) and blacks (*listed second*) where the path is not restricted or fixed.]

DISCUSSION

The potentially damaging health and social consequences of racism, homophobia, and financial hardship on individual well being are well established in the research literature (Diaz et al., 2001; Finch et al., 2001; Klonoff, Landerine, & Ullman, 1999; Waldo, 1999; DiPlacido, 1998; Meyer, 1995; Jones, 1992; Williams, 1990; Rosser & Ross, 1989; Schuman, Steeh, & Bobo, 1985). Social discrimination and the strategies used by Latino MSM to cope with and minimize exposure to such discrimination can shape both opportunities an individual has to meet sexual partners as well as meanings attached to those relationships (Ayala & Diaz, 2001). For example, social structures supportive of racial/ethnic identity and important sources of connectedness may exert gender-role conformity pressure driven by homophobic attitudes, whereas social structures supportive of gay identities may fail to support Latino men under the weight of race-based stereotyping and sexual objectification that take place in the gay sexual market place (Paul, Ayala, & Choi, 2010; Wilson & Miller, 2002; Contrada et al., 2000; Greene, 1997; Hildalgo, 1995; Walters, 1998). In this regard, issues associated with multiple marginalization (i.e., being the target of both racism and homophobia) faced by Latino MSM, including how Latino gay men manage competing loyalties they sometimes feel to their families and communities of origin versus their families and communities of choice, are poignantly relevant to their sexual health and wellness. In addition, how racism and homophobia are enacted and experienced may vary as a function of skin color (as in the case for black or dark-skinned Latinos) and/or immigration, socioeconomic, and HIV serostaus, factors that were not systematically explored in the studies present in this chapter.

Until recently, the disproportionate impact of the HIV/AIDS epidemic on Latino gay men and other men who have sex with men was largely attributed to higher, individual-level behavioral risk for HIV among this population (i.e., low level of knowledge, inaccurate assessments of risk, low perceptions of personal vulnerability to HIV, and a lack of motivation or personal intentions to practice safer sex) (Fisher, Fisher, & Harman, 2003; Fisher & Fisher, 2000; Fishbein et al., 1991; Catania, Kegeles, & Coates, 1990). However, it is becoming increasingly clear that the context of behavioral risk must be better understood if we are to continue to lower risk levels for vulnerable populations. With regard to men in the studies presented here, sexual risk for HIV is influenced by at least three forms of social discrimination highly salient to Latino MSM and MSM of color more generally—homophobia, racism, and financial hardship.

Research has shown powerful associations between experiences of discrimination and social alienation, depression, and personal shame, which in turn were positively correlated with sexual risk behavior among Latino MSM (Ayala & Diaz, 2001; Diaz et al., 2001; Diaz, 1998). As this line of research evolves (as seen in the three studies presented above), we are now learning that the sources and types of discrimination matter, are cumulative, and may have differential salience for different men of color. For example, homophobia from family and racism from gay peers may be more salient for Latino gay men who may view these sources of discrimination as also possible sources of social support, and hence with mixed feelings. In addition, experiences of discrimination add up—experiencing two or three cooccurring forms of discrimination leads to worse sexual health outcomes (i.e., unprotected anal intercourse with a casual partner of unknown HIV status) than experiencing one or no discrimination. Moreover, the impact that homophobia and racism have on the sexual risk for HIV is mediated by lack of social support and difficult or riskier sexual situations. In the case of Latino gay men, it may be that homophobia and racism heighten the sexual risk for HIV by decreasing social support and increasing the likelihood of participation in riskier sexual situations. This may be especially true for poor, immigrant black (or darker skinned men living with HIV who, for example, may have greater difficulty accessing services if they are undocumented and working illegally or in hazardous working environments). These men may also be encountering racism in both the mainstream gay community and labor market. The racial, immigration, socioeconomic, and HIV serostatus of these men may be impacting their HIV risk in ways that remain unexplored. Furthermore, experiences of social discrimination vary by type and source across groups of MSM of color as suggested in the third study presented above. This finding is corroborated by new research showing that (1) African American, followed by Latino MSM experience harsher and more explicit forms of racism from broader society than Asian and Pacific Islander (API) MSM; (2) API MSM were more likely to report racism in the mainstream gay community than other MSM of color; (3) Latino MSM were least likely to report racism in the mainstream gay community (in Los Angeles) but more likely to report having experienced homophobia in the past year; (4) MSM of color who reported financial difficulties and incarceration histories were more likely to report experiences of racism; (5) self-identified gay men, HIV-positive men, men with greater financial difficulties, and men with incarceration experiences were more likely to report homophobia; and (6) men who had been married to a woman and had less formal education were less likely to report experiences of homophobia (Ayala, Paul, Boylan, Gregorich, & Choi, 2011).

IMPLICATIONS FOR FUTURE RESEARCH AND INTERVENTION DEVELOPMENT

The above findings imply two important loci for possible future interventions— social supports and difficult sexual situations. We may be able to buffer the effects of discrimination by supporting and enhancing social support, particularly from family and friends. In addition, HIV preventionists may need to challenge traditional conceptualizations of HIV risk, which assume risk to be an individual-level or intrapsychic characteristic that in turn therefore implies intervention with the individual. If risk is situational or context specific, interventions may also need to be redirected to the interpersonal situations and contexts that compromise men's capacity to participate in health-promoting behaviors. Carlos Caceres (2000) underscores this point when he wrote:

An overly superficial focus on sexual practices as defined by medical and behavioral science categories, rather than as understood and enacted by the individuals concerned, will inevitably lead to naive formulations of behavior change and to associated problems with intervention and program development. (p. 251)

Finally, the direct effect of racism and financial hardship for black and Latino gay men, respectively, remains unexplained by the mediating variables explored in the studies presented above. More research is needed to understand more clearly the differential impact of racism and homophobia on Latino and other MSM of color. Future research should explore other factors such as skin color, immigration status, and financial hardship given that each is intimately tied to how Latino gay men and other MSM of color experience these forms of discrimination.

REFERENCES

Ayala, G., Bingham, T., Kim, J., Wheeler, D., & Millet, G. A. (2012). Modeling the impact of social discrimination and financial hardship on the sexual risk for HIV among Latino and Black MSM. *American Journal of Public Health*. [Epub ahead of print].

Ayala, G., & Diaz, R. M. (2001). Racism, poverty and other truths about sex: race, class and HIV risk among Latino gay men. *Revista Interamericana de Psicologia, 35*(2), 59–77.

Ayala, G., Paul, J., Boylan, R., Gregorich, S., & Choi, K. H. (2011). Variations and correlates of discrimination among racial/ethnic minority MSM living in Los Angeles. Oral presentation given at the 2011 U.S. National HIV Prevention Conference, Atlanta, GA.

Ayala, G., Paul, J., & Choi, K. H. (2011). Sources and types of social discrimination experienced by African American, Asian and Pacific Islander, and Latino MSM in Los Angeles. Unpublished manuscript.

Baron, R. M., & Kenny, D. A. (1986). The moderator-mediator variable distinction in social psychological research: Conceptual, strategic, and statistical considerations. *Journal of Personality and Social Psychology, 51*(6), 1173–1182.

Bruce, D., Ramirez-Valles, J., & Campbell, R. T. (2008). Stigmatization, substance use, and sexual risk behavior among Latino gay and bisexual men and transgender persons. *Journal of Drug Issues, 38*(1), 235–260.

Caceres, C. F. (2000). Afterword: The production of knowledge on sexuality in the AIDS era: Some issues, opportunities and challenges. In R. Parker, R. M. Barbosa, and P. Aggleton (Eds) Framing the Sexual Subject: The Politics of Gender, Sexuality and Power, (pp. 241–260). University of California Press: Berkeley and Los Angeles, CA.

Cain, V. S., & Kington, R. S. (2003). Investigating the role of racial/ethnic bias in health outcomes. *American Journal of Public Health, 93*, 191–192.

Catania, J. A., Kegeles, S. M., & Coates, T. J. (1990). Towards an understanding of risk behavior: An AIDS risk reduction model (ARRM). *Health Education Quarterly, 17*(1), 53–72.

CDC. (2005). H IV prevalence, unrecognized infection, and HIV testing among men who have sex with men—five U.S. cities, June 2004—April 2005. *Morbidity and Mortality Weekly Report, 54*(24), 597–601.

CDC. (2008a). HIV prevalence estimates—United States, 2006. *Morbidity and Mortality Weekly Report, 57*(39), 1073–1076.

CDC. (2008b). Subpopulation estimates from the HIV incidence surveillance system—United States, 2006. *Morbidity and Mortality Weekly Report, 57*, 985–989.

CDC. (2009). HIV AIDS surveillance report, 2007. Atlanta: U.S. Department of Health and Human Services, Centers for Disease Control and Prevention. http://www.cdc.gov/hiv/topics/surveillance/resources/reports/.

Contrada, R., Ashmore, R., Gary, M., Coups, E., Egeth, J. D., Sewell, A., Ewell, K., Goya, T. M., & Chasse, V. (2000). Ethnicity-related sources of stress and their effects on well-being. *Current Directions in Psychological Science, 9*(4), 136–139.

Diaz, R. M. (1998). *Latino gay men and HIV: Culture, sexuality, & risk behavior.* New York: Routledge.

Diaz, R., & Ayala, G. (2001).*The impact of social discrimination on health outcomes: The case of Latino gay men.* A monograph of the National Gay and Lesbian Task Force. New York City.

Díaz, R. M., Ayala, G., & Bein, E. (2004). Sexual risk as an outcome of social oppression: Data from a probability sample of Latino gay men in three US cities. *Cultural Diversity and Ethnic Minority Psychology, 10*(3), 255–267.

Diaz, R. M., Ayala. G., Bein, E., Henne, J., & Marin, B. (2001). The impact of homophobia, poverty, and racism on the mental health of gay and bisexual Latino men: findings from 3 U.S. cities. *American Journal of Public Health, 91*(6), 927–932.

DiPlacido, J. (1998). Minority stress among lesbians, gay men, and bisexuals: A consequence of heterosexism, homophobia, and stigmatization. In G. Herek (Ed.), *Stigma and sexual orientation: Understanding prejudice against lesbians, gay men, and bisexuals* (pp. 138–159). Thousand Oaks, CA: Sage Publications.

Finch, B., Hummer, R., Kolody, B., & Vega, W. (2001). The role of discrimination and acculturative stress in the physical health of Mexican-origin adults. *Hispanic Journal of Behavioral Sciences, 23*(4), 399–429.

Fishbein, M., Bandura, A., Triandis, H. C., Kaufer, F. H., & Becker, M. H. (1991). Factors influencing behavior and behavior change. *Final Report of Theorists' Workshop.* Unpublished manuscript.

Fisher, J. D., & Fisher, J. D. (2000). Theoretical approaches to individual-level change in HIV risk behavior. In J. L. Peterson & R. J. DiClemente (Eds.), *Handbook of HIV prevention* (pp. 3–48). New York: Kluwer Academic/Plenum Publishers.

Fisher, W. A., Fisher, J. D., & Harmen, J. (2003). The information-motivation-behavioral skills model as a general model of health behavior change. In J. Suls & K. Wallston (Eds.), *Social psychological foundations of health,* (pp. 82–106). London: Blackwell Publishing.

Greene, B. (1997). Lesbian women of color: Triple jeopardy. *Journal of Lesbian Studies, I*(1), 109–147.

Hidalgo, H. (1995). *Lesbians of color: Social and human services.* New York: Harrington Park Press/Haworth Press, Inc.

Jones, J. (1992). Understanding the mental health consequences of race: Contributions of basic social psychological processes. In D. Ruble, P. Costanzo, & M. Oliveri (Eds.), *The social psychology of mental health: Basic mechanisms and applications* (pp. 199–240). New York: Guilford Press.

Klonoff, E., Landrine, H., & Ullman, J. (1999). Racial discrimination and psychiatric symptoms among Blacks. *Cultural Diversity & Ethnic Minority Psychology, 5*(4), 329–339.

Krieger, N. (2003). Does racism harm health? Did child abuse exist before 1962? On explicit questions, critical science and current controversies: An ecosocial perspective. *American Journal of Public Health, 93*(2), 194–199.

Krieger, N., Rowley, D., Hermann, A., Avery, B., & Phillips, M. (1993). Racism, sexism, and social class: Implications for studies of health, disease, and well-being. *American Journal of Preventive Medicine, 9,* 82–122.

Kuzel, A. J. (1999). Sampling in qualitative inquiry. In B. F. Crabtree & W. L. Miller (Eds.), *Doing qualitative research* (pp. 33–45). Thousand Oaks, CA: Sage Publications.

Laumann, E., & Youm, Y. (1999). Racial/ethnic group differences in the prevalence of sexually transmitted diseases in the United States: A network explanation. *Sexually Transmitted Diseases, 26*(5), 250–261.

Mays, V., & Cochran, S. (2001). Mental health correlates of perceived discrimination among lesbian, gay, and bisexual adults in the United States. *American Journal of Public Health, 91,* 1869–1876.

Meyer, I. H. (1995). Minority stress and mental health in gay men. *Journal of Health Social Behavior, 36,* 35–56.

Mizuno, Y., Borkowf, C., Millet, G. A., Bingham, T., Ayala, G., & Stueve, A. (2011). Homophobia and racism experienced by Latino men who have sex with men in the United States: Correlates of exposure and associations with HIV risk behaviors. *AIDS Behavior*, June 1, 2011, DOI 10.1007/s10461-011-9967-1.

Nakamura, N., & Zea, M. C. (2010). Experiences of homonegativity and sexual risk behavior in a sample of Latino gay and bisexual men. *Culture, Health, & Sexuality, 12*, 73–85.

Paul, J. P., Ayala, G., & Choi, K. C. (2010). Internet sex ads for MSM and partner selection criteria: The potency of race/ethnicity online. *Journal of Sex Research, 47*(6), 528–538.

Rosser, S., & Ross, M. (1989). A gay life events scale (GALES) for homosexual men. *Journal of Gay & Lesbian Psychotherapy, 1*(2), 87–101.

Schuman, H., Steeh, C., & Bobo, L. (1985). *Racial attitudes in America: Trends and interpretations.* Cambridge, MA: Harvard University Press.

Valleroy, L. A., MacKellar, D. A., Karon, J. M., Rosen, D. H., McFarland, W., Shehan, D. A., Stoyanoff, S. R., LaLota, M., Celentano, D. D., Koblin, B. A., Thiede, H., Katz, M. H., Torian, L. V., & Janssen, R. S. (2000). HIV prevalence and associated risks in young men who have sex with men. Young men's survey study group. *Journal of the American Medical Association (JAMA), 284*(2), 198–204.

Waldo, C. (1999). Working in a majority context: A structural model of heterosexism as minority stress in the workplace. *Journal of Counseling Psychology, 46*(2), 218–232.

Walters, K. (1998). Negotiating conflicts in allegiances among lesbians and gays of color: Reconciling divided selves and communities. In G. Mallon (Ed.), *Foundations of social work practice with lesbian and gay persons* (pp. 47–75). Binghamton, NY: Harrington Park Press/Haworth Press, Inc.

Williams, D. (1990). Socioeconomic differentials in health: A review and redirection. *Social Psychology Quarterly, 53*(2), 81–99.

Williams, D. R., Neighbors, H. W., & Jackson, J. S. (2003). Racial/ethnic discrimination and health: Findings from community studies. *American Journal of Public Health, 93*, 200–208.

Wilson, B., & Miller, R. (2002). Strategies for managing heterosexism used among African American gay and bisexual men. *Journal of Black Psychology, 28*(4), 371–391.

Wilson, P. A., Valera, P., Ventuneac, A., Balan, I., Rowe, M., & Carballo-Dieguez, A. (2009). Race-based stereotyping and sexual partnering among men who use the internet to identify other men for bareback sex. *Journal of Sex Research, 46*, 1–15.

9 Contextual Influences of Sexual Risk among Latino Men Who Have Sex with Men

Maria Cecilia Zea, Carol A. Reisen, Fernanda T. Bianchi, and Paul J. Poppen

INTRODUCTION

As the opening chapter of this book points out, environmental and situational factors influence the way a person behaves, and therefore they should be incorporated into theoretical and practical approaches to HIV risk and prevention (Organista, Worby, Quesada, Kral, Diaz, Neilands, & Arreola, Chapter 1, this volume). The structural-environmental (SE) model proposed by Organista and colleagues examines risk behavior within the context of the individual's life. That context can include conditions that are proximal to the potential HIV-risk behavior, such as the use of alcohol or drugs during sex, or conditions that are more distal. Distal factors can be related to macro, structural conditions (i.e., the cultural, social, or economic context that shapes sexual risk behavior).

In this chapter, we will discuss research illustrating a number of different ways in which characteristics and conditions of the larger environmental context, as well as of the sexual encounter itself, can influence sexual risk behavior of Latino men who have sex with men (MSM). The findings stem from a 5-year, mixed-method study of immigrant MSM from three countries (Brazil, Colombia, and the Dominican Republic) performed by the Latino Health Research Center at George Washington University and funded by the National Institute of Child Health and Development (NICHD). We focused on these three groups of Latinos because they were under-represented in research on Latinos in the United States. Colombians and Dominicans constitute the largest of the "New Latino Groups" (Logan, 2001), and they have received much less research attention than the long-established U.S. populations of Mexicans, Puerto Ricans, and Cubans. We also included Brazilians, who, as Portuguese speakers, are often excluded from studies of Latinos.

Our thinking was influenced by Ewart's (1991) Social Action Theory, which posited the importance of the immediate social, emotional, and physical circumstances, as well as personal characteristics, in shaping an individual's self-protective behavior. When applied to HIV prevention, this approach would suggest that behaviors such as condom use are influenced not only by characteristics of the person, but also by the context of the partnership (e.g., emotional relationship, seroconcordance or discordance) and the physical circumstances of the people in the encounter (e.g., level of sexual arousal, state related to substance use). Moreover, characteristics at these two levels may interact with each other: for example, the impact of being drunk on the likelihood of having unprotected sex could differ for younger and older MSM.

Examining the circumstances of the specific encounter is valuable because sexual risk behavior not only varies between individuals, but may also be inconsistent within an individual: the same person may use a condom in one situation, but not in another. Conditions of the sexual encounter may be responsible for such variation in a given person's behavior from one situation to the next. We use the term *situational* to refer to these characteristics that can vary from one sexual encounter to another.

Our conceptualization of the contextual influences on sexual risk has also been shaped by a social epidemiological model of HIV/AIDS population incidence proposed by Poundstone, Strathdee, and Celentano (2004). Although this model addresses the prediction of HIV incidence within a population, the conceptual organization can be adapted and applied to individual risk behavior. Poundstone and colleagues created a heuristic framework that included three levels of factors influencing HIV incidence. The structural level relates to the legal and policy environment, demographic features of a population such as migration or urbanization, and structural violence or discrimination; the social level relates to the cultural context, social networks, and neighborhood effects; the individual level relates to personal characteristics, socioeconomic situation, and behaviors. In this chapter, we refer to the levels with these same terms: *structural, social, and individual* levels (see Figure 9.1). In both the SE model and the social epidemiological model, the different levels are seen as interrelated and permeable.

In summary, we view sexual risk behavior as shaped by four levels of influence, the three discussed above plus the situational level described earlier. The structural and social levels represent the broader social context in which sexual relationships occur. The individual level concerns a given person's characteristics, whereas the situational level addresses the particular circumstances of the sexual encounter.

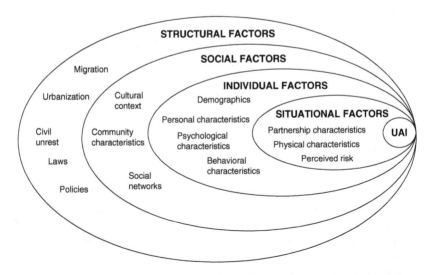

FIGURE 9.1 Theoretical model of multiple levels of influence on sexual risk behavior.

The latter enables us to examine a person's varied behavior under different conditions of specific sexual encounters.

In the following sections, we will first describe the 5-year research project that was the source of all the data described in this chapter. Then we will give examples of a variety of ways in which contextual factors at different levels can influence sexual risk behavior among Latino MSM. We will discuss four papers derived from the research project. The first was based on qualitative data only, whereas the remaining three reflect quantitative analyses. In discussing the quantitative papers, however, we also incorporate quotations from participants in the qualitative phase, because the perspectives and experiences described by the men serve to enrich our understanding.

METHODS OF THE STUDY

The research project examined sexual risk behavior among Brazilian, Colombian, and Dominican MSM living in the New York City metropolitan area. The study had two phases. The qualitative phase was designed to elucidate the context of sexual encounters of Dominican, Colombian, and Brazilian MSM in New York City; to identify aspects of the context of social and sexual encounters that lead to various forms of protected and unprotected sex; and to describe similar and different patterns of beliefs, norms, and behaviors in the three groups. We obtained descriptions of the context of sexual encounters, as well as the broader social context in which Brazilian, Colombian, and Dominican MSM live. The quantitative phase followed, and was designed to refine a theoretical model and to administer a computerized survey to test hypotheses concerning the effect on sexual risk behavior of sociocultural and psychosocial factors that characterize the individual, and of situational factors that characterize sexual encounters.

The qualitative data were collected in the New York metropolitan area from 2003 to 2004. The data consisted of key informant interviews, focus groups, and in-depth interviews. The qualitative sample included 25 participants in three separate focus groups—9 in the Brazilian group, 11 in the Colombian group, and 5 in the Dominican group. In addition, there were 36 other participants for in-depth interviews: 10 Brazilians, 14 Colombians, 12 Dominicans (three of whom were later dropped when we discovered that they did not meet inclusion criterion of being an immigrant). Participants for the focus groups and in-depth interviews were recruited through snowball sampling, advertisements in gay publications and on Internet websites, flyers, and referrals made by staff at Latino gay community organizations. Details concerning the qualitative methods can be found in Bianchi, Reisen, Zea, Poppen, Shedlin, and Montes-Penha (2007).

There were two samples used for quantitative data collection: first, 120 for the pilot test of the quantitative survey and then 482 for the full administration. The pilot test was used to refine measures, language, and Audio-enhanced Computer Assisted Self-Interview (A-CASI) procedures. The full quantitative sample consisted of 146 Brazilian, 169 Colombian, and 167 Dominican immigrant MSM. Targeted sampling approaches similar to those in the qualitative phase were used, with flyers, advertisements on websites, referrals from some participants, and recruitment at gay venues, community organizations, and Latino cultural events. Eligibility criteria included having been born in Brazil, Colombia, or the Dominican Republic, residing in the New York metropolitan area, being at least 18 years of age, having had sex with men, and having had sex in the last 6 months. Data collection in both phases took place in Spanish, Portuguese, or English, depending on the preference of the participant.

A survey was administered via computer assisted self-interview technology with audio enhancement (A-CASI) and touch-screen responding. The survey included many questions about specific types of sexual encounters, including encounters involving condom use, no condom use, substance use, different types of settings, and partners. In addition, the survey covered sexual behavior over the previous 3 months, depression, self-efficacy for safer sex, experiences of discrimination, Latino cultural beliefs, acculturation, and involvement in the gay community. Details of the quantitative methods used can be found in Zea, Reisen, Poppen, and Bianchi (2009).

In the conceptualization of this research, we anticipated that Brazilian, Colombian, and Dominican MSM would differ in their sexual behavior patterns, because cultural background can be an important social factor shaping sexual scripts and practices. The three groups did vary on some demographic characteristics: Dominicans were younger, had immigrated to the United States at a younger age, were less educated, were more likely to identify as bisexual, and were less likely to identify as gay than the other two groups, whereas Brazilians reported higher incomes than the Colombian or Dominican MSM. There were no differences among the three groups in HIV status or having a main partner. As can be seen in the findings described below, we failed to find differences based on country of birth on a variety of sexual behavior patterns, including risk-taking. It seems possible that relative to sexual behavior among MSM, the influence of gay culture supersedes that of national culture for MSM in a gay epicenter such as New York.

SOCIAL AND STRUCTURAL INFLUENCES ON IMMIGRATION AND SEXUAL RISK

The first phase of the study involved qualitative data collection and illustrated ways in which the social and structural context in the country of origin, as well as in the New York metropolitan area, affected the behavior of Latino MSM from Brazil, Colombia, and the Dominican Republic (see Bianchi et al., 2007). Migration itself is frequently a response to conditions in the country of origin. On a structural level such conditions could include poverty, political instability or violence, and lack of economic or educational opportunity. For Latino MSM, migration may also be motivated by social conditions related to gay discrimination, family rejection, and a desire to find a gay community or greater opportunity to find partners (Carrillo, 2004; Díaz, 1998; Parker, 1997).

Among the MSM in our qualitative sample, the reasons given for moving to the United States included the traditional economic and political conditions, as well as the perceived climate for gay men in both the sending and receiving countries. Consistent with the findings of Diaz et al. in Chapter 7, experiences of homonegativity and of hostility arising from HIV stigma were especially evident among men from rural or conservative areas. For example, one Colombian noted,

I was young, they teased me a lot, I knew that life was going to be chaotic for me, it already was. And I said, 'The only way I can solve this problem is to get out of here.'

Another motivation for migration was more positive: some men came in order to achieve fuller expression of themselves and their sexuality. The image of New York as a city with a vibrant gay life was particularly attractive.

The social context encountered by the men in New York City shaped their behavior in ways that had implications for sexual risk. The sexual freedom, opportunity to find partners, and anonymity in the urban area was a thrilling combination for many of the men. A key informant described the situation in this way:

You come to New York City, I think it happens to all of us. It's like a playground: if you want to have sex every night, you can have sex every night. And sometimes I do think that it's so available and the drugs, the parties, all that stuff, that if you come from a culture where you were so in the closet or didn't want to talk about your sexuality, your whole family was against it, religion was against it. You come here and nobody knows what you're doing and it more, like, it opens up for you.

Participants spoke of the ways in which their sexual practices and behavior changed after arriving in New York. Some participants—especially those who immigrated as young men—reported that their newly found sexual freedom led to an almost compulsive pursuit of sexual partners and exploration of gay spaces, as well as to a perception that having a very large number of casual sexual partners was normative. Other participants spoke of enlarging their sexual repertoires and a willingness to try many things. In some cases, the newfound freedom within the gay social context led to behaviors that placed the men at increased risk for HIV and other STIs. One participant described his own behavior this way: "I arrived in the United States today, let us suppose, and the following day . . . I was being passive, and the next day I was being passive without a condom."

The influence of structural factors on sexual behavior was also evident in the participants' descriptions of their use of public sex settings during the early period after immigration. Several noted that they frequently had sex in cruising areas such as parks and public rest rooms, because in these environments there was no need to speak English, to be familiar with the social norms of gay bars or nightclubs, or to spend money. In addition, the lack of privacy in the shared living situations of many new immigrants precluded sexual encounters at home.

Although we had originally expected to find substantial differences among the experiences of the MSM from the three countries, for the most part, this was not the case. For example, the themes described above applied to men from all three groups. One way in which country-of-birth differences emerged in the qualitative data concerned stereotypes that the men encountered concerning their own groups. For example, participants reported that potential partners tended to expect Brazilians to be sexy and sensual and to expect that all Dominicans would have big penises (Bianchi et al., 2010).

SEXUAL BEHAVIOR IN PUBLIC AND PRIVATE SETTINGS

The qualitative data revealed how the experience of being an immigrant made public sex venues particularly attractive. We used quantitative data from a subsample of participants ($N = 315$ from the total sample of 482) who reported on sexual encounters in both public and private places in order to explore how physical setting shaped sexual behavior (see Reisen, Iracheta, Zea, Bianchi, & Poppen, 2010). Previous research has indicated a greater likelihood of low-risk practices and lower likelihood of unprotected anal intercourse (UAI) in public than in private settings (Tewksbury, 2002; Van Beneden et al., 2002; Woods et al., 2007) due to a variety of factors including intimacy with partners and privacy. We performed within-person comparisons and also found that individuals tended to have more UAI in their encounters that occurred in private (23%) compared to those that occurred in public venues (14%). Moreover, the MSM in this study were more likely to report other behaviors involving the anus in their encounters that took place at home or in other private settings. Thus, there was greater likelihood not only of UAI, but also of any anal intercourse and stimulation of the anus with a tongue or fingers.

There are many factors that contribute to the difference in behaviors in different places. Whereas sex in public settings is often between unknown and novel partners, sex in private settings frequently occurs between partners with some level of established intimacy, including primary relationships. As one of the participants in the qualitative phase of the study explained:

If I meet someone at a party in which I have the opportunity to see the person, pay attention to details, to get to know them better, person to person, you understand, I am going to go all the way. That is, I will have full sex [anal sex]. When it comes to saunas and theaters, well, things are different there because, even if I would want to, I have too much control in that regard. And the only thing that I allow to happen there is that someone gives me oral sex.

In our sample, about three quarters of the encounters in public settings involved no emotional relationship, in contrast to one quarter of those in private settings. The emotional bond in private settings can have the psychological effect of providing a sense of safety and increasing a desire for the physical intimacy associated with unprotected sex (Elford, Bolding, McGuire, & Sherr, 2001; Poppen, Reisen, Zea, Bianchi, & Echeverry, 2004) and with other anal sexual practices. Moreover, structural features also contribute to the difference in behaviors: the greater privacy, safety, and opportunity for nudity in home settings may be more conducive to anal sex practices than the conditions in public cruising areas such as parks or public bathrooms.

We and others have previously found that emotionally intimate partners are more likely to know each other's serostatus (Poppen et al., 2004; Poppen, Reisen, Zea, Bianchi, & Echeverry, 2005), and consistent with this earlier work, we found covariation of emotional intimacy and HIV-status knowledge in this sample. There was a greater likelihood of discussion of HIV status and of known seroconcordance in encounters that occurred in private compared to those that occurred in public settings, probably because the partners were more likely to know each other well in private settings. This greater knowledge of and intimacy with the partner have been widely associated with unprotected sex (e.g., Poppen et al., 2004). As a participant in the qualitative phase said:

I never say my status in one of those [public] places. . . I talk about my status when I have intimacy with the person, and then I can tell them about me. . . .

The more common practice of UAI in private settings may have been partially due to the strategy of risk management through serosorting (Kippax et al., 1993), in which partners seek to decrease risk by having unprotected sex only with seroconcordant partners. Obviously, this approach is possible only when partners are aware of each other's status.

In addition to a contrast between public and private settings, there is also variation in the environments of different types of public venues. Structural characteristics differ for commercial venues and free public spaces, such as parks and public restrooms (Parsons & Vicioso, 2005). Furthermore, a distinction has been made been between commercial settings that have the apparent purpose of providing a place for MSM to have sexual encounters (e.g., gay bathhouses or sex clubs) and those that have another ostensible purpose (e.g., gay bars, adult bookstores, pornographic movie houses) (Binson et al., 2001). Therefore, we examined sexual behaviors reported by a subsample of participants ($N = 182$) who went to at least one of these three types of public venues in the previous 6 months. We selected the most recent encounter in a public venue for each participant.

We found that oral sex was common in all types of public settings, but that manual stimulation of a partner's penis occurred more frequently in public cruising areas such as parks or public bathrooms than in either of the commercial venue types. We believe that characteristics of the physical setting are at least partially responsible for this behavioral difference. As a participant in the qualitative phase noted:

I have done it many times in parks. One is with the anxiety that the police will come, that someone will see me, and such and such.

The vulnerability to arrest, harassment, or embarrassment posed in cruising places would promote sexual activities, such as manual stimulation, that allow greater facility for dressing quickly and breaking away from the encounter.

Results also indicated that anal intercourse, anal stimulation with the tongue, or anal insertion with a finger or hand were most common in bathhouses. Again, the influence of structural factors is evident, as bathhouses afford a greater measure of privacy, safety, and comfort than other public settings (Tewksbury, 2002). In addition, communal steam rooms and showers provide a physical structure conducive to group sex, a behavior that we found in over half of the encounters occurring in bathhouses—a significantly greater proportion than in the other types of public sex venues. The duration of the visit and the social atmosphere in bathhouses (Tewksbury, 2002; Woods et al., 2007) could also promote group sex. A participant in the qualitative interviews also noted the role of nudity in defining a sexual setting:

What happens when you go to a sex place, that they tell you that this is a "sex party," this is a sauna, or this is. . . You arrive there and the first thing they say to you is, "Leave your clothes outside." The simple act of taking off your clothes means that you are entering a totally different environment. The fact that you go inside a place, a room, and that you are naked with other naked people, that is totally different.

It is interesting that despite the greater likelihood of anal intercourse in bathhouses, we failed to find a difference in the incidence of UAI in the three types of venues. This finding is in contrast to previous research reporting more UAI in bathhouses than in public cruising areas (Binson et al., 2001). It is possible that the lack of a significant effect in the current study is due to the success of recent prevention campaigns that seek to make condom use normative in bathhouses (Binson et al., 2005; Tewksbury, 2002).

Due to concerns about power, the analyses described above collapsed over the men born in the three countries, but we also explored whether sexual behaviors performed in public settings differed for Brazilian, Colombian, and Dominican MSM. There were no differences on any of the behaviors, which included protected and unprotected anal intercourse, anal stimulation with the tongue, anal stimulation with the hand, and oral or manual stimulation of the penis. Although the effect was not significant ($p < 0.08$), Dominican MSM were more likely to have sex in public cruising areas than were Brazilian or Colombian MSM.

SEXUAL ORIENTATION, RELATIONSHIP BETWEEN PARTNERS, AND BEHAVIOR

The social context of a sexual encounter stems in part from the identity and roles of the individuals involved. Using pilot data for the quantitative survey ($N = 120$), we examined sexual behavior in the context of partnerships between our Latino gay-identified participants and their non-gay-identified partners (Reisen, Zea, Bianchi, Poppen, Shedlin, & Montes-Penha, 2010). Over two-thirds of our participants reported having sex at some time with men who identified as heterosexual, and this proportion did not differ among the Brazilian, Colombian, and Dominican MSM. Of the participants who reported sex with a non-gay-identified man, about half had sustained relationships with these men, the majority of whom were also Latino.

Although there were no differences found in the likelihood of UAI in sexual encounters between our participants and the gay, straight, or bisexually identified partners, the men in our sample were significantly more likely to take an insertive role for anal intercourse and oral sex when their partners saw themselves as gay than as either straight or bisexual. Indeed, insertive anal sex was twice as likely to be performed by our participants with their gay partners than with their straight ones. Moreover, with gay partners, oral sex was typically given and received, but in contrast, participants gave oral sex more frequently and received oral sex less frequently with straight partners. These findings may stem from an unequal power dynamic, due to the privileged sexual orientation of the straight-identified man. It is possible that our gay participants may service their straight partners and relegate their own sexual needs as less important in the context of partnerships with non-gay-identified men.

It is also possible that the behavioral patterns stem from the Latino cultural context. There is a belief among some Latinos that "homosexuals" take a receptive role in anal intercourse, whereas "men" (i.e., heterosexuals) take an insertive role, regardless of the gender of the partner (Carballo-Diéguez et al., 2004; Carrillo, 2002; Díaz, 1998; Finlinson, Colón, Robles, & Soto, 2006). As one of the participants in the qualitative phase explained:

In Colombia, in the region where I live, there is the belief that the man who penetrates is not homosexual. In short, I had many adventures, many, beyond number, with men who remain 'straight,' to put it that way, socially, married men, men (with) females who, nevertheless, played with gays.

A similar belief about the correspondence between role and identity has been noted for oral sex among some Latino MSM (Tabet et al., 1996). Among our participants who had ongoing relationships with straight men, only about half reported that their non-gay-identified partner took the insertive sexual role in anal intercourse, but the others did not. Thus, it is evident that this culturally derived perception that role defines sexual orientation identity is far from universal among Latinos and may be rapidly changing.

PERSONAL AND SITUATIONAL FACTORS IN SEXUAL RISK

Exploring the context in which sexual behavior occurs reveals the complexity of potential influences at multiple levels. As we saw above, a person's actions may be affected by structural conditions (e.g., safety, physical circumstances) and social conditions (e.g., emotional intimacy, seroconcordance) that characterize specific sexual encounters. A person may have a general tendency to behave in a certain manner in sexual situations, presumably shaped by a variety of traits (e.g., age, tendency toward sensation-seeking); however, behavior is not always consistent for a person across situations. Furthermore, individuals may not be aware of how circumstances affect their behavior. For example, a participant in our qualitative interviews described having unprotected sex in a sexual encounter with two other men in a sauna:

We did it without a condom and I, frankly, I tell you that I do not remember why I did that because I never. . .I always protect myself. . .and that day I forgot to use a condom.

Using multivariate and multilevel methods, we examined the impact of individual-level and situational-level characteristics, as well as the ways in which they interact, on sexual risk behavior (see Zea et al., 2009). We collected data about UAI during the previous 3 months, as well as during multiple specific sexual encounters. In this way, we had indicators of both general patterns of risk behavior, as well a risk behavior in situation-specific conditions.

First we investigated general patterns of sexual risk behavior with an ordinal variable reflecting the number of instances of UAI during the previous 3 months. There were two sets of predictors in a hierarchical set logistic regression (see Table 9.1). Set 1 included characteristics reflecting the individual's cultural background (country of birth and U.S. acculturation), as well as education, income, age, and HIV status; Set 2 included the psychological characteristics of self-efficacy for safer sex and depression. Both sets contributed significantly to the explanation of UAI over the 3-month period. In the final model containing all variables, several individual-level characteristics were linked to a person's sexual risk history of the previous 3 months. Greater acculturation in the United States, older age, lower income, and greater self-efficacy were associated with less UAI.

Next we examined how individual-level and situational-level characteristics affected UAI in the most recent sexual encounter. Again, we used hierarchical set regression, and the individual-level characteristics of Sets 1 and 2 were identical to those described for the previous analysis. In addition, Set 3 included situational-level characteristics describing specific conditions of the sexual encounter: emotional closeness to the partner, concern about transmission of STIs, drug use, sexual desire, and seroconcordance with the partner (see Table 9.2). Results indicated that Set 1 did not provide significant explanation of UAI, but the addition of each of the next sets (psychological and situational) did. In the final model,

Table 9.1 Logistic Set Regression: UAI in the Previous 3 Months (N = 482)

Model	−2 log L	Overall Model	Change in −2 log L	
Set 1: Demographic and cultural set	1217.19	$X^2(7) = 32.21$**		
Set 2: Psychological set	1182.06	$X^2(9) = 67.34$**	35.13**	
Final model	**Coefficient**	**Wald X²**	**Odds Ratio**	**95% CI**
Set 1: Demographic and cultural characteristics				
Intercept 4	0.16	0.06		
Intercept 3	0.98	2.35		
Intercept 2	1.81	7.94**		
Intercept 1	2.61	16.24**		
Education level	0.14	0.50	1.15	0.78–1.68
Income	0.23	12.77**	1.26	1.11–1.44
Age	−0.04	10.77**	0.97	0.94–0.99
HIV-positive status	0.44	3.78	1.56	1.00–2.43
Brazilian	−0.42	3.24	0.66	0.41–1.04
Dominican	0.32	2.14	1.38	0.90–2.13
U.S. Acculturation	−0.30	4.50*	0.74	0.56–0.98
Set 2: Psychological characteristics				
Self-efficacy for safer sex	−0.61	32.05**	0.55	0.44–0.67
Depression	0.06	0.18	1.06	0.81–1.40

*$p < 0.05$; **$p < 0.01$.

the only significant individual-level variable was self-efficacy for safer sex, which was again associated with a lower likelihood of UAI. Several situational variables were significant: known seroconcordance, a closer relationship with the partner, and less concern about STIs in that situation were associated with a higher probability of UAI.

The influential role of seroconcordance and the emotional relationship between partners—findings that are consistent with previous research (e.g., Crepaz et al., 2000; Poppen et al., 2005; Semple et al., 2003)—illustrated the importance of the social-interpersonal context in shaping behavior, as suggested by Social Action Theory. UAI was also more likely to occur when there was less concern about the risk of STIs. Traditional psychological theories have often emphasized risk perception as a personal characteristic (e.g., Janz & Becker, 1984; Rogers, 1975); our findings illustrate a role for perception of risk posed by a specific person in a given sexual encounter.

Taken together, these two analyses provided some support for a point made by Ajzen and Fishbein (1977), who argued that prediction of behavior is often dependent on having corresponding levels of specificity of the predictor and outcome measures—in other words, similar contextual levels. When applied to the case of sexual risk, this assertion would imply that sexual risk behavior in a specific encounter would be best explained by conditions in that encounter, whereas a person's general pattern of sexual risk behavior would be best explained

Table 9.2 Logistic Set Regression: UAI at the Most Recent Encounter (N = 413)

Model	−2 log L	Overall Model	Change in −2 log L		
Set 1: Demographic and cultural set	400.28	$X^2(7) = 8.57$			
Set 2: Psychological set	390.60	$X^2(9) = 18.26^*$	9.68*		
Set 3: Situational set	359.24	$X^2(14) = 49.62^{**}$	31.36**		
Final model	**Coefficient**	**Wald X²**	**Odds ratio**	**95% CI**	
Set 1: Demographic and cultural characteristics					
Intercept	−1.13	1.28			
Education level	−0.15	.26	0.86	0.48–1.54	
Income	0.14	2.04	1.15	0.95–1.39	
Age	−0.00	0.01	1.00	0.97–1.03	
HIV-positive status	−0.01	0.00	0.99	0.48–2.05	
Brazilian	0.01	0.00	1.01	0.50–2.03	
Dominican	0.47	1.98	1.60	0.83–3.08	
U.S. acculturation	−0.15	0.47	0.86	0.56–1.32	
Set 2: Psychological characteristics					
Self-efficacy for condom use	−0.57	14.05**	0.57	0.42–0.76	
Depression	0.03	0.02	1.03	0.67–1.59	
Set 3: Situational characteristics					
Closeness with partner	0.31	6.17*	1.37	1.07–1.75	
Concern about STIs	−0.62	4.30*	0.54	0.30–0.97	
Drug use in encounter	0.55	2.77	1.74	0.91–3.33	
Sexual desire in encounter	0.21	1.57	1.23	0.89–1.70	
Seroconcordance	0.70	5.58*	2.02	1.13–3.63	

$^*p < 0.05$; $^{**}p < 0.01$.

by characteristics of that person, rather than a structural characteristic such as poverty or urbanization, for example. We found that personal characteristics of U.S. acculturation, age, income, and self-efficacy were important in the model concerning risk behavior during the previous 3 months. However, of these variables, only self-efficacy for safer sex was also a strong predictor in the model concerning risk in the most recent sexual encounter. In that analysis, the situational characteristics, which, like the outcome, are reflective of conditions at the most recent sexual encounter, provided greater explanatory power.

Although this argument concerning the importance of corresponding specificity between predictors and outcomes appears to contradict a conceptual approach stressing influences from multiple levels (structural, social, individual, and situational), we believe that the two are not incompatible. Rather, we argue that it is easier to demonstrate the links between predictors and outcomes measured at the same level, and that influences arising from other levels are more difficult to detect due to their more distal positions and to possible complex interactions within and across levels.

We examined one type of cross-level interaction (i.e., individual level by situational level) using Hierarchical General Linear Modeling (HGLM; Raudenbush & Bryk, 2002). Because our participants had each reported on several sexual encounters, we had two levels of data—sexual encounter and person, with sexual encounters nested within the person. We investigated interactions of the individual-level variable self-efficacy for safer sex with two situational variables. We expected that situational states fostering disinhibition, such as greater sexual desire or drug use at the time of the sexual encounter, would have differing impact on the probability of UAI in that encounter depending on the person's self-efficacy for safer sex. Analysis with HGLM revealed a significant interaction: among those individuals with low self-efficacy, increased sexual desire was associated with a greater likelihood of unprotected sex, but the effect of desire on UAI was minor for individuals with high self-efficacy for safer sex (see Figure 9.2). We failed to find a significant effect in a similar model examining the cross-level interaction between self-efficacy and drug use during the encounter.

The personal characteristic of self-efficacy for safer sex was linked to UAI aggregated over the previous three months, at the most recent sexual encounter, and over multiple encounters reported by each participant. Moreover, self-efficacy moderated the impact of sexual desire on unprotected sex. The findings are consistent with traditional psychological theories that have concluded self-efficacy influences risk behavior (e.g., Bandura, 1986; Fishbein & Azjen, 1975), as well as with previous research on Latinos showing the importance of this variable (e.g., Fernandez-Esquer et al., 2004; Marín et al., 1997). However, results also demonstrate the complexity of influences across levels, a concept that was missing from some earlier psychological conceptualizations. It is evident that individuals characterized by different levels of self-efficacy reacted differently to different situational conditions.

We performed a similar HGLM analysis examining the interaction between age at the individual level and closeness to partner at the situational level. Results indicated that for younger men, there was more UAI in encounters characterized by closer relationships between partners (see Figure 9.2). For older men, however, emotional closeness had little impact on sexual risk behavior.

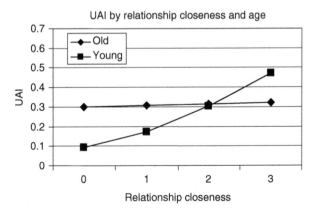

FIGURE 9.2 Cross-level interactions predicting the probability of UAI.

Taken together, the results concerning the effect of age on UAI from the three types of analysis illustrate the complexity of influences on sexual risk. The model predicting UAI over a 3-month period included only individual-level variables, and age was significant, with younger men reporting more UAI. Thus, summarizing risk behavior over the sexual encounters that occurred during that period, we see that age has an impact on sexual risk. Next, we look at the model predicting UAI at the most recent sexual encounter and including individual-level and situational-level variables. In this case, the individual-level characteristic of age was not significant, but the situational variable of closeness to the partner was. Thus, in examining behavior in one specific encounter, we failed to find an effect of the individual-level variable of age. Finally, we performed a multilevel analysis that included individual-level characteristics and multiple encounters for each person. In this analysis, which allowed for assessment of variance both within and between people, we found a significant interaction across the two levels. The likelihood of unprotected sex increased as intimacy increased for younger men, but not for older men. Thus, we see that the role of age is actually more complex than it initially appeared.

This example can serve as an illustration of the complications involved in assessing multiple influences on sexual risk behavior. Our current conceptual models posit that conditions at the structural, social, individual, and situational levels can all affect behavior. Moreover, conditions at the different levels can alter the impact of conditions at other levels. When we consider possible moderation or mediation within and across the levels, the difficulty of identifying causal paths becomes evident.

CONCLUSIONS

So where does all this complexity leave us? First of all, we acknowledge that the multilevel models of influence on HIV risk behavior are appealing precisely because of their complexity. In considering the lives of the Latino immigrant MSM in this research project, we can see not only the impact of conditions at different levels, but also the interconnections among levels. For example, we saw how structural circumstances related to economics in the home country and the United States resulted in migration, and that migration then resulted in drastic changes in the social and cultural context for these men (as discussed in Chapters 3 and 7). The open and active gay life in New York City presented opportunities and a variety of venues for meeting potential partners, who in turn brought their own characteristics and expectations. The resulting social context of the partnership then affected sexual practices. We also saw how the structural position of English as the standard language could cause a new immigrant to choose one type of sex venue over another, and we noted differences in behaviors found in different physical settings. We noted how a person's own characteristics, such as self-efficacy for safer sex, could influence sexual risk, not only directly but also by moderating the impact of characteristics in a given sexual encounter. Thus, this study provides evidence that conditions at multiple levels affect sexual behavior and risk in Latino immigrant MSM.

Second, we recognize that the task of capturing the multilevel influences is not easy. We have seen evidence supporting the contention that associations between predictors and outcomes are more easily detected when they are measured as the same level. For example, we would expect that the structural context of the society would be more predictive of prevalence of HIV than of a specific person's serostatus or risk behavior. This is not to suggest that structural factors do not affect individual behavior, but rather that they often do so in a more indirect manner. Structural poverty may result in an individual having lower self-efficacy, which could affect sexual risk behavior, but we are more likely to detect the relationship statistically by measuring the person's socioeconomic situation than that of the state or country in which he lives.

Third, we realize that the moderation and mediation within and across levels contribute to the difficulty of detecting the effects from the different levels. Therefore, it is imperative for the field to include studies that incorporate multilevel approaches to measurement and analysis, which can directly test for direct and indirect relationships, including moderation and mediation. In addition, other research needs to continue to focus on the models at any given level, so that we can better understand the dynamics occurring within levels. We believe that it would also be helpful if researchers came to use a common terminology in labeling the levels. For example, in this chapter we used the terms suggested by Poundstone and colleagues (2004) to label the structural, social, and individual levels, and we added the label situational for the encounter level.

Finally, we appreciate the value of multiple methods in elucidating the complex relationships among the influences on sexual risk behavior that arise from the structural, social, individual, and situational levels. For example, the descriptions provided by the Latino MSM who participated in the qualitative phase of our research enabled us to understand the findings of our quantitative data concerning sex in public venues. In speaking about their behavior and experiences in various circumstances, we were able to ascertain how different factors affected each other, as well as the outcome of sexual risk. Qualitative research can not only elucidate complex relationships, but also suggest interactions that could be explored in subsequent quantitative studies.

Identifying contextual and personal influences of sexual risk behavior of Latino MSM is a difficult task. Moreover, the need to understand the relationships among those influences, as well as the ways that the relationships alter the impact on sexual risk behavior, renders the task even more daunting. However, by pulling together results from a variety of approaches and methods, the field can continue to move toward greater knowledge of sexual behavior and risk, and consequently toward more effective approaches to supporting people's health and well-being.

REFERENCES

Ajzen, I., & Fishbein, M. (1977). Attitude-behavior relations: A theoretical analysis and review of empirical research. *Psychological Bulletin, 84*, 888–918.

Bandura, A. (1986). *Social foundations of thought and action: A social cognitive theory.* Englewood Cliffs, NJ: Prentice Hall.

Bianchi, F. T., Reisen, C. A., Zea, M. C., Poppen, P. J., Shedlin, M., & Montes-Penha, M. (2007). The sexual experiences of Latino men who have sex with men who migrated to a gay epicentre in the U.S.A. *Culture, Health and Sexuality, 9*, 505–518.

Bianchi, F. T., Shedlin, M. G., Brooks, K. D., Montes-Penha, M., Reisen, C. A., Zea., M. C., & Poppen, P. J. (2010). Partner selection among Latino immigrant men who have sex with men. *Archives of Sexual Behavior, 39*, 1321–1330.

Binson, D., Woods, W. J., Pollack, J., Paul, J., Stall, R., & Catania, J. A. (2001). Differential HIV risk in bathhouses and public cruising areas. *American Journal of Public Health, 91*, 1482–1486.

Binson, D., Blea, L., Cotten, P. D., Kant, J., & Woods, W. J. (2005). Building an HIV prevention program in a gay bathhouse: A case study. *AIDS Education and Prevention, 17*, 386–399.

Carballo-Diéguez, A., Dolezal, C., Nieves Rosa, L., Díez, F., Decena, C., & Balan, I. (2004). Looking for a tall, dark, macho man. . . Sexual-role behaviour variations according to partner characteristics in Latino gay and bisexual men. *Culture, Health, and Sexuality, 6*, 159–171.

Carrillo, H. (2002). *The night is young: Sexuality in Mexico in the time of AIDS.* Chicago: University of Chicago Press.

Carrillo, H. (2004). Sexual migration, cross-cultural sexual encounters, and sexual health. *Sexuality Research and Social Policy, 1*, 58–70.

Crepaz, N., Marks, G., Mansergh, G., Murphy, S., Miller, L. C., & Appleby, P. R. (2000). Age-related risk for HIV-infection in men who have sex with men: Examination of behavioral, relationship, and serostatus variables. *AIDS Education and Prevention, 12*, 405–415.

Díaz, R. (1998). *Latino gay men and HIV: Culture, sexuality, and risk behavior.* Boston: Routledge Kegan Paul.

Elford, J., Bolding, G., McGuire, M., & Sherr, L. (2001). Gay men, risk and relationships. *AIDS, 15*, 1053–1055.

Ewart, C. K. (1991). Social action theory for a public health psychology. *American Psychologist, 46*, 931–946.

Fernandez-Esquer, M. E., Atkinson, J., Diamond, P., Useche, B., & Mendiola, R. (2004). Condom use self-efficacy among U.S.- and foreign-born Latinos in Texas. *Journal of Sex Research, 41*, 390–399.

Finlinson, H. A., Colón, H. M., Robles, R. R., & Soto, M. (2006). Sexual identity formation and AIDS prevention: An exploratory study of non-gay-identified Puerto Rican MSM from working class neighborhoods. *AIDS & Behavior, 10*, 531–539.

Fishbein, M., & Ajzen, I. (1975). *Belief, attitude, intention and behavior: An introduction to theory and research.* Reading, MA: Addison-Wesley.

Janz, N. K., & Becker, M. H. (1984). The health belief model: A decade later. *Health Education Quarterly, 11*, 1–47.

Kippax, S., Crawford, J., Davis, M., Rodden, P., & Dowsett, G. (1993). Sustaining safe sex: A longitudinal sample of homosexual men. *AIDS, 7*, 257–263.

Logan, J. R. (2001, September 10). The new Latinos: Who they are, where they are. http://www.albany.edu/munford/albany.edu/census/report.html.

Marín, B, V., Gomez, C. A., Tschann, J. M., & Gregorich, S. (1997). Condom use in unmarried Latino men: A test of cultural constructs. *Health Psychology, 16*, 458–467.

Parker, R. G. (1997). Migration, sexual subcultures, and HIV/AIDS in Brazil. In G. Herdt (Ed.), *Sexual cultures and migration in the era of AIDS* (pp. 55–69). Oxford: Clarendon Press.

Parsons, J. T., & Vicioso, K. (2005). Brief encounters: The roles of public and commercial sex environments in the sexual lives of HIV-positive gay and bisexual men. In P. N. Halkitis, C. A. Gómez, & R. J. Wolitski (Eds.), *HIV + sex: The psychological and interpersonal dynamics of HIV-seropositive gay and bisexual men's relationships* (pp. 183–200). Washington, DC: American Psychological Association.

Poppen, P. J., Reisen, C. A., Zea, M. C., Bianchi, F. T., & Echeverry, J. J. (2004). Predictors of unprotected anal intercourse among HIV-positive Latino gay and bisexual men. *AIDS & Behavior, 8*, 379–389.

Poppen, P. J., Reisen, C. A., Zea, M. C., Bianchi, F. T., & Echeverry, J. J. (2005). Serostatus disclosure, seroconcordance, partner relationship, and unprotected anal intercourse among

HIV-positive Latino men who have sex with men. *AIDS Education and Prevention, 17*, 227–237.

Poundstone, K. E., Strathdee, S. A., & Celentano, D. D. (2004). The social epidemiology of human immunodeficiency virus/acquired immunodeficiency syndrome. *Epidemiologic Reviews, 26*, 22–35.

Raudenbush, S. W., & Bryk, A. (2002). *Hierarchical linear models: Applications and data analysis methods,* 2nd ed. Thousand Oaks, CA: Sage.

Reisen, C. A., Iracheta, M. A., Zea, M. C., Bianchi, F. T., & Poppen, P. J. (2010). Sex in public and private settings among Latino MSM. *AIDS Care, 22*, 697–704.

Reisen, C. A., Zea, M. C., Bianchi, F., Poppen, P. J., Shedlin, M. G., & Montes Penha, M. (2011). Latino gay and bisexual men's relationships with non-gay-identified MSM. *Journal of Homosexuality, 57*, 1004–1021.

Semple, S. J., Patterson, T. L., & Grant, I. (2003). HIV-positive gay and bisexual men: Predictors of unsafe sex. *AIDS Care, 15*, 3–15.

Tabet, S. R., de Moya, E. A., Holmes, K. K., Krone, M. R., Rosado de Quinones, M., Butler de Lister, M., Garris, I., Thorman, M., Castellanos, C., Swenson, P. D., Dallabetta, G. A., & Ryan, C. A. (1996). Sexual behaviors and risk factors for HIV infection among men who have sex with men in the Dominican Republic. *AIDS, 10*, 201–206.

Tewksbury, R. (2002). Bathhouse intercourse: Structural and behavioral aspects of an erotic oasis. *Deviant Behavior: An Interdisciplinary Journal, 23*, 75–112.

Van Beneden, C. A., O'Brian, K., Modesitt, S., Yusem, S., Rose, A., & Fleming, D. (2002). Sexual behaviors in an urban bathhouse 15 years into the HIV/AIDS epidemic. *Journal of Acquired Immune Deficiency Syndromes, 30*, 522–526.

Woods, W. J., Binson, D., Blair, J., Han, L., Spielberg, F., & Pollack, L. M. (2007). Probability sample estimates of bathhouse sexual risk behavior. *Journal of Acquired Immune Deficiency Syndromes, 45*, 231–238.

Zea, M. C., Reisen, C. A., Poppen, P. J., & Bianchi, F. T. (2009). Unprotected anal intercourse among Latino MSM: the role of characteristics of the person and the sexual encounter. *AIDS & Behavior, 13*, 700–715.

10 Clean Sweeps and Social Control in Latino Bisexual Male Sex Markets in New York City

Edgar Rivera Colón, Miguel Muñoz-Laboy, and Diana Hernández

INTRODUCTION

Jesus was in the bar of an Atlantic City casino after having spent most of his evening with his new girlfriend, Alicia. She moved there to work as a bartender.[1] They met in New York and when she found this job, Jesus decided to follow her. One evening, Jesus decided to go to another bar before returning to their apartment. The bartender brought Jesus a drink and said that this was from the gentleman sitting across the way. Jesus had some curiosity about men before that night, but never acted on it. He accepted the drink and after that night, he continued seeing this person for brief encounters that led to his first sexual intercourse with a man. For many young Latino men, the bar scene represents the initial sex marketplace to find their first male partners.

ON SEX MARKETS AND MARKETPLACES

In the field of HIV, we often overlook how sex marketplaces regulate the practices of young men who are there to shop for sex or find sexual partners. In their study of the sexual organization of Chicago, Laumann and his colleagues (2004) articulated two key notions that we use to frame our data: *sex markets* and *sexual marketplaces*. Laumann et al. define sex markets "as a subsystem of a community whose participants are mutually relevant to one another and generally share some common orientation by observing each other's strategies and evaluative criteria regarding sexual partnering" (pp. 12–13). Thus, the notion of a sex market is relational and grounded in behavioral observation as a means of social control. Sexual marketplaces are spatial units in which the interactions associated with sex markets take place. Sexual marketplaces index the local nature of the information and social control that drive sex markets. It is this idea of "local (bi)sexual culture(s)" that allows us to do a comparative analysis of sexual marketplaces over time and across space.

In this chapter, we conduct a comparative analysis of the sex marketplaces of Latino bisexual men in New York City between 2000 and 2009. Our aims are to identify the role that sexual marketplaces play in the sexual lives of Latino bisexual young men, particularly the impact of historical and geographic differences in the partnering and sex practices of bisexual Latino men as well as their implications for

HIV prevention research and interventions. Our ethnographic research on Latino male same-sex markets in New York City between the years of 2000 and 2009 led us to investigate the following key question: what are the political, technological, and social enabling conditions that have produced the behavioral differences over time that we have observed? More specifically, how do male friendship groups function as mechanisms of "intimate surveillance" vis-à-vis sexual partner selection in these marketplaces, and what are the digital platforms (i.e., cell phones, mobile technology, and Internet cruising) that enable these interactions? How might we frame these "local sexual cultures" within two macrodynamics of what we refer to as "intimate/participatory surveillance" (Rivera Colón, 2010, p. 3), and what social philosopher Gilles Deleuze (1992) has called "societies of control"?

Brief Historical Context of Same-Sex Marketplaces

To complicate the situation more, studying Latino bisexual spaces in New York City requires a clear understanding of the historical context of the city as a palimpsest of erotic spaces (Delany, 1999). Chauncey (1994) has documented how public spaces in New York City have been the center of heteroerotic and homoerotic interactions since as early as 1904. Streets, parks, and beaches have served for more than a century as areas for cruising, which was defined in the 1920s as gathering in places to meet other friends or to search for sexual partners and to have sex (Chauncey, 1994). Since the turn of the twentieth century, massive police efforts to control public sex have characterized New York City and this continues to be true today. As Chauncey (1994) demonstrates, in the 1940s and 1950s, men interested in erotic interactions with other men managed to develop strategies to avoid police interventions, including negotiating their way in the streets (e.g., manner of dress, eye contact, asking for a match, avoiding verbal solicitation of sex).

Another element that transformed the landscape of public sex in New York City was male prostitution. Male prostitution invaded spaces of traditional female prostitution. But it was the proliferation of gay bars during the early 1930s that changed the hustler scene, bringing male sex workers and potential clients under the shelter of bars and cheap cafeterias (Chauncey, 1994). Although this did not stop police persecution, it altered the landscape of male-centered public sex in New York City.

Public parks and other spaces were also widely used by heterosexual couples to engage in one-night stands or to have sex with lovers, friends, or co-workers. Both homosexuals and heterosexuals found in the parks secluded spots where couples could find privacy from their families and other people (Chauncey, 1994). Since the 1930s, subway station washrooms, movie theaters, and bathhouses became centers for homoerotic interactions in New York City, adding a new dimension to the landscapes of public sex between men. Activity became concentrated in those areas and, as a result, the parks were less frequented locales for public sexual encounters (Chauncey, 1994). However, the streets and parks of New York City played an essential role in the formation of New York's gay culture. As Chauncey (1994) indicates: "The streets and parks served them [gay men] as social centers as well as sites of rendezvous, places where they could meet others like themselves and find collective support for their rejection of the sexual and gender roles prescribed them. The mysterious bond between gay men that allowed them to locate and communicate with one another even in the settings potentially most hostile to them attests to the resiliency of their world and to the resources their subculture had made available to them" (Chauncey, 1994, pp. 204–205).

Through discussions on mapping male bisexuality, it has been demonstrated that there is a complex relationship between sexuality and space, both physical and social, in the construction of homoerotic relations among Latino men. Part of this can be explained by the complexity of bisexuality itself as an erstwhile "betwixt and between" (Turner, 1970, p. 93) category that functions as a deconstructive force relative to more established categories such as straight, gay, or even men who have sex with men (MSM). Consumer market dynamics and state-funded initiatives have facilitated the emergence of gay consumers, straight "metrosexuals,"[2] and MSM research funding: the relative institutional weight and discursive stability of these social actors/consolidated subjectivities stand in stark contrast to the paucity of bisexual institutions and the attending relative fluidity of bisexual identities and practices. That is to say, our ethnographic research indicates that Latino male bisexuality lives in the interstices of "gay" and "straight" subjectivities, discourses, sex markets, cultures, and institutions. Yet Latino male bisexuality remains significantly understudied and poorly understood, hence the purpose of the current study to contribute to the development of this field of study using ethnographically grounded social theory relevant to the ongoing HIV/AIDS epidemic among Latino communities in general and Latino male bisexual populations within a community in particular.

METHODS
Study Design

The data analyzed in this chapter emerged from two sources of data collected over a 9-year time span. Both are ethnographic studies on bisexual Latino men in New York City, the first of which was conducted in 2000, and the other is an ongoing study initiated in 2009. The studies incorporated three methods of inquiry including *key informant interviews* (interviews with individuals who have a broad knowledge of Latino male bisexuality from a historical, personal, service, or community-level perspective), *sexual histories* (detailed descriptions of sexual identity and behavior over the life course), as well as *field observations* of sexual marketplaces.

PROCEDURES
Sources of Data

The first study was conducted from 1998 to 2001 (*The Sexual Organization of Bisexually Active Latino Men*, NIMH Grant P50-MH43520: PI: A. Ehrhardt— Minority Supplement). As part of this first study we conducted 18 sexual histories with Latino bisexual men and 25 key informant interviews (Columbia University Department of Psychiatry and the New York State Psychiatric Institute Institutional Review Board IRB No. 3905; Federal Certificate of Confidentiality No. MH-00-07),[3] and systematic ethnographic observations for a period of 12 months in a variety of settings in which study participants found sexual partners including bars, nightclubs, street corners, and public parks. During the ethnographic work conducted in 2000, we observed that New York City parks and police were targeting the homoerotic place within a park in Washington Heights. These efforts to alter the landscape of the park characterize government in the truest sense of the word, that is, "the conduct of others' conduct" (Foucault, 1990). The state attempted to shape the patterns of action within the park by shaping the landscape of the park, which was expected to curtail certain behaviors via the threat of social control by outsiders. These renovation efforts were, in effect, a power technique deployed by the state in its effort to conduct others' conduct. It was an attempt to shape local practice through directing self-governance. Through spatial changes, the city attempted to shape the present and future practice of participants in the local sexual culture. The increase in traffic by recreational visitors effectively policed the sexual culture of the men in this space.

Our data from this early study suggest that by analyzing ethnographic case studies, we can begin to understand the complexities of sexuality, and in particular, how place provides the context for the nexus of societal structure and individual agency. This study reinforces other studies that have found sexual behavior to be contingent upon the context of sex. If the spatial context of sex changes, the configuration of erotic and sexual interactions also changes, which demonstrates that place and context should not be considered static, but rather fluid through space and time. Thus, having the capability to change the sexual milieu through spatial changes poses inevitable questions about intervention from the perspectives of the state and public health.

This initial ethnography laid the foundation together with two other pilot studies for a large scale study to examine the sexual market and geography of HIV/STI risk among Latino bisexual men in New York and New Jersey (*Gender, Power and Latino Men's HIV Risk*, 1R01HD056948-01A2: PI: M. Muñoz-Laboy). In this ongoing study, as of August 2009, we have conducted 60 sexual histories, interviewed 20 key informants, and conducted ethnographic observations in 10 bars and nightclubs (Columbia University IRB No. AAAE0494; Federal Certificate of Confidentiality No. CC-HD-09-84). Participants in both projects were identified in the sites where field observations were conducted as well as through snowball sampling techniques.

ANALYSIS OF DATA

Our analytical approach consisted of five steps: (1) to present an environmental description of the sex marketplaces; (2) to document the types of interactions between patterns; (3) to identify the sex that takes place in the marketplace and outside of it; (4) to compare the differences and similarities in sex marketplaces between the two cohorts; and (5) to apply the theoretical concepts of sex markets and intimate surveillance to identify the implications of changes in sex marketplaces for situational and individual-level HIV/STI risk for bisexual Latino men.

The authors independently examined the fieldnotes, key informant interviews, and sexual history transcripts and conducted open coding following the first three analytical steps above. Together with the larger research team from the R01 team noted above, they conducted steps 4 and 5. It is important to note that because this is not an individual-level analysis, we do not present data on the sample characteristics of both samples. However, suffice it to note that the total number of respondents, 123 (43 from the 2000 study and 80 from the 2009 study) participants, ranged in age from 18 to 63 years old, and ethnic background including immigrants and native-born Latinos included the Dominican Republic, Puerto Rico, Cuba, Mexico, Ecuador, and other Central and South American countries. Although the importance of individual background characteristics is taken for granted in HIV prevention research, there is an urgent need to study structural-environmental factors related to HIV risk and mediated by spaces and situations as advocated in

Chapter 1. Hence the focus here on an analysis of space or settings at the nexus of social structures and individual agency.

To conduct the main analysis, the authors selected two key sex marketplaces from the fieldnotes of both studies that represented the typical club experience of each interview cohort. We selected fieldnotes from two well-established Latino gay night clubs, Gargoyle and Eso Es! (pseudonyms), from the Spring/Summer 2000 and Fall 2009, respectively. Then we selected the sexual histories that best capture the common experiences of patrons in those two spaces.

RESULTS
Latino Nights at the Gargoyle: 2000

In the middle of New York's West Village, there was a gay nightclub that sponsored the biggest Latino nights in the area, the Gargoyle. We visited it first on a cold night during February 2000. The first floor was bright with an oval bar that served as the center of the floor. Around the bar, there were smaller areas at different levels with couches. Opposite the main entrance, there was a large piano. Patrons played the piano. The bar was packed with people, clean-shaven young and middle-age men. All the clubgoers were men. None appeared to be women or male-to-female transgender women. The decoration was mostly white, old wood and golden fixtures. The music from the piano dominated most of the floor, although a low beat music could be heard from the ceiling speakers. However, louder than any type of music were the voices of men speaking and laughing with each other. There were very few Latino men on the floor, either as staff or as patrons. Latinos were dancing on the basement floor.

Whether there was a Latino night or not, Latino men dominated the Gargoyle's basement dance floor. Latino men danced with each other, in groups, with people they just met, or by themselves. The dance area was rectangular. On one side, there was a small bar serving drinks. On the other side, there was a wall-length mirror. The north side of the room had a couch along the wall where people sat in the dark. In the south side of the room, there was a small elevated stage with three lowered stages with polls. Male dancers took the stage late at night. On Latino nights, the main attractions were not the dancers, but the patrons' dancing to techno-Latin music mixes and merengue songs.

Latino nights attracted a large number of Latino men, but also a number of white and African American men interested in Latino men. Most of the cruising did not happen through standing, making eye contact, or walking up and talking to someone. That occurred in the upper floor of the Gargoyle. In the basement, the cruising happened on the dance floor through dancing and making eye contact or simply bumping into someone. The Gargoyle's basement was the "making out" area. There was no dark or back room. However, Latino men and other patrons kissed, engaged in heavy petting, jerked each other off (mostly through their pants without pulling their penises out), or sat on each other's laps. The male dancers were more decorative than anything else and largely limited themselves to the stage. Latino male hustlers were usually at the bottom of the stairs, but they were four or five per night in a space that accommodated more than 70 people. The bathrooms were strictly monitored by two staff members. Large signs were posted restricting stall occupancy to one per person only.

The Gargoyle was the first nightclub that Hector (25 years old, college-educated, Puerto Rican financial planner) visited. He went there with a female friend of his. It was not atypical to see Latina young woman accompanying their male Latino gay or bisexual friends to the Gargoyle. After telling his friend that he was bisexual, she said: "Oh, I'm going to take you to this club." His reaction was:

But, my whole idea of being gay was I always thought it was older men with leather and chains, the butt part cut out. That was my vision of what a gay man was. So, I was always scared that I'm never going to go out. I'm never going to try and meet anybody. Because if this is what it's like, I don't want to have nothing to do with it. So, she told me, it's not like that. She says, "You've got to come out with me." And, she took me to [the Gargoyle]. I was nervous, completely nervous, because it was the first time I was in a gay bar and I didn't realize there were other guys like me. (BP005, 06/23/2000, 25 years old)

On that first night out, Hector did not dance. He sat on the couches and kept looking at the people dancing while having a few drinks.

There was this guy dancing that I was attracted to, and he kept looking at me. So, finally he approached me and started talking and he asked me, "Are you new here? I've never seen you before." So, he walked me to the car at the end of the night and something was telling me, I have to know if I'm gay, I have to know if I'm gay. That was my whole goal that night of going out with my friend, just to find out if I was gay. So, I told him, I said, "Look, don't think of me as a pervert, don't think of me as being sick. I need to know if this lifestyle is for me." He starts laughing, "Why what do you want to do?" I said, "I need to hold you." He was like, "Go ahead, hold me." I was like, "No, you don't understand." He's like, "Why is that?" "I need to hold your dick to see if it's something that I'm comfortable with." So, I did. It was just something that was real stupid and he just laughed about it. He was like, "Okay . . ." I was like, "I guess." He said, "Did you feel uncomfortable?" I was like, "Not at all." "Did you like it?" I was like, "Yeah." So, that was my first encounter, my first real encounter with another gay man. (BP005, 06/23/2000, 25 years old)

A week later Hector met him again in the Gargoyle, and went to his apartment and had sex for the first time with a man.

Well, he's a D.J. He was showing me his equipment and stuff like that and teaching me how to spin records and stuff like that. So, he's behind me, kissing up on my neck and I already knew at that time what I wanted. So, we got into it. We went on his bed and we started. He went down on me. I went down on him for the first time ever on anybody. And, then, I ended up fucking him, completely naked this time. We were completely naked and I ended up having sex with him. And, I loved it. The feeling that was going through my mind, I knew it was different than that first time, then when I had with the first time with my ex-girlfriend. And, I was comparing, as I'm having sex with him, oh my God, it's different, it is so much better, more relaxed and you know, it was only comparing the first time with each. Because now, today, I can honestly say that it really doesn't matter. I'm more selective of girls than with guys. With guys, not that it doesn't matter what they look like, but I'm more prone to have sex with a guy than I am with a girl because I already know what kind of girl I'm looking for. Do you understand what I'm saying? And, it's a certain look that I go for in a girl and when I find her, then it's completely different. (BP005, 06/23/2000, 25 years old)

175

Clean Sweeps and Social Control in Latino Bisexual Male Sex Markets in New York City

The social scene of the Gargoyle, like other clubs that would emerge in the first decade of the twentieth century primarily in Manhattan, was constructed in many ways in opposition to the gay bars and nightclubs of the 1980s and 1990s that were generally characterized by having backrooms and darkrooms for sex to take place in the premises. During his municipal administration, Rudolph Giuliani implemented closures of gay bath houses, sex clubs, and public sex spaces in New York City.[4]

Clubs like the Gargoyle were *"sanitized"*[5] and reconfigured to become spaces of social, erotic (not necessarily sexual) entertainment and as primary venues for meeting potential sexual partners. Other clubs, like the West Village's now defunct Uncle Charlie's or Chelsea's still open Splash, served as models for "cleaned-up" homoerotic sexual cultures in Manhattan's gay bars and clubs. Splash even featured a large bar behind which a black-tiled shower and male dancers under the faucet soaping up, but rarely interacting with the patrons. Splash's public shower referenced the sexual freedom of the now shuttered gay bathhouses while retaining a very controlled and literally "washed up" version of antecedent homoerotic sexual cultures of the 1960s, 1970s, and 1980s.

For Latino bisexual young men, visiting clubs like the Gargoyle, Splash, or Uncle Charlie's was their initiation in mapping out their sex marketplaces to find male partners. Other same-sex marketplaces were through social events organized by more traditional social networks (e.g., friends, work, and school) of Latino bisexual young men, but also public spaces such as areas of public parks in Latino neighborhoods. These other same-sex marketplaces have not changed dramatically between the years 2000 and 2010. However, the sex marketplace scenes such as the Gargoyle have changed significantly over the past 10 years. In the next section, we will describe a current sex marketplace for Latino bisexual young men in 2009 illustrated by excerpts of fieldnotes from the Eso Es! Club in Washington Heights.

The Eso Es! Club: Halloween 2009 (Fieldnotes Written on November 2, 2009)

"It was Halloween in New York City. The city was alight with the distracted mirth that diffuses throughout its street on a day of sanctioned transformations and inversions. The night air had a cool lift to it and brushed against the manic pace of people and cars that made Washington Heights, a sprawling Dominican enclave in Upper Manhattan, the very definition of urban immigrant motion and conviviality. Midnight took its regal mantle to lord over the best remnants of Halloween in this part of the city: when the children were slumbering after a day of mostly sugary treating, with a few tricks added in for good measure, and the adult revelers come out to play. Eso Es! is a Latino gay club located a few blocks from the steel majesty of the George Washington Bridge. Tonight definitely had an added playfulness to the usual drinking, dancing, chatting, and cruising that typify Saturday nights at the Eso Es! bar."

"This Halloween a jungle theme dominated the décor at Eso Es! The 'jungles vines' were actually large strips of fabric hanging from the ceiling. The vines came in a plethora of colors, but green was the predominant one. Along the north wall of the club were a series of small skulls hung up at equidistant intervals. The skulls were laced with fake spider webs. Perhaps, it was a little memento from the club staff to its patrons on a night where the lines between the living and the dead, as well as humans and animals, were blurred. On the opposite wall, a life-sized Frankenstein doll occupied a whole window pane. The bartenders were dressed up in animal costumes consistent with the jungle theme (e.g., cats, lions, cheetahs, panthers). Their makeup jobs had an elaborate and professional quality to them. The bartenders had not been shy about using body paint either. They were all sporting tails and are wearing sexy bikini briefs colored to match their beastly avatars."

"The D-shaped bar has a white top upon which two go-go boys and a go-girl undulated their bodies in search of the next bill and a friendly patron's testing of the wares. Tucked into the northeast corner, the D.J. booth sits atop a small stage area where people stood to get a more global view of the crowd. Closer to the southeast corner, the bathroom has two individual toilets and two urinals in the back separated by a half-wall. There are three hand washing basins opposite the doors to the individual toilets and a large mirror that frames the basins. There is a bowl also in the bathroom full of Department of Health subway-themed condoms for the taking. In the southwest corner of the bar, there is a small stage and a rather large screen playing music videos. The World Series game was on one of the smaller monitors and many patrons intermittently took notice of the ongoing game."

"The crowd itself was predominantly made up of Latino men in their 20s and 30s. Given its location in Washington Heights, many of the patrons are, in fact, first and second generation Dominicans, but Eso Es! was not exclusively Dominican or male for that matter. There was a significant group of Latinas who are mostly in their 20s and 30s as well. There was also a group of black men some of whom seem to be in their 40s. There were a few Asian and white male club-goers as well as some black and white women. Although Eso Es! was partially segregated spatially by race, gender, and age, the segregation was very porous and shifted throughout the night."

"The bar's south side was a real hot spot and where the most dancing went on during the night and, consequently, always a bit crowded. On this Halloween night, any location in the bar was a site of dancing. Most of the dancing couples appeared to be friends having a go at it. Most of the dirty dancing looked like friends testing each other's skills at hip-gyrating provocations, which seemed to end with laughter and finger pointing at who might be considered the most shameless "sucia" [dirty female] for the moment. Opposite one side of the bar was a long bench where many men sat or stood to get a good look at the crowd. At various points as the night progressed, different groups of men yelled or made hand signals to go outside for a smoke or simply to get a breath of fresh air as the air conditioning struggled to keep Eso Es! cool as the amount of bodies multiply dramatically and heated up the place. The music was loud to the point of distraction, but by no means unusually so for this kind of venue" (Excerpts from Fieldnotes, Eso Es! Club, Washington Heights, NYC, Fall 2009).

As the night progressed, it became clear to us that the Latino men at Eso Es! were part of friendship networks that may or may not overlap with sexual partnering networks. The friendship networks tended to be fairly stable groups that sat, stood, drank, and danced together throughout the night at the bar. They also went to the bathroom together in groups of two and three and went out for smoking breaks and bodega runs as well. These breaks or store runs disaggregated members from the mass of bar patrons that allowed for more animated conversations by friendship network members. There were interesting gender dynamics at play here as well. The friendship networks were comparatively denser among Latino men who presented as more feminine in their gender expressions. Many of the more "butch" presenting men tended to come alone or in duos or maybe groups of three. A few more "butch" presenting men were integrated into the larger friendship networks, but the majority of the members were feminine presenting men. Many of these Latino men had navel rings that were exposed by virtue of their costumes.

We watched the men at Eso Es! look at each other and cruise: there was very little actual "hooking up" in terms of physical closeness, caressing, dirty dancing, kissing, etc. Or to put it another way, given the hypersexualized character of adult Halloween social play, we expected to see more of that behavior. Those expectations were not realized.

What was very visible that night at Eso Es! was an array of hand-held digital communications devices and the constant messaging that went on as people danced, talked, and drank. People showed text messages and photos to each other and many patrons took pictures of the go-go dancers using their cell phones or smart-phones. Groups of friends posed as another friend took a photo of their Halloween night out. We can only imagine how many of these photos from that night at Eso Es! made their way to photo galleries on social networking sites. The use of digital communications platforms was one key difference from our ethnographic research at the Gargoyle a decade ago and what we observed at the Eso Es! club that night.

Sex Marketplaces for Female Partners: Now and Then

In spite of these technological and social changes, female sex marketplaces for Latino bisexual men have remained practically unchanged. The nightclub scene of 2000 or 2009 has not served as the main sex marketplaces for finding female partners for bisexual Latino men. Among our sample of Latino bisexual men in 2000, women partners were met mostly through work, school, or social events organized by members of other social networks (e.g., friends, relatives, or neighbors).

A subgroup of bisexual men also had sex with female sex workers. For example, Marcos (39 years old) has been in a relationship with another man in New York City for 3 years. He periodically (i.e., about once a month) had sex with women whom he met through work or his female friends. However, when he visited the Dominican Republic, his friends, cousins, and he frequented weekend establishments where customers can select a woman with whom to spend the night and/or the weekend. This pattern of visiting sex work establishments during return trips to their respective Latin American countries of origin, where commercial sex service is cheaper than in New York City, has remained consistent for some of our sample at present as it did for our prior group of research participants.

Reflecting an overall secular trend in American society, our present research subjects are deeply engaged in using Internet sex and dating sites and cellular phones of all kinds to find and connect with potential sex partners. In comparing the straight venues we visited with a club like Eso Es!, we observed a much more marked use of mobile phone devices in these Latino same-sex sex marketplaces. Of course, bisexual Latino men in nightclubs use the same codes and cues of cruising as their straight counterparts (e.g., casually starting up or breaking into conversations at the bar with someone they are interested in or being introduced by a third party who might know a potential sex partner).

Although female sex work establishments remain a sex marketplace for a number of bisexual Latino men in our sample, there have been enormous transformations in the ways transactional sex is practiced since 2000. In brief, we can describe this transformation as a shift from clients wanting to experience sexual pleasure and release to now seeking, what some scholars have termed, "the girlfriend experience." In effect, the client spends longer periods of time establishing a form of temporary intimacy with the female sex worker(s) he patronizes. Although a minority of bisexual Latino men in both our samples visited female sex workers, these transformations in this particular sex marketplace are relevant when examining HIV risk in this population.

Our data on Latino bisexual men confirm that work, school, and the Internet are the main types of female sex marketplaces and that nightclubs, church, or sex work establishments are relatively marginal venues for female sex partners. Thus, our participants' marketplaces for female partners are much more diversified and have a much wider social ambit. In contradistinction, our participants' sex marketplaces for male partners are constricted to a number of specified venues wherein nightclubs and specific sections of public parks play key roles in their spatial organization of their same-sex sexuality. Of course, this is not to say that they do not have sex with male partners outside the parameters of the above sex marketplaces.

Intimate/Participatory Surveillance

Technological innovations that eventually become consumer items reflect and transform a set of subtending social relations. Our research at Eso Es! led us to wonder how these digital platforms sanitize (see footnote 5) Latino male same-sex sexual marketplaces. This sanitizing process is also a mechanism for distributing and managing stigma. Parker and Aggleton (2003, p. 448) have argued: "Stigma and stigmatization function, quite literally, at the point of intersection between culture, power and difference—and it is only by exploring the relationship between these different categories that it becomes possible to understand stigma and stigmatization not merely as an isolated phenomenon, or expressions of individual attitudes or of cultural values, but as central to the constitution of the social order." How was stigma being managed that night at Eso Es! and what parts of the social order were being constituted through behaviors that were observable and those that were noticeably absent? Why was there such little physical sexual display in Eso Es! in the fall of 2009 as compared to the Gargoyle just a decade earlier? What did our respective ethnographic projects on Latino male same-sex marketplaces tell us about the sanitizing of these spaces in the past decade? What were the underlying factors that made our fieldnotes in 2009 less descriptive of sexual behavior than just 10 years ago in the same city with very similar populations of Latino men? What social factors could account for such a shift?

Part of the answer to the above set of queries can be found in the Latino gay argot term "sucia" mentioned in the previous section, which literally means "dirty woman," but would probably be better translated into something like "nasty girl" or "dirty slut." The first thing to notice about this term, which we heard a number of times at Eso Es!, is the gender play at work: the "sucia" usually references a feminine presenting Latino man. Clearly, organizing sexual and gender inequality among Latino men entails assigning subordinate sexual and gender roles to some men and not others (Lancaster, 1994). Part of this reproduction of inequality is marking some men as different or, more to the point, morally degraded via their easy sexual availability and ostensibly having a large number of male sexual partners. The moral degradation that we are referring to here is in the register of selling damaged or very used goods in a given same-sex marketplace. It is not a direct equivalent to more religiously based notions of moral degradation. Thus, what is dirty about the Latino male "sucia" in the context of a Latino male same-sex marketplace such as Eso Es! is that the "sucia" is perceived as more likely to be seropositive because he is so easily available for sex and shameless about it. Our argument is that the trope of the "sucia" is animated by sex negativity, which informs the attitudes and behaviors of the friendship groups at clubs such as Eso Es! The comparative lack of sexual display between Latino men at this club is indicative of two dynamics: (1) a desire not to play one's hand too early in a public space where as the night goes on better options might materialize, and (2) a desire to not be seen as a "sucia" by potential male sexual partners. Both these desires are part of a sanitizing impression management that has increased in the past decade in response to state-level repression of sexual marketplaces, such as the bathhouses and sex clubs of a decade ago, and an attending HIV phobia that materializes as a restrictive sexual behavior repertoire compared to a sex marketplace such as the Gargoyle during an earlier period. Although we did not document changes in levels of sex phobia between these two time periods (defined here as the irrational fear and subsequent rejection of public sexual expression), our data suggest a historical trend toward the sanitation of the public space. In this way, public sexual expressions are equated to and are as much a target for public scrutiny as public smoking, sidewalk spitting, or shooting drugs.

Moreover, digital forms of communication via cell phones that provide access to the Internet and mobile applications are a mediating influence in sexual partner selection resulting in the reduction of potential embarrassment for friendship network members by *not* making those sexual plays in a public space in front of their friends, enemies, or potential sex/romantic partners. In fact, the immediate connection created by mobile technologies such as Grinder®, Facebook®, Flickr®, and gay cruising sites facilitates local hookups that do not require a public meeting space as was the case in the past. We argue that these new digital platforms have reduced some socially pricey transactions that were available for public scrutiny in pre-internet gay clubs. This also means that part of this selection process has been privatized. It is this privatization of cruising and sex partner selection that helps mitigate the "sucia effect" and decreases the stigma to those who cruise by other means than the kind of public sex we observed in the Gargoyle a decade ago. These digital platforms are embedded in the friendship groups we observed and the policing of displays of physical sexuality as well as partner selection in Latino male same-sex marketplaces or what we mean by "intimate surveillance." It is a form of surveillance that presents itself as a concern for a friend's reputation and health and an attempt to offer a respite from the burdens of HIV stigma or "sucia" stigma. Nonetheless, it is a form of micropolicing that empowers itself through digital means, but uses the tried and true forces of stigma to "clean up" the self-images of Latino men who engage in same-sex practices and especially those whose sexual lives are produced in the interstices of gay and straight erotic and social worlds (i.e., Latino bisexual men).

We contend as well that "intimate surveillance" is part of a larger dynamic that we have conceptualized as "participatory surveillance" (Rivera Colón, 2010, p. 3). Building on Foucault's notion of the panopticon (Foucault, 1995) and the ideal of 1960s and 1970s social movements of bringing all minoritarian subjects (Muñoz, 1999) into a "participatory democracy" (Hayden, 2005), we argue that the emergence of hand-held digital communications devices with photo, video, and Internet capacities and the rise of reality television in the past decade as the television genre of choice signal the convergence of surveillance and entertainment as the cultural forms of choice for the coming period.

The asymptotic theoretical scenario that informs our formulation is that the ultimate dystopian outcome of social control will be an American society in which there are as many television channels as they are people and that everyone will be a star of his or her own reality show while being a spectator to the reality shows of all the other members of the U.S. population, that is to say, a population that is constantly under surveillance and is entertained simultaneously. It is this digital, dystopian ideal that informs this preliminary conceptualization of "participatory surveillance" (Rivera Colón, 2010, p. 3). One potentially empowering aspect of technology is the prenegotiation that occurs prior to physical contact. Issues such as HIV status, condom use, and a myriad of other characteristics can be discussed prior to meeting in ways that may reduce stigma and promote discussion of these matters. Furthermore, we see both "intimate surveillance" and "participatory surveillance" (Rivera Colón, 2010, p. 3) as partial dynamics within what social philosopher Gilles Deleuze has called "societies of control" (Deleuze, 1992). Extending Foucault's work on disciplinary societies wherein institutions are built in tandem with forms of socially sanctioned knowledge (e.g., mental asylums and psychiatric discourses), Deleuze argued that Western advanced capitalist societies were moving beyond this disciplinary model toward a new model that is more flexible and in little need of overarching institutions. Deleuze writes: "The disciplinary man was a discontinuous producer of energy, but the man of control is undulatory, in orbit, in continuous network. Everywhere surfing has replaced the older sports" (Deleuze, 1992, p. 5).

Contemporary Latino same-sex marketplaces have shifted to this undulation, networking, and surfing modality. State repression provided the political and economic impetus for the narrowing of behaviors that we have observed in the past decade. The digital revolution has literally put stigma management into the hands of the friendship groups we have described while wider social logics (e.g., "intimate surveillance," "participatory surveillance") have provided the productive pleasures that not being identified as a "sucia" can afford. However, the relationship is not exactly linear in that the digital revolution to which we refer here can at once frustrate and recapitulate state social control. Nevertheless, these technological advancements and shifting social interactions have important implications for risk management in safety and HIV as discussed in more detail below.

DISCUSSION

Our field observations are most useful in their ability to make inferences on the implications for public health. Most importantly, through this work we have identified sex marketplaces and gaps in structural approaches to HIV risk for bisexual Latino men. In our analysis, we compare two sex marketplaces at two time points to demonstrate how historical and social environment changes influence the ways bisexual Latino men seek sexual partnerships. At first glance, it may seem that these changes are simply a reflection of changes in cruising and courtship (i.e., this is how things were in the past and these are the rules now) with no implications to HIV/STI risk. However, if we look carefully at the above case study we see four implications for HIV/STI risk and prevention:

1. *Sanitization of sex marketplaces may lead to HIV/STI risk.* As the same-sex marketplaces become sanitized by state repression and ideological/moral forces, there appears to be less sex, comparatively speaking, on the premises. We argue

that this lack of public sex is managed by our research subjects through utilization of technological devices to prenegotiate sexual encounters and that this engenders a higher impetus to move faster into anal intercourse, which may lead to higher HIV/STI risk. Face-to-face interactions often require more time to build connections and extract pertinent information; however, using digital technology allows people to "cut to the chase" and fast forward to riskier behavior in less time. According to our ethnographic research, sex on the premises of nightclubs is regulated by the conditions of the space where in fact anal sex is least likely to occur. Even when anal sex takes place, the provision of condoms at these sites could serve as a structural protective factor. The question that remains in abeyance is, "what impact does providing condoms *in situ* actually have on condom usage beyond the space of the nightclubs?" There is no doubt that condom provision is a positive, proactive public health strategy. Thus, prevention campaigning should also begin to focus on sex that takes place after the nightclub or that is initiated as a result of social networking sites (using social media as an intervention tool is discussed in greater detail below).

2. *Same-sex marketplaces may potentially lead to HIV risk.* For bisexual Latino men, their sex marketplaces with women partners is diversified, with ample traditional and nontraditional spaces from which to find female partners and establish, if so desired, long-term relationships with them. In other words, if they want a one night stand, they can go to a bar or a party hosted by any of their friends. But if they are interested in dating and having a long-term relationship, they can meet partners through friendship and kinship networks. In contrast, the sex marketplaces for bisexual Latino men are regulated by the social structure of a heterosexist system of relations in which same-sex relationships are not sanctioned and long-term relationships are stigmatized through social policy (e.g., the prohibition of same-sex marriage) and ingrained social norms of proper masculinity (e.g., real men are not in erotic/romantic relationships with other men). The same-sex marketplaces for bisexual Latino men are limited, restricted, and opportunistic because these spaces are accessed and carved out within their dominant heterosexual lives. Thus, with few exceptions, male partners become time-bounded commodities of "pleasure," "sexual release," or "short-term love" (phrases used by many of our participants when referring to sex with males) with limited capacity for long-term intimacy. Future research should establish whether the nature of these types of encounters lead to higher HIV risk than if the sex marketplaces were, in fact, structured in parallel ways to the sex marketplaces for finding women.

3. *Heterosexual marketplaces are also sources of sexual risk.* If for the most part men are commodified as pleasurable goods, women are also commodified by our participants because of their social value and their reproductive capacity. Having girlfriends, wives, and children is a well-documented social expectation of traditional Latino men's masculinity. The masculinity of the men in both cohorts is under constant surveillance by kinship and friendship networks. From a cost-benefit perspective, Latino bisexual men's public relationships with women reduce the burden of this ubiquitous heteronormative surveillance and increase their male privilege in their home communities. That is not to say that bisexual men make rational, calculated decisions about their partnership choices, but rather that this cost-benefit dynamic might be operating in the background when they are accessing sex marketplaces for women. Furthermore, because their relations with women can be long term and socially desirable, men allow themselves

to fall in love and create intimate bonds in ways that are more difficult to do with their male partners. This social reality is combined with the fact that at the advent of the third decade of the AIDS epidemic, many men in our study still associate HIV risk with sex with men and not sex with women. In the absence of the threat of pregnancy, bisexual men in the study do not regularly use condoms during vaginal intercourse. Men in both cohorts were prone to have unprotected vaginal sex with women that they met through their workplace, school, or through family and friendship networks. Moreover, men in our sample exhibited much more consistent condom use with partners they met in nightclubs or in sex work venues. Nonetheless, we still have a limited understanding of how pregnancy intentions and the social structure of fatherhood may lead to HIV/STI risk or protective decision-making.

4. *High demand and low offer dispositions bisexual Latino men to be risk-takers.* Openly identified bisexual men are often stigmatized and considered to be untrustworthy or closeted gay men. However, "straight-looking guys" (i.e., individuals who conform to ideal images of masculinity) are viewed as "hot," desirable commodities by other men in the club scene. Bisexual Latino men in our study often, but not always, conform to this performative image, and are in high demand by other Latino and non-Latino men in the club scene. As documented by Ayala et al. (2001) and other scholars, the need to perform a risk-taking masculinity among Latinos was a critical aspect of the ways the men we studied interacted sexually with other men in both club scenes as well as with women in their respective sex marketplaces. This seems to be more evident across racial-ethnic sexual interactions where racialized images of sexual performance are expected and it was up to the men in our study to live up to those images.

CONCLUSIONS

Our observations of the shifts and differences in sex marketplaces lead us to conclude that the digital revolution provides an opportunity to capitalize on social media as an HIV prevention and intervention tool for Latino bisexual men. Research on the impact of such interventions has demonstrated favorable results on the part of increased condom use and self-efficacy among at-risk populations (Noar, 2008). The development of such interventions for Latino bisexual men would require particular cultural foci along with messaging geared toward a sexually diverse group.

From the state perspective, intervening in club scenes serves to sanitize the public sphere by eliminating spaces in which "undesirable" behavior is practiced; by increasing perceived and actual levels of safety, given that environments such as nightclubs and surroundings could serve as spaces to commit crimes ranging from indecent exposure and solicitation to violent acts; and/or by improving property values through gentrification and perceived beautification of city spaces. Repression of sexual expression by the State can promote internationalization of stigma (the unacceptability of bisexuality) and sexual transgression (unplanned sexual encounters under unsafe conditions for condom use). A form of structural intervention is to promote the acceptance of sexual diversity and sexual solidarity.

In the world of technology, new applications are created, marketed, and implemented constantly. Yet, innovative interventions are still lacking. As such, many opportunities exist for constructive partnerships between information technology specialists and social networking researchers to generate mapping applications for harm reduction purposes. For example, a "safe clubbing" application might encourage users to have fun while minimizing risks by use of harm reduction messages. Clubs might also utilize this application to stream messages about their club's location, promotions, and amenities including the location of condom bowls for example. Mapping functions can be installed on mobile devices to search nearby locations that sell or provide free condoms and lubrication, together with maps of the best locations to engage in lower level risk behavior such as kissing, cuddling, or oral sex. Mapping applications can also be devised to locate testing sites and to support centers and other technologies that facilitate access to care. Users can also find and network with individuals who are committed to safe sex and/or creating dialogues for support on living bisexual lives through social networking technologies.

The incorporation of these innovative technology-based intervention methods would be consistent with lifestyle behaviors of the target population as well as today's society. Developing an intervention of this sort will allow us to integrate the voices of Latino bisexual men in the design and streamlining of the HIV/AIDS continuum of care. Moreover, intervening in this mode can create strategies and greater accessibility with higher population impacts than creating a series of human-facilitated individual-level interventions. In the interim of the development of more policy-relevant research on bisexuality and HIV, Internet-based and cell phone-based interventions can function as urgently needed stepping stones to create sustainable solutions for bisexual Latino men's vulnerabilities and lives.

NOTES

1. The names of the study respondents cited in this chapter are pseudonyms to protect informants' privacy in compliance with human subject and institutional review board procedures.
2. The term "metrosexual," coined by Mark Simpson, is often associated with straight men who devote considerable attention to their physical appearance. It is often used to distinguish heterosexual men from their gay counterparts. http://www.salon.com/entertainment/feature/2002/07/22/metrosexual.
3. Miguel Muñoz-Laboy, the principal investigator on both projects, is affiliated with the HIV Center and the Department of Sociomedical Sciences in the Mailman School of Public Health. IRB clearance at both institutions is required of all researchers at Columbia University Medical Center.
4. This occurred in part as a response to the growing HIV/AIDS epidemic but also in his broader effort to convert New York City to a "revanchist" state where sex and poverty were criminalized and heavily sanctioned in order to sanitize the city and accommodate the gentrification process (Smith, 1996),
5. "Sanitized" in this context refers to a narrowing of public sex and displays of physical affection, particularly in gay clubs where this was once quite commonplace.

REFERENCES

Asencio, M. (2002). *Sex and sexuality among New York's Puerto Rican youth.* Boulder, CO: Lynne Reiner Publishers.

Ayala, G., & Diaz, R. (2001). Racism, poverty and other truths about sex: Race, class and HIV risk among Latino gay men. *Revista Interamericana de Psicologia/Interamercan Journal of Psychology, 35,* 59–77.

Chauncey, G. (1994). *Gay New York: Gender, urban culture and the making of the gay male world, 1890–1940.* New York: HarperCollins.

Decena, C. U. (2008). Tacit subjects. *GLQ: Journal of Lesbian and Gay Studies, 14*(2–3), 339–359.

Delany, S. (1988). *The motion of light in water: Sex and science fiction writing in the east village:* Minneapolis: University of Minnesota Press.

Delany, S. (1999). *Times Square red, Times Square blue.* New York: New York University Press.

Deleuze, G. (1992). *Postscript on Societies of Control.* October, 59, 3–7.

Diaz, R. M. (1997). *Latino gay men and HIV: Culture, sexuality, and risk behavior.* New York: Routledge.

Foucault, M. (1990). *The History of Sexuality: An Introduction.* Vol. I. Trans. by Robert Hurley. New York: Vintage Books.

Foucault, M. (1995). *Discipline and punish: The birth of the prison.* New York: Vintage.

Guttman, M. C. (1996). *The meanings of macho: Being a man in Mexico City.* Berkeley: University of California Press.

Hayden, T. (2005). *The Port Huron statement: The vision call of the 1960s revolution.* New York: Avalon.

Lancaster, R. (1994). *Life Is hard: Machismo, danger, and the intimacy of power in Nicaragua.* Berkeley: University of California Press.

Laumann, E. O., Ellingson, S., Mahay, J., Paik, A., & Youm, Y. (2004). *The sexual organization of the city.* Chicago: The University of Chicago Press.

Muñoz, J. E. (1999). *Disidentifications: Queers of color and the performance of politics.* Minneapolis: University of Minnesota Press.

Noar, S. M. (2008). Behavioral interventions to reduce HIV-related sexual risk behavior: Review and synthesis of meta-analytic evidence. *AIDS Behavior, 12,* 335–353.

Parker R., & Aggleton, P. (2003). HIV and AIDS-related stigma and discrimination: A conceptual framework and implications for action. In R. Parker & P. Aggleton (Eds.), *Culture, society, and sexuality: A reader* (pp. 443–458). New York: Routledge.

Rivera Colón, E. (2010). Participatory surveillance: Incarnational techniques in American dystopias in the making. Talk given at New York City's new museum's projects for a revolution in New York: Experiments in Collective Research and Action, 3.

Smith, N. (1996). *The new urban frontier—gentrification and the revanchist city.* New York: Routledge.

Turner, V. (1970). *The forest of symbols: aspects of ndembu ritual.* Ithaca, NY: Cornell University Press.

11 Latina Transgender Women

The Social Context of HIV Risk and Responsive Multilevel Prevention Capacity Building

Frank Galvan and JoAnne Keatley

This chapter focuses on one population greatly impacted by HIV, Latina transgender women. It consists of two major sections. The first section provides an overview of how HIV has disproportionately affected transgender women and examines specific factors that contribute to the spread of HIV among Latina transgender women. The second section provides a personal reflection on how capacity building in one community has led to the creation of local, state, and national programs and services that address the needs of transgender women in culturally responsive and affirming ways and that can serve as models for other transgender communities. This approach to the chapter was followed to emphasize that the problems faced by Latina transgender women that elevate their risk for HIV infection can be successfully addressed through capacity-building efforts that involve the participation of transgender women in the planning and implementation of programs directed to them.

The structural-environmental (SE) model presented in Chapter 1 provided the theoretical context through which the structural-environmental factors that contribute to HIV risk are examined. Some of these factors include stigma, discrimination, limited employment opportunities, physical and sexual violence, immigration issues, and racism. These examples parallel some of the factors provided in the model.

The model also identified individual factors contributing to HIV risk. Some of the individual factors examined in this chapter include mental health problems, social isolation, and incarceration, oftentimes due to engagement in commercial sex work. The use of alcohol and other substances, partially as a way of coping with the stress of *transphobia*, is also covered.

Consistent with the SE model's incorporation of HIV-related sexual risk behaviors and resilience, both are also covered in this chapter. Unsafe sexual practices and commercial sex work are examined in some depth. Resilience is covered in two ways. First, in the "personal reflection" section, the capacity building that resulted in the development of programs for the transgender community can be seen as a way of promoting resilience in that it fosters active coping to improve one's community's situation, and as a result, one's own situation as well, and also it creates environmental resources that subsequently can be used by transgender women. Second, in "Recommendations for Future Research," a form of resilience, "collective self-esteem," is described. This final section also makes the argument that future research should identify additional ways to increase resilience among transgender women.

CHALLENGES IN COLLECTING INFORMATION ON LATINA TRANSGENDER WOMEN

Individuals in search of information on Latina transgender women in the research literature will immediately be faced with several challenges. The first is that there is very little scholarly research that includes Latina transgender women. A review of the literature through PsychInfo using the key term "transgender" yields 2309 citations. However, combining the term "transgender" with either "Latina," "Latinas," "Hispanic," Hispanics," "Latino," or "Latinos" yields, at the most, only 27 citations. Thus it is necessary to rely primarily on the published literature that describes the experiences of transgender women in general in order to obtain an understanding of the variety of issues that may be faced by Latina transgender women.

A second challenge is that scholarly articles often include Latina transgender women combined with other groups that are believed to share common experiences with them. However, these articles often do not attempt to explore any differences that may exist between the Latina transgender women and the members of the other subgroups. For example, Latina transgender women are included in articles that also include Latino gay or bisexual men, but with no separate descriptions of the Latina transgender women as compared to the Latino men (Ramirez-Valles et al., 2008). As a result of combining findings of Latina transgender women with those of the other groups, there is limited information regarding the extent to which Latina transgender women may actually be similar to or different from these other groups.

In the reports of the studies described in this chapter, whenever possible, information is provided using data that specifically describe the experiences of Latina transgender women. However, it will be necessary to supplement this with information based on transgender women in general for the reasons described above. Table 11.1 lists all the journal articles used in this chapter to describe the experiences of transgender women living in the United States. Information is provided on the extent of participation by Latina transgender women in each study.

Another challenge worth noting is the fact that individuals who are transgender are referred to and also refer to themselves by different terms. Such terms include but are not limited to the following: *transsexual, transvestite, woman, drag queen, cross-dresser,* and *gender queer* (Bockting et al., 2005; Herbst et al., 2008; Melendez & Pinto, 2009; Rosser, Oakes, Bockting, & Miner, 2007). Among Latina transgender women, a variety of terms also exists. In addition to *homosexual,* others include *hombres muy afeminados* ("very feminine men") and *mujeres completas* ("complete women") (Infante, Sosa-Rubi, & Magali Cuadra, 2009), as well as *vestidas* ("the ones who dress up," using the Spanish feminine ending) (Diaz, 1998, p. 56; Prieur, 1998, p. 25). Although the variety of terms used does allow for individuals to use the descriptions that they feel are most appropriate for themselves, one result of not using consistent terminology to identify transgender women is that this can lead to confusion.

Table 11.1 Percent of Latina Transgender Women in the Cited Studies from the United States

Author	Number of Participants	Percent Latina Transgender Women
Bockting et al. (2005)	181	Information not provided
Clements-Nolle et al. (2001)	392	27.0
De Santis (2009)	1757	Information not provided
Edwards, Fisher, and Reynolds (2007)	2126	41.0
Garofalo et al. (2006)	51	16.0
Harawa and Bingham (2009)	128	39.0
Herbst et al. (2008)	Approximately 3300	Approximately 18.0
Hwahng and Nuttbrock (2007)	Information not provided	Information not provided
Kenagy (2005)	182	6.1
Koken, Bimbi, and Parsons (2009)	20	40.0
Melendez and Pinto (2007)	20	80.0
Melendez and Pinto (2009)	20	80.0
Nemoto et al. (2004)	332	33.1
Nuttbrock et al. (2009)	517	47.6
Operario, Soma, and Underhill (2008)	6405	Information not provided
Ramirez-Valles et al. (2008)	94	100.0
Reback et al. (2005)	244	49.2
Reisner et al. (2009)	11	36.4
Rosser et al. (2007)	1229	4.1
Sanchez and Vilain (2009)	53	0.0
Sausa, Keatley, and Operario (2007)	48	31.3
Schulden et al. (2008)	559	42.0
Sevelius et al. (2009)	153	27.0
Wilson et al. (2009)	151	38.0

Although the word *transgender* has been used primarily only in the past 10–20 years to refer to an individual who takes on a gender different from the sex assigned to them at birth, this same term has also been used to refer to a broader range of "gender-variant practices and identities" (Stryker, 2008, p. 19). This broader definition of *transgender* is based on the belief that gender variance is not limited to only one particular expression (Stryker, 2008). It may include individuals who change their physical appearance through hormones or surgery; it may also include others who do not change their physical bodies but instead express themselves through different behaviors or ways of presenting themselves (Herbst et al., 2008).

Yet another challenge is that, as noted above, gender identity is sometimes conflated with sexual orientation, although they are not the same constructs, with the former term referring to the gender to which one feels he or she pertains and the latter term referring to the gender to which one is sexually attracted. An example of such conflation is found in the book *Mema's House, Mexico City: On Transvestites, Queens, and Machos* (Prieur, 1998). The study participants were individuals who were assigned a male sex at birth but who underwent breast implants, hormone injections, and injections of oils to give their buttocks and hips a feminine appearance. In addition, they identified as females, took on female names, and, in some cases, even desired sex change operations. Yet they are referred throughout the book as *transvestic homosexuals*, and even they refer to themselves as *homosexuals*. Such conflation of gender identity and sexual orientation contributes to the confusion already noted above that may occur when consistent terminology is not used to describe transgender women.

A final challenge deals with trying to describe the experiences of transgender women from epochs or times that occurred before the current understandings of gender identity existed. For example, in previous time periods, Latin Americans who were described as being homosexual or transvestite may in fact have been more accurately described as being transgender. We are left having to infer this from all the best possible information available and, as stated by Stryker (2008), "apply(ing) it to people who might not (have applied) it to themselves" (p. 24). All of these challenges demonstrate the very real difficulties that exist in exploring the lives of Latina transgender women.

PREVALENCE OF HIV INFECTION AMONG TRANSGENDER WOMEN

HIV prevalence rates among transgender women in the United States are often alarmingly high, ranging from 8% to 78% (Clements-Nolle et al., 2001; De Santis, 2009; Kenagy, 2005; Garofalo et al., 2006; Melendez & Pinto, 2007; Operario, Soma, & Underhill, 2008; Reback et al., 2005; Reisner et al., 2009; Sevelius et al., 2009; Schulden et al., 2008). Rates of HIV prevalence are higher among transgender women who engage in commercial sex work compared to those who do not (Operario et al., 2008; Reback et al., 2005) and also higher compared to male sex workers (Operario et al., 2008). Furthermore, rates of infection among transgender women are reportedly higher than those among men who have sex with men or partners of people living with HIV (Herbst et al., 2008; Reisner et al., 2009). To understand why the prevalence of HIV is so disproportionately high among transgender women, we need to consider the compelling social context in which they live.

THE SOCIAL CONTEXT OF LATINA TRANSGENDER WOMEN
Experiences from Latin America

Many Latina transgender women in the United States immigrated from Latin America and most likely had experiences related to being transgender in their home countries prior to their arrival in the United States. Thus in order to better understand the experiences of Latina transgender women living in the United States, it is important to take into account the social contexts of transgender women in Latin American countries and the historical roots of their experiences.

In Mexico, as far back as the nineteenth century, men who appeared outwardly as women (referred to as *transvestites*) were presented in a derogatory manner in newspapers and political cartoons (Dominguez-Ruvalcaba, 2007, pp. 33–52; Irwin, 2003, pp. 66–91). One example of this was the case of the "Famous 41." In November

1901, a police raid occurred in a private party and resulted in the arrest of 41 men, half of whom were dressed as women. These individuals were ridiculed in the press, and it was implied that they belonged to the upper classes. The famous Mexican artist, José Guadalupe Posada, painted four etchings of the "41" in 1901 as a political critique of the ruling bourgeoisie class during the presidency of Porfirio Diaz (Dominguez-Ruvalcaba, 2007) (see Figure 11.1).

Although greater visibility of transgender people in Latin America is currently occurring through networks they have developed for themselves such as *La Red de Personas Trans de Latinoamérica y el Caribe* [The Network of Trans Persons from Latin America and the Caribbean], for the most part, much stigma and discrimination toward transgender individuals continue to exist in Latin American countries. At times this takes the form of violence against transgender women (Prieur, 1998) or even murder (Sente, 2006). Sometimes the violence is perpetrated by police authorities (Sotelo, 2008).

As a result, to escape the stigma and discrimination that transgender Latinas experience in Latin America (expressed as social rejection, isolation, gossiping, and even violence), in particular from their families, many move from their home towns of origin to larger cities (Infante, Sosa-Rubi, & Magali Cuadra, 2009; Prieur, 1998). Upon arrival in the city, many take jobs as sex workers, hairdressers, or entertainers in shows or bars.

Because of limited employment opportunities, sex work becomes for many a way of gaining financial independence and economic survival (Smallman, 2007). However, transgender sex workers also report experiencing rejection, stigma, discrimination, physical and emotional violence, and unemployment (Infante, Sosa-Rubi, & Magali Cuadra, 2009; Prieur, 1998). In fact, transgender sex workers in Mexico City have been found to work within a more violent street environment compared to young men (both heterosexual and gay) living in the streets because their physical transformations result in more abuse and violence (Infante et al., 2009). Such abuse is experienced from different sources including sex clients, the police, and even the gay community. The despair that many transgender individuals

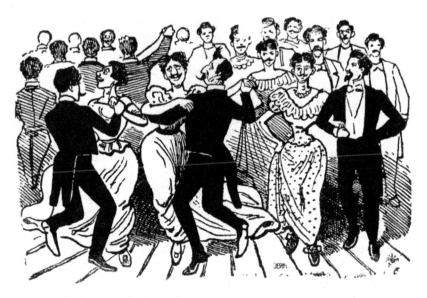

FIGURE 11.1 José Guadalupe Posada, *Corrido "los 41" (Ballad "the 41")*. Courtesy of Benson Latin American Collection, The University of Texas at Austin.

experience can also lead to substance abuse with alcohol and/or drugs (Smallman, 2007).

This, then, is the social context of many Latina transgender women who end up migrating to the United States. In many ways, however, they experience similar forms of stigma and discrimination following their arrival to their new country.

Experiences from the United States

"Transphobia" has been defined as discrimination toward transgender people (Wilson et al., 2009), and most or all of transgender women in the United States report having experienced this type of discrimination (De Santis, 2009; Melendez & Pinto, 2007; Sanchez & Vilain, 2009). It can come from different societal sources, including family members, work associates, health and social services providers or complete strangers, or be internally experienced.

Discrimination is often experienced from gay and lesbian people (Garofalo et al., 2006; Melendez & Pinto, 2009). Despite the fact that organizations developed by the gay community often serve transgender people and the two communities are considered allies in many respects, there are also occasions when their political goals have been in conflict (Linthicum, 2010). For example, some gay and lesbian political initiatives exclude transgender people for fear that such an inclusion would weaken support for the initiative. As a result, transgender people at times perceive gay and lesbian people as not being fully supportive of them.

Studies of transgender women in the United States confirm the extent to which transphobia has limited their opportunities and contributed to a lifetime of marginalization (De Santis, 2009; Nemoto et al., 2004). These have occurred principally in the areas of employment, education, housing, and access to services (De Santis, 2009; Herbst et al., 2008). For example, the *National Transgender Discrimination Study: Employment and Economic Insecurity,* a survey of 6450 transgender people conducted by the National Gay and Lesbian Task Force (NGLTF) (2009) and the National Center for Transgender Equality (NCTE), found that 15% lived on $10,000 per year or less. Forty-seven percent had negative job experiences such as being fired, not hired, or denied a promotion, and almost all (97%) reported being harassed or mistreated on the job. In addition, 13% reported being unemployed. For the Latino transgender participants, the unemployment rate was 18%. Other research has found an even higher rate of unemployment (23%) among transgender individuals in general (Herbst et al., 2008).

Many transgender women are also at risk for lower levels of education. In a study of 244 multiethnic transgender women in Los Angeles, the mean number of years of education was 11 (Reback et al., 2005). Lower education is reported by some transgender women as a result of dropping out of school because of being harassed and discriminated (Wilson et al., 2009).

Housing is another problem area for transgender women. Forty-one percent of a sample of 153 transgender women in San Francisco described their housing situation as having been unstable within the previous year (Sevelius et al., 2009). In addition, the extent of homelessness among transgender individuals has been reported as being between 12.9% and 19% (Herbst et al., 2008; Garofalo et al., 2006; National Gay and Lesbian Task Force, 2009). Homelessness, in turn, can contribute to engaging in commercial sex work as a means of survival, especially when exacerbated by a lack of formal employment (Schulden et al., 2008; Wilson et al., 2009).

In addition, many transgender women do not obtain adequate health care and needed social services. Thirty-six percent of the sample of 141 transgender women in Minnesota reported having had difficulty obtaining health care services because of their gender identity or presentation (Bockting et al., 2005). Many transgender individuals fail to seek care because of previous discriminatory experiences in medical settings (De Santis, 2009; Herbst et al., 2008).

Social isolation is experienced by many transgender individuals due to reports of feeling uncomfortable or unsafe in public settings or a fear of rejection or actual rejection by family members or others (Herbst et al., 2008; Koken, Bimbi, & Parsons, 2009; Wilson et al., 2009). Other factors contributing to social isolation include a lack of cohesiveness within the transgender community itself and a lack of connection to the gay, lesbian,and bisexual community (Herbst et al., 2008).

Incarceration is high among transgender individuals, with estimates of between 7% and 81% reporting a history of prior incarceration (Clements-Nolle et al., 2001; Herbst et al., 2008; Wilson et al., 2009). These high rates have been attributed at least in part to a lack of employment opportunities for the transgender population, resulting in resorting to commercial sex work as a form of income ("survival sex") and subsequently being incarcerated for this (Herbst et al., 2008).

Up to 60% report having been harassed or having experienced violence during their lifetime (De Santis, 2009; Melendez & Pinto, 2007). The extent of violence experienced by transgender people is higher than that of many other at-risk populations. For example, transgender people experience hate crimes at proportionately higher rates than gay, lesbian, and bisexual people (Sanchez & Vilain, 2009).

In many cases, transgender people are also murdered (Glionna, 2005). Murders are so common among transgender people (on average one death per month worldwide) that November 20 has been designated as an annual Transgender Day of Remembrance. It commemorates those who have lost their lives as a result of anti-transgender hatred.

Sometimes the violence is of a sexual nature, including rape or other types of forced sexual activity, such as during a sex work encounter (Garofalo et al., 2006; Kenagy, 2005; Reisner et al., 2009). The estimates of sexually related violence are high. Among female transgender youth, aged 16 to 25 years, 52% of 51 individuals reported having been forced to have sex against their will in the previous 12 months (Garofalo et al., 2006). In a sample of 392 adult transgender females, 59% reported having had forced sex or having been raped in their lifetime (Clements-Nolle et al., 2001).

When the violence is experienced from intimate or sexual partners, the perpetrators are more likely to be the primary partners of transgender women rather than casual partners (Herbst et al., 2008). However, among transgender women engaged in commercial sex work, the risk of violence from clients is ever-present (Sausa, Keatley, & Operario, 2007). Violence can also occur when a transgender woman is discovered to be transgender during or following a sexual encounter (Glionna, 2005; Reisner et al., 2009). Violence or the threat of violence during a sexual encounter, regardless of who the partner is, can result in an inability to negotiate safer sex behaviors by the transgender woman because of fear of her partner (De Santis, 2009).

For many, the experience of being physically abused because of a transgender identity began in the family home with aggressive reactions on the part of parents and other close family members (Kenagy, 2005; Koken, Bimbi, & Parsons, 2009; Sausa et al., 2007). In a sample of 20 transgender females, 71% reported having been beaten as a child, and 50% indicated that they had been sexually abused as children (Kenagy, 2005).

Given the many negative effects of transphobia in the lives of transgender women, it is not at all surprising that many report having various mental health problems such as feeling depressed and having poor self-esteem (De Santis, 2009; Nemoto et al., 2004). In fact, fears related to being transgender have been found to be positively associated with psychological distress (Sanchez & Vilain, 2009). In a study conducted with 392 transgender females in San Francisco, nearly two-thirds were depressed at the time of the interview, based on the Center for Epidemiologic Studies Depression Scale of Radloff (1977) (Clements-Nolle et al., 2001). This estimate of the prevalence of depression among transgender women is similar to that found in other studies: 63.6% in a study conducted in Boston of transgender females (Reisner et al., 2009) and 61% in a study from Minnesota that included 181 both male-to-female and female-to-male transgender individuals (Bockting et al., 2005).

In the same study from San Francisco mentioned above, 32% reported having had a history of a suicide attempt (Clements-Nolle et al., 2001). A similar rate of suicide attempts (32.4%) was reported by a sample of 111 transgender women in Philadelphia (Kenagy, 2005). When asked further if their suicide attempts were related to their being transgender, three-quarters answered in the affirmative. A review of other studies in the United States by Herbst et al. (2008) revealed a lifetime rate of suicide attempts of 31.4%, consistent with the above figures.

In addition to the challenges described above that Latina transgender women share in common with transgender women of other ethnic groups, Latinas have unique experiences that can also contribute to their further marginalization. For example, many Latinas may be of undocumented residency status in the United States and fear that accessing services could jeopardize their stay in the country (Melendez & Pinto, 2009). Many also may experience language barriers that could impede their advancement in several areas of their lives. In addition, many may experience racism as another type of systemic oppression above and beyond that experienced from transphobia (Sausa et al., 2007).

However, as transgender women, Latinas also share much in common with other transgender women, including stigma and discrimination, violence, problems with mental health, social isolation, economic marginalization, incarceration, and unmet transgender-specific health care needs. All of these have been found to be associated with increased risk of HIV infection among transgender people (De Santis, 2009; Herbst et al., 2008).

HIV-RELATED RISK BEHAVIORS OF TRANSGENDER WOMEN

For many of the reasons outlined above, transgender women engage in a number of activities that can increase their risk of becoming infected with the HIV virus. Chief among these is engaging in unsafe sexual practices (De Santis, 2009). In a sample of 392 transgender females in San Francisco, receptive anal sex was more commonly reported than insertive anal sex, with a large percentage of the study participants reporting having had unprotected anal intercourse (Clements-Nolle, 2001). The rate of those reporting unprotected anal sex was found to vary by their choice of sexual partner. Among those reporting having had receptive anal intercourse, 62% reported having done so without the use of a condom with their main partners, 44% with casual partners, and 28% with exchange partners (an exchange partner was defined as someone with whom one had sex in exchange for money, drugs, shelter, or food). This same trend (highest rate of unprotected sex with main partners, lowest with commercial partners, with casual partners somewhere in between) has been confirmed by other studies (Nemoto et al., 2004).

The reasons often given by transgender women for not using condoms are the inconvenience of using them and the fear of a negative response on the part of their sexual partners (Garofalo et al., 2006). Another reason for not using condoms is wanting to affirm one's feminine gender identity and attractiveness, as well as to increase sexual intimacy (Herbst et al., 2008; Nemoto et al., 2004; Reisner et al., 2009), a factor in need of serious study.

Another HIV-related risk behavior of transgender women is commercial sex work, which is considerably high among this population, with estimates of from 24% to 75% engaging in this activity (Herbst et al., 2008). A study of 128 transgender female adults conducted in Los Angeles found that two-thirds reported having engaged in commercial sex work in the previous 12 months (Harawa & Bingham, 2009). Commercial sex work also was reported by 59% of transgender females aged 16 to 25 years living in Chicago (Garofalo et al., 2006).

The primary reasons for engaging in commercial sex work are the poverty, unemployment, and discrimination faced by transgender females (Clements-Nolle, 2001; Edwards, Fisher, & Reynolds, 2007; Reisner et al., 2009). Other reported reasons include drug and alcohol addictions (Reisner et al., 2009). Engaging in commercial sex work places transgender women at high risk for HIV infection (Edwards, Fisher, & Reynolds, 2007), especially when clients pay extra for sex without condoms (Melendez & Pinto, 2007; Nemoto et al., 2004; Reisner et al., 2009).

Some ethnic differences have been reported among transgender women who engage in commercial sex work. In a study comparing female transgender communities from different ethnicities in New York City, Latina and African American transgender women were found to engage in survival sex work that involved the most risk (e.g., as streetwalkers exposing themselves to the possibilities of HIV infection, other sexually transmitted diseases, violence, and rape) compared to the other ethnic groups (Hwahng & Nuttbrock, 2007). Asian sex workers often described the use of condoms as being absolutely necessary in their sexual transactions, in contrast to the reports of the Latinas and African Americans. White transgender (cross-dressing) females in the New York sample did not have to depend on sex work for their livelihood, but when they did engage in sex work, they engaged in very low-risk sex.

Another high-risk activity reported by transgender women is substance abuse (Garofalo et al., 2006; Harawa & Bingham, 2009; Herbst et al., 2008). A meta-analysis of studies of transgender women found that 43.7% reportedly consumed alcohol, 26.7% used crack or other illicit drugs, and 20.2% smoked marijuana (Herbst et al., 2008). This may be a way of coping with the stress of transphobia (Hwahng & Nuttbrock, 2007; Sevelius et al., 2009) or with the stress specifically associated with sex work (Hwahng & Nuttbrock, 2007; Wilson et al., 2009). Substance use becomes a risk factor for HIV, especially when combined with sexual activity.

The extent of substance use during sexual activity appears to be high. A study of 51 transgender female youth found that 53% reported having had sex while under the influence of drugs or alcohol (Garofalo et al., 2006). A similar rate has been reported among adult transgender women (Harawa & Bingham, 2009). The combination of sex and drug use also appears to vary with the choice of sexual partner.

A study of transgender women in San Francisco found that the use of drugs during sex was more common when having sex with primary partners (53.5%), followed by casual partners (31.5%) and commercial sex partners (14.8%) (Nemoto et al., 2004). The use of substances during sexual activity may result in impaired judgment and hence increase one's risk of HIV infection (De Santis, 2009). It has been found among transgender women to be a significant predictor of unprotected receptive anal sex, in particular with primary and casual partners (Nemoto et al., 2004).

Finally, transgender women often use needles for administering female hormones and silicone (De Santis, 2009). About a quarter of transgender women report engaging in these activities (Herbst et al., 2008). This becomes a risk factor for HIV when needles are shared among individuals because of a lack of access to sterile needles and syringes (Edwards et al., 2007; Lombardi, 2001). However, actual needle sharing for this purpose appears to be low at around 6% (Herbst et al., 2008). In addition, one study concluded that the impact of intramuscular injections on HIV infection was "either extremely weak or nonexistent among Hispanic or African American MTFs" (Nuttbrock et al., 2009, p. 420). Of course, HIV transmission can also occur when needles are shared for the purposes of injecting street drugs. However, the sharing of needles for this purpose has been found to be low among transgender women, at 2% (Herbst et al., 2008), and this should be further studied.

As this brief overview of the social contexts and HIV-related risk behaviors of transgender women has demonstrated, transgender communities, including Latinas, share similarities as well as experience differences with one another. It is important, then, when developing programs for transgender women, to take into consideration the circumstances and needs of the particular community being served. What follows is an example of a sensitive needs assessment research that resulted in programs targeting a specific transgender community. It demonstrates successful capacity building within a community and can serve as a model for similar efforts at the local, state, and national levels to meet the needs of transgender women in general and Latinas in particular. The next two sections, "Developing Transgender Programs: Personal Reflections and Insights" and "Responding to Transgender Women: Multilevel HIV Prevention in Context," were written by the second author of this chapter, JoAnne Keatley, a transgender Latina woman, to describe the development of programs that successfully addressed the needs of her San Francisco community.

DEVELOPING TRANSGENDER PROGRAMS: PERSONAL REFLECTIONS AND INSIGHTS

In 1998 while beginning a graduate course of study at the School of Social Welfare at the University of California, Berkeley, I reviewed the scant literature on transgender women that suggested that they may be at highest risk for HIV when compared to other high-risk groups. It was clear that the literature and social service field were in dire need of developing a greater understanding of the factors driving health and mental health disparities among transgender people. I sought out and obtained a position at the University of California, San Francisco (UCSF), Center for AIDS Prevention Studies (CAPS), in order to understand the risk factors impacting transgender people and design and deliver prevention intervention programs that would address HIV risk in a culturally responsive and affirming way.

Formative Research to Understand the Experiences of Transgender People of Color

In partnership with a research team we called Health Studies for People of Color (HSPC) housed at CAPS, we conducted formative research with funding from the National Institute on Drug Abuse (Grant DA11589) with a community sample of 332 transgender women of color living in San Francisco. This study focused on health issues and HIV risk behaviors among transgender women of color because research had demonstrated that minorities in San Francisco were at disproportionate risk for negative health outcomes (San Francisco Department of Public Health, 1999). Between November 2000 and July 2001, a team of transgender female interviewers recruited participants from a range of venues including health clinics, bars, beauty parlors, and other social venues identified through community mapping.

Four San Francisco AIDS service organizations with transgender-specific programs referred 46% of the sample utilizing a snowball sampling methodology. To be considered eligible for the study, each participant had to (1) identify as a transgender female; (2) identify as African American, Asian, and/or Pacific Islander or Latina; (3) have a history of exchanging sex for money, drugs, or shelter; and (4) be 18 years of age or older. We used a two-stage approach. The first involved conducting qualitative research in order to develop a quantitative survey instrument for individual interviews. We conducted a series of focus groups with 48 transgender women of color, interviewed key informants in the San Francisco transgender women's community, and mapped social spaces frequented by transgender women. On the basis of qualitative research findings, we developed a survey that was sensitive to the experiences of transgender women of color in San Francisco. For example, instead of utilizing the standard male/female gender binary, we provided participants multiple options to self-report gender identity. Additionally, the research team paid close attention to the language used for participants' body parts so as to be respectful of how transgender people refer to their own anatomy. Latinas completed the survey in Spanish or English with a bilingual Latina interviewer.

Preliminary Findings of Significance

Ninety-eight percent of the transgender sample reported having tested for HIV, and 91% reported having tested for tuberculosis (TB). Of those who had tested for HIV, 26% reported a positive result on their last test, 4% were not sure of their status, and 1% declined to report it. Fourteen percent of the sample reported having tested positive for TB, and 11% reported testing positive for hepatitis C. Latinas were the most likely to report a positive TB result.

Transgender respondents reported high levels of alcohol use (56%) and other drug use including marijuana (38%) and noninjection amphetamines (24%). More than 40% of the transgender women sampled reported sex under the influence of alcohol, and 50% reported sex under the influence of illicit drugs in the past 30 days. Latinas reported the highest levels of depression (65%), 46% reported suicide ideation, and 30% reported at least one suicide attempt. Participants experienced high levels of stigma associated with transphobia in society, and almost 80% reported having been made fun of or ridiculed as a child, hearing that transgender people were abnormal as an adult (63%), and being targeted for harassment by the police (61%). These data documented HIV-related and other risk factors and were used as a basis for developing programmatic and service-related capacity building to begin

Table 11.2 Multilevel Initiatives to Prevent HIV and Promote Health in Transgender People

	Initiative	*Purpose*
Local	HIV risk behavior among transgender women of color in San Francisco	To investigate risk behavior and document protective factors among transgender people in San Francisco
	Transgender Resources and Neighborhood Space (TRANS)	To develop the first federally funded transgender HIV and substance use intervention program in the country
	Transgender Life Care	To implement a free mental health intervention for transgender people in San Francisco
State	Center of Excellence for Transgender HIV Prevention	To increase access to HIV prevention services and health care for transgender people in California
	Primary Care Protocols Project	To develop and disseminate best practices for transgender health care providers
National	Center of Excellence for Transgender Health	To increase access to HIV prevention services and increase capacity to provide health care for transgender people in the United States
	Transitions Project	To increase the capacity to adapt, implement, and evaluate evidence-based HIV prevention interventions for transgender communities
	Coalitions in Action for Transgender Community Health (CATCH)	To promote provider networking and transgender community utilization of existing health care and HIV prevention services

to support transgender women of color and to reduce their risk for HIV and related problems. These multiple level efforts and initiatives are described below and are depicted in Table 11.2.

RESPONDING TO TRANSGENDER WOMEN: MULTILEVEL HIV PREVENTION IN CONTEXT
Local Capacity Building

As the primary facilitator of all of the focus groups conducted in the qualitative phase of the study, "HIV Risk Behaviors among Male-to-Female Transgender Persons of Color in San Francisco," (Nemoto et al., 2004) it was immediately apparent to me that the transgender community was in critical need of a transgender-specific space where they could obtain effective and culturally relevant intervention services. It had also become clear that transgender people would likely respond best to services that were delivered by members of their own community and, when possible, in a language familiar to them. Thus, our team explored the development of the first transgender-specific health intervention space in the nation, the Transgender Resources and Neighborhood Space project, or TRANS, of San Francisco.

TRANS, a collaborative effort among researchers, community-based organizations, health and recovery service providers, and the community, was launched in October 2000 with support from the Substance Abuse and Mental Health Services Administration (SAMHSA) (Grant H79TI12592). TRANS was located in the Tenderloin area of San Francisco (where many transgender women call home) and provided a safe space for a living room, education area, private offices for the health educators, a private shower, and a resource closet. TRANS offered a series of 18 health education classes designed by the transgender team of health educators in English and in Spanish.

In the first several years of existence, TRANS reached close to 500 unique participants and quickly became a critical component of the service delivery system for transgender people in San Francisco. One of the most successful elements of TRANS was working with the community to address the full range of social service needs. For example, in response to the continued lack of employment opportunities for transgender people, in 2004 TRANS collaborated with a number of service providers and the San Francisco LGBT Center to organize the first transgender-specific job fair in history. TRANS has continued to exist outside of the university as TRANS:THRIVE (Transgender Resource and Neighborhood Space and Transgender Health & Resource Initiative for Vital Empowerment) and receives ongoing support from various sources, including the AIDS Healthcare Foundation, the San Francisco Department of Public Health, and private foundations. It has been in existence now for over 10 years.

We also partnered with Walden House (WH), a large residential drug treatment program, and created the Transgender Recovery Program (TRP), the first residential treatment program for transgender people in the country. With newly designed policies, the goal was to improve treatment outcomes by increasing transgender clients' retention and improving awareness and acceptance of transgender people by other residents and staff. WH was able to demonstrate that, with consideration of cultural and privacy issues and careful integration into a therapeutic community, transgender people could successfully complete treatment and recover from alcohol and drug use. TRP has been able to continue to provide services with support from the San Francisco Department of Public Health and is considered a model program to this day.

Mental health services were also identified early on as a critical service need among transgender women. To that end, a partnership was sought with the San Francisco Behavioral Health Services, and a collaborative effort, Transgender Life Care (TLC), was formed to respond to those needs. The SAMHSA-funded project provided free transgender mental health services at both the TRANS site and at the Castro Mission Health Center, a clinic of the Community Health Network in San Francisco. After recruiting a psychiatrist and a marriage and family therapist, TLC staff provided case management, emotional support, support groups, and hormonal care at a primary care site.

A unique element of the TRANS project was the development of the *Costura y Charla* (Sewing and Chatting) workshop for transgender Latinas. As a result of the lack of employment opportunities for many of the monolingual participants at TRANS, many felt that they needed some form of economic empowerment and an ability to discuss issues in a space with their specific needs addressed. To that end, we identified volunteer staff to teach participants sewing and pattern-making skills

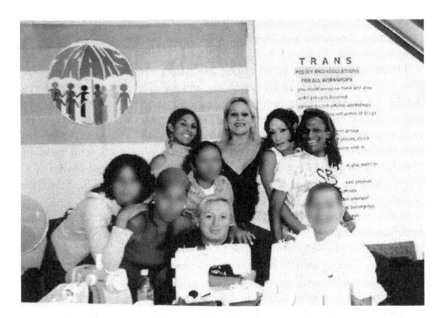

FIGURE 11.2 Participants at *Costura y Charla* (Sewing and Chatting) Workshop at Transgender Resources and Neighborhood Space (TRANS), University of California, San Francisco. (Blurred faces indicate participants who could not be reached for permission to use photo.)

that could lead to some form of income generation and purchased a number of sewing machines for participants to use. During these sewing circles, our Spanish-speaking health educators would engage participants in safer sex discussions, safer sex negotiation skills building and strategizing, and other important topics driven by a participant's identified need. These sessions proved immensely popular and were always very well attended (see Figure 11.2).

It took a long-term vision to develop the above range of programs to begin to address the needs of transgender people of color in San Francisco. HSPC no longer exists at UCSF, but the programs that were put in place by the initial research team continue to thrive, and as a result transgender peoples' lives have been supported. As a social worker, it has been very rewarding to see macrolevel results emerge from this close and personal commitment to a community and other successes that have come along as a result of the early work in San Francisco.

Statewide Capacity Building

In 2007, with a grant from the California Department of Public Health, Office of AIDS, we were able to develop and launch the Center of Excellence for Transgender HIV Prevention (CoE). The CoE combined the unique strengths and resources of a nationally renowned training and capacity building institution, the Pacific AIDS Education and Training Center (PAETC), and an internationally recognized leader in HIV prevention research, the Center for AIDS Prevention Studies (CAPS), both of which are housed at the University of California, San Francisco.

The tasks before us were to provide leadership, capacity building, professional training, policy advocacy, research development, and resources to increase access to culturally competent HIV prevention services for transgender people in California.

The CoE identified the need to synthesize information about existing programs that address HIV prevention needs among transgender people in California in order to identify service needs both met and unmet. To achieve this goal, we compiled a resource inventory and service gap analysis of transgender HIV prevention programs in California. While collecting and analyzing resources and services, the CoE was able to identify, publish, and disseminate best practices for HIV prevention with transgender populations, develop coursework for providers interested in increasing their capacity to serve transgender people, and provide technical assistance to service providers, health departments, and researchers.

One example of building provider capacity was when the East Valley Community Health Center, a service provider in Southern California, needed to expand its ability to provide care and prevention services to the transgender community; the CoE was able to provide direct technical assistance by providing three different on-site trainings to all of their clinical and support staff. Another example of building provider capacity is the Primary Care Protocols project currently under development at the CoE. Working with a medical advisory board, we have developed protocols that will guide physicians interested in delivering primary care to transgender patients. These capacity building trainings were developed specifically for agency-identified needs and addressed the clinical, cultural, and legal issues that needed to be considered.

National Capacity Building

In 2009, the Centers for Disease Control and Prevention awarded the CoE with a 5-year grant to expand its service delivery nationally. At the same time, the CoE changed its name to the Center of Excellence for Transgender Health (www.transhealth.ucsf.edu). The CoE's ultimate goal is to improve the overall health and well-being of transgender individuals by developing and implementing programs in response to community-identified needs across the country. We include community perspectives by actively engaging a national advisory body (NAB) of 14 transgender-identified leaders from throughout the country. The collective experience of our diverse talent pool of NAB members maximizes the probability that our programs address issues that are timely and relevant to the community.

Currently the national CoE is focused on the following four distinct programs: (1) Coalitions in Action for Transgender Community Health (CATCH), a transgender community mobilization for increasing health care access, (2) the Transitions project, a capacity building assistance project for organizations delivering HIV/AIDS prevention services for transgender people, (3) research and development of evidence-based HIV interventions for transgender people, and (4) the Primary Care Protocols project working on the development and dissemination of transgender primary care treatment information for clinicians. We continue to identify and challenge barriers to services for transgender people, with the goal of reducing and hopefully one day eliminating those barriers.

This year the seemingly impossible occurred when I was honored with an invitation to speak on transgender HIV issues at a White House meeting held by the Office of National AIDS Policy. With an administration that understands the need for transgender inclusion in the National HIV/AIDS Strategy, I believe we can finally begin to address the significant needs of the transgender community in a meaningful way on a larger scale. However, we must be diligent and ensure that the steps outlined in the National Strategy are followed. Data collection must reflect transgender identities in order to more accurately understand the full scope of the HIV epidemic among higher priority populations.

Yet, there are many urgent continued service needs to be addressed and other barriers to overcome. We must continue to focus on addressing the immense stigma that leads so many transgender people into risk-taking behavior in the first place and provide a means for the community to empower itself. We must advocate for employment policies that will support gender-variant people, provide education and employment opportunities, and create safer living environments. We must work toward eliminating transphobia in health care. Only then will we be able to claim a true level of success in enhancing transgender health and wellbeing.

RECOMMENDATIONS FOR FUTURE RESEARCH

Transphobia is pervasive in the United States and beyond. Acceptance of the rights of transgender people has not reached the same level of acceptance as gay and lesbian people (Linthicum, 2010). Given that transphobia is associated with an increased risk of HIV infection among transgender people, it would seem prudent and wise, then, to identify ways of confronting transphobia on both personal and community levels in order to lower the prevalence of HIV infection among transgender women in general and Latinas in particular.

Despite the high level of transphobia experienced by transgender women, there continues to be a dearth of information in the literature about how transgender women cope with stress in a positive manner and the resources that are available to help them to do this. Coping in a positive manner can be described as a "stabilizing factor that can help individuals maintain psychosocial adaptation during stressful periods" (Holahan et al., 1996, p. 25). Such coping can include cognitive and behavioral efforts, as well as community and cultural resources, which can diminish or eliminate the conditions that contribute to distress and its negative emotional consequences. Examples of positive ways of coping can include thinking of different ways to deal with a problem, seeking guidance and support from others, and taking problem-solving actions.

One positive way of coping that could potentially be used to lower the rate of HIV infection among transgender women is by promoting "collective self-esteem" (Sanchez & Vilain, 2009). Collective self-esteem is defined as positive identification with one's social group. In a non-HIV-related study that looked at the association between psychological distress and a positive identification with the transgender community, it found that the more positively the women felt about the transgender community, the less psychological distress they reported. Future research could examine the extent to which programs that promote collective self-esteem among Latina transgender women can be effective in lowering their risk of HIV infection.

Other possible positive coping resources that could also be examined in relation to HIV risk among Latina transgender women include personal self-esteem, social support (from family, friends, partners, and transgender support groups) and religiosity/spirituality. Further research should be conducted on issues related to resilience among transgender women to identify and promote ways of coping with stigma and discrimination in a positive manner in order to lower their risk of HIV infection (Wilson et al., 2009).

In addition to identifying individual-level factors that could be used by transgender women to lower their HIV risk, it is also important to conduct research to identify ways of altering the social context and environments in which they live.

This is an essential component to accomplish the overall goal of lowering the prevalence of HIV among this population because, as noted above, experiences of transphobia, such as stigma and discrimination, have been found to be associated with increased risk of HIV infection among transgender people (De Santis, 2009; Herbst et al., 2008).

Altering the social context of the lives of transgender women requires the development of structural-level interventions that result in the greater acceptance of transgender people by institutions with which they interact and by society in general. Structural interventions seek to change the context in which health-related behaviors are shaped (Blakenship et al., 2006). One example of a structural intervention is a policy change that decreases discrimination in the workplace or improves the economic opportunities available for transgender people. Having more economic opportunities would decrease the need of many transgender women to engage in commercial sex work as a dangerous form of economic survival and thereby also reduce their likelihood of becoming infected by HIV.

Further research is necessary to identify how to promote structural-level changes that have a positive impact in the lives of transgender women. For example, there are no known evidenced-based structural-level interventions to promote a successful transition from commercial sex work to the formal employment sector (Operario, Soma, & Underhill, 2008). Once such interventions are developed or identified, it would be important then to examine their impact as well as to conduct a systematic evaluation of how they were implemented in order to identify successful components for duplication in other programs (Blakenship, Friedman, & Dworkin, 2006).

The structural-environmental model presented in Chapter 1 provides a framework of how the creation of programs for the transgender community can lead to lower HIV-related risk behaviors and also foster resilience. Programs such as TRANS:THRIVE (formerly called TRANS or the Transgender Resources and Neighborhood Space project), the Transgender Recovery Program, and the Center of Excellence for Transgender Health play an important role for a community in great need of services. Such programs can serve as models for the rest of the country and should also be evaluated. By providing greater opportunities for transgender women, these programs can contribute to lowering the disproportionately very high prevalence of HIV among this community in general and among Latina transgender women in particular.

ACKNOWLEDGEMENTS

Support for Dr. Frank Galvan was provided by the Institute for Community Health Research of Charles Drew University of Medicine and Science sponsored by the California HIV/AIDS Research Program (CHRP) of the University of California Office of the President (CH05-DREW-616) and the UCLA/Drew/RAND Center for HIV Identification, Prevention and Treatment Services (CHIPTS) sponsored by the National Institute of Mental Health (P30MH-58-107).

REFERENCES

Blankenship, K. M., Friedman, S.R., Dworkin, S., & Mantell, J. E. (2006). Structural interventions: Concepts, challenges and opportunities for research. *Journal of Urban Health: Bulletin of the New York Academy of Medicine, 83*(1), 59–72.

Bockting, W. O., Robinson, B. E., Forberg, J., & Scheltema, K. (2005). Evaluation of a sexual health approach to reducing HIV/STD risk in the transgender community. *AIDS Care, 17*(3), 289–303.

Clements-Nolle, K., Marx, R., Guzman, R., & Katz, M. (2001). HIV prevalence, risk behaviors, health care use, and mental health status of transgender persons: Implications for public health interventions. *American Journal of Public Health, 91*(6), 915–921.

De Santis, J. P. (2009). HIV infection risk factors among male-to-female transgender persons: A review of the literature. *Journal of the Association of Nurses in AIDS Care, 20*(5), 362–372.

Diaz, R. M. (1998). *Latino gay men and HIV: Culture, sexuality and risk behavior.* New York: Routledge.

Dominguez-Ruvalcaba, H. (2007). *Modernity and the nation in Mexican representations of masculinity.* New York: Palgrave Macmillan.

Dominguez-Ruvalcaba, H. (2009). From fags to gays: Political adaptations and cultural translations in the Mexican gay liberation movement. In L. Egan & M. K. Long (Eds.), *Mexico reading the United States* (pp. 116–134). Nashville: Vanderbilt University Press.

Edwards, J. W, Fisher, D. G., & Reynolds, G. L. (2007). Male-to-female transgender and transsexual clients of HIV service programs in Los Angeles County, California. *American Journal of Public Health, 97*(6), 1030–1033.

Garofalo, R., Deleon, J., Osmer, E., Doll, M., & Harper, G. W. (2006). Overlooked, misunderstood and at-risk: Exploring the lives and HIV risk of ethnic minority male-to-female transgender youth. *Journal of Adolescent Health, 38*, 230–236.

Glionna, J. M. (2005). 2 guilty of killing transgender teen. *Los Angeles Times* (September 13). Available at http://articles.latimes.com/2005/sep/13/local/me-gwen13. Accessed February 17, 2010.

Harawa, N, T., & Bingham, T. A. (2009). Exploring HIV prevention utilization among female sex workers and male-to-female transgenders. *AIDS Education and Prevention, 21*(4), 356–371.

Herbst, J. H., Jacobs, E. D., Finlayson, T. J., McKleroy, V. S., Neumann, M. S., & Crepaz, N. (2008). Estimating HIV prevalence and risk behaviors of transgender persons in the United States. *AIDS & Behavior, 12*, 1–17.

Holahan, C. J., Moos, R. H., & Schaefer, J. A. (1996). Coping, stress resistance, and growth: Conceptualizing adaptive functioning. In M. Zeidner & N. S. Endler (Eds.), *Handbook of coping: Theory, research, applications* (pp. 24–43). New York: John Wiley & Sons.

Hwahng, S. J., & Nuttbrock, L. (2007). Sex workers, fem queens, and cross-dressers: Differential marginalizations and HIV vulnerabilities among three ethnocultural male-to-female transgender communities in New York City. *Sexuality Research and Social Policy, 4*(4), 36–59.

Infante, C., Sosa-Rubi, S. G., & Magali Cuadra, S. (2009). Sex work in Mexico: Vulnerability of male, *travesty*, transgender and transsexual sex workers. *Culture, Health & Sexuality, 11*(2), 125–137.

Irwin, R. M. (2003). *Mexican masculinities.* Minneapolis: University of Minnesota Press.

Kenagy, G. P. (2005). Transgender health: Findings from two needs assessment studies in Philadelphia. *Health & Social Work, 30*(1), 19–26.

Koken, J. A., Bimbi, D. S., & Parsons, J. T. (2009). Experiences of familial acceptance-rejection among transwomen of color. *Journal of Family Psychology, 23*(6), 853–860.

Linthicum, K. (2010). Small victories for transgender rights. *Los Angeles Times* (May 26).

Lombardi, E. (2001). Enhancing transgender health care. *American Journal of Public Health, 91*(6), 869–872.

Melendez, R. M., & Pinto, R. (2007). "It's really a hard life": Love, gender and HIV risk among male-to-female transgender persons. *Culture, Health & Sexuality, 9*(3), 233–245.

Melendez, R. M., & Pinto, R. M. (2009). HIV prevention and primary care for transgender women in a community-based clinic. *Journal of the Association of Nurses in AIDS Care, 20*(5), 387–397.

National Gay and Lesbian Task Force/National Center for Transgender Equality (November 2009). *National Transgender Discrimination Study: Employment and Economic Insecurity.* Available at http://www.thetaskforce.org/downloads/reports/fact_sheet/transsurvey_prelim_findings.pdf. Accessed November 1, 2010.

Nemoto, T., Operario, D., Keatley, J., Han, L., & Soma, T. (2004). HIV risk behaviors among male-to-female transgender persons of color in San Francisco. *American Journal of Public Health 94*(7), 1193–1199.

Nuttbrock, L., Hwahng, S., Bockting, W., Rosemblum, A., Mason, M., Macri, M., & Becker, J. (2009). Lifetime risk factors for HIV/sexually transmitted infections among male-to-female transgender persons. *Journal of Acquired Immune Deficiency Syndrome, 52*(3), 417–421.

Operario, D., Soma, T., & Underhill, K. (2008). Sex work and HIV status among transgender women: Systematic review and meta-analysis. *Journal of Acquired Immune Deficiency Syndromes, 48*(1), 97–103.

Prieur, A. (1998). *Mema's house, Mexico City: On transvestites, queens, and machos.* Chicago: The University of Chicago Press.

Radloff, L. S. (1977). The CES-D scale: A self-report depression scale for research in the general population. *Applied Psychological Measures, 1*, 385–401.

Ramirez-Valles, J., Garcia, D., Campbell, R. T., Diaz, R. M., & Heckathorn, D. D. (2008). HIV infection, sexual risk behavior, and substance use among Latino gay and bisexual men and transgender persons. *American Journal of Public Health, 98*(6), 1036–1042.

Reback, C. J., Lombardi, E. L., Simon, P. A., & Frye, D. M. (2005). HIV seroprevalence and risk behaviors among transgendered women who exchange sex in comparison with those who do not. *Journal of Psychology & Human Sexuality, 17*(1/2), 5–22.

Red de Personas Trans de Latinoamérica y el Caribe. Available at www.redlactrans.org.ar/home.htm. Accessed August 11, 2010.

Reisner, S. L., Mimiaga, M. J., Bland, S., Mayer, K. H., Perkovich, B., & Safren, S. A. (2009). HIV risk and social networks among male-to-female transgender sex workers in Boston, Massachusetts. *Journal of the Association of Nurses in AIDS Care, 20*(5), 373–386.

Rosser, B. R. S., Oakes, J. M., Bockting, W. O., & Miner, M. (2007). Capturing the social demographics of hidden sexual minorities: An Internet study of the transgender population in the United States. *Sexuality Research & Social Policy, 4*(2), 50–64.

San Francisco Department of Public Health. (1999). *The transgender community/health project.* San Francisco: City and County of San Francisco.

Sanchez, F., & Vilain, E. (2009). Collective self-esteem as a coping resource for male-to-female transsexuals. *Journal of Counseling Psychology, 56*(1), 202–209.

Sausa, L. A., Keatley, J., & Operario, D. (2007). Perceived risks and benefits of sex work among transgender women of color in San Francisco. *Archives of Sex Behavior, 36*, 768–777.

Schulden, J. D., Song, B., Barros, A., Mares-DelGrasso, A., Martin, C. W., Ramirez, R., Smith, L. C., Wheller, D. P., Oster, A.M., Sullivan, P. S., & Heffelfinger, J. D. (2008). Rapid HIV testing in transgender communities by community-based organizations in three cities. *Public Health Reports, 123*(3), 101–123.

Sente, J. R. (2006). Mujer embarazada herida y travesti asesinado. *La Hora.* Guatemala de la Asunción (October 14).

Sevelius, J. M., Grinstead Reznick, O., Hart, S. L., & Schwarcz, S. (2009). Informing interventions: The importance of contextual factors in the prediction of sexual risk behaviors among transgender women. *AIDS Education and Prevention, 21*(2), 113–127.

Smallman, S. (2007). *The AIDS pandemic in Latin America.* Chapel Hill: The University of North Carolina Press.

Sotela, J. (2008). Estudio de seroprevalencia de VIH en personas trans. In *Salud, VIH-SIDA y sexualidad trans* (pp. 49–59). Buenos Aires: Coordinación SIDA del Gobierno de la Cuidad de Buenos Aires.

Stryker S. (2008). *Transgender History.* Berkeley, CA: Seal Press.

Wilson, E. C., Garofalo, R., Harris, R. D., Herrick, A., Martinez, M., Martinez, J., & Belzer, M. (2009). Transgender female youth and sex work: HIV risk and a comparison of life factors related to engagement in sex work. *AIDS & Behavior, 13,* 902–913.

12 HIV Risk and Prevention for Latinos in Jails and Prisons

Megan Comfort, Carmen Albizu-García, Timoteo Rodriguez, and Carlos Molina III

INTRODUCTION

I first went to prison years ago. I wanted to go. I thought I would be around people of respect, killers. . . . [But] there was a lot of misuse of authority [among Latino prison mafia members]. I was down for my crime and found myself just catching more time. . . I really started losing everything and hurting my family and myself. . . Others told me that I was going to die in prison . . . I started using [heroin] inside. . . I thought that "this is where I am going to be for the rest of my life" and I didn't know a way out. . . And it was eating me up inside. . . . I caught everything: hep C, the virus [HIV]. . . (Rodriguez, interview with formerly incarcerated Latino)[1]

As Organista et al. describe in the opening chapter of this volume, there is an urgent need to focus on structural and environmental factors when investigating and addressing HIV risk and prevention among Latino populations in the United States. Prisons and jails are among the most extreme environments in our society: designed to contain, isolate, and punish, they operate under policies that differ—at times substantially—from those that govern "life on the outside." Within correctional environments, people are denied certain rights, are limited in or cut off entirely from contact with family members and friends, are subjected to intense bodily surveillance and social control, learn to operate within a specific and often violent social world, have no access to goods and materials commonly available in free society, and are continually reminded directly and indirectly of their skewed power relations, lack of autonomy, and distorted status. All of these factors affect HIV risk and prevention within the carceral sphere and in the communities that bear the burden of intensive incarceration policies.

In recent years, an edifying literature has developed focusing on how correctional environments contribute to risk of HIV infection for people while they are behind bars and after they are released, as well as for people who are not incarcerated but experience the incarceration of their loved ones, family members, and neighbors (Freudenberg, 2001; Comfort & Grinstead, 2004; Hammett, 2006). Research has also grown on HIV counseling, testing, and treatment for incarcerated people and their linkage to care after they leave correctional institutions (Rich, Holmes, et al., 2001; Baillargeon, Giordano, et al., 2009). However, the specific issues faced by Latinos in the criminal justice system have been less well addressed, and there exists a notable dearth of research on incarcerated Latinas (Díaz-Cotto, 2006). This chapter provides a review of HIV risk for incarcerated people and for their kin and community members, as well as HIV testing and treatment inside of correctional facilities. Throughout, we highlight what has been studied specific to Latino populations and indicate areas in need of further research for a fuller understanding of Latinos' experiences with the criminal justice system relative to HIV risk and prevention. To complement this discussion, we delve in more depth into the existing literature on California Latino prison mafias, and consider the role these groups may play in HIV prevention and risk. We also examine the context of injection drug use (IDU) in Puerto Rico, where IDU remains a primary means of HIV infection in contrast to the mainland United States (Centers for Disease Control and Prevention, 2009), and the consequences of this for Puerto Rican drug users behind bars.

People experience contact with the criminal justice system in a variety of ways: in addition to jails and prisons, people may be held in police lock-ups or immigration detention centers; individuals may be placed on probation or parole supervision; and many undergo stops-and-searches or raids by police as well as arrests, whether or not these activities lead to charges being filed. In this chapter we focus on incarceration in jail and prison because these are critical HIV risk environments on which research exists, but all forms of criminal justice involvement have important consequences and can cause harm that merits further study regarding HIV and health outcomes. For example, having a warrant out for one's arrest can result in anxiety, depression, and possible physical injury (Goffman, 2009), and children or family members who observe this event may also be traumatized and experience mental health repercussions (Kampfner, 1995). Our hope is that this chapter will inspire others to think broadly about how involvement with the criminal justice system can affect the health and well-being of individuals, families, and social networks, and to undertake research in the many understudied areas related to incarceration, Latino populations, and HIV risk and prevention. In that spirit we urge readers to use what we present here as a springboard for new ideas and directions, and we acknowledge that many important issues will fall outside of the scope of what we are able to cover.

INCARCERATION IN THE UNITED STATES

They [correctional administrators] kept moving me around. My offense was minor but I ended up. . . in a high-security unit with these crazy ass fools. . . There was no bunks, so the C.O. [correctional officer] gave me this flimsy mattress to sleep on the floor with, and there was like four other guys on the floor too. . . ("Nico," describing his experience in county jail)

The United States has experienced a massive and now-infamous expansion of its correctional population over the past four decades: from the 1920s through the 1970s, the incarceration rate held steady around 100 jail and prison inmates per 100,000 residents, and then jumped spectacularly from 221 in 1980 to 762 per 100,000 in 2008 (Western & Pettit, 2010). This scale of punishment has earned the United States its standing as the world's top incarcerator, with rates of confinement at six to twelve times higher than western European countries and Canada. Puerto Rico, at 303 inmates per 100,000 residents, confines members of its population at less than half of the rate of the mainland, but still well above Europe and Canada (Tonry, 2001; International Centre for Prison Studies, 2010).

Nationwide in 2009, U.S. law enforcement authorities carried out an estimated 14 million arrests for all offenses except traffic violations (Federal Bureau of Investigation, 2005: data are not available on the total number of unique individuals arrested).[2] That same year, there were 4.2 million probationers and 819,308 parolees under active supervision in the United States, as well as 2.37 million people confined in the country's jails and prisons (Glaze & Bonczar, 2006; Harrison & Beck, 2006: this count excludes those held in juvenile facilities and police lockups). Correctional supervision disproportionately affects men, and particularly men of color. Males constituted 87% of jail detainees and 93% of state and federal prisoners in 2007 (Glaze & Bonczar, 2006; Harrison & Beck, 2006), as well as 76% of those on probation and 88% of those on parole in 2008 (Glaze & Bonczar, 2009); females composed the remaining percentage in each of these populations, with transgender people rarely if ever being accounted for in the data.

The American Community Survey Demographic Estimates for 2005–2009 report Latinos as 15% of the U.S. population (U.S. Census Bureau, 2010), yet in 2007 Latinos comprised 32% of the U.S. federal prison population and 18% of the total U.S. inmate population (Sabol & Couture, 2008), as well as 19% of the parolee population in 2008 (Glaze & Bonczar, 2009). As shown in Figure 12.1, in 2009 non-Hispanic black men were imprisoned at a rate six times higher than non-Hispanic white men and almost three times higher than Latino men; non-Hispanic black women were imprisoned at nearly three times the rate of non-Hispanic white women and just under two times the rate of Latina women (Sabol & West, 2010). Non-U.S. citizens accounted for 4.1% (94,498 inmates) of the inmates held in custody in state or federal prisons in 2009, and U.S. Immigration and Customs Enforcement (ICE) facilities held an additional 9957 people in 2008 (Sabol & West, 2010; Sabol et al., 2009).

At year end 2008, 21,987 inmates held in state or federal prisons (1.5% of the total custody population) were reported to be HIV-positive or had confirmed AIDS, with Florida, New York, and Texas accounting for 24% of the state custody population but 46% of those reported to be HIV positive (Maruschak, 2009). Because HIV testing policies in correctional facilities vary by jurisdiction and not all

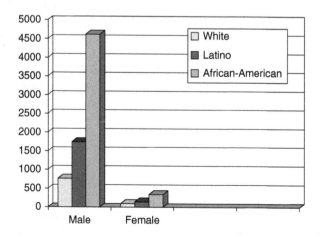

FIGURE 12.1 Incarceration rates per 100,000 United States residents.
Source: Sabol & West, 2010.

Table 12.1 HIV Prevalence among Jail Inmates, 2002

Gender	Latino	Black, Non-Hispanic	White
Male	2.9%	1%	0.6%
Female	2.9%	3%	1.6%

Source: Maruschak (2004).

inmates are required to test for HIV, the actual percentage of HIV-positive inmates is likely to be higher than reported in the official statistics (Lanier & Paoline, 2005). Interviews conducted in 2002 determined that nearly two-thirds of jail inmates had ever tested for HIV, and 2.5% of inmates who had tested after admission to jail were HIV positive (Maruschak, 2004). Importantly, among jail inmates who had ever been tested, Latinos were more than three times as likely as whites and twice as likely as African Americans to report being HIV-positive (2.9% for Hispanics, 0.8% for whites, and 1.2% for African Americans) (Maruschak, 2004). Potential reasons for the elevated number of Latino jail detainees who report being HIV-positive merit further investigation, and are likely to have vital implications for culturally specific prevention interventions and testing protocols both inside and out of correctional environments. Likewise, as shown in Table 12.1, there are prominent differences in the prevalence of HIV when stratified by gender and ethnicity, and the high prevalence among Latinos and Latinas signals another key area for further research.

In general, the prevalence of HIV infection is notably higher among female inmates: in 2002 1.2% of male jail inmates and 2.3% of female jail inmates were known to be HIV positive (Maruschak, 2004) and at year end 2008 1.5% of male state prisoners and 1.9% of female state prisoners were known to be HIV positive (Maruschak, 2005). Nearly 12% of female prisoners and 5.6% of male prisoners were known to be HIV positive in New York state, which estimates the number of HIV and confirmed AIDS cases using data from blind seroprevalence studies conducted biannually (Maruschak, 2005). The overall elevated HIV prevalence among women may be attributable to higher proportions of women inmates having histories of injection drug use, sexual relationships with injection drug users, histories of sexual abuse, or involvement in sex work (Braithwaite, Treadwell, et al., 2005; Hammett & Drachman-Jones, 2006). Transgender people are not accounted for in official statistics on HIV in correctional institutions, despite the fact that they are particularly vulnerable to HIV infection both when incarcerated and when not in correctional custody due to social marginalization, survival sex work, hormonal injections, and sexual victimization (Bockting, Robinson, et al., 1998; Clements-Nolle, Marx, et al., 2001; Kenagy, 2002).

HIV TRANSMISSION RISK FACTORS IN THE CORRECTIONAL SETTING

Although a large number of individuals admitted to U.S. prisons and jails have a history of injection drug use and a higher prevalence of infection with blood-borne viruses prior to incarceration, incident cases of HIV have been reported in U.S. correctional facilities. For example, the Georgia Department of Corrections identified 88 cases of HIV known to have become positive while in prison that were associated with injection drug use, tattooing, or men having sex with men during confinement (MMWR, 2006; see also Krebs & Simmons, 2002).

A large proportion of the U.S. prison population has used an illegal drug within the 30 days prior to arrest (Karberg & James, 2005). Many studies have documented considerable levels of risky drug injection among inmates [Toepell, 1992; Expert Committee on AIDS and Prison (ECAP), 1994; Braithwaite, Hammett, et al., 1996; Dufour, Alary, et al., 1996; Luekefeld, Logan, et al., 1999] and drug overdose events have been reported in at least one prison setting (Albizu-Garcia et al., 2009). However, drug use inside correctional facilities is prohibited and any associated paraphernalia such as syringes, needles, or bleach are considered contraband (Hammett, Harmon, et al., 1999). Although needle-exchange programs have been successfully implemented in some European prisons since the late 1990s (Dolan, Rutter, et al., 2003), no American jurisdiction allows syringe distribution or exchange. This policy means that inmates who inject drugs typically reuse and share smuggled or makeshift syringes (Muller, Stark, et al., 1995; Darke, Kaye, et al., 1998), as vividly described by a Latino prisoner:

We'd pull the cartridges out of the pen, remove the little ball from the tip, and sharpen the shaft to a point. It would look similar to the needle device used to pump up a basketball. Then we'd fill an eye dropper with liquid heroin as if it were a syringe and fit the sharpened pen cartridge tightly into the open end of it. Now we had a clear eye-dropper tube attached to the needle. We'd then jam it into a vein, squeeze the rubber bulb at the end of the eye dropper, and shoot the heroin into our bloodstream. It was brutal, like injecting yourself with a nail, but it worked. The blood squirted out of your arm and I'd have to grab my arm and apply pressure for about ten minutes before the bleeding stopped. (Quoted in Blatchford, 2009, p. 159)

Lack of availability of opioid substitution therapy (OST) in many institutions may also contribute to risky injection practices: studies of inmates in prisons that provide OST found decreases in injection drug use and in needle and syringe sharing (Larney, 2010). Furthermore, the mechanisms by which incarceration affects injection drug use in the community may be associated with the persistence of drug use while in confinement. In a longitudinal study that followed young hepatitis C-negative injection drug users in San Francisco to identify predictors of injection cessation, Evans and collaborators (2009) found that incarceration was negatively associated with change in injecting behavior.

Likewise, despite the cultural importance and centrality of tattooing in prison and jail gang culture (see Phillips, 2001), standard policies prohibit this activity behind bars and therefore inmates reuse and share "homemade" tattoo needles (Doll, 1988; Demello, 1993). Researchers have hypothesized that tattooing involves a greater number of inmates than injection drug use and accounts for a primary means of HIV and HCV transmission or coinfection in correctional facilities (Doll, 1988). Notably, the significant health risks posed by in-prison tattooing prompted the Correctional Service of Canada to undertake a pilot program of supervised tattoo parlors in six prisons (Krauss, 2005); program evaluation determined that this initiative resulted in enhanced knowledge among staff and prisoners regarding blood-borne infectious disease prevention and potential to reduce exposure to health risk among staff and prisoners (Nafekh et al., 2009). Latinos may be at elevated risk for HIV infection in correctional institutions through unsafe tattooing practices. Several studies report that in the general population, Latinos acquire tattoos in greater proportion compared to non-Hispanic whites and African Americans. For instance, a telephone survey conducted in 2004 with a national probability sample of adults 18 to 50 years of age found that tattoos were twice as common among respondents of Hispanic ancestry (Laumann & Derick, 2006). Similar differences in prevalence have been reported for individuals in correctional institutions, and indeed, as will be discussed later in this chapter, tattooing is a key component of the organization of Latino prison mafias. In a study with incarcerated individuals in the Northeastern United States, the proportion of Latino inmates with tattoos was nearly twice that of African Americans and 33% greater than that for whites (Bryan et al., 2006). A forensic study in New Mexico of victims of homicide or accidents found statistically significant differences in tattoo frequencies by ethnicity (52% Hispanic compared to 29.5% non-Hispanic) and a greater proportion of Hispanics with multiple tattoos (Komar & Lathrop, 2008). The potential contribution of in-prison tattooing practices to HIV infection in U.S. penal institutions by ethnicity requires further exploration. If incarcerated Latinos are more likely than other ethnic groups to acquire tattoos during confinement, they also face increased risk of infection with HIV and other blood-borne pathogens.

The correctional environment can increase the likelihood that people will engage in certain behaviors in which they do not participate when not incarcerated, as well as escalate the risk associated with these behaviors. One example of this is consensual sex among men (Nacci & Kane, 1983; Solursh, Solursh, et al., 1993; Wohl, Johnson, et al., 2000). Although this subject is difficult to systematically document due to stigma, reports from inmates indicate that voluntary male-to-male sex is common in correctional facilities, often among men who identify as heterosexual and have only female partners when not incarcerated (Stephens, Cozza, et al., 1999; Lichtenstein, 2000; Koscheski, Hensley, et al., 2002; Taussig, Shouse, et al., 2006). Because state laws explicitly prohibit the distribution of condoms in prisons in every state except Mississippi and Vermont (Polonsky, Kerr, et al., 1994; LRP Publications, 2005) and the distribution of condoms in jails is permitted only in New York City, Philadelphia, Washington, D.C., Los Angeles, and San Francisco, the vast majority of inmates do not have the option to choose protected sex. Even materials such as latex gloves or plastic bags can be difficult to obtain in correctional facilities, further limiting harm reduction possibilities.

In addition, sexual violence and rape are ritualized elements of carceral culture and may be perpetrated against people who are not targets of such violence when outside of correctional walls (Rideau & Wikberg, 1992; Kupers, 1999; Sabo, Kupers, et al., 2001). Situational factors such as overcrowding in facilities can increase stress among inmates and decrease officers' ability to maintain security, which may translate into escalated sexual violence (King, 1992). A Bureau of Justice Statistics survey of over 81,500 inmates found that 2.1% of prisoners and 1.5% of jail inmates reported at least one incident of sexual victimization involving another inmate in the prior year, and 2.8% of prisoners and 2% of jail inmates reported having had sexual contact with the correctional staff (Beck, Harrison, et al., 2010). The first-ever survey of administrative records on sexual violence in adult and juvenile facilities found that males comprised 90% of victims and perpetrators of inmate-on-inmate nonconsensual sex acts (Beck & Hughes, 2005). However, in the recent Bureau of Justice Statistics survey, female prison and jail inmates were more than twice as likely as male inmates to report sexual victimization by another inmate (Beck, Harrison, et al., 2010). Women and transgender inmates have also been found to be at risk of sexual assault by or coercive sexual relationships with male correctional officers (The Members of the ACE Program of the Bedford Hills Correctional Facility, 1998; LeBlanc, 2003), and sexual abuse of women has been documented to occur at the hands of correctional staff during routine medical examinations (Braithwaite, Treadwell, et al., 2005).

Finally, the dearth of drug treatment, mental health services, and other rehabilitative programs in jails and prisons may lead to increased vulnerability to HIV infection. Among state prisoners in 2004, just 34% of people categorized as having been drug dependent or abusing in the year prior to their arrest reported taking part in self-help groups, peer counseling, or drug abuse education programs, and only 14% reported taking part in drug treatment programs with a trained professional (Mumola & Karberg, 2006). Similarly, a mere 34% of state prisoners and 17% of jail inmates who had a mental health problem received treatment during their incarceration; taking a prescribed medication was the most common form of treatment received (James & Glaze, 2006). Untreated substance use or mental health issues may place people at greater risk for HIV infection. For example, in one study of juvenile arrestees, those who indicated symptoms of clinical depression reported significantly greater sexual risk taking (Tolou-Shams, Brown, et al., 2008). Poor mental health or the need to obtain drugs while incarcerated could also make people more vulnerable to trading sex or to being the victim of forced sex (Kupers, 1999).

Although not systematically reported, it is likely that the majority of any services available in correctional facilities are provided in English, with little or no adaptation to cultural factors. As reported by Bryan et al. (2006), in an evaluation of an HIV-prevention intervention delivered to prisoners, Latinos showed a slight *decrease* in condom use self-efficacy, whereas African American and white participants showed increases. Similarly, Latinos showed a decrease in positive attitudes about not sharing needles, whereas African Americans and whites showed an increase in positive attitudes to avoid needle sharing. Bryan and co-authors posit that these outcomes may have been due to "deficits in the cultural relevance and appropriateness of the intervention material related to condom use" (2006, p. 171) and needle sharing.

Furthermore, incarceration involves prolonged separation from home and family. Many of the factors affecting Latino day laborers described in Chapters 1 and 18 of this volume also affect men and women in jail and prison: they are far from their loved ones and they suffer from a lack of social, recreational, and romantic outlets. This is particularly exacerbated for people whose family is not in the United States and for people whose family cannot afford to stay in contact (for example, to pay for collect phone calls or send packages to an incarcerated relative), as well as for people whose family cannot visit them in the correctional institution because they are undocumented. Further research investigating these factors among Latino and Latina inmates and their families could greatly expand our understanding of the links between the maintenance of family ties, HIV risk behaviors, and other health outcomes.

For those who remain behind in the community, the forced removal of large numbers of men creates a shortage of male sexual partners, which has been linked to increases in concurrent partnerships. Indeed, one's own incarceration and the incarceration of one's partner have been repeatedly associated with a greater prevalence of concurrent sexual partnerships (Gorbach, Stoner, et al., 2002; Manhart, Aral, et al., 2002; Adimora, Schoenbach, et al., 2003a, 2003b; Johnson & Raphael, 2005; Thomas & Sampson, 2005). Sexual contact is typically forbidden during the incarceration period. Although some state prisons permit conjugal visits, eligibility requirements (including the necessity of the couple being legally married and the prisoner having a low security status) and logistics result in only a tiny fraction of prisoners being able to participate. The prohibition of intimacy for extended periods of time leads to sexual frustration (Comfort, Grinstead, et al., 2005), which may lead to sexual relations outside of the primary partnership. Similarly, disruption of continuity in a primary relationship (Johnson & Raphael, 2005; Stephenson, Wohl, et al., 2006), a desire to "make up for lost time" (Seal, Margolis, et al., 2003), or the need to assert a sense of masculinity (Sabo, Kupers, et al., 2001) can also lead to concurrent partnerships upon release from prison (see also Khan et al., 2009).

For partners who reunite after a prison sentence, unprotected sexual intercourse (UPI) has emotional and practical importance within a larger context of romantic connectedness and societal reintegration for couples coping with cycles of freedom and confinement (Comfort, 2002; Comfort, Grinstead, et al., 2005). For those who also experienced a separation across a border, the significance of UPI may be particularly strong as a means of reestablishing a relationship. When inmates are released before the end of their sentence, they are required to serve out the remainder of that sentence under the supervision of a probation or parole agent. During this time, people must meet a variety of requirements: for example, parolees in California are not allowed to carry weapons or to travel more than 50 miles from their residence, and they must submit to their person, residence, or vehicle being searched at any time by police or parole agents (Petersilia, 1999). Failure to meet any parole condition is considered a "violation" and can result in an immediate return to prison. People may feel that the encroachment on their and their partner's privacy in the form of surveillance and searches inhibits the feelings of relaxation and intimacy needed to discuss sensitive issues such as HIV risk (Comfort, Grinstead, et al., 2005). In addition, the possibility that someone might be abruptly reincarcerated discourages couples who desire pregnancy from waiting 6 months to confirm negative HIV test results before having unprotected sex, as is generally recommended by HIV prevention practitioners.

HIV TESTING AND TREATMENT IN CORRECTIONAL FACILITIES

Early HIV diagnosis is essential for effective treatment to deter disease progression and curtail transmission. Centers for Disease Control and Prevention surveillance data from 2006 indicate that a larger proportion of male and female Latinos receive a late diagnosis when compared to whites (CDC, 2009). It is not known whether the same is true for incarcerated Latinos. Testing policies for HIV and hepatitis C virus (HCV) are determined at the county level for jails and at the state or federal level for prisons. Testing in jails is often less systematic because jails hold pretrial detainees and people sentenced to less than 1 year of confinement, which results in high population turnover rates and the possibility that individuals may not be held in the facility long enough to receive a test result if rapid testing is not being used or to see an HIV specialist or begin treatment if necessary. The prison system incarcerates people with sentences longer than 1 year and those who are returned to custody for violating the conditions of their parole. In 2008, a total of 24 state departments of corrections reported testing all inmates for HIV either at admission or sometime during the incarceration period, while all 50 states and the federal system provided HIV testing upon request or if inmates presented clinical indication of infection. Regardless of the HIV testing policies, people often have their blood drawn and tested for certain diseases, such as syphilis, upon entry to the facility. If medical procedures are not well explained or an inmate is not conversant in English, people may believe that they are being tested for HIV when this is not the case. Budget limitations frequently necessitate a "no news is good news" policy, meaning that only those whose results show infection receive a follow-up appointment to discuss their status. Consequently, an inmate who never receives HIV test results might assume that he or she tested negative, when in fact the test might not have been performed.

In addition, the rigorous protection of the confidentiality of medical information that is considered paramount for most U.S. residents does not exist for inmates who test HIV positive or voluntarily disclose their positive status while behind bars. Standing in line daily for medication, requesting to see the designated HIV doctor, or having a correctional officer discuss information obtained through a monitored phone call or letter quickly spreads talk of one's serostatus throughout the correctional microcosm, and possibly beyond, if any fellow inmates or officers know one's family or associates in the outside world (Murphy, 2004). People may choose to forego testing or conceal their already-known positive status while incarcerated in order to preserve their medical privacy, particularly if they are serving a relatively short sentence and prefer to test or receive treatment upon release (McTighe, 2005).

Physicians and nurses working behind bars find their efforts to provide care complicated by prison-specific impediments such as outdated medical records and documentation systems,[3] mandatory racial segregation (which can prevent inmates of different races/ethnicities from being in the infirmary simultaneously, purportedly to avoid gang violence), lack of equipment and supplies, high costs for security when transporting inmates to and from outside hospitals, and severe understaffing (Sterngold, 2005). Furthermore, serious errors, neglect, and incompetence can impede diagnosis and treatment for HIV-positive inmates because doctors and other medical personnel who have been sanctioned for poor standards of practice and who have had their general licenses revoked are at times allowed to continue to work in correctional facilities (Pollack, Khoshnood, et al., 1999; Hylton, 2003). Recent lawsuits filed by or on behalf of ill inmates are bringing questions of state liability for medical malpractice and neglect to the fore: in 2005 federal judge Thelton Henderson cited "horrifying" and "abysmal" conditions in his decision to place California's prison health care system under receivership (Bee, 2005; Sterngold, 2005). Even in less egregious situations in which adequate general care is available, it is critical for HIV-positive jail detainees and prisoners to have access to HIV specialists in order to ensure proper treatment and to avoid errors (Cusac, 2000). Excellent models of providing comprehensive medical care for HIV-positive incarcerated people do exist (see Farley et al., 2000; Flanigan et al., 2009); enhancing these services by providing culturally sensitive and Spanish-speaking medical providers available is imperative.

Whatever treatment inmates may receive while incarcerated, new challenges face them upon release from custody. One study of HIV-positive prisoners in Texas found that only 5.4% filled an initial prescription for antiretroviral therapy medications within 10 days of release from custody, and only 17.7% had done so by 30 days postrelease (Baillargeon, Giordano, et al., 2009). For Latinos who are not fluent in English and are not connected with a Spanish-speaking provider, one would imagine that this percentage would be even smaller; for those who face deportation upon release from jail or prison, the probability of connecting to adequate HIV care in a timely manner could be hypothesized to drop dramatically. Once again, these are critical areas for additional research in helping to build a fuller understanding of HIV-positive Latinos' experiences leaving correctional custody and connecting to care upon release.

As noted in the Introduction, given the relative scarcity of Latino-focused research on the issues of HIV risk behaviors in correctional settings, motivations for and barriers to testing in the carceral environment, and facilitators of and impediments to connecting to care in the community, we decided to focus on two specific issues about which more information is available. We now turn to these case studies, first Latino prison mafias in the California state prison system, and then injection drug use among Puerto Rican inmates. In harmony with our overall goals for this chapter, we hope that these case studies will stimulate thinking about avenues for future research by drawing on existing literature.

CASE STUDY 1: THE CALIFORNIA PRISON MAFIAS

In thinking about the distinct contexts of HIV risk that may be faced by incarcerated Latinos, it is crucial to consider how inmates organize themselves during incarceration (Rodriguez, 2010), and how those internal carceral structures influence people in barrios and communities outside of prison (Garcia, 2010). Once a Latino becomes an inmate in California, he enters a structured field of carceral power relations that can potentially affect HIV risk behavior, specifically engagement in sexual and physical violence, tattooing, and intravenous drug use. Latinos in jails and prisons have constrained choices regarding specific behaviors; upon incarceration, they face significant pressure to "click up" or claim allegiance to internal inmate organizations. Sometimes referred to as "prison gangs" (Rafael, 2007), these internal inmate organizations are not divided strictly by ethnicity for Latinos, as they are for other ethnic groups, but rather are also stratified by territorial affiliation (i.e., Southsiders or Northerners).

In our framing of how inmates organize themselves, we identify two primary forms of internal organization: *prison clicks* and *prison mafias*. Prison clicks (like the Aryan Brotherhood, Paisas and Black Guerilla Family) are groups of inmates that function primarily within prisons and jails. In contrast, prison mafias such as Nuestra Familia [Our Family] and La eMe [The M] have a significant presence inside of the prison as well as distinct influence in neighborhoods and communities on the outside. Furthermore, penal institutions serve as headquarters for the prison mafias, as elite mafia members or "shot callers" maintain control on the outside through their power base from inside the penitentiaries. The prison mafias' direct and indirect influence rests on the fact that Latino street gang members more often than not will end up in prison. Thus, over the past 50 years, California Latino prison mafias have devised an inmate organizational structure that protects and unifies rival Latino street gangs inside prisons and jails. As such, Latino prison mafias depend on a symbiotic relationship between carceral institutions and *prison-pathway* neighborhoods, barrios, and communities (Wacquant, 2001; Rodriguez, 2010; Molina, 2010).

Furthermore, these prison mafias have set up a sophisticated structure with specific modes of governance, discipline, and reward that operate within and outside of the penal system. There is a clear hierarchy consisting of mafioso elites, mid-range officers, and thousands of soldiers in prison yards, county jails, juvenile correctional facilities, and on the streets. Like other criminal organizations, one primary purpose of the prison mafias is to make an economic profit. Through Latino mafias' extensive networks of street soldiers, associates, lieutenants, *carnales* [blood brothers], *camaradas* [comrades], and homeboys, these organizations have a significant degree of power in neighborhoods and communities hundreds of miles away from the penitentiaries that house the shot callers. This barrio/prison symbiosis (Rodriguez, 2010; see also Wacquant, 2001) is a unique and defining characteristic of Latinos in prisons and may be related to HIV risk behavior, for the reason that Latino mafias control very profitable criminal enterprises that potentially involve HIV risk: in-prison sex-worker rings, drug distribution, and extortion through extreme violence.

Through a robust network of mafia associates and street gang soldiers, prison mafias conduct and control criminal businesses through a series of individuals earning promotions; importantly, these promotions occur exclusively *in prisons*, and thus in order to be promoted, an individual must be serving hard time. Once a mafia promotion is made, the individual's status does not directly relate to the institution in which he is being held. Instead, his mafia ranking is associated with him and is carried by him to the streets and to any prison or jail to which he is sent. This allows him to return from correctional facilities to the streets as a higher-ranking member of the organization with a power position that usurps that of regular street gang members. As status elevation is primarily acquired within the penitentiary, many young street gang members aspire to become elite mafia members, and thus desire to go to prison in order to earn a higher status. This trajectory consequentially involves entering and inhabiting a potentially higher HIV risk sociopenal environment. As the formerly incarcerated person quoted at the beginning of this chapter emphasizes: "*I first went to prison years ago. I wanted to go. I thought I would be around people of respect, killers*" (emphasis added). Upon incarceration, a basic requirement of survival in jails or prisons is to "click up" for protection. Paradoxically, this leads to potentially increasing one's HIV risk. When earning a prison-mafia promotion a Latino will receive tattoos signifying his higher rank. Members of clicks will share needles if participating in intravenous drug use. And even with the protection of a click, an inmate who is perceived as weak may be "turned out" as a sex worker. Give this context, we consider: *How have Latino prison mafias developed and what is their relationship to HIV risk?*

Prison Mafia Origins of Protection and Violence

During the 1940s and 1950s, racial minority inmates did not have a critical mass to challenge the prevalence of the white convict code. In correctional facilities, inmates of color had to adhere to the request and demands of white inmates as well as prison guards. In the late 1950s the earliest formations of Latino prison mafias in California brought together young Mexican Americans inmates who sought to protect themselves against inmate predators and prison guards (Rafael, 2007). The span of the 1960s dramatically reconstituted relationships among ethnic/racial groups in prisons and shaped the current prison mafia ethos. First, the Civil Rights movements outside prison walls, such as United Farm Workers, the Black Panthers, and the Brown Berets, coalesced with internal inmate organization schemas. Furthermore, police brutality and the prison were connected as a major platform of dissent for these civil rights movements [Salazar, 1998; Jackson, 1994 (1970)]. Second, the population of prisoners of color grew into a sizable force that could challenge forms of violent oppression, be it by whites, other inmates groups, or prison guards. Given the correctional institutions' inability to provide adequate protection, racial minorities could now mobilize united fronts in response to violence and oppression.

Third, although the ideological underpinnings of Latino mafias are predicated upon civil rights and self-determination, in vying for power and respect Latino prison mafia members use violence to achieve their aims. The mafias' historic origins mandated resorting to extreme violence as a form of protection in warding off predators, and this persists today as a fundamental structure in the Latino prison mafia code of conduct. One example of the magnitude of collective violence occurred in February 2000 on the prison exercise yard of Pelican Bay State Penitentiary, located on the California-Oregon border, when a Latino prison mafia attacked black inmates. Dozens of inmates were stabbed or shot by correctional officers, and several were killed. In the end, correctional officers recovered about 50 prison-made knives and weapons from the yard (Wallace, Podger, et al., 2000). It is likely that the majority of these knives and weapons were concealed from correctional officers by being hidden in inmates' rectums (a practice called "keystering"). This practice has possible implications for HIV risk as men's rectums are likely to suffer tears and cuts through the process of keystering, which would render them highly vulnerable to infection if they were subsequently to engage in receptive anal sex and would also increase the risk of transmission of blood-borne pathogens during acts of violence since the knives used would be bloody from these internal injuries.

Placas and Cultural Pride

California Latino prison mafias adopted Chicano cultural iconography, such as images of Aztec warriors and ancient Mesoamerican temples. Prison mafias and clicks have symbolic tattoos that are awarded in prison and most often have to be tattooed on one's body while incarcerated. A person cannot obtain these specific tattoos on the outside, and thus potential HIV risk is increased because prison tattoos are given clandestinely in unsanitary conditions. In addition, prison tattoos illustrate status within the prison social environment and serve as a form of defense and respect by signaling to others that this inmate has committed violent acts to earn tattooed badges of honor, such as the "black hand" of la eMe (Blatchford, 2009). In prison, gang members have an incentive to be tattooed. Tattoos show loyalty to the prison mafia and signify to other inmates one's willingness to engage in extreme violence if necessary, and further an alliance to the protective organization of the mafia. Refusing to be tattooed may be taken as a form of disrespect or the sign of an uncommitted member.

Tecatos and Intravenous Drug Users

Prison mafias tend to look down upon drug use, but some organizations are more effective in enforcing a prohibition on the use of hard drugs. A major source of revenue comes from selling drugs, so nonaffiliates (called "fish" or "punks") are encouraged to use drugs by prison dealers with an eye to the potential profit they can bring to the mafia. However, mafia "tax collectors" are expected to not engage in substance use because they handle the transactions and must be trusted not to use the drugs themselves. Although some mafia members may engage in substance use, they are often able to avoid the exchange of sex for drugs because the mafia controls the flow of drugs in prisons (Rafael, 2007). However, active members who are serving life or very long sentences tend to burn out after decades of incarceration and may become addicted to their own distribution supply of heroin. Blatchford's account of a high ranking mafia member ("Boxer") who became an addict and then an informant explains that when Boxer and a fellow inmate named "Jacko" received the news that Boxer's brother had been diagnosed with rapidly advancing AIDS, hepatitis C, and cirrhosis after years of sharing dirty needles and having sex in prison, Boxer and Jacko did not stop their own in-prison substance use, but practiced a form of harm reduction by starting to sniff heroin instead of injecting it. Boxer remarks that "we thought it was classier and had this false perception, a focused moral standard that we weren't shooting up. . . we were still heroin addicts" (Blatchford, 2009, p. 160).

Sexual Taboos

Men having sex with men is officially condemned by both La eMe and Nuestra Familia, although this is difficult to enforce among the mafia's soldiers. Mafia members tend to be from barrios that have strong informational networks within the prison. Before a mafia promotion will be made, there will be a "background check" and sexual orientation is a major point of interest within the promotion criteria. If a mafia member engages in prohibited sexual activities, he is likely to be ostracized (Molina fieldnotes, 2010; Rodriguez fieldnotes, 2010). Unlike mafia members, nonaffiliates do not have the advantage of a protective organization that can decrease their chances of being raped or being forced to exchange sex for physical protection. In addition, nonaffiliates or punks are not only used for sex, but also as "mules" to transport weapons and drugs. Therefore, being a member of a prison mafia may have some protective benefits with regard to the risk of HIV infection resulting from sexual victimization or exploitation and forced keystering (Molina fieldnotes, 2010; Rodriguez fieldnotes, 2010).

Overall, we conclude that the norms enforced by Latino prison mafias require further study to assess their role in risk behaviors in prison and their potential for involvement in prison-based prevention programs. Of note, the role of prison mafia involvement and its effects on HIV risk behaviors may differ for inmates in the Puerto Rico prison system. Although this is a topic that has not received extensive research attention, data suggest that gang norms in Puerto Rico are associated with less sharing of drug preparation equipment (Kang et al., 2005). In recognition of the fact that different factors from those on the mainland may contribute to HIV risk for Puerto Ricans living on the island, we turn to examining the Puerto Rican context in more depth.

CASE STUDY 2: DISAGGREGATING HIV IN PRISON BY LATINO NATIONALITY: INJECTION DRUG USE AND THE BURDEN OF HIV INFECTION AMONG PUERTO RICAN INMATES

Disaggregating risk factors for HIV by Latino origin is necessary to understand the dynamics of the HIV epidemic and to develop cultural and contextually appropriate prevention interventions in prison and in the community. Data reported in 2008 by the Centers for Disease Control and Prevention indicate that males in Puerto Rico are more likely to acquire HIV as a result of IDU or high-risk sexual contact with women in contrast to men born in Central America, South America, Cuba, Mexico, or in the United States, who are more likely to become HIV infected through sexual contact with men (see Chapter 19 for a review of the literature on HIV and injection drug use in Puerto Ricans; as well as Chapter 13 for an in-depth study of serodiscordant Puerto Rican couples). The burden of the HIV epidemic also differs by national origin. Puerto Ricans exhibit a higher death rate from HIV when compared to Latinos of Cuban, South/Central American, and Mexican origin (Selik et al., 2003). These differences extend to the prison population.

Incarcerated island Puerto Ricans experience a large disparity in HIV prevalence when compared to the aggregate U.S. inmate population that is primarily driven by IDU. Whereas in 2006 the largest prevalence of HIV/AIDS cases among people in custody reported for a region of the United States was 3.6% (Maruschak, 2009), the HIV/AIDS prevalence in incarcerated populations in Puerto Rico is 6.9% (Rodríguez-Díaz, Reece, et al., 2011). In a study commissioned in 2005 by the Puerto Rico Department of Corrections (PRDCR) to assess the need for drug treatment among sentenced inmates, 4% of male and 11% of female inmates reported that they were infected with HIV. Self-reported HIV prevalence was significantly greater among inmates who injected drugs in prison (Albizu-García et al., 2005). Addressing the needs of this subgroup requires understanding the factors that contribute to the disproportionate prevalence of HIV in Puerto Rico. HIV incidence in the Puerto Rican prison population has not been studied. Although risky IDU and tattooing practices take place in this setting (Albizu-Garcia et al., 2005), it is likely that the higher prevalence of HIV in Puerto Rican prisons primarily reflects the burden of infection among drug users in the community, who are at greater risk of arrest and incarceration.

Puerto Rico is a major site of the U.S. HIV epidemic and the only jurisdiction in the Caribbean in which IDU still prevails as the major route of infection (UNAIDS, 2009). In 2006, with an estimated 45 cases per 100,000 population, Puerto Rico had the second highest HIV incidence among the 33 U.S. states and five territories that report HIV infection (CDC, 2009). This is twice the rate for the 50 U.S. states and District of Columbia (DC). Although Puerto Ricans comprise about 9% of the U.S. Latino population, 23% of new HIV cases among Latinos were contributed by Puerto Ricans. Injection drug use (39%) and high-risk heterosexual contact (37%) constitute the most frequent modes of infection.

Several factors have been identified that help explain the disparities in HIV prevalence in the island and the higher prevalence of HIV among IDUs, among which those that are contextual or structural in nature are of particular importance. A study exploring factors associated with cessation of injecting among New York Puerto Rican IDUs and those residing on the island reported that the proportion of cessation among Puerto Rican IDUs in New York at a 6-month follow-up was twice that of their island counterparts (Deren et al., 2007). The higher rate of cessation was associated with a 5-fold greater access to methadone maintenance treatment for Puerto Ricans in New York. The authors conclude that "differences in the significant relationships found in the two locations points to the importance of examining social and structural differences as part of studying and planning methods to enhance HIV prevention methods" (Deren et al., 2007, p. 297; see also Kang et al., 2005). The frequency of IDU in prison reported by island Puerto Rican IDUs was 10 times greater than that reported by those in New York (53% vs. 5%). It is possible that in Puerto Rico, which has been designated as a High Intensity Drug Traffic Area (HIDTA) since 1994 (Rosa, 2005), there may be readier access to heroin in prison, which accounts for the differences observed.

That existing barriers to prevention of HIV infection are predominantly related to the scarcity of important prevention services in the island and less so to the disposition of at-risk individuals to engage in risk behaviors is also emphasized by findings from a study of Puerto Rican out-of-treatment IDUs (Colon et al., 1992) conducted during the first decade of the epidemic. Comparable to their counterparts in Western Europe and the United States exposed to injecting risk-reduction interventions, Puerto Rican injectors showed a substantial reduction in all sharing behaviors, from 33% in shared use of cookers to 74.2% in sharing equipment with strangers. Discontinuation rates of sharing needles, renting needles, sharing with sexual partners, and sharing with strangers were all larger than 50% . Among protective behaviors, use of new needles was increased almost twice as much as use of bleach (20.6% vs. 11.3%, respectively).

In a recent review of prison-based HIV prevention interventions, Jurgens, Ball, and Verster (2009) discuss evidence that supports the effectiveness of needle and syringe programs and opioid substitution therapies at reducing HIV risk behaviors in diverse prison contexts worldwide. In 2002 the PRDCR initiated a small pilot program of prerelease methadone maintenance treatment for opiate-addicted inmates that curtailed heroin use among participants by nearly 100% at 1 year (Heimer et al., 2006). In 2006, the PRDCR facilitated a study funded by the National Institute on Drug Abuse to assess the feasibility of initiating an opiate agonist treatment program with buprenorphine-naloxone that demonstrated acceptability for staff and inmates as well as a significant retention in treatment at 1 month postrelease and reduction of heroin use (Garcia et al., 2007). In spite of these efforts, the enormous treatment gap existing in the community contributes to a continued flow of opiate-dependent inmates into the island's correctional facilities. Data from a community survey conducted in the island in 2008 indicate that there is treatment capacity for less than 8% of the island's subpopulation with a diagnosis of abuse or dependence to an illicit drug (Colón et al., 2009).

Given the centrality of injected drug use and unprotected sex between injectors and their partners in the spread of HIV in Puerto Rico, interventions to reduce drug use in prison and upon release are essential to curtail the epidemic. This will require a continuum of care that includes a prominent role for expansion of medication-assisted treatment for opiate dependence, testing for HIV and STDs, and providing appropriate counseling and antiretroviral treatment to those who are eligible. The disparities observed for island Puerto Rican injectors when compared to their compatriots who reside in New York City highlight the prominence of structural rather than cultural factors as determinants of HIV risk-reducing behaviors. Oversight of the status of the epidemic in the prison setting needs to be assumed by the island's public health authorities and policies facilitating implementation of strategies based on harm reduction measures should become a priority in HIV prevention for the island.

CONCLUSIONS

Throughout this chapter, we have noted areas of need for future studies to identify, expand, and deepen our understanding of the experiences of incarcerated and formerly incarcerated Latinos in relation to HIV risk behavior, testing, and linkage to care. We have also focused on two bodies of existing literature as a means to stimulate our thinking about the ways in which context and culture may affect HIV risk and prevention for incarcerated Latinos. The potential avenues for further research are vast, and include many additional topics, such as:

- The role of religion in coping, resiliency, and substance-use recovery for HIV-positive Latino inmates and former inmates;
- Experiences of monolingual Spanish speakers in jail and prison, and how these relate to their HIV risk behaviors;
- Formerly incarcerated Latinos' access to housing, drug treatment, mental health services, educational programs, and employment assistance, and how the provision or lack of provision of these social services affects risk behaviors for HIV-negative people or continuity of care for HIV-positive people;
- Incarcerated Latinas' experiences of consensual and nonconsensual sex, tattooing, and injection drug practices;
- Stigma and discrimination against Latinos with criminal records, and the relationship between these factors and HIV risk.

In spite of effective interventions to curtail the HIV epidemic and to reduce morbidity and mortality among those living with HIV, disparities exist for Latinos that are likely compounded by their greater likelihood of facing arrest, incarceration, and its accompanying social isolation. Identifying the extent to which these social determinants contribute to infection risk and act as barriers to effective prevention and treatment services demands prompt attention. There is much work to be done. But together we can get there: *¡Juntos adelante!*

NOTES

1. The qualitative data presented in this chapter come from two ongoing ethnographic investigations: Timoteo Rodriguez's *Religious Conversions Among Latino Male Heroin Users* (CALM) study, funded by the National Institute of Mental Health (supplement to R01MH 078743, M. Comfort, PI) and Carlos Molina's *Born Suspect Study: How Civil Gang Injunctions Influence Perception of Law, Self, and Community* (funded by the U.C. Berkeley McNairs Scholars Program). These two projects investigate the social dynamics between the barrio and penal relationship on individual Latinos and Latino communities.

2. The figures in this chapter are the most recent available at the time of this writing. Readers are encouraged to consult the Bureau of Justice Statistics website (www.ojp.usdoj.gov/bjs) for the most up-to-date reports.

3. As Sufrin (2010) notes, these antiquated paper-based or dated computer systems for tracking medical information can still provide opportunities for generating social relationships between medical providers and inmates. As such, seemingly incidental objects of bureaucracy in a correctional medical clinic can potentially facilitate relationships of care and rehumanization.

REFERENCES

Adimora, A. A., Schoenbach, V. J., et al. (2003a). Concurrent partnerships among rural African Americans with recently reported heterosexually transmitted HIV infection. *Journal of Acquired Immune Deficiency Syndrome, 34*(4), 423–429.

Adimora, A. A., Schoenbach, V. J., et al. (2003b). Concurrent sexual partnerships among African Americans in the rural South. *AIDS Education and Prevention, 14*(3), 155–160.

Albizu-García, C. E., Hernández-Viver, A., Feal, J., & Rodríguez-Orengo, J. F. (2009). Characteristics of inmates witnessing overdose events in prison: Implications for prevention in the correctional setting. *Harm Reduction Journal, 6*, 15.

Albizu-García, C. E., Román-Badenas, L., et al. (2005). Estudio de necesidades de tratamiento para el uso de sustancias y la prevención de VIH y hepatitis B/C en las prisiones de Puerto Rico, San Juan.

Baillargeon, J., Giordano, T. P., et al. (2009). Accessing antiretroviral therapy following release from prison. *Journal of the American Medical Association, JAMA, 301*(8), 848–857.

Beck, A. J., Harrison, P. M., et al. (2010). *Sexual victimization in prisons & jails reported by inmates, 2008–2009*. U.S. Department of Justice Bureau of Justice Statistics (August 2010). Available at http://bjs.ojp.usdoj.gov/content/pub/pdf/svpjri0809.pdf. NCJ 231169.

Beck, A. J., & Hughes, T. A. (2005). *Sexual violence reported by correctional authorities, 2004*. Washington, DC: Bureau of Justice Statistics.

Bee, C. C. (2005). Prison health care seized: Citing some "outright depravity," U.S. judge will pick overseer. *Sacramento Bee*, July 1, p. A1.

Blatchford, C. (2009). *The black hand: The bloody rise & redemption of "Boxer" Enriguez, a Mexican mob killer*. New York: HarperCollins Publishers.

Bockting, W., Robinson, B., et al. (1998). Transgender HIV prevention: A qualitative needs assessment. *AIDS Care, 10*(4), 505–525.

Braithwaite, R., Hammett, T., et al. (1996). *Prisons and AIDS: A public health challenge*. San Francisco: Jossey-Bass.

Braithwaite, R. L., Treadwell, H. M., et al. (2005). Health disparities and incarcerated women: A population ignored. *American Journal of Public Health, 95*(10), 1679–1681.

Bryan, A., Robbins, R. N., Ruiz, M. S., & O'Neill, D. (2006). Effectiveness of an HIV prevention intervention in prison among African Americans, Hispanics, & Caucasians. *Health Education & Behavior, 33*(2), 154–177.

Centers for Disease Control and Prevention. Incidence and diagnoses of HIV infection— Puerto Rico, 2006. (2009). *Morbidity and Mortality Weekly Report, 58*(21), 589–591.

Centers for Disease Control and Prevention. (2010). *Diagnoses of HIV infection and AIDS in the United States and Dependent Areas, 2008*. HIV Surveillance Report, Volume 20. Retrieved from http://www.cdc.gov/hiv/surveillance/resources/reports/2008report/.

Clements-Nolle, K., Marx, R., et al. (2001). HIV prevalence, risk behaviors, health care use, and mental health status of transgender persons: Implications for public health intervention. *American Journal of Public Health, 91*(6), 915–921.

Colón, H., Reyes Pulliza, J. C., et al. (2009) Trastornos de Substancias y Uso de Servicios en Puerto Rico Encuesta de Hogares—2008. Administración de Servicios de Salud Mental y Contra la Adicción, Puerto Rico.

Colón, H. M., Rivera Robles, R., Sahai, H., & Matos, T. (1992). Changes in HIV risk behaviors among intravenous drug users in San Juan, Puerto Rico. *British Journal of Addiction to Alcohol and Other Drugs, 87*(4), 585–590.

Comfort, M. L. (2002). "Papa's house": The prison as domestic and social satellite. *Ethnography, 3*(4), 467–499.

Comfort, M., & Grinstead, O. (2004). The carceral limb of the public body: Jail detainees, prisoners, and infectious disease. *Journal of the International Association of Physicians in AIDS Care, 3*, 45–48.

Comfort, M., & Grinstead, O., et al. (2005). "You can't do nothing in this damn place!": Sex & intimacy among couples with an incarcerated male partner. *Journal of Sex Research, 42*(1), 3–12.

Cusac, A. M. (2000). The judge gave me ten years. He didn't sentence me to death. Inmates with HIV deprived of proper care. *The Progressive*. Retrieved from http://www.progressive. org/amc0700.htm.

Darke, S., Kaye, S., et al. (1998). Drug use & injection risk-taking among prison methadone maintenance patients. *Addiction, 93*(8), 1169–1175.

Demello, M. (1993). The convict body: Tattooing among male American prisoners. *Anthropology Today, 9*(6), 10–13.

Deren, S., Kang, S-Y., et al. (2007). Predictors of injection drug use cessation among Puerto Rican drug injectors in New York & Puerto Rico. *The American Journal of Drug and Alcohol Abuse, 33*, 291–299.

Díaz-Cotto, J. (2006). *Chicana lives and criminal justice: Voices from el Barrio.* Austin: University of Texas Press.

Dolan, K., Rutter, S., et al. (2003). Prison-based syringe exchange programmes: A review of international research and development. *Addiction, 98*(2), 153–158.

Doll, D. C. (1988). Tattooing in prison & HIV infection. *Lancet, 2*(9), 66.

Dufour, A., Alary, M., et al. (1996). Prevalence and risk behaviours for HIV infection among inmates of a provincial prison in Quebec City. *AIDS, 10*(9), 1009–1015.

Expert Committee on AIDS and Prison (ECAP). (1994). *HIV/AIDS in prisons: Summary report and recommendations of the expert committee on AIDS and prisons* (Catalogue No. JS82–68/81–1994E). Ottawa, Canada, Correctional Service of Canada: Ministry of Supply and Services Canada.

Evans, J. L, Hahn, J. A., Lum, P. J., Stein, E. S., & Page, K. (2009). Predictors of injection drug use cessation & relapse in a prospective cohort of young injection drug users in San Francisco, CA (UFO Study). *Drug and Alcohol Dependence, 101*, 152–157.

Farley, J. L., Mitty, J. A., et al. (2000). Comprehensive medical care among HIV-positive incarcerated women: The Rhode Island experience. *Journal of Womens Health & Gender-Based Medicine, 9*(1), 51–60.

Federal Bureau of Investigation. (2010). *Uniform crime reports: Crime in the United States.* Washington, DC.

Flanigan, T. P., et al. (2009). HIV and infectious disease care in jails and prisons: Breaking down the walls with the help of academic medicine. *Transactions of the American Clinical Climatol Association, 120*, 73–83.

Freudenberg, N. (2001). Jails, prisons, and the health of urban populations: A review of the impact of the correctional system on community health. *Journal of Urban Health, 78*(2), 214–235.

Garcia, A. (2010). The pastoral clinic: Addiction & dispossession along the Rio Grande. Berkeley: University of California Press.

Garcia, A. C., Correa, G. C., et al. (2007). Buprenorphine-naloxone treatment for pre-release opioid-dependent inmates in Puerto Rico. *Journal of Addiction Medicine, 1*, 126–132.

Glaze, L. E. (2010). *Correctional populations in the United States, 2009.* Washington, DC: Bureau of Justice Statistics.

Glaze, L. E., & Bonczar, T. P. (2006). *Probation and parole in the United States, 2005.* Washington, DC: Bureau of Justice Statistics.

Glaze, L. E., & Bonczar, T. P. (2009). *Probation and parole in the United States, 2008.* Washington, DC: Bureau of Justice Statistics.

Goffman, A. (2009). On the run: Wanted men in a Philadelphia ghetto. *American Sociological Review, 74*(2), 339–357.

Gorbach, P., Stoner, B., et al. (2002). It takes a village: Understanding concurrent sexual partnerships in Seattle, Washington. *Sexually Transmitted Diseases, 29*, 453–462.

Hammett, T. M., & Drachman-Jones, A. (2006). HIV/AIDS, sexually transmitted diseases, and incarceration among women: National and Southern perspectives. *Sexually Transmitted Diseases, 33*(7), S17–S22.

Hammett, T., Harmon, P., et al. (1999). *1996–1997 Update: HIV/AIDS, STDs and TB in correctional facilities.* Cambridge, MA: Abt Associates.

Harrison, P. M., & Beck, A. (2006). *Prison and jail inmates at midyear 2005.* Washington, DC: Bureau of Justice Statistics, U.S. Department of Justice.

Heimer, R., Catania, H., et al. (2006). Methadone maintenance in prison: evaluation of a pilot program in Puerto Rico. *Drug Alcohol & Dependence Journal, 83*, 122–129.

Hylton, W. S. (2003). Sick on the inside: Correctional HMOs and the coming prison plague. *Harper's Magazine*, August, 43–54.

International Centre for Prison Studies. (2010). *World prison brief.* Retrieved August 31, 2006, from http://www.kcl.ac.uk/depsta/rel/icps/worldbrief/world_brief.html.

Jackson, G. (1994). *Soledad brother: The prison letters of George Jackson.* New York: Lawrence Hill Books.

James, D. J., & Glaze, L. E. (2006). *Mental health problems of prison & jail inmates.* Washington, DC: Bureau of Justice Statistics, U.S. Department of Justice.

Johnson, R. C., & Raphael, S. (2006). *The effects of male incarceration dynamics on AIDS infection rates among African-American women & men.* National Poverty Center working paper, volume 06-22.

Jürgens, R., Ball, A., & Verster, A. (2009). Interventions to reduce HIV transmission related to injecting drug use in prison. *Lancet Infectious Diseases, 9*(1), 57–66.

Kampfner, C. J.(1995). Post-traumatic stress reactions of children of imprisoned mothers. In K. Gabel & D. Johnston (Eds.), *Children of incarcerated parents* (pp. 59–88). New York: Lexington.

Kang S-Y., Deren, S., et al. (2005). HIV transmission behaviors in jail/prison among Puerto Rican drug injectors in New York & Puerto Rico. *AIDS and Behavior, 9*, 377–386.

Karberg, J. C., & James, D. J. (2005). *Substance dependence, abuse, and treatment of jail inmates, 2002.* Washington, DC: U.S. Department of Justice, Office of Justice Programs, Bureau of Justice Statistics.

Kenagy, G. (2002). HIV among transgendered people. *AIDS Care, 14*(1), 127–134.

Khan, M. R., Doherty, I. A., et. al. (2009). Incarceration & high-risk sex parterships among men in the United States. *Journal of Urban Health, 86*(4), 584–601.

King, M. (1992). Male rape in institutional settings. In G. Mezey & M. King, (Eds.), *Male victims of sexual assault.* New York: Oxford University Press.

Komar, D., & Lathrop, S. (2008). Tattoo types & frequencies in New Mexican white Hispanics & white Non-Hispanics: Autopsy data from homicidal & accidental deaths, 2002–2005. *American Journal of Forensic Medicine & Pathology, 29*, 285–289.

Koscheski, M., Hensley, C., et al. (2002). Consensual sexual behavior. In C. Hensley (Ed.), *Prison sex: Practice & policy* (pp. 111–131). Boulder, CO: Lynne Rienner Publishers, Inc.

Krauss, C. (2005). A prison makes the illicit & dangerous legal & safe. *New York Times*, November 24, p. 4.

Krebs, C. P., & Simmons, M. (2002). Intraprison HIV transmission: An assessment of whether it occurs, how it occurs, and who is at risk. *AIDS Education and Prevention. 14*(5), S53–S64.

Kupers, T. (1999). *Prison madness: The mental health crisis behind bars & what we must do about it.* San Francisco: Jossey-Bass Publishers.

Lanier, M. M., & Paoline, E. A. (2005). Expressed needs and behavioral risk factors of HIV-positive inmates. *International Journal of Offender Therapy and Comparative Criminology, 49*(5), 561–573.

Larney, S. (2010). Does opioid substitution treatment in prisons reduce injecting-related HIV risk behaviours? A systematic review. *Addiction, 105*(2), 216–223.

Laumann, A. E., & Derick, A. (2006). Tattoos & body piercings in the United States: A national data set. *Journal of American Academy Dermatology, 55*(3), 413–421.

LeBlanc, A. N. (2003). *Random family: Love, drugs, trouble, & coming of age in the Bronx.* New York: Scribner.

Lichtenstein, B. (2000). Secret encounters: Black men, bisexuality, & AIDS in Alabama. *Medical Anthropology Quarterly, 14*(3), 374–393.

LRP Publications. (2005). California chamber approves measure to give inmates condoms: Cost of AIDS care weighs heavy on decision. *Corrections Professional, 10*(18).

Luekefeld, C., Logan, T. K., et al. (1999). Drug dependency and HIV testing among state prisoners. *Population Research and Policy Review, 18*, 55–69.

Macalino, G. E., Vlahov, D., et al. (2004). Prevalence and incidence of HIV, hepatitis B virus, and hepatitis C virus infections among males in Rhode Island prisons. *American Journal of Public Health, 94*(7), 1218–1223.

Manhart, L. E., Aral, S. O., et al. (2002). Sex partner concurrency: Measurement, prevalence, & correlates among urban 18–39-year-olds. *Sexually Transmitted Diseases, 29*(3), 133–143.

Maruschak, L. (2004). *HIV in prisons and jails, 2002.* Washington, DC: Bureau of Justice Statistics.

Maruschak, L. M. (2005). *HIV in prisons, 2003.* Washington, DC: Bureau of Justice Statistics.

Maruschak, L. M. (2009). *HIV in prisons, 2007–8.* Washington, DC: Bureau of Justice Statistics.

McTighe, L. (2005). Prison health crisis—What you can do. *The Body*: www.thebody.com Retrieved December 14, 2005.

Mele, C., & Miller, T. A. (Eds.). (2005). *Civil penalties, social consequences.* New York: Routledge.

MMWR. (2006). HIV transmission among male inmates in a state prison system—Georgia, 1992–2005. *Morbidity and Mortality Weekly Report, 55*(15), 421–426.

Molina, C. III. (2010, August). *The unusual suspect.* Paper presented at the Eighteenth Annual California McNair Scholars Symposium at the University of California, Berkeley.

Muller, R., Stark, K., et al. (1995). Imprisonment: A risk factor for HIV infection counteracting education & prevention programmes for intravenous drug users. *AIDS, 9*(2), 183–190.

Mumola, C. J., & Karberg, J. C. (2006). *Drug use & dependence, state & federal prisoners, 2004.* Washington, DC: Bureau of Justice Statistics, U.S. Department of Justice.

Murphy, T. (2004). Getting out alive. *POZ, 4*, 34–41.

Nacci, P. L., & Kane, T. R. (1983). The incidence of sex & sexual aggression in federal prisons. *Federal Probation, 47*(4), 31–36.

Nafekh, M., et al. (2009). *Correctional service Canada's safer tattooing practices pilot initiative.* Retrieved January 20, 2011. http://www.csc-scc.gc.ca/text/pa/ev-tattooing-394-2-39/index-eng.shtml.

Petersilia, J. (1999). Parole & prisoner reentry in the United States. In M. Tonry & J. Petersilia (Eds.), *Prisons* (pp. 479–529). Chicago: University of Chicago Press.

Phillips, S. A. (2001). Gallo's body: Decoration & damnation in the life of a Chicano gang member. *Ethnography, 2*(3), 357–388.

Pollack, H., Khoshnood, K. et al. (1999). Health care delivery strategies for criminal offenders. *Journal of Health Care Finance, 26*(1), 63–77.

Polonsky, S., Kerr, S., et al. (1994). HIV prevention in prisons & jails: Obstacles & opportunities. *Public Health Reports, 109*(5), 615–626.

Rafael, T. (2007). *The Mexican mafia.* New York: Encounter Books.

Rich, J. D., Holmes, L., et al. (2001). Successful linkage of medical care and community services for HIV-positive offenders being released from prison. *Journal of Urban Health, 78*(2), 279–289.

Rideau, W., & Wikberg, R. (1992). *Life sentences: Rage & survival behind bars.* New York: Times Books.

Rodiguez, T. (2010). Bio-pistis: Conversion of heroin addicts in prisons, on medicine, & with God. In J. Adkins, L. Occhiinti, & T. Hefferan (Eds.), *Not by faith alone: Social services, social justice, & faith-based organizations in the United States.* Lanham, MD: Lexington Books.

Rodríguez-Díaz, C. E., Reece, M., Rivera-Alonso, B., Laureano-Landrón, I., Dodge, B., & Malow, R. M. (2011). Behind the bars of paradise: HIV and substance use among incarcerated populations in Puerto Rico. *Journal of the International Association of Physicians in AIDS Care, 10*(4), 248–259.

Rosa, 2005Rosa, T. (2005). With the highest murder rate in the U.S., Puerto Rico needs immediate solutions. *Caribbean Business.* San Juan, Puerto Rico. 8–14.

Sabo, D., Kupers, T. A., et al., (Eds.) (2001). *Prison masculinities.* Philadelphia: Temple University Press.

Sabol, W. J., & Couture, H. (2008). *Prison inmates at midyear 2007.* Washington, DC: Office of Justice Programs, U.S. Department of Justice.

Sabol, W. J., & West, H. C. (2010). *Prisoners in 2009.* Washington, DC: Office of Justice Programs, U.S. Department of Justice, Bureau of Justice Statistics.

Sabol, W. J., & West, H. C., et al. (2009). *Prisoners in 2008.* Washington, DC: Office of Justice Programs, U.S. Department of Justice.

Salazar, R. (1998). In. M. T. Garcia (Ed.), *Border correspondent: Selected writings 1955–1970.* Los Angeles: University of California Press.

Seal, D. W., Margolis, A. D., et al. (2003). HIV & STD risk behavior among 18- to 25-year-old men released from U.S. prisons: Provider perspectives. *AIDS & Behavior, 7*(2), 131–141.

Selik, R. M, Anderson, R. N., McKenna, M. T., & Rosenberg, H. M. (2003). Increase in deaths caused by HIV infection due to changes in rules for selecting underlying cause of death. *Journal of Acquired Immune Deficiency Syndrome, 32*(1), 62–69.

Solursh, L. P., Solursh, D. S., et al. (1993). Is there sex after the prison door slams shut? *Medicine & Law, 12*(3–5), 439–443.

Spaulding, A. C., Seals, R. M., et al. (2009). HIV/AIDS among inmates of & releasees from US correctional facilities, 2006: Declining share of epidemic but persistent public health opportunity. *PLoS ONE, 4*, 1–8.

Stephens, T., Cozza, S., et al. (1999). Transsexual orientation in HIV risk behaviors in an adult male prison. *International Journal of STD and AIDS, 10*, 28–31.

Stephenson, B., Wohl, D., et al. (2006). Sexual behaviors of HIV-seropositive men & women following release from prison. *International Journal of STD & AIDS, 17*, 103–108.

Sterngold, J. (2005). Overhaul of prison health system delayed. (November 3). *The San Francisco Chronicle*, p. B1.

Sufrin, C. (2010) *Paper and electronic incarcerated identities: Personalized processing in a jail medical system.* Paper presented at the American Anthropological Association Annual Meetings in New Orleans, LA.

Taussig, J., Shouse, R., et al. (2006). HIV transmission among male inmates in a state prison system: Georgia 1992–2005. *Morbidity and Mortality Weekly Report, 55*(15), 421–426.

The Members of the ACE Program of the Bedford Hills Correctional Facility. (1998). *Breaking the walls of silence: AIDS & women in a New York state maximum-security prison.* Woodstock & New York: The Overlook Press.

Thomas, J., & Sampson, L. (2005). High rates of incarceration as a social force associated with community rates of sexually transmitted infection. *Journal of Infectious Diseases, 191*(1), S55–S60.

Toepell, A. (1992). *Prisoners and AIDS: AIDS education needs assessment.* Toronto, Canada: John Howard Society of Metropolitan Toronto.

Tolou-Shams, M., Brown, L., et al. (2008). The association between depressive symptoms, substance use, & HIV risk among youth with an arrest history. *Journal of the Study of Alcohol and Drugs, 69*(1), 58–64.

Tonry, M. (2001). Punishment policies and patterns in Western countries. In M. Tonry & R. S. Frase (Eds.),. *Sentencing and sanctions in western countries* (pp. 3–28). New York: Oxford University Press.

United the World Against AIDS. (2009). *UNAIDS annual report 2009.* Retrieved from http://data.unaids.org/pub/Report/2010/2009_annual_report_en.pdf.

Wacquant, L. (2001). Deadly symbiosis: When ghetto & prison meet & mesh. *Punishment & Society, 3*(1), 95–133.

Wallace, B., Podger, P. J., & Van Derbeken, J. (2000). Guards kills prisoner in brawl at Pelican Bay/12 other inmates shot in knife-wielding melee. *San Francisco Chronicle,* February 24.

Western, B., & Pettit, B. (2010). Incarceration and social inequality. *Daedalus: the Journal of the American Academy of Arts & Sciences, 139*(3), 8–19.

Wohl, A., Johnson, D., et al. (2000). High risk behaviors during incarceration in African-American men treated for HIV at three Los Angeles public medical centers. *Journal of Acquired Immune Deficiency Syndromes, 24*(4), 386–392.

13 Puerto Rican Heterosexual Serodiscordant Couples

Cultural Challenges for Healthy Dyads[1]

Sheilla Rodríguez-Madera and
Nelson Varas-Díaz

INTRODUCTION

The HIV/AIDS epidemic is strongly influenced by the contexts in which it is manifested. This includes the social, cultural, and political dimensions that can serve to foster the spread of infection throughout the population. As of September 2011, more than 32,000 AIDS cases have been reported in Puerto Rico and it is estimated that 1% of the population has HIV (Puerto Rico AIDS Surveillance Report, 2011). This situation imposes a great challenge for primary and secondary prevention. And yet, these numbers by themselves and out of context do not help to foster a clear understanding of the implications of the epidemic for Puerto Ricans living in a small island in the Caribbean, the second epicenter of the epidemic after Sub-Saharan Africa.

The Island of Puerto Rico was a possession of Spain from 1493 to 1898, when it became a nonincorporated territory of the United States at the end of the Spanish-American War. After more than 400 years of colonial rule, Spain's cultural heritage still holds a strong presence in the everyday lives of Puerto Ricans that is manifested in the use of Spanish as the main language, strong religious life-perspectives, and traditional gender roles, among many other cultural practices. Puerto Ricans are currently United States citizens who still hold strong to their cultural identities firmly rooted in a mix of Spanish, Indian, and African traditions. As a nonincorporated territory of the United States, Puerto Rico is poorer than any of the 50 states of the Union. In this scenario of poverty and cultural differentiation from the continental United States, Puerto Rico faces an ever-growing HIV/AIDS epidemic mainly through unclean needle exchange (51%) and unprotected heterosexual activity (25%). Puerto Ricans in the Island are categorized as Latinos within the United States, and yet are citizens embedded in a context of poverty and lack of political self-determination, and are without political representation in mainland decision-making political spheres. In this context, the HIV epidemic continues to grow unchallenged. For example, prevention strategies have systematically ignored infection through needle sharing for intravenous drug use and state policies have tended to criminalize individuals with HIV (Varas-Díaz & Toro-Alfonso, 2002). See Chapter 19 by Zerden, López, and Lundgren for an extended discussion of HIV prevention with Puerto Rican injection drug users.

One of the most taxing issues in the prevention of heterosexual transmission of HIV in Puerto Rico is culture itself. Researchers have pointed to the need to change cultural norms related to gender and sexuality in order to reduce HIV transmission (Ortiz Torres, Serrano-García, & Torres-Burgos, 2000). Some of these norms are related to traditional gender roles that dictate the need for unprotected sex as a measure of trust in a relationship, understanding monogamy as an HIV prevention strategy, and the role of religion in discouraging condom use as a prevention effort. Although these issues are complex enough when addressing individuals, they become even more multifaceted when taken into consideration among couples that tend to feel protected from the HIV epidemic, just by having a steady partner. However, when one partner of the dyad is already HIV positive, the implications for prevention are even more daunting. The purpose of this chapter, within the overall framework of this edited book, is to contribute to a better understanding of those challenges among serodiscordant couples in Puerto Rico, a significant yet highly underresearched area.

Serodiscordant Couples: Particular Considerations for the HIV Epidemic

People with HIV/AIDS (PWHA) not only deal with the stress associated with a life-threatening illness, but also cope with the inherent uncertainty and psychological factors (Santos, 2002), including concerns related to the impact of HIV status on their relationships (Canada HIV/AIDS Information Centre, 2006; Van der Straten, Vernon, Knight, Gómez, & Padian, 1998). The impact of HIV on relationships has been evident in different dimensions such as perceived and internalized stigma, difficulties in status disclosure, and sexual practices (The California Partner Study, 1999).

Interpersonal dynamics have not been well explored among serodiscordant couples (Stevens & Galvao, 2007). Research has shown that the realities of relationships between men and women are critically important in shaping their health-related behaviors (Manfrin-Ledet & Porche, 2003). Studies have found that serostatus imposes pressure and feelings of alienation within relationships (Stevens & Galvao, 2007). Fear of HIV transmission, shifts in emotional intimacy, barriers to communication, dilemmas regarding how HIV will impact their lives, and lack of reproductive alternatives have been identified as the most commonly experienced issues for serodiscordant couples (Beckerman, 2002; Grinstead, Gregorich, Choi, & Coates, 2001). Other challenges include rejection, abandonment, practicing safer sex, serostatus disclosure, and financial planning (Persson, 2008).

It is not surprising that the needs of serodiscordant couples have not been well addressed in the epidemic. One of the major difficulties in HIV prevention studies is related to male's lack of involvement in initiatives that target heterosexual transmission (Burton, Darbes, & Operario, 2008). This difficulty helps to explain why women were primarily addressed in prevention interventions. Researchers have emphasized that couples should be brought into the picture, recommending the conscientious involvement of both partners in secondary prevention strategies (Jemmot, 2007; Roth, Stewart, Clay, Van der Straten, Karita, & Allen, 2001). This call is particularly important for serodiscordant couples given the two main challenges they face: (1) safer sexual practices to protect the seronegative partner, and (2) adherence to highly active antiretroviral treatment (HAART) by the seropositive partner.

Safer Sex and Adherence to Treatment: Intertwined Challenges in Secondary Prevention

Safer sex practices and adherence to treatment are two important issues to address in the context of serodiscordant couples. Furthermore, they are important to overall public health, because partial or poor HAART adherence can lead to rapid viral replication and the development of mutant viral strains that are resistant to available antiretroviral drugs (Castro, 2005). This, in turn, is worsened when unsafe sexual practices are present among PWHA who can transmit the virus. In this scenario, serodiscordant couples are a key factor for secondary prevention because the issues of sexuality and adherence to treatment are intertwined.

Engaging in safer sexual practices is not easy, particularly when those practices are related to condom use. Factors such as motivation and positive attitudes toward condoms have been documented among Puerto Ricans as important variables to address when promoting safer sex (Pérez-Jimenez, Serrano-García, & Escabí Montalvo, 2007). Negative attitudes toward condom use, which lead to risky sexual behaviors, can be related to social norms that govern heterosexual relationships. Rigid social meanings attached to what is considered "good" and "bad" sexuality are related to unprotected sex. Research carried out among Puerto Ricans show that good sexuality is interpreted as being achieved through unprotected penetration, which has a direct implication for risky behaviors (Rodríguez Madera & Marqués Reyes, 2006). In the context of couples, abstinence seems to be an impossible and unreasonable demand, and condom use is complicated by social factors that link condoms to unfaithfulness (Hirsch, Meneses, Thomson, Negroni, Pelcastre, & del Río, 2007). For example, research has shown that women with HIV/AIDS in serodiscordant couples report resistance from their partners to the idea of using condoms, which in turn propitiates their feelings of guilt and concern (Stevens & Galvao, 2007).

Even more concerning is the growing evidence indicating that the proliferation of HIV treatment options over the past decade may have decreased individuals' concerns about HIV transmission (Stevens & Galvao, 2007). Findings from studies in the United States suggest that PWHA engage in more unprotected sexual intercourse after they are on HAART (Buchacz, Van der Straten, Saul, Shiboski, Gómez, & Padiau, 2001; Wilson, Gore, Greenblatt, Cohen, Minkoff, Silver, et al., 2004). For example, researchers have found that PWHA in couple relationships frequently practice unprotected sexual intercourse with their partners, independent of their serostatus (Bova & Durante, 2003; Weinhardt, Kelly, Brondino, Rotheram-Borus, Kirshenbaum, Chesney, et al., 2004). Still, gaps remain in specific knowledge about the factors that impede or facilitate their capacity to reduce risky sexual behaviors and adopt healthy strategies within the couple dyad (Stevens & Galvao, 2007).

Adherence to HAART among serodiscordant couples is another major area of concern. It is widely known that adherence to HAART is a strong predictor of the progression to AIDS and death (Machtinger & Bangsberg, 2006). Although HAART represents great progress in the fight against HIV/AIDS, one of the most important challenges facing this epidemic is adherence to treatment. Studies that have identified variables related to adherence to treatment among PWHA reveal the importance of addressing psychosocial factors that foster it, including positive experiences within the partner relationship (Catz, Kelly, Bogart, Benotsch, & McAuliffe, 2000; Toro-Alfonso, Andújar-Bello, Amico, & Fisher, 2002). Still, little is known about how the perceptions of experiences within the dyad may influence PWHA's adherence to treatment (Lichtenstein, 2006; Roberts & Mann, 2000).

Research indicates that many patients have difficulty adhering. A meta-analysis of 59 studies conducted in the United States reported that only 55% of patients demonstrated high levels of HAART adherence (Mills, Nachega, Bangsberg, Singh, Rchliz, Wu, et al., 2006). Other studies have shown that up to 84% of participants miss medication doses (Dunbar, Madigan, Grohskopf, Revere, Woodward, Minstrell, et al., 2003; Erlen, Sereika, Cook, & Hunt, 2002). Several factor are associated with nonadherence including alcohol and drug use (Murphy, Greenwell, & Hoffman, 2002), difficulty of medication regimens (Roberts & Mann, 2000), fear of side effects (Dunbar et al., 2003), depression (Starace, Ammassar, Trotta, Murri, De Longis, Izzo, et al., 2002), lack of social support, and self-efficacy problems (Safren, Otto, Worth, Salomon, Johnson, Mayer, et al., 2001).

Research related to HIV status among couples and its impact on adherence to treatment for the infected person is scarce. Studies that do exist suggest that barriers in adherence are related to psychological factors such as negative perception of the relationship, absence of emotional support, and having an unsupportive partner (Murphy, Greenwell, & Hoffman, 2002; Wagner, Remien, Carballo-Dieguez, & Dolezal, 2002). Remien and Stirratt (2002) found in a study of 42 serodiscordant couples that there was a relationship between adherence to HAART and safer sex practices. In addition, poor adherence was significantly associated with increased unprotected anal/vaginal sex with the primary partner. Other studies have suggested that the seronegative partner's engagement in the treatment of the seropositive member of the dyad is related to good adherence (Mitrani, Prado, Feaster, Robinson-Batista, & Szapocznik, 2003). Still, it is important to note that none of these studies included Puerto Ricans.

Considering the importance of understanding the dynamics of serodiscordant couples for secondary prevention, and the intertwined role of adherence to treatment and safer sexual practices, relationship experiences within these dyads need attention. Understanding the dynamics of such relationships and how members of the dyad interpret them can yield important information to develop interventions for serodiscordant couples. In light of the challenges posed by the HIV/AIDS epidemic in Puerto Rico for individuals in general, and serodiscordant couples in particular, our study aimed to explore (1) variables related to relationship experiences among Puerto Rican heterosexual serodiscordant couples, and (2) the perceived influence of these variables on safe sexual practices among couples and adherence to treatment of the PWHA, from the perspective of both members of the dyad.

METHOD

To achieve the aims of the study we carried out an exploratory qualitative design. We implemented in-depth interviews with 20 heterosexual serodiscordant couples ($n = 40$). The couples were balanced with regard to the HIV-infected partner (male or female) in order to explore gender variations. We initially interviewed participants individually, and afterward conducted a joint interview.

The total sample for our study included 40 participants (20 couples) who engaged in qualitative interviews. All met the following criteria in order to participate: (1) of Puerto Rican nationality who live in the Island at the time of the study, (2) adults (at least 21 years of age), (3) being a seropositive person with a seronegative partner (or vice versa), (4) receiving HAART or having a partner who does, and (5) being in a heterosexual relationship within the previous 6 months in which both partners are informed of each other's serostatus. Furthermore, both members of the couple needed to be willing to participate in the qualitative interviews. These criteria were implemented in order to ensure that the findings of the study are of pertinence to Puerto Ricans PWHA, that participants are of legal age to engage in the study, and that both partner perspectives were considered.

Participants were residents of the San Juan metropolitan area with a mean age of 44 years. Most (73%) had not completed a high school diploma and were unemployed at the moment of the study (62%).[2] Seventy percent lived with their partners at the time of the interview and 68% identified them as the primary source of social support.

Data-Gathering Forms

Participants completed several data-gathering forms as part of their participation. These included a screening form that addressed all the inclusion criteria described above, an informed consent form detailing the study objectives, and a demographic data questionnaire. Our main data-gathering forms were our qualitative interview guides. We developed three interview guides: two versions for seropositive and seronegative individuals, respectively, and a third one for the couple interviews. They served to maintain a minimum level of uniformity across participant interviews. Questions addressed issues related to overall experiences with HIV, the perceived impact on couple dynamics, sexual practices, and adherence to treatment. Guides for seronegative participants included questions about their perception of the partner's adherence to his or her treatment. The interview guide for couples included questions that were asked of both partners simultaneously, placing emphasis on the couple's perspective. A panel of five experts in HIV-related research reviewed all the interview guides before using them in the field in order to ensure their appropriateness to the Puerto Rican context. We conducted a pilot study with two couples to test their understanding of the questions in the developed forms.

Procedures

Participants were recruited from Puerto Rico's largest facility complex for treating PWHA. This facility is composed of eight government-operated centers that provide health-related services to approximately 10,000 PWHA in Puerto Rico. At the time of the study, we met with the contact person from the facility prior to participants' recruitment in order to fully explain the study. We asked him to identify potential participants according with the inclusion criteria, and familiarize them with the nature of the study. If they were interested in participating, their contact information was given to us. Afterward, a member of the research team invited them to participate without the presence of the contact person. We administered the screening form to ensure that individuals complied with the selection criteria.

We informed participants immediately if they were eligible to participate. If the partner was present, we gave him or her the screening form. If this was not the case, we provided the participant with information on the study and set up a scheduled meeting in which he or she could bring the partner in order to carry out the invitation. We provided him or her with our phone numbers in case they had problems explaining the study to the partner or needed to change the scheduled meeting. We gathered consent individually in order to avoid coercion by one member of the dyad. Only two of the recruited couples decided not to participate in the study.

All interviews were carried out at the recruitment sites in private rooms. Once participants were interviewed individually, we engaged in a couple interview in which both participants and interviewers were present. Each interview lasted approximately 1 hour. Total participation entailed 3 hours considering the recruitment process. Once they finished their participation, we provide each participant with a $50 incentive for their participation.

Data Analysis

To maintain the quality of our analysis, we started with a supervised transcription process to ensure fidelity (Poland, 2002). Research assistants were trained by the investigators on the appropriate way to transcribe an audio interview. After transcriptions were carried out, the team read the transcriptions while listening to the audiotapes in order to identify inconsistencies between them. The team met and corrected all errors in the transcriptions. Once this process was completed for each audiotape, the data analysis procedures began.

The research team met on a weekly basis to identify themes or patterns that emerged from our transcriptions. The team developed a master list of these themes to keep for the analysis. These themes continued to be modified throughout the reading of all the transcriptions. Once those general themes were identified for all the interviews, the team searched for texts that evidenced them in the transcriptions. All selected texts for each theme were discussed in weekly meetings to ensure that they were appropriately selected by all members of the team (Phillips & Ardí, 2002). This consensus-based dispute resolution procedure will generate an interrater reliability of 100% for the analysis (Miller, 2001). This step was carried out in order to ensure that the analysts agreed on the final interpretation of the coded passages and to avoid the inclusion of verbalizations that are unclear in their phrasing or overall meaning. The text selection and coding process were carried out with the use of qualitative analysis computer software Nudist Nvivo (V.8.). Throughout the process several steps were taken in order to ensure the trustworthiness of the data (Lincoln & Guba, 1985; Schwandt, 2001). These included (1) supervising the overall transcription process of the audio taped interviews and focus groups, (2) meeting with members of the research team to discuss the quality of these transcriptions, and (3) establishing group discussions throughout the data collection and analysis process so that team members could discuss concerns and findings. The results obtained from this process are presented in the following section.

RESULTS

Findings from this study highlight issues of pertinence for couples that need to be addressed in preventive initiatives in the Puerto Rican context. Throughout our analysis we were able to document multiple areas that could potentially negatively affect PWHA, their health-related behaviors, and overall quality of life. To facilitate the analysis of participants' narratives, we will present four of the categories that to our understanding reflect major challenges for serodiscordant couples. These are (1) social stigma and serostatus disclosure, (2) social support and adherence to treatment, (3) gender discourse and condom use, and (4) religion and protective sexual behaviors.

Social Stigma and Serostatus Disclosure

HIV/AIDS continues to be a highly stigmatized condition among Puerto Ricans. Multiple research studies have documented how stigma is perceived by individuals with HIV/AIDS in everyday life activities (Varas-Díaz, Serrano-García, & Toro-Alfonso, 2004). Furthermore, research has also documented how social stigma is manifested through media (Varas-Díaz & Toro-Alfonso, 2003), policies (Varas-Díaz & Toro-Alfonso, 2002), and the medical establishment (Varas-Díaz, Malavé-Rivera, & Cintrón-Bou, 2008). Due to its strong hold on local culture, stigma continues to be a major challenge for disclosure of serostatus.

Research has suggested that this decision-making process results from a consideration of the pros and cons associated with the serostatus disclosure (Armistead, Tannenbaum, Forehand, Morse, & Morse, 2001; Black & Miles, 2002; Serovich, 2001). According to Ostrom et al. (2006), disclosure to others also decreases the ability to control secondhand disclosure by others. In this sense, gossip is a practice of concern for PWHA. This is of particular relevance to Puerto Ricans as research has documented the central role of this social communication process in local culture (Roldán, 2007).[3] Gossip's main objective is to discredit a person based on a particular characteristic that has been previously identified as immoral or a transgression of a social normative (Velázquez Sánchez, 2002). It serves as a vehicle for social stigma that can have negative effects for the seropositive person and her or his partners.

Participants in our study were concerned with the potential implications of gossip throughout the process of disclosure. Almost all of the participants of our study (90%) knew each other after the HIV diagnosis of one member of the dyad. With few exceptions, they described serostatus disclosure to their partners as a highly stressful experience due to the fear of being rejected. Some of them withheld this information from partners to avoid rejection, even when they were aware of the potential implications. Rejection and fear of subsequent gossip were catalysts for this decision.

— *It is sad, but I lied to him. I had to . . . I hid it [serostatus], until one day he found the paper on the desk [lab result]. (P6-A)[4]*

— *I was hiding it [the serostatus] for a year . . . but I couldn't take it anymore and decided to tell him. (P17-A)*

— *It took me two years [to tell him]. He was asking about the amount of pills that I had to take. He said: "why do you have to take so much medicine?" At that time, the treatment for HIV required a lot of pills . . . to be stable, you know . . . And he said: "Ahh, you have not said anything to me." He accepted me. I was not the first woman he knew with the condition, because he had friends . . . (P4-A)*

— *She didn't know [the serostatus]. I was afraid when having sexual relations with her . . . you know. Sometimes I had sex with her without protection. Then, I thought of what I was doing. When I was going to come, I pulled out and ejaculated outside of her. Then, she asked why did I do that. I said: "you know, before we got back together I was crazy in the streets. You never know what can happen." (P2-A)*

— *It had a terrible effect on me [to know her serostatus]. When we started, she did not say, "Look, I have been in a difficult situation, etc." Thus, I could have taken alternative ways . . . Maybe she thought she was going to be rejected by me. That's not who I am. I told her: "you did something bad, you never told me, you didn't trust me . . . Now, what do you think is my opinion of you? (P6-B)*

Secrecy was not an exclusive experience in the relationship context. Ninety-five percent of participants had not disclosed their serostatus to others (family or friends) in order to avoid negative effects and gossip. Problems with disclosure continue to be documented in Puerto Rico 30 years into the epidemic because individuals who do so can experience personal rejection and stigmatization from partners and family members (Varas-Díaz, Serrano-García, & Toro-Alfonso, 2004).

— *My in-laws don't know about it. We have decided not to tell them. Those two oldies would die if they know I am positive. They are crazy about me. (P14-A)*
— *Her children don't know [my serostatus]. It affects me. I don't know. I would like them to know it, but I fear they might reject me. Anyways, she does not want me to tell because they will oppose our relationship. (P2-A)*
— *In my house, we don't talk about the condition. I have forbidden it. My family doesn't know. Once they know, everybody will eventually know . . . That's how they are. His family doesn't know either. Nor my children, that now are grownups. They don't know. (P4-A)*
— *He says: "but I don't care what people say about us," and I tell him: "but I do care." I am always . . . Oh my God, they are looking at me. I say: "you are going to have a bad time when you visit my barrio." They are going to say: "she has the condition" . . . even if I don't have a label on my forehead. (P7-A)*

Participants who had revealed their serostatus to family members identified stigmatizing experiences. Some participants stated:

— *It affects us [HIV] because there is rejection. We feel it even from his family. We have decided to stop visiting them because it's not easy to deal with that. (10-C)*
— *My mother used to tell me: "you cannot have [sexual] relations with others because you will get them sick." My mother's words are here [pointing to her head]. I thought: "coño, I am a human being of flesh and bones." Then she said: "if you get pregnant your children are going to be sick." Wow, I had the illusion [of being a mother] as any other woman. (P7-A)*

Throughout the interviews some participants mentioned positive effects of discloure, although these were minimal. Interestingly, some participants avoided mentioning HIV altogether, preferring to mention it as "it" throughout the interviews. These difficulties naming HIV may be a reflection of a social stigma manifested through everyday language. It could also reflect an avoidance of what Sinyemu and Baillie (2005) describe as the process by which HIV becomes one's name. If HIV is the identity ascribed after infection, then avoiding its name could entail some kind of control over everyday discourse.

— *Knowing that she has it, I have been more supportive. (P1-B)*
— *At the beginning I was scared knowing that he had it. (P12-B)*
  I have never discriminated against him because you have it . . . I don't know. (P19-B)
— *People fear you when you tell them that you have it. They ask themselves: "what am I doing with this person if I am healthy? It is better to find a healthy person." Maybe the person can be disgusted with you, or even worse they feel fear . . . because people usually are scared when you say that you have it. Fear, disgust, and everything else. (P 7-A)*

The verbalizations presented here encompass a challenge for serodiscordant couples in our study as rejection by a member of the dyad continues to be present and therefore a potential barrier for healthy relationships (Poindexter & Linsk, 1999; Santana & Dancy, 2000). Stigma-free disclosure has the potential to foster social support, buffer the effects of stress, and reduce mental health discomfort (Chin & Kroesen, 1999).

Social Support and Adherence to Treatment

Adherence to treatment is of vital importance for PWHA because it can foster healthier living. Still, even though medication regimens have become simpler in recent years, adherence can be challenging (Toro-Alfonso, Andújar-Bello, Amico, & Fisher, 2002). According to participants' responses, difficulties with adherence to treatment were associated with oversights, the complexity of the regime, side effects, and depression. Thirty-five percent of participants reported having trouble with adherence. Partners also described such difficulties.

— *I forget because I usually get involved in other activities. Times go by rapidly. (P5-A)*
  It's not easy and she [seropositive partner] gets indisposed with meds. The side effects make her sick. (P6-B)
— *To take pills every day . . . one gets tired of thinking that's it for the rest of my life. When having breakfast, I start looking at the pillbox . . . and I say "Hell." (P9-A)*
— *It's like laziness. She doesn't want to deal with medicines, even when I try to makes thing easier for her. (P4-B)*
— *At night, when I take the pills they give me side effects . . . I can't sleep. It's awful. (P15-A)*

Even when facing the challenge of adherence to treatment, partners seem to provide a crucial source of support for the task. Studies with PWHA have shown that good social support levels contribute to a better quality of life, adequate understanding of the illness, and benefits for mental and physical health (Olamakinde Olapegba, 2005). Social support networks can include multiple sources such as health care providers, family, and friends. Research in Puerto Rico has stressed the need to focus on primary partners due to the way these relationships are culturally constructed (Ortiz-Torres, Serrano-García, & Ortiz-Burgos, 2000). A strongly patriarchal background and the legacy of Judeo-Christian religion stress the importance of monogamous and formal relationships among Puerto Ricans. Although these ideals are not always met, social expectations place them as the desired norm. Participants

(68%) considered their partners as the main source of social support. This echoed previous studies carried out with serodiscordant couples in Puerto Rico (Rodríguez Madera & Marqués Reyes, 2006). Most participants identified their partners, irrespective of their gender, as supportive in having a good adherence to treatment through consistent follow-up and reminders.

— *She is always taking care of me . . . She reminds me: "Did you bring your pills?" I am very happy with her support. Definitively it is making a difference. (P12-A)*
— *I am her nurse. More or less . . . as if I was a nurse. I follow her every step of the way . . . I never leave her alone and she is well. The virus load is very low. (P1-B)*
— *I am used to it [taking medicines]. I think of them [pills] as if they were vitamins. If I want to be healthy, I have to take my medicine. Anyways, he does his part . . . always asks me: "did you take your pills?" (P17-A)*
— *I go with her to the doctor's appointments. I remind her every day to take her meds and I give my support in the house. (P11-B)*
— *I have to be involved, because I have to remind her of the pills and the appointments with doctors. Sometimes if I can't go with her to the doctor, she doesn't go by herself. She doesn't have anyone else to help her with her daughter. (P16-B)*

Evidently social support from partners seems to be an important factor for those who identified themselves as being adherent to HAART. Although adherence is part of a healthy lifestyle and a preventive approach, condom use to prevent infection seemed more of a challenge and an area in which support in the dyad was less clear.

Gender Discourse and Condom Use

Condom use among heterosexual couples in Puerto Rico has multiple obstacles that include women's lack of self-efficacy in negotiating its use with partners and religious morality regarding what is "good" and "bad" sex (Rodríguez Madera & Marqués Reyes, 2006). Research in Puerto Rico has evidenced that women face serious difficulties negotiating condom use, particularly in long standing relationships (Ortiz-Torres, Serrano-García, & Torres-Burgos, 2000). In addition, there is evidence that men, in general, have negative attitudes toward condoms use (Pérez-Jimenez, Serrano-García, & Escabí Montalvo, 2007).

Participants in our study revealed interesting information regarding condom use. Half of them were using condoms because they wanted to protect their partners, even when they dislike them.

— *Well, I wish I did not need to be protected [with condoms] and use it [the penis] as intended by God. He created humans to have intercourse with nothing done by men . . . but this disease is transmitted to the partner if one is not protected. If there were no condoms . . . you can imagine that you will infect your partner. We are lucky that we have condoms to avoid placing your partner at risk. (P15-A)*
— *There are a lot of things that you can't do. I don't like to use condoms . . . but I use them. Always. Every time that we have sex, I use condoms and it bothers me because I don't like them. (P18-B)*
— *Yes, we use condoms because we have to protect me. At the beginning I was scared because he was sick. Then he explained to me: "Hey, babe . . . that's how we are going*

> to do it. If we use condoms you will not be infected." So he always uses protection, and I have them [condoms] with me also . . . just in case. (P12-B)
> — If there are no condoms, we don't have sex. She says that condoms bother her . . . that it's not the same. I understand her because I am allergic to condoms [laughs out loud]. Mentally allergic! Of course it's not the same, no, no, no. But I have to deal with that. (PP6-B)

Unprotected sexual intercourse was common among participants who delayed informing their partners of their serostatus. The consequences of these actions encompass psychological anxiety and guilt, as described by some participants:

> — For me it was a shock . . . thinking that he had not told me anything about his condition. Wow, you can be infected if you are not protected! During that time that we were together, without me knowing that fact, we had sex. I wanted to kill him because I believed that I was also going to be sick. After that we used condoms. (P17-B)
> — I felt bad and guilty because I made her suffer. I didn't tell her [regarding serostatus] at the beginning. I was also scared because I thought that maybe she could have it too. When I told her, she started to cry. Later she accepted me because everything in life is possible if there is love. (P20-A)
> — There have been changes. Yes, because there are [sexual] activities that before . . . Before I told him about my condition I dared to do things that now are not possible, because he knows. (P14-A)
> — I believe he is afraid [of being infected]. Once I told him I started to think that. Now he always wants to use condoms because he thinks badly about me. He is scared, you know, after I told him . . . (P6-A)

Several other participants reported not using condoms during sexual activity. The narratives reflect how women were particularly flexible regarding stopping condoms use and a concerning lack of information on how to use them and in which context they are necessary.

> — She usually says: "You're stepping over the line. You are wrong. You get me all involved until you penetrate me." It is like trying to get your way. (P5-A)
> — We don't use condoms because we were tired of them, but he has his labs results every three months. (P 9-A)
> — Poor thing! He doesn't use them because they slip off. You can imagine? It is OK with me. (P16-A)
> — I have condoms there [in the house], but she says: "why do you have to use condoms if I had surgery [to avoid pregnancy]. I could use them . . ." (P20-A)
> — I have penetrated her on several occasions without condoms because she agreed with it. Then I used it . . . I am scared for her. I told her that she must go to the doctor. Sometimes I don't use her [sexually], because I am having sex with other people. It is with people that she knows. (P3-A)

Religion and Protective Sexual Behaviors

Worrisome information was provided by participants regarding the role of religion in their lives, risk, and health activities. Although there is a general perception that religion is a protective factor for health, it seems that within the HIV prevention arena the story is more complicated. The role of religion in Puerto Rican culture, and its relation to health, has been rarely addressed in previous studies. Still, the few studies that exist have documented how religious practices and beliefs foster manifestations of HIV/AIDS stigma (Varas-Díaz, Torsten, Malavé Rivera, & Betancourt, 2010). It is important to recognize the strong influence of organized religion on Puerto Rican culture due to its Spanish cultural roots[5]

Traditionally the negative stands toward condom use, and HIV in general, taken by Judeo-Christians have been detrimental to HIV prevention. For example, these beliefs have been shown to foster erroneous perceptions and attitudes that can affect participation in treatment and other protective behaviors (Zou, Yamanaka, Muze, Watt, Ostermann, & Thielman, 2009). Researchers have also determined that religion can influence married couple's low HIV risk perception, which can in turn lead to risky behaviors (Bekele & Nichols, 1998; Trinitapoli & Regnerus, 2006).

Participants of our study verbalized several instances that revealed how religious beliefs influenced their behavior related to HIV prevention and adherence to treatment. For example, some participants explained their unsafe sexual practices based on religion.

— *At the beginning we protected ourselves, but then he did not want to use it [condom] anymore. What happens is that he is very into religion with God . . . and he says that God will not allow something bad to happen to us. (P11-A)*
— *We usually use condoms, but once when we weren't, I told her that she should have some tests done. I don't know if she did it. She told me she did. She is very Christian and she says that nothing is going to happen to me because I have God protecting me. She is into her faith. But that was a long time ago and thank God, until now she is well. (P2-A).*

Research has also shown how it is common among religious groups to conceptualize HIV/AIDS as a punishment from God (Zou et al., 2009). In the same manner, God can be interpreted as a source of healing from illness. Two participants in our study echoed this position:

— *In my church they don't talk about HIV like that . . . you know, "it is a plague in this world." Remember? It is like cancer. Who heals it? The only one who can heal it is God. There is no medicine, and no one who can cure cancer. The one who heals is God. This is told [in church] to the people that have the condition [HIV]. That God is the one who can cure them. For all purposes, I am cured . . . For all purposes, I feel cured. I know that I have to take my pills but I have to testify in the name of God . . . I think this way. I feel healed and for the church, I am cured. For the rest of the people I still have the condition, and I have my pills with me and I have to take them. But it will be until God says: "You will not take more pills. Lab tests will be negative." Well then, God did what he had to do and that's it. Meanwhile I know that I still have to take my pills until he does what he has to, but I am already healed. Nothing else . . . (P11-C)*
— *That's when I met him [the physician] and he said: "Lets do some tests on him [seronegative partner]." Every three months, the doctor ran the tests and he was well . . . and I said: "Oh, Lord." I prayed a lot and asked him for help. I told the Lord: "God, help him. I don't want to be guilty if he is sick." I felt guilty . . . I felt guilty of having sex without condoms. Well, we continued like that and after a while I went to the doctor and he told me: "Well, he is still negative." I could not believe it.*

I said: "How it is possible?" The doctor said: "because you prayed a lot and asked a lot for God's mercy, He is helping you."

DISCUSSION

During the last months of the year 2010, while this chapter was under development, an event of significance happened in the Island of Puerto Rico that can serve to highlight how HIV is interpreted in this Caribbean land mass. A famous baseball player was accused by his wife, who he was divorcing, of exposing her to HIV without her knowledge (Rivera Arguinzoni, 2009). It was argued that he knew of his condition, and yet withheld information from her during their marriage. The accusation was made public through local gossip television shows and even ended up on the front page of one of the most widely circulated and respected newspapers in the Island, *El Nuevo Día* [The New Day]. The baseball player's previous girlfriend was publicly identified as a potential HIV carrier, and therefore preceded to engage in tests to confirm the opposite. She revealed her negative tests to the media spectacle and publicly thanked God for protecting her from the disease. As if by a stroke of luck, during the month of December of the same year the Governor's wife told the media of the importance of being tested for HIV, because this was a curable disease (Marrero, 2010). It would be hard to make up a story like this, and yet it is a reflection of the context in which the HIV epidemic continues to spread in Puerto Rico, with more than three new infections every day.

The story described above serves as an excellent example of triangulation for our qualitative findings with serodiscordant couples. The story evidences several issues that reflect how HIV is interpreted in light of (1) fear of being socially stigmatized by the community, (2) the use of gossip as a mechanism to discuss health-related issues and values, (3) how traditional gender roles can promote unprotected sex that places women in particular at a high risk for infection, and (4) the way highly religious communities interpret having/not having HIV as related to divine intervention. Serodiscordant couples in Puerto Rico face the same situations entrenched in local culture, with the added challenge of doing so on a daily basis with the potential implications for their health and quality of life.

Serodiscordant couples need to be understood and addressed with the understanding that they, just as any social individual, are influenced by their local culture, social values, and norms. Such structural-environmental and societal factors serve to control what is possible in each setting, including control over individuals' bodily practices related to health and sexuality. Couples in which a member of the dyad is HIV positive face these social norms and expectations with a highly stigmatized disease in the midst of their everyday dynamics. After 30 years of the HIV/AIDS epidemic, the social response to HIV has become polarized. On one hand, there are still crude manifestations of stigma such as discrimination, marginalization, rights violations, and other forms of social violence against PWHA. These are manifested in the denial of quality services by governmental agencies, among other instances. On the other, there is tacit stigma hidden by a politically correct discourse as evidenced, for example, on public health campaigns that completely exclude transmission through needle exchange. These socially sensitive subjects are strategically ignored. Serodiscordant couples face both levels of stigma as part of their dyadic dynamics.

The challenge of social stigma seems to be faced by these couple dyads through mechanisms of social support they provide to each other. These instances of collaborative functioning in the dyad may be the most important factor for adherence to treatment of the person with HIV. This is vital because adherence to treatment and social support within the couple dyad can better serve to foster health-related practices. Social support has long been established in the scientific literature as an important factor for health maintenance and general well being. Efforts to foster health practices among serodiscordant couples need to take advantage of the cultural importance placed on close-knit extended families in Puerto Rican culture (i.e., familismo), because members can serve as vital sources of support. This can also be manifested within the greater Puerto Rican barrio or community, of course, when stigma is less of an obstacle.

Although culture is a vital protective factor when discussing adherence to treatment, it is immensely complex and can also be the opposite when addressing safe sex practices. Puerto Rican culture is not exempt from the Victorian morality of the Western world, which has had serious implications for gender construction and the sexual activities repertoire. The legacy of Victorian era sexuality, characterized by rigid norms on sexuality, delineates the frontiers of what is permissible and acceptable for males and females. Female social scenarios, although challenged today, still seem to highlight their role in the marital bed and the kitchen (Quesada Monje, 2001). Thus, social discourses regarding "good" (i.e., procreation) versus "bad" (i.e., pleasure) sexuality are still present. This conceptualization of bad sexuality and female roles allows for frequent lack of control in the process of protecting oneself during sexual intercourse. Condom use among the dyads is mediated by (1) lack of knowledge of HIV infection, (2) lack of control over the decision-making process regarding their use, and (3) religiomagical thoughts regarding divine protection from the disease. See Chapters 4, 16, and 17 for extended discussions of Latinas and HIV risk and prevention.

This last issue is of vital importance for understanding the process through which partners in serodiscordant dyads are influenced by culture in their decision-making process. In a highly religious social context, participants mentioned the protective role of God during intercourse and the negative serostatus of the partner. It is not farfetched to suggest that couples believe that a divine entity watches over them and protects them from infecting the negative partner, even when not using condoms. This fact is of concern because it clearly reflects how cultural beliefs in Puerto Rican society, this time related to religion, can foster the spread of HIV infection. Couples seemed to manifest some sort of religiomagical thought process through which infection was averted. Although this thought process might seem rudimentary at best, it is a clear reflection of a context that places such high importance on religion, while at the same time neglecting basic sexual education in public schools and medical facilities.

It is commonplace to suggest that the HIV epidemic in Puerto Rico has impacted society in general. It has affected those who have become infected and those who can potentially be exposed in the future. Serodiscordant couples in this context seem to be even more affected than most, as they live in the midst of being infected and avoiding a new infection. They are not only faced with personal challenges within their couple dynamics, but as our findings suggest, are simultaneously embedded in a cultural context that can be at times beneficial and at times detrimental. It can serve to highlight the role of social support, and at the same time foster high-risk behaviors. HIV prevention strategies that focus on serodiscordant couples need to address Puerto Rican culture as it is manifested in these couple dynamics, with both its positive and negative implications. This central role of culture on HIV prevention stresses the need for the development and application of the Structural-Environmental Model proposed in Chapter 1 of this book as a way to move forward. Failure to do so will yield only generic HIV prevention efforts that are a poor reflection of the realities and challenges faced by serodiscordant couples in Puerto Rico.

NOTES

1. This study was funded by a grant from the National Institute of Child Health and Human Development (5R03HD060448). The authors can be contacted through regular mail at University of Puerto Rico, Center for the Study of Social Differences and Health, Graduate School of Social Work, P.O. Box 23345, San Juan, PR 00931-3345 or by e-mail at sheillalrm@me.com.

2. These numbers reflect an even worse socioeconomic scenario than the one faced by the general population in Puerto Rico, where approximately 50% do not complete high school and unemployment fluctuates to 15% of the potential working force.

3. As a testament to the cultural importance of gossip in Puerto Rico, it should be stated that the most watched television show in the Island is called "Xclusivo" (Exclusive in English) and it is solely based on providing gossip about local and international figures. Although faced with heavy fines and legal challenges, Puerto Rican audiences have kept it on the air for more than a decade. This fact is of significance as negative references to HIV, homosexuality, and drug use are commonly manifested through it. It is, in fact, a cultural artifact of importance in Puerto Rican society.

4. Each verbalization is presented with the following code to help identify its source: P = Participant; Number = the identification number assigned to each couple; Letter = type of interview [A—seropositive person; B—seronegative person; C—couple).

5. As an example of the importance of religion on the everyday lives of Puerto Ricans we should point out that there are more religious television and radio stations than secular ones, and therefore these are very influential in everyday lives. Furthermore, the expansion of churches has grown exponentially in the past decade, so much so that the government does not have an updated and reliable list of how many exist.

REFERENCES

Armistead, L., Tannenbaum, L., Forehand, R., Morse, E., & Morse, P. (2001). Disclosing HIV status: Are mothers telling their children? *Journal of Pedriatic Psychology, 26,* 11–20.

Beckerman, N. L. (2002). Couples coping with discordant HIV status. *AIDS Patient Care and STDs, 16,* 55–59.

Bekele, M., & Nichols, K. (1998). Religion and HIV risk perception among African immigrants living in New York City. International Conference on AIDS, 12: 658 [Abstract no. 33333].

Black, B., & Miles, M. S. (2002). Calculating the risks and benefits of disclosure in African American women who have HIV. *Journal of Obstetric, Gynecologic and Neonatal Nursing, 31,* 688–697.

Bova, C., & Durante, S. (2003). Sexual functioning among HIV-infected women. *AIDS Patient Care, 17,* 75–83.

Buchacz, K., Van der Straten, A., Saul, J., Shiboski, S. C., Gomez, C. A., & Padiau, N. (2001). Sociodemographic, behavioral, and clinical correlates of inconsistent condom use in HIV-serodiscordant heterosexual couples. *Journal of Acquired Immune Deficiency Syndrome, 28,* 289–297.

Burton, J., Darbes, L. A., & Operario, D. (2008). Couples-focused behavioral interventions for prevention of HIV: Systematic review of the state if evidence. *AIDS & Behavior, 14*, 1–10.

Canada HIV Information Centre. (2006). *Serodiscordant relationships.* Accessed on November 24, 2010 at http://library.catie.ca/PDF/P16/21260e.pdf.

Castro, A. (2005) Adherence to antiretroviral therapy: Merging the clinical and social course of AIDS. *PLoS Med, 2*(12): e338. doi:10.1371/journal.pmed.0020338.

Catz, S. L., Kelly, J. A., Bogart, L. M., Benotsch, E. G., & McAuliffe, T. L. (2000). Patterns, correlates, and barriers to medication adherence among persons prescribed new treatments for HIV disease. *Health Psychology, 19*, 124–133.

Chin, D., & Kroesen, K. (1999). Disclosure of HIV infection among Asian/Pacific islander American women: Cultural stigma and support. *Cultural Diversity and Ethnic Minority Psychology, 5*, 222–235.

Dunbar, P. J., Madigan, D., Grohskopf, L. A., Revere, D., Woodward, J., Minstrell, J., et al. (2003). A two-way messaging system to enhance antiretroviral adherence. *Journal of American Medical Information Association, 10*, 11–15.

Erlen, J. A., Sereika, S. M., Cook, R. L., & Hunt, S. C. (2002). Adherence to antiretroviral therapy among women with HIV infection. *Journal of Obstetric Gynecology Neonatal Nursing, 31*, 470–477.

Grinstead, O. A., Gregorich, S. E., Choi, K. H., & Coates, T. (2001). Positive and negative life events after counseling and testing: The voluntary HIV-1 counseling and testing efficacy study. *AIDS, 15*, 1045–1052.

Hirsch, J., Meneses, S., Thomson, B., Negroni, M., Pelcastre, B., & del Río, C. (2007). The inevitability of infidelity: Sexual reputation, social geographies, and marital HIV risk in rural Mexico. *American Journal of Public Health, 97*, 986–996.

Jemmot, J. B. (2007). HIV/STD risk reduction for African American couples. Accessed December 14, 2010 at http://www.annenbergpublicpolicycenter.org/Downloads/FishbeinLectures/Jemmott_102110.pdf.

Lichtenstein, B. (2006). Domestic violence in barriers to health care for HIV/AIDS women. *Aids Patient Care and STDs, 20*, 122.

Lincoln, Y. S., & Guba, E. G. (1985). *Naturalistic inquiry.* Beverly Hills, CA: Sage.

Machtinger, E., & Bangsberg, D. (2006). Adherence to HIV Antiretroviral therapy. *HIV InSite.* Accessed December, 14, 2010 at http://hivinsite.ucsf.edu/insite?page=kb-03-02-09.

Manfrin-Ledet, L., & Porche, D. J. (2003). The state of science: Violence and HIV infection in women. *Journal of the Association on Nurses in AIDS Care, 14*, 56–58.

Marrero, R. (2010). Primera Dama dice que el SIDA tiene cura. *Primera Hora.* San Juan, Puerto Rico.

Miller, R. L. (2001). Innovation in HIV prevention: Organizational and intervention characteristics affecting program adoption. *American Journal of Community Psychology, 29*, 621–647.

Mills, E. J., Nachega, J. B., Bangsberg, D. R., Singh, S., Rachlis, B., Wu, B., et al., (2006). Adherence to HAART: A systematic review of developed and developing nation patient-reported barriers and facilitators. *PLoS Med, 3*, e438. doi:10.1371/journal.pmed.0030438.

Mitrani, V. B., Prado, G., Feaster, D. J., Robinson-Batista, C., & Szapocznik, J. (2003). Relational factors and family treatment engagement among low-income, HIV-positive African American mothers. *Family Process, 42*, 31–45.

Murphy, D. A., Greenwell, L., & Hoffman, D. (2002). Factors associated with antiretroviral adherence among HIV-infected women with children. *Women Health, 36*, 97–111.

Olamakinde Olapegba, P. (2005). Predicting mental health of people living with HIV/AIDS (PLWHA): The role of psychological factors. *Journal of Human Ecology, 18*, 69–72.

Ortiz-Torres, B., Serrano-García, I., & Torres-Burgos, N. (2000). Subverting culture: Promoting HIV/AIDS prevention among Puerto Rican and Dominican women. *American Journal of Community Psychology, 28*, 859–881.

Ostrom, R. A., Serovich, J. M., Lim, J. Y., & Mason T. L. (2006). The role of stigma in rehaznos for HIV disclosure and non-disclosure to children. *AIDS Care, 19*, 28–33.

Perez-Jimenez, D., Serrano-Gracía, I., & Escabí Montalvo, A (2007). Men's role in HIV/AIDS prevention for women: exploring different views. *Puerto Rico Health Sciences Journal, 26*, 13–22.

Persson, A. (2008). Sero-silence and sero-sharing: Managing HIV in serodiscordant hetero-sexual relationships. *AIDS Care, 20*, 503–506.

Phillips, N., & Ardí, C. (2002). *Discourse analysis: Investigating processes of social construction.* Thousand Oaks, CA: Sage.

Poindexter, C. C., & Linsk, N. (1999). HIV-related stigma in a sample of HIV-affected older female African American caregivers. *Social Work, 44*, 46–61.

Poland, B. (2002). Transcription quality. In J. F. Gubrium, & J. A. Holstein (Eds.), *Handbook of interview research: Context and method* (pp. 629–649). Thousand Oaks, CA: Sage.

Puerto Rico AIDS Surveillance Report. (2011). San Juan, P.R.: Department of Health.

Quesada Monje, R. (2001). El reinado de Victoria (1837–1901): Imperialismo y civilización. Accessed November 15, 2010 at http://www.escaner.cl/escaner24/perfiles.htm.

Remien, R. H., & Stirratt, M. (2002). Research with couples of mixed HIV status identifying mutual concerns, fostering mutual care-taking. *Body Positive, 1*, 1–2.

Rivera Arguinzone, A. (2009, February). Alomar y el SIDA. *El Nuevo Día.* San Juan, Puerto Rico.

Roberts, K. J., & Mann, T. (2000). Barriers to antiretroviral medication adherence in HIV-infected women. *AIDS Care, 12*, 377–386.

Rodríguez Madera, S., & Marqués Reyes, D. (2006). Partner relationships as contexts of lack of control in the HIV epidemic. *Behavioral Sciences, 21*, 97–128.

Roldán, I. (2007). AIDS stigma in the Puerto Rican community: An expression of other stigma phenomenon in Puerto Rican Culture. *Interamerican Journal of Psychology, 41*, 41–48.

Roth, D. L., Stewart, K. E., Clay, O. J., Van der Straten, A., Karita, E., & Allen, S. (2001). Sexual practices of HIV discordant and concordant couples in Rwanda: Effects of a testing and counseling programme for men. *International Journal of STD and AIDS, 12*, 181–188.

Safren, S. A., Otto, M. W., Worth, J. L., Salomon, E., Johnson, W., Mayer, K., et al. (2001). Two strategies to increase adherence to HIV antiretroviral medication: Life-steps and medica-tion monitoring. *Behavior Research Therapy, 39*, 1151–1162.

Santana, M. A., & Dancy, B. L. (2000). The stigma of being named "AIDS carriers" on Haitian-American women. *Health Care for Women International, 21*, 161–171.

Santos, D. (2002). *Psychological distress and doping of women with HIV/AIDS living in the west coast of Puerto Rico.* Presentation at the Public Health and Environment Conference. Washington, DC.

Schwandt, T. A. (2001). *Dictionary of qualitative inquiry.* Thousand Oaks, CA: Sage.

Serovich, J. M. (2001). A test of two: HIV disclosure theories. *AIDS Education and Prevention, 13*, 355–364.

Sinyemu, E., & Baillie, M. (2005). *HIV becomes your name: A report on the issues facing Africans living in Scotland who are HIV positive.* Accessed December 1, 2010 at http://www.waver-leycare.org/userfiles/file/publications/HIV%20becomes%20your%20name.pdf.

Starace, F., Ammassari, A., Trotta, M. P., Murri, R., De Longis, P., Izzo, C., et al. (2002). Depression is a risk factor for suboptimal adherence to highly active antiretroviral therapy. *Journal of Acquired Immune Deficiency Syndrome*, 15, 136–139.

Stevens, P., & Galvao, L. (2007). "He won't use condoms": HIV-infected women's struggles in primary relationships with serodiscordant partners. *American Journal of Public Health*, 97, 1015–1022.

The California Partners Study. (1999). *The management of HIV, sex and risk among serodiscordant heterosexual couples*. Presentation at the National Conference of Women & HIV. Los Angeles, CA.

Trinitapoli, J., & Regnerus, M. D. (2006). Religion and HIV risk behaviors among married men: Initial results from a study in rural Sub-Saharan Africa. *Journal for the Scientific Study of Religion*, 45, 505–528.

Toro-Alfonso, J., Andujar-Bello, I., Amico, R., & Fisher, J. D. (2002). *Psychosocial implications and level of adherence to treatment in a sample of people living with HIV/AIDS in Puerto Rico*. Presentation at the International Conference on AIDS, July 7–12. Abstract no. B10436.

Van der Straten, A., Vernon, K. A., Knight, K. R., Gómez, C. A., & Padian, N. S. (1998). Managing HIV among serodiscordant heterosexual couples: Serostatus, stigma and sex. *AIDS Care*, 10, 533–548.

Varas-Díaz, N., & Toro-Alfonso, J. (2002). Juggling individual and collective concerns in HIV/AIDS policies: A view from Latin America. *Canadian HIV/AIDS Policy and Law Review*, 7, 2/3, 106–107.

Varas-Díaz, N., & Toro-Alfonso, J. (2003). Incarnating stigma: Visual images of the body with HIV/AIDS. *Forum Qualitative Social Research [On-line Journal]*, 4, 3. Accessed December 16, 2010 at http://www.qualitative-research.net/fqs-texte/3-03/3-03varastoro-e.htm.

Varas-Díaz, N., Malavé Rivera, S., & Cintrón Bou, F. (2008). AIDS stigma combinations in a sample of Puerto Rican health professionals: Qualitative and quantitative evidence. *Puerto Rico Health Sciences Journal*, 27, 147–157.

Varas-Díaz, N., Serrano-García, I., & Toro-Alfonso, J. (2004). AIDS related stigma and social interaction: Puerto Ricans living with HIV/AIDS. *Qualitative Health Research*, 15(2), 169–187.

Varas Díaz, N., Torsten, B. N., Malavé Rivera, S., & Betancourt, E. (2010). Religion and HIV/AIDS stigma: Implications for health professionals in Puerto Rico. *Global Public Health*, 19, 109–118.

Velásquez Sanchez, F. M. (2002). Los chismes y difamación en los medios de comunicación. *Focus*, 1, 81–87.

Wagner, G. J., Remien, R. H., Carballo-Dieguez, A., & Dolezal, C. (2002). Correlates of adherence to combination antiretroviral therapy among members of HIV-positive mixed status couples. *AIDS Care*, 14, 105–109.

Weinhardt, L. S., Kelly, J. A., Brondino, M. J., Rotheram-Borus, M. J., Kirshenbaum, S. B., Chesney, M. A., et al. (2004). HIV transmission risk behavior among men and women living with HIV in 4 cities in the United States. *Journal of Acquired Immune Deficiency Syndrome*, 36, 1057–1066.

Wilson, T. E., Gore, M. E., Greenblatt, R., Cohen, M., Minkoff, H., Silver, S., et al. (2004). Changes in sexual behavior among HIV-infected women after initiation of HAART. *American Journal of Public Health*, 94, 1141–1146.

Zou, J., Yamanaka, Y., Muze, J., Watt, M., Ostermann, J., & Thielman, N. (2009). Religion and HIV in Tanzania: Influence of religious beliefs on HIV stigma, disclosure, and treatment attitudes. *BioMedCentral Public Health*, 9, 75.

14 HIV/STI Risk among Latino Migrant Men in New Receiving Communities

A Case Study of Postdisaster New Orleans

Patricia J. Kissinger and
Michele G. Shedlin

LATINO IMMIGRANTS AND HIV RISK IN THE UNITED STATES
Introduction

Understanding and addressing the causes of health disparities among the Latino population in the United States are increasingly important as the size of immigrant and migrant populations from Latin America and the Caribbean continues to grow. It has been estimated that if U.S. demographic trends continue, the Latino population, already the nation's largest minority group, will triple in size and make up nearly one-third of the U.S. population by 2050 (Passel & Cohn, 2008). This trend is largely driven by ongoing immigration and high birth rates among immigrants. Of the nearly 47 million Latinos in the United States in 2008, over one-third (38%) were foreign born and birth rates among foreign born Latinas were 44% higher than the general U.S. population (Pew Hispanic Center, 2010). Thus, Latino immigrants are an important and rapidly growing demographic group in the United States.

Migration has long been implicated in the spread of HIV/STI by bridging populations with low and high prevalence (Bronfman, Sejenovich, & Uribe, 1998; Herdt, 1997; UNAIDS/IOM, 1998). The study of HIV/STI risk behaviors among mobile and immigrant groups, particularly those in new receiving communities, has not received adequate attention in public health. In this chapter, we synthesize the literature on what is known regarding sex and drug-related HIV risk and morbidity in this group and on individual, cultural, and environmental factors that have been identified as barriers or facilitators of this risk. We focus on risk networks as an important environmental factor that can either promote or prevent HIV risk behavior and illustrate this concept by presenting data from a cohort of Latino migrants in postdisaster New Orleans.

The Importance of New Receiving Communities

Migrant workers are a significant and vulnerable subgroup of Latinos. There are presently an estimated 8.8 million undocumented Latinos in the United States, representing 3% of the population and 4.2% of the work force (Passel & Cohn, 2009). Close to 4 million Latin American migrants entered the United States between 1990 and 2000, doubling the number of foreign born Latinos in just a decade (United States Census Bureau, 2006). Prior to 1990, most immigration from Mexico and Central America had been confined to about 10 states. Between 1990 and 2000, the number of Latinos in selected southern states (i.e., Alabama, Arkansas, Georgia, North Carolina, South Carolina, and Tennessee) that had no or small Latino communities increased by more than 300% on average (Painter, 2008). Many of these rapid growth states also have high existing HIV/STI rates. Compared to Latinos who migrate to more established Latino communities, Latinos migrating to these new receiving states are more often young, male, foreign born, and unaccompanied by women (Kochhar, Suro, & Tafoy, 2005), a demographic group at higher risk for drugs and HIV than the general population of Latino men.

Migrant workers are particularly vulnerable because of their undocumented status, clandestine and mobile lifestyle, economically disadvantaged backgrounds, and language barriers. They frequently migrate without their families, and this separation from family, friends, and familiar environments can lead to loneliness and loss of social capital, social control, and the creation of new social networks (Organista, 2007).

Latino migrants in new receiving communities may be even more vulnerable than other migrants. One factor contributing to this is that they may be less protected by the "barrio effect" than their counterparts who move into more traditional receiving areas (Gallo, Penedo, Espinosa de los Monteros, & Arguelles, 2009). The "barrio effect" refers to a health benefit described by some scientists for immigrants that are living in areas that are more densely populated by persons of their own culture (Eschbach, Ostir, Patel, Markides, & Goodwin, 2004). The "barrio" can also help to insulate language nonfluency, which has been associated with a higher likelihood of victimization and abuse (Shihadesh & Barranco, 2010). The lack of a Latino receiving community may result in migrants living in isolated environments that lack the cultural and community infrastructure needed. Isolation often leads to patronage of sex workers and substance abuse, placing migrants at higher risk for HIV and other sexually transmitted infections (STIs) (Decena & Shedlin, 2005)

In post-Katrina New Orleans, the environment was particularly harsh. Because the infrastructure for the indigenous residents was destroyed and scant infrastructure existed for newly arrived Latinos. Latino migrant workers, consequently, were forced to live in substandard housing including tents or the houses they worked on, often sharing rooms with multiple other workers. They accepted jobs that were risky (such as gutting houses and removing asbestos material) and were rarely offered protection (Rabito et al., 2010). Migrants were often victims of crime and discrimination, with no rights or protections in place (Nossiter, 2009).

To date, most studies have concentrated on Latino populations in established receiving areas and not in new receiving communities and have focused mostly on Mexicans rather than rapidly increasing Central American groups (Fernandez-Kelly, 1983; Sorensen, 2004) and on Latino men who have sex with men (MSM) rather than heterosexuals. Heterosexual HIV transmission is more common among Latino men compared to white men (16% vs. 6%) (CDC, 2005), and the majority of Latino migrants are heterosexual. Because our case study of postdisaster New Orleans examines a group of migrant men in a new receiving area who are mostly from Central America and who are mostly heterosexual, it can help to fill this gap in the literature.

STI/HIV Epidemiology among Latinos in the United States

The Latino population in the United States is disproportionately affected by AIDS (CDC, 2008), HIV (Hall et al., 2008), and many STIs (CDC, 2004). Although Latinos represent approximately 15% of the U.S. population, in 2006 they accounted for 19% of the AIDS cases, 17% of new HIV infections, and nearly 18% of people living with HIV disease (Hall et al., 2008). In the United States, the rates of chlamydia, gonorrhea, and syphilis were two to four times higher among Latinos compared to non-Latino whites in 2003 (CDC, 2004) and in 2008 the rate of HIV infections was three times higher for Latinos than for non-Latino whites (CDC, 2010).

Although Latino migrants are considered to be at high risk for HIV/STI, few prevalence studies among them have been conducted (Ferreira Pinto, Ramos, & Shedlin, 1996). Among studies involving biological testing for HIV/STI, morbidity was low despite high rates of HIV/STI risk behavior (Levy et al., 2005; Martínez-Donate, 2005; Wong, 2003). A venue-based study of Latino migrant men in New Orleans found no cases of HIV or syphilis and only 3.2% were infected with *Chlamydia trachomatis* (Kissinger et al., 2008). A subsequent prospective study of this target group also found a low prevalence of chlamydia and gonorrhea and no cases of gonorrhea, HIV, or syphilis (Kissinger et al., 2012). These low rates of HIV/STI morbidity are incongruous with the high rates of risk behavior, such as high female sex worker (FSW) patronage, binge drinking, and drug use. Possible explanations for this paradox include self-medication for the treatable STIs, increased condom use with high-risk partners, and drug use is that is mostly non-injection.

The potential for HIV/STI infection among Latino migrants, however, does exist. An outbreak of syphilis in Morgan County, Alabama, found that half of those infected were Latino migrants (Paz-Bailey, Teran, Levine, & Markowitz, 2004). The existing literature indicates that in the early phase of immigration migrants may be at lower risk, but this risk increases with time (Ojeda, Patterson, & Strathdee, 2008). Thus, it is imperative to understand how risk evolves and how resilience can be maintained and built upon to prevent an HIV epidemic in this subgroup.

STI/HIV Epidemiology among Latino Sending Communities

Central America and Mexico, once thought to be areas with low HIV prevalence, have seen a steady rise in the rates of HIV. Prevalence rates of HIV in Central America and Mexico range from a high of 2.1% in Belize to a low of 0.2% in Nicaragua (UNAIDS, 2008). In these areas, the prevalence of HIV is higher in regions with significant emigration to the United States, especially among women, and the spread is often attributed to mobility from the United States and back (Magis-Rodriguez et al., 2004), suggesting that circular migration serves as a vehicle of spread. Root causes of HIV subepidemics within and between countries are indeed complex processes.

Whereas overall country rates may be low to mid-range, among certain subgroups within countries rates are high. For example, in Mexico the rate of HIV in the general population is 0.3% (UNAIDS/WHO, 2006), however, rates among injection drug users (16%) (Patterson et al., 2006, pp. 13–18) and male sex workers (25%) (Gayet et al., 2006) are much higher. In Honduras, HIV rates are mid-range 0.7% (UNAIDS, 2008), but are much higher among subgroups such as Garífunas (4.5%) (Paz-Bailey et al., 2009). And although 75% of HIV found in Mexico and Central America occurs among MSM, some countries such as Honduras exhibit a male-to-female ratio of 1:1, indicating that the epidemic is largely a heterosexual one. Rates of early sexual debut, high risk sexual activity during adulthood, and homosexuality–bisexuality patterns were found to be heterogeneous between and within countries in Central America and Mexico (Bozon, Gayet, & Barrientos, 2009).

DRUGS, ALCOHOL AND STI/HIV: A WEB OF RISK

Scientists now recognize that there is a constellation of individual, environmental, and cultural factors that places migrant men at higher risk (Aguilar-Gaxiola et al., 2006). Individual factors include poverty, limited education, language barriers, and undocumented status (Apostolopoulos, 2006). The overrepresentation of men in migration streams, family separation, disruption of established channels of social control, and a sense of anonymity often facilitate the use of drugs and risky sexual practice (Alaniz, 2002).

Basing our model on Bronfenbrenner's Ecological Theory and Sweat and Denison's model of HIV causation (Sweat & Denison, 1995), we posit that contextual, social, and cultural factors interplay with environmental factors to influence the individual to engage or not engage in HIV/STI and drug risk behaviors (Figure 14.1). This will eventually lead, or not lead, to STI/HIV infection.

Drug and Alcohol Use among Latino Migrants

Injection drug use is an important transmission vehicle for HIV and other blood-borne diseases. It promotes HIV transmission directly through the sharing of infected needles or equipment and indirectly by decreasing condom use and increasing participation in transactional sex (Dolezal, 2000; Ramirez-Valles, Garcia, Campbell, Diaz, & Heckathorn, 2008; Ramirez-Valles, Heckathorn, Vázuiz, Diaz, & Campbell, 2005). Non injection drugs also increases HIV risk. Several studies have shown that substance use increases high-risk sexual behavior (Dolezal, 2000; Ramirez-Valles et al., 2008; Ramirez-Valles, Heckathorn, Vázuiz, Diaz, & Campbell,

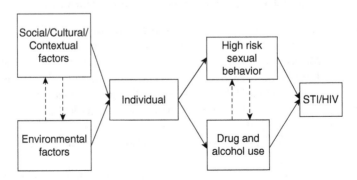

FIGURE 14.1 Factors influencing STI/HIV risk.

2005). Various hypotheses have been offered to explain the association between substance use and sexual risk behavior, including disinhibiting pharmacological effects, social context (including increased transactional sex), situation-specific rituals, cognitive escapism, expectancy effects, and personality traits (Dolezal, 2000). These hypotheses, however, have yet to be verified and some have failed to find event-level associations (Leigh & Stall, 1993).

Whereas drugs, alcohol, and sexual risk behavior share similar risk factors, some scientists believe that the behaviors cluster but do not cause one another (i.e., they are coincidental rather than causal) (Dolezal, 2000; Leigh & Stall, 1993; Temple, Leigh, & Schafer, 1993; Weatherburn et al., 1993).

Studies with Latinos that have found associations between substance use and high-risk sexual behavior were conducted primarily among men who have sex with men (MSM) (Diaz, Ayala, & Bein, 2004; Dolezal, 2000; Ramirez-Valles et al., 2008) and less is known about the association among heterosexual Latinos, who represent the majority of migrant men (Inciardi, 1999). The aforementioned syphilis outbreak in Morgan County Alabama among Latino migrants found crack cocaine use and increased commercial sex use in close proximity to the Latino community to be associated with infection (Paz-Bailey et al., 2004). One study found that the prevalence of mental health illness and substance use among immigrants was lower than among nonimmigrant Latinos, but that variations by country of origin were found, suggesting it is not a universal trend (Alegria et al., 2008)

For alcohol, the literature indicates that newly arrived Latino migrants may have lower drinking rates compared to U.S. Latino and non-Latino residents, but that protection deteriorates with acculturation and time (Worby, 2007). Research on migrant farm workers demonstrates high rates of alcohol use and identifies environmental factors that may serve as risk factors such as isolation from family, stress, lack of alternative recreation; the desire for social acceptability, friendship, and male bonding through sharing alcohol; self-medication for aches and injuries caused by harsh working conditions; and the need to relieve boredom and stress (Organista, 2007). High rates of alcohol use among newly arrived migrants in New Orleans, a particularly liberal environment for alcohol use, underscores the potential influence of environment on alcohol behavior.

Prevalence studies have demonstrated wide ranges of drug use (7.3%–60%) (Inciardi, 1999; Kissinger et al., 2008) largely because nonprobability sampling was used or a single area was studied. Furthermore, even among those studies that found low rates of drug use, risky behavior was noted among those who did use drugs. For example, one study of Mexican immigrants reported a low prevalence of injection drug use (IDU) (7%) but also found frequent sharing of needles and equipment without bleach cleaning among men who did engage in IDU (Organista & Kubo, 2005).

Although there is a good deal of literature on alcohol use among Latino migrant workers, far less research has been devoted to the sexual risk behaviors among Latino migrants who use drugs, and much of it has been limited to descriptive epidemiology studies (Aguilar-Gaxiola et al., 2006). More research is needed on how substance use influences HIV risk among Latino migrants, as advocated in migrant-focused Chapters 1 and 18 of this book.

Patronage of Commercial Sex Workers and Condom Use

Commercial sex workers fill a void that is created by migration because many men migrate without their families (Passel, 2006). Studies of Latino migrant men in the

U.S. report a wide range of commercial sex patronage ranging from 26% to 69% (Galvan, Ortiz, Martinez, & Bing, 2009; Kissinger et al., 2008; Parrado, Flippen, & McQuiston, 2004; Sena, Hammer, Wilson, Zeveloff, & Gamble, 2010). Variability may be attributed to the characteristics of the study sample. A study of mostly Mexican Latino migrants in North Carolina demonstrated that unaccompanied men reported more lifetime sexual partners, more partners in the previous year, more extramarital partners, and more contact with FSWs than accompanied married men (Viadro, 2000). There is evidence that commercial sex patronage is common during early migration and as migrant men settle and find partners, FSW use declines (Levy et al., 2005)(Kissinger et al., 2012).

Yet while commercial sex patronage is common, so is condom use, suggesting that, paradoxically, sex worker patronage may not necessarily be a risk factor for HIV for these men (Denner, Organista, Dupree, & Thrush, 2005; Caballero-Hoyos et al., 2008). Over time, there appears to be a relaxation of condom use with FSWs (Parrado et al., 2004), and married men may be less likely than unmarried men to use condoms with FSWs (Parrado et al., 2004; Organista, Balls Organista, Garcia de Alba, Castillo Moran, & Ureta Carrillo, 1997).

Contextual factors, such as drug-using environments, may also play a role in reduced condom use (Magis-Rodriguez et al., 2009; Paz-Bailey et al., 2004; Ibanez, Van Oss Marin, Villarreal, & Gomez, 2005), so the conditions under which condoms are used with FSWs need further study. Type of sex is also a factor for consideration as illustrated by a study of Mexican migrants that indicated that condom use with FSWs was frequent for anal but not vaginal sex (Organista & Kubo, 2005).

In our 2006 cross-sectional study of Latino Migrants in New Orleans, we found that only 50% of the men reported consistent condom use (Kissinger et al., 2008). In our on-going cohort study that began in 2007, consistent condom use with FSWs ranged from 61% to 100%, but was far less common with non-FSW partners (range 23–41%). Qualitative work suggested that condoms were used because FSW demanded it. One random-digit dial telephone survey of heterosexually active, unmarried Latino men found that those who reported having a condom available, engaging in conversation about condoms, and having a nonsteady, casual, or one-time partner were more likely to have used condoms at their last sex act (Ibanez et al., 2005). They were also more likely to use condoms to avoid pregnancy when no other form of birth control was being used. These findings were true of both low and highly acculturated men. Studies of the prevalence of condom use and factors associated with nonuse among Latino migrants have shown inconsistent results, suggesting that contextual factors may be influential.

Risk-Related Acculturation Factors

The relationship between acculturation, drug use and HIV sexual risk behavior is complex (Alaniz, 2002). Acculturation brings about social, economic, and personal challenges and adjustments that can influence mental health, and acculturative stress is often cited as a risk factor for substance use (Alaniz, 2002; Amaro, Whitaker, Coffman, & Heeren, 1990; Conway, Swendsen, Dierker, Canino, & Merikangas, 2007; Vega, 1998). Acculturation may reduce the protective effects of traditional norms, such as expectations for close extended family relationships and responsibilities, which may directly or indirectly buffer the effects of stress and prevent the development of mental health sequelae including drug use (De La Rosa, 2002).

The reasons why and how Latino migrants use illicit drugs are also not well understood. It has been postulated that the process of migration and the subsequent changes in lifestyle contribute to drug use, namely through acculturation (De La Rosa, 2002; Finch, Reanne, & Vega, 2004; Finch, Catalano, Novaco, & Vega, 2003). Some studies have found that recent immigrants are less likely to use drugs than more established immigrants (Ojeda et al., 2008) and that substance use tends to increase with the time spent in the United States (Alaniz, 2002; De La Rosa, 2002; Ojeda et al., 2008) (Gfroerer & Tan, 2003) and with availability (Valdez, Cepeda, Negi, & Kaplan, 2009). These studies suggest that acculturation may be a factor in increased substance use.

Separation from family and lack of a community are the most often-cited stressors for new immigrants (Caplan, 2007), and studies have documented that acculturative stress is elevated in the absence of social support and language capability (Finch et al., 2003, 2004; Finch & Vega, 2003). Almeida et al. (2009) found that Latinos in the United States, specifically foreign born Mexicans, rely on family ties for support more than do non-Latino whites (Almeida, Molnar, Kawachi, & Subramanian, 2009). Immigration laws that foster separation of families, therefore, may play an important role in increasing migrant's risk for drug use.

Risk-Related Social and Cultural Factors

As the HIV/STI epidemic takes different forms in distinct communities, understanding the role that cultural factors play in shaping risk for new immigrants becomes increasingly crucial. This is an especially complex task because processes of cultural adaptation and change affect both the communities and the immigrant populations residing in them (Handwerker, 2002).

There are countless studies that cite *machismo, marianismo, familismo*, etc., as specific cultural factors that may contribute to HIV risk among Latinos. These cultural constructs in certain contexts also influence "social risk," specifically individuals' concerns about how they are perceived and their reputation in the community (Hirsch, 2009). Thus *machista* attitudes influence mens' needs to be seen as virile and have multiple partners, whereas *familismo* influences their concern with protection and respect for partners and family, consequently the need to hide extramarital sexual relations whether with a new partner here in the United States or relations with an FSW. Concern about social risk and reputation can, in fact, outweigh concerns about health and HIV/STI risk.

The construct of *machismo,* or male power, is especially salient in any examination of Latino cultural norms because it organizes social and power relations between men and women and structures power between and among men. A direct impact of *machismo* and *familismo*, the strong identification and attachment to nuclear and extended family, was clearly illustrated on behaviors such as HIV testing and care-seeking in a Ryan White assessment by Shedlin and Shulman (2001). Social service agency staff serving new Latino immigrants in New York stated that the use of condoms was very low among immigrant men who perceive them as undermining their *machismo*. Providers also reported that most Latino immigrant men with whom they interacted thought oral sex was safe and thus condoms were unnecessary (Shedlin & Shulman, 2004).

Yet we still know little about the experiences and adaptations that lead to specific attitudinal and behavioral changes in host countries, and how migrants influence the cultures and subcultures into which they move (Ortiz-Torres). We do know, however, that both bear critically on health behavior. The influence of Latino gender norms and the role of changing gender dynamics as men and women adapt and acculturate must also be considered, especially how economic stress and possibilities for women's employment affect power dynamics (Decena, Shedlin, & Martínez, 2006).

It is important as well to pay specific attention to these cultural factors that influence the patterns, networks, and character of social interaction through which culture and high-risk environments shape behavior change, specifically as it applies to new options and opportunities for drug use and risky sex. For example, because many migrant workers do not have family members living with them, they may lack their normal form of social control and therefore may be more likely to engage in risky sex. Heavy use of alcohol and drugs has been associated with masculinity or *machismo* among Latino men (Dolezal, 2000; Singer, Valentin, Baer, & Jia, 1992) and focus groups have revealed beliefs that alcohol and drugs contribute to an inability to control sexual urges (Diaz et al., 2004) (see the discussion of this topic in Chapter 5). However, adding to the complexity of the issue, differences in the use of alcohol and drugs among Latino subgroups have also been reported (De La Rosa, Khalsa, & Rouse, 1990; Shedlin, 2005).

The absence of cross-cultural understanding and misinterpretations of language and behavior can also cause stress for migrant workers and their families. For example, the Latino culture emphasizes *personalismo*, or interpersonal relationships, which values respectful behavior and the personal dimension in both business and personal relationships. Day labor pick up sites do not foster such relationships; men must aggressively compete for a day of work that can ultimately make the difference in their ability to provide food for themselves or their families. Other values such as *respeto* (or an expectation of appropriate deferential behavior on the basis of a position of authority, race, or economic status) may be seen as weakness or subordination in other cultures and foster abuse. This could also inhibit migrants from demanding appropriate wages or treatment from employers. Wage theft among migrant workers in New Orleans is commonplace (Foley, 2010).

These cultural norms are often cited as obstacles to health care utilization and preventive behaviors. *Machismo*, for example, has been an easy explanation for lack of condom use. However, this simplistic explanation does little to inform interventions or address health disparities. Studies such as that presented by Caballero-Hoyos et al. (2008) provide more insight into the interactions of context and traditional norms and suggest. For example, the complexities of the coexistence of a traditional cultural orientation that does not support condom use with another one that does, provided the sex partner is formally employed.

Risk-Related Environmental Factors

Although there is a growing understanding of individual factors associated with drugs and high-risk sexual behavior among Latinos, environmental influences that may serve as root causes of these behaviors are not well understood. Among the environmental factors are physical/social/cultural isolation, long work hours, constant mobility, hazardous work conditions, crowded and substandard housing, limited leisure activities, and limited access to health care and legal protection (International Conference on Auditory Display, 2004). Crowded housing as well as too much leisure between jobs promote and provide the opportunity for the use of alcohol, drugs, and commercial and/or casual sex (Apostolopoulos, 2006). Migrants in new communities may experience social and sexual norms that are different from those in their community of origin and these discrepencies can be magnified in new receiving communities. In addition, an understanding of the environments from which mobile and migrant groups come and the impact of immigration and the "journey" (in all senses of the word) itself are needed. Poverty, repressive governments, lack of education/literacy, ethnicity, class, color-based stigma, and cultural norms are crucial factors in determining their attitudes, motivations, decisions, and behavior in their new U.S. receiving environments (Shedlin & Shulman, 2004).

Some risky environments have been identified. One study of Latino day laborers found that 38% reported being solicited for sex by other men, and that 9.4% accepted, and that accepting was associated with more time in the United States (Galvan et al., 2009). Construction work, for example, has been associated with cocaine use (Hersh, McPherson, & Cook, 2002; Parrado et al., 2004).

Migrant workers are also more vulnerable to violence and discrimination, particularly in new receiving environments in which communities are largely unfamiliar with these populations and their communication and behavioral norms. Fear that migrants may take jobs, among myriad other concerns, causes expressions of xenophobia and discrimination. In postdisaster New Orleans, many migrants were the victims of crime. They are known to carry cash and to underreport crime, prompting reference to day laborers as "walking ATM machines" (Nossiter, 2009).

Results from our pilot cohort study further support the importance of environmental influences on drug behavior. In a case-control study of drug users and non-drug users, 71.9% of drug users reported experiencing at least one discriminatory event in the past 3 months compared to 35.2% of non-drug users. Although environmental risk factors have been individually associated with HIV acquisition in New York City and Tijuana, no studies have compared risk environments in more rural areas to those of urban areas. Migration also heightens individual risk by creating environmental changes that increase vulnerability. Studies have found that the availability of drugs is considered to be a risk factor for drug use (Gillmore, 1990).

Transmission of HIV, like that of other behaviorally mediated infections, is influenced by the particular environment in which risk is produced (Poundstone, Strathdee, & Celentano, 2004; Ramos et al., 2009; Rhodes et al., 1999; Sanchez, 2008). Risk environments are comprised of risk factors exogenous to the individual, such as social, cultural, economic, and political factors (Rhodes, 2002) and understanding these factors is key to developing relevant prevention strategies (Rhodes, Singer, Bourgois, Friedman, & Strathdee, 2005). New migrants may engage in more risky drug transactions because they have no established social networks for obtaining drugs (Paschane & Fisher, 2000; Tori, 1989). It is crucial to understand the nature of illicit drug use among this group and the factors surrounding it, because illicit drug use can lead to addiction (Rosen, 2008), high-risk sex (Dolezal, 2000; Ramirez-Valles et al., 2008; Ramirez-Valles, Heckathorn, Vázuiz, Diaz, & Campbell, 2005), and death (Cherpital, 2008; Rosen, 2008). A growing body of research demonstrates that social and structural processes shape an individual's risk for acquiring HIV/STIs and drug use (Barnett & Whiteside, 1999; Bourgois et al., 2006; Deren, 2005; Friedman & Reid, 2002; Latkin & Knowlton, 2005; Neaigus et al., 1994; Organista, 2007; Rhodes, 2009; Rhodes & Simic, 2005; Strathdee et al., 2006, 2008; Wasserheit, 1994). More exploration of the link between drugs, alcohol, and HIV sexual risk is needed in this rapidly increasing group.

Social networks, defined as alliances between people who have some common interest, are an important part of the environment. Networks have been employed in epidemiological research to help understand how patterns of human contact aid or inhibit the spread of diseases such as HIV in a population. Sexual networks, in which individuals are connected to each other either directly or indirectly by sexual contact, and drug networks, in which people are linked by drug-using behavior, are subsets of social networks. Either can transmit HIV or other infections because social networks transmit social influence, shaping norms and behaviors such as drug use (Friedman et al., 2007; Valente, 2006; Valente & Fosados, 2006). For example, having a child or woman in the household has been associated with decreased sexual risk behavior (Parrado et al., 2004; Viadro, 2000), yet about 54% of married, undocumented migrant men in the United States are unaccompanied by their spouse or primary partner (Passel, 2006). Consistent condom use among male partners of FSWs in the Dominican Republic was associated with a perception that some or all of their social network members were using condoms (Barrington et al., 2009).

Sexual partnering behaviors have been linked to HIV/STI transmission, specifically sexual concurrency and dissortative mixing. Sexual concurrency, defined as having two or more sexual partnerships that overlap in time, amplifies the spread of sexually transmitted infections (STIs) and has been shown to increase transmission of STI epidemics (Morris & Kretzschmar, 1997). Sexual mixing can be disassortative or assortative. Disassortative mixing refers to individuals who demonstrate a preference for partners in other groups and an aversion to partners in their own groups, whereas in assortative mixing individuals tend to have sex with partners that are like them (Hertog, 2007). Disassortative sexual mixing patterns tend to spread epidemics more widely in a community (from network to network) whereas assortative patterns tend to maintain epidemics within networks (Morris & Ferguson, 2006; Morris, Kurth, Hamilton, Moody, & Wakefield, 2009). Given the highly mobile nature of Latino migrants and the evidence that infection has already entered some communities, it is important to measure transmission factors such as concurrency and sexual mixing to gain a better understanding of the vulnerability of Latinos and how they may or may not contribute to the spread of HIV/STIs.

Migration can interrupt existing social networks in sending communities as well as shaping the formation of new networks or the incorporation of individuals into existing receiving community networks that may involve new risk options. For an epidemic to occur, infected and susceptible people need to mix and engage in risk behavior that facilitates infection (Rothenberg, 2001). Thus, identifying the network characteristics and the behaviors of members of these networks is key to understanding the potential for an epidemic to occur in any group (Friedman, Rossi, & Braine, 2009).

The configuration of these new networks, the position of the individual in the network, and the infection status of its members can serve to facilitate or impede transmission (Fichtenberg et al., 2009; Rothenberg, Potterat, et al., 1998). Several network measures have been associated with transmission and risk including partner concurrency (Morris & Kretzschmar, 1997), bridge positioning (Bettinger, Adler, Curriero, & Ellen, 2004), information centrality (Stephenson & Zelen, 1989), the size of connected components (or a set of people who are linked to one another), nodal degree (or the number of connections one has to others), the size and frequency of microstructures (Cook et al., 2007; Friedman et al., 1997;

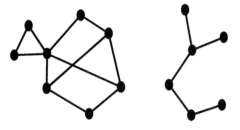

FIGURE 14.2 Two network components: one cyclic with eight persons (left) and one dendritic with six (right). Cyclic is more likely to transmit infection.

Rothenberg, Sterk, et al., 1998; Seidman, 1983), and density (Doherty, Shiboski, Ellen, Adimora, & Padian, 2006) of the network. Characteristics of these measures can be used to adapt interventions. For example, cyclic microstructures facilitate the spread of HIV and STIs more readily than dendritic (tree-like) shapes (see Figure 14.2) (Potterat et al., 2002; Potterat, Rothenberg, & Muth, 1999). Fragmented or disconnected network structures consisting of many small components may respond more efficiently to targeted screening than to contact tracing, or the practice of having public health workers find, test, and refer people who have been exposed to HIV and other STIs. Densely connected structures may be more efficiently fragmented by contact tracing. Contract tracing is a public health approach to STD control in which a specially trained outreach worker finds contacts of infected persons in the community and encourages them to get tested. In this way, network informed interventions may be more effective than traditional risk factor monitoring. Individuals in core and bridge positions tend to have lower risk perceptions (Bettinger et al., 2004), leading to less condom use and more risky sexual and drug-using behaviors.

The majority of all infections occur in the core group of a network and this is an important group to identify and target for interventions (Keeling & Eames, 2005). Mixing between core, high-risk populations and peripheral, lower-risk populations (disassortative mixing) is known to spread disease within the general population, whereas assortative mixing (i.e., sex with individuals in the same group) tends to compartmentalize infection within specific groups (Laumann & Youm, 1999). Highly mobile migrants have the potential to serve as bridges between low and high prevalence groups by reducing the path distance between individuals, both between different subgroups and geographic locations (Nordvik, Liljeros, Osterlund, & Herrmann, 2007), leading to an increased transmission between groups with different risk levels and prevalence (e.g., migrants who move between the United States and Mexico) (Jolly & Wylie, 2002; Keeling & Eames, 2005; Nordvik et al., 2007; Wylie, Cabral, & Jolly, 2005).

Spatial bridging, when individuals travel, is associated with high-risk behavior including higher numbers of partners and partnership concurrency (Kerani et al., 2003), defined as the number of temporally overlapping partnerships (Kretzschmar & Morris, 1996). Networks can be analyzed as egocentric or sociometric. In an egocentric study, the individual is asked about his or her contacts but these contacts are not followed. Whereas egocentric approaches are logistically more appealing, they likely underestimate risk (Fichtenberg et al., 2009). This could lead to lack of attention to this group and ultimately could lead to a major epidemic. A sociometric study, on the other hand, entails the recruitment of the identified partners to further elaborate on the network structure and risk factors (Doherty, Padian, Marlow, & Aral, 2005). Looking at social connections through sociometric studies can lead to the discovery of otherwise untraced infections (Sena et al., 2007) and is needed to understand the dynamics of risk and resilience in this population.

CASE STUDY OF SEXUAL AND DRUG-RELATED HIV/STI RISK: New Orleans, Louisiana, after Hurricane Katrina

Although the pre-Katrina Orleans' population included Latinos, it can be considered a truly new migratory destination. Until 2002, Louisiana was considered among the least frequent destinations for migrants (Passel, 2006). The first wave of Latinos was composed of Spanish explorers who arrived in the 1700s. The next major wave was that of Latinos from Central America, mostly Hondurans, to New Orleans in the 1930s with the Standard Fruit Company, later Dole. The third wave represented Cubans escaping the Castro regime in the 1950s, mainly settling in suburban areas of the greater metropolitan New Orleans area. By 2005, despite these waves of Latino immigrants, only 4.4% of metropolitan New Orleans was Latino.

On August 29, 2005 New Orleans experienced a Category 3 hurricane named Katrina that resulted in the breaching of the levees and the flooding of over 80% of the city. In postdisaster New Orleans, a large influx of Latino workers arrived to assist with rebuilding efforts, facilitated, in part, by a Department of Homeland Security directive to suspend employment immigration enforcement in the area immediately following the storm. Although precise numbers are not available, some estimate that this wave of immigrants constituted as much as 20% of the population in the year after the storm (Bordelon, 2006; Donato, 2006). Census data show the percentage of Latinos in the metropolitan area increased by 50% (from 4.4% prehurricane to 6.6% posthurricane) (Plyer & Ortiz, 2010). Most estimates of the numbers of Latinos in New Orleans are likely underestimates of the true population because they likely do not include newcomer migrants who are undocumented, have irregular housing arrangements, have limited language skills, and are not usually captured by traditional population estimating techniques such as sewerage bills and electric and land telephone hookups (Louisiana Public Health Institute, 2006). In our sample of 68 migrant men, for example, only 63% filled out a census form in 2010.

Prior to Hurricane Katrina, services for Spanish-speaking populations were limited since the Latino population was relatively small. After Katrina, not only were these services even more limited, but the City's infrastructure was heavily damaged by the hurricane and subsequent flooding creating a very unfavorable environment for the migrants. This imbalance in the need- to-availability ratio resulted in serious disparities for the new Latino migrants. Eventually, an increase in the infrastructure for Latinos, including grocery stores, taco stands, clubs, churches, radio stations, television stations, and schools, started to appear, indicating that at least some of these newly arrived migrants were going to stay.

New Orleans as a Risk Environment for Substance Use and HIV/STIs

Compared to other new migratory destinations in the United States, New Orleans has always represented an extreme. Prior to Katrina, rates of crack and heroin use and market participation were comparable to New York. There was a precipitous drop in availability immediately after the storm, which appeared to rebound shortly thereafter (Dunlap, Johnson, & Morse, 2007). After the Katrina disaster in 2005, violent and nonviolent crime in the City skyrocketed, much of which was attributed to the drug trade (Foster, 2006; Johnson, 2007; Kaste, 2006). There are thousands of drug busts every year in metropolitan New Orleans (Perlstein, 2010). High-profile cases have included major drug seizures of heroin (Fox, 2008; WWLTV, 2008b), prescription narcotics (WWLTV, 2008a), and crack cocaine (Sparacello, 2008). Systemic irregularities in the New Orleans Police Department (NOPD) served further to exacerbate the problem. Although drug availability immediately after the storm was low (Valdez et al., 2009), federal agents have indicated that the quantity of drugs seized at drug busts has become larger since the storm (Fox, 2008; WWLTV, 2008b), suggesting that the market for use has increased.

New Orleans, with its vibrant sex and drug industry, is a high-risk HIV/STI environment. In 2006, compared to other states, Louisiana ranked first for syphilis, second for gonorrhea, and sixth for HIV. There was also a dramatic increase in the HIV statistics for Latinos. In 2005, of all newly diagnosed cases of HIV in metropolitan New Orleans, 4% were among Latinos; in 2010 that rate jumped to 9% (Louisiana Office of Public Health, 2008). This is, in part, due to the increased numbers of Latinos, yet it serves to illustrate the magnitude of the problem. Although Louisiana generally is considered to be conservative, the New Orleans area is a popular adult entertainment area. The New Orleans French Quarter, a 78 square block area, has 131 bars, 22 gentlemen's clubs, and 3 known brothels, and local laws allow the bars to remain open all night with revelers carrying open alcohol containers in the streets. Throughout the greater New Orleans area there are also over 100 available escort services, more than 50 adult entertainment stores and services, and well-known "sex clubs." After Hurricane Katrina, echoing the influx of migrant workers, there was an influx of commercial sex workers and sex managers, making sexual entertainment in the city even more readily available. The availability of drugs, alcohol, and sex was widespread in the postdisaster New Orleans area, available as well to migrant men without the constraints of their families and with the availability of disposable income.

Thus, the complex risk environment that Katrina compounded presented an ideal natural experiment for a longitudinal study of Latino migrant workers. It offered a concrete, identifiable start date for the influx of workers, clear risks for HIV/STI transmission for large numbers of unaccompanied men, availability of sex workers and illicit drugs, and a hobbled infrastructure.

Venue-Based Cross-Sectional Study

For our first pilot study, we conducted a venue-based sample of Latinos who came to New Orleans post-Hurricane Katrina (Kissinger et al., 2008). The venues included locations of day labor pick-up sites within the city such as home improvement stores and other areas where migrant men congregated, a soccer field, and a Latino church. Participants were administered an anonymous, structured interview in Spanish in a mobile unit and urine tested for *Chlamydia trachomatis* (CT) and *Neisseria gonorrhea* (GC) using the nucleic acid amplification technique—and HIV. Recruited were 180 men with a mean age of 33 (range, 18–79) who did not speak or understand English well (93.9%), were undocumented (91.2%), were married (63.5%), and had children (67.4%), although the low percent living with a spouse and children was 6.1% and 4.9%, respectively. Although most men were born in Honduras (49.7%) and Mexico (25.4%), 61.9% came to New Orleans via another U.S. state.

The majority of respondents drank alcohol in the past week (75.5%), and of those, 68.7% engaged in binge drinking. A lower percentage used marijuana (16.6%) and cocaine (5.5%) at least once in the prior week. None reported injection drug use. The self-reported history of HIV was 10%, however, because this is much higher than reported in the literature, it is possible that the participants misunderstood the question. No men tested positive for GC and five (2.8%) tested positive for CT. In the past month, 68.9% engaged in sex with high-risk sex partners, 30.0% were in potential bridge position (i.e., a person who has sex with persons in infected and uninfected networks), 50.0% used condoms inconsistently, 30.6% did not use a condom the last time they had sex, and 21.1% were abstinent. Since arriving, 9.4% reported leaving and returning to New Orleans, usually from other U.S. states.

Latino migrant workers in this study reported risky sexual behaviors and low condom use within a potential bridge position. Although a low prevalence of CT and GC was found, there was a high percent of self-reported HIV infection. We concluded that the cultural and contextual factors that place these migrant workers and their sex partner(s) at risk for HIV/STI infection needed further investigation.

Prospective Cohort Study

To further explore the cultural and contextual factors associated with substance use and HIV/STI risk among Latino migrants, we embarked on a cohort study in 2007. Latino men ($N = 125$) were recruited using respondent-driven sampling, a sampling technique that can simulate a population-based sample for hidden populations. Formative research identified four nationalities (Honduran, Mexican, Salvadoran, and Dominican) and eight recruitment sites. Eight initial recruits ("seeds") who represented the nationalities identified were consented and each given three coupons to distribute to persons in their social network that met the eligibility criteria [i.e., 18 years or older, arrived in New Orleans after Hurricane Katrina (August 29, 2005) for the purpose of work, born in Mexico or Latin America, and native Spanish speaking]. Latino men who contacted study personnel within the time allowed, presented a coupon, and met the eligibility criteria were offered admission into the study, consented, and were given three coupons to recruit additional persons. Waves of recruitment continued until 125 were enrolled in the study. Six of the eight seeds produced large heterogeneous chains (see Figure 14.3).

Participants were contacted monthly and interviewed quarterly for 30 months and HIV/STI was tested annually. Individual, environmental, and cultural factors by partner type and condom use were explored. Twenty-six men from this cohort also participated in either focus groups or in-depth interviews to provide qualitative data that were used to further elucidate the quantitative findings. These interviews and focus groups were conducted in the second half of the cohort study period.

Demographics in this second group studied were remarkably similar to the prior cross-sectional group. The mean age of participants was 30.1 (std 7.81). Most men were born in Honduras (71%) and Mexico (11%); other countries of origin were Guatemala (6%), El Salvador (6%), Nicaragua (6%), and the Dominican Republic (< 1%) . Just over half (55%) migrated to New Orleans from their home country

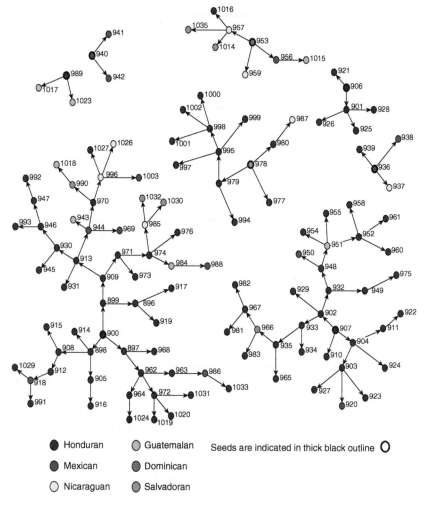

Honduran   Guatemalan   Seeds are indicated in thick black outline ◯

Mexican   Dominican

Nicaraguan   Salvadoran

FIGURE 14.3 Migrant recruitment chains using respondent driven sampling (Rds).

while 44% arrived from another U.S. state. Men reported being in New Orleans an average of 1.26 years (std 0.69). Forty-four percent were married and 72% reported having children, with 4.8% and 5.6% living with their spouse and children, respectively. The majority could not speak or understand English very well (98%) and had 6 years of education or less (59%).

We noted significant trends for sexual partnering over the 18-month study period. Sex with FSWs and multiple partners decreased and sex with main partners and abstinence increased, whereas the number of casual partners remained stable. Consistent condom use was highest with FSWs, lowest with main partners, and midrange with casual partners, with no trends over time. STI morbidity was low; no HIV was detected. High mobility was associated with inconsistent condom use with both FSW and casual partners. Drug use and high mobility were associated whereas having family in the home was protective for inconsistent condom use with FSWs. Migrant men who belonged to a social organization were more likely to use condoms consistently with casual partners than those who did not belong to such organizations (Kissinger et al., 2012).

Drug Behavior among Latino Migrant Men in New Orleans

At baseline, of the 125 sampled, 77.6% reported drinking alcohol and of those that drink (n = 97) 96% reported binge drinking in the past month. Lifetime use of marijuana, cocaine, and crack was 70%, 50.4%, and 22.4%, respectively. Nearly half (47%) reported any illicit drug use during follow-up with 42% reporting cocaine use and 18% reporting crack use. One in five (20%) reported initiating drug use in New Orleans, including a 47-year-old man from Honduras. Alcohol was by far the most common substance used (62%–89%), followed by marijuana (5–22%), then cocaine (5–20%) and crack (1–8%). Although there were fluctuations in use over time, no statistical trends were found. Figure 14.4 depicts these trends.

Few participants reported injection drug use. Factors associated with crack and/or cocaine use were younger age, having more friends in New Orleans upon arrival, having no family members living in the household, greater mobility, and working in construction.

An analysis of illicit drug use among the cohort used both quantitative and qualitative findings. Quantitative data indicated that the individual risk factors associated with illicit drug use were less years of education, migrating to New Orleans from within the United States, patronage of female sex workers, incorrect use of condoms, multiple sexual partners, binge drinking, higher endorsement of sensation-seeking personality, and loneliness. Qualitative data illustrated that the patronage of FSWs was related to drug use because men would either buy drugs directly from FSWs or share or trade drugs for sex. Some men described taking drugs so that they could drink longer.

Having a wife or long-term partner was protective for past month drug use. Participants discussed changes in their drug behavior if a family member was present in the household or if they began a relationship with a woman who discouraged drug use. Countering the role of family and partners, relationships with drug users also influenced drug use. Drug networks were drug specific and networks

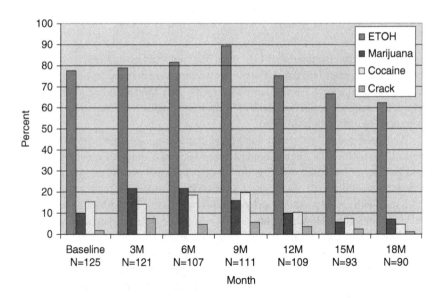

FIGURE 14.4 Percentage of Latino migrant workers using drugs and alcohol.

influenced the initiation of new drugs. Men pooled resources to purchase drugs, a behavior that can indicate a possibility of future sharing of drug paraphernalia as well. Men were more likely to use drugs if they lived in Latino-dense neighborhoods. Participants discussed drug use as a *vicio* (vice), making it difficult for them to stop. This was corroborated in the quantitative analysis; two components of the Fatalism scale that represent external forces were associated with drug use. Our data are also corroborated by Valdez et al. (2009), who found that the presence of a flourishing drug market in New Orleans facilitated and maintained patterns of crack cocaine use including initiation and daily use. Isolation and constant exposure to victimization due to day laborers' marginal status were seen as contributing to this drug use as well (Valdez et al., 2009).

High-Risk Sexual Behavior among Latino Migrant Men in New Orleans

Although high at baseline, sex with FSWs and multiple partners decreased, whereas sex with main partners and abstinence increased over time for men in the Cohort study. The number of casual partners remained stable over time (Figure 14.5). Consistent condom use was highest with FSWs, lowest with main partners, and midrange with casual partners with no trends over time (Figure 14.6). STI morbidity was low; no HIV was detected. Drug use and high mobility were associated with inconsistent condom use; belonging to a social organization and having family in the household were protective. Men were more likely to have sex with an FSW if they engaged in binge drinking or used cocaine or crack, had come to New Orleans more recently, were more mobile, and scored higher on the HIV fatalism (Hess, 2007) and sensation-seeking personality (Zuckerman, 2004) scales. They were also at more risk if they did not belong to any clubs and did not have family or children living in their home, suggesting that social networks are highly influential.

Sexual concurrency (having two or more sexual partners overlapping in time) and multiple partnership (two or more sexual partners over the study period not overlapping in time) was evaluated longitudinally midway through the study. Overall concurrency was observed to decrease along with multiple partnership whereas steady sexually monogamous relationship was observed to increase over time (see Figure 14.6)

Factors associated with sexual concurrency were using drugs; self-reporting their sexual partners as "casual" only; having a wife or long-term partner in their home country; living in crowed housing conditions; having children; working in construction; and patronage of female sex workers. Belonging to a social organization or club was a highly protective factor in preventing sexual concurrency. We did not find a protective effect of having a women or child living in the home for this high-risk behavior. This lack of concurrence with other studies may be attributable to the specific environmental contexts (i.e., lack of barrio effect and little family support/ties) and the removal of traditional protective norms.

This Cohort case study of migrant workers in a new receiving location known for high-risk drug and sex options not only documents migrant behavior over time and their decisions and risks, but also provides insight into the importance of the context/environment in which they live and work. In this case, in which migrants had no established receiving communities and where the microenvironments into which they moved were varied (shipyards, inner city housing, trailer parks, and a Vietnamese housing project), a study of risk networks provided crucial information

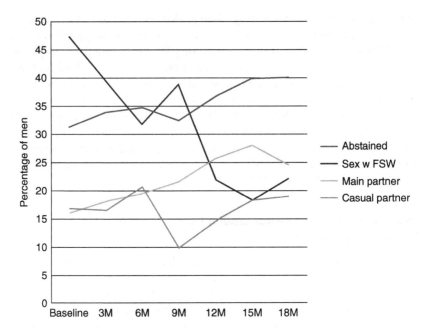

FIGURE 14.5 Trends in sexual partnership over time, N = 125.
Note: Trends over time: FSW (p< 0.001), Main, Casual (p< 0.01), abstained (p< 0.05).

on their drug and commercial sex patterns. More longitudinal research is needed to describe the evolution of risk behaviors over time. The ability to follow mobile population is often described as a barrier to such research. However, over the 3-year period, we were able to retain approximately 50% of our cohort. We continue to examine the influence of drug and sexual networks on Latino migrant men's risk for substance use and HIV/STI infection in the hopes of gaining an even greater understanding of how the environment shapes HIV/STI risk.

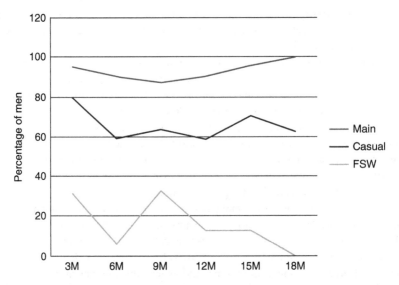

FIGURE 14.6 Inconsistent condom use by partner type, N = 125.
Note: All trends were not statistically significant.

As advocated in Chapters 1 and 6, a greater understanding of environments that promote or prevent risk is needed so that better intervention strategies can be developed. Together with their demographic growth, the recent attention garnered by the rising number of HIV diagnoses among Latino groups in the United States (Hall et al., 2008) challenge researchers, advocates, and policymakers to identify prevention and care priorities that address the contexts and needs of these populations. However, researchers, advocates, and policymakers might benefit from conceptualizing concentrations of new immigrants in ways that reflect their composition, social dynamics, economic and health status, and permanency.

It will be important, as well, to examine the use of the term "community" as epidemiological and social researchers begin to define and locate new immigrant groups (Decena & Shedlin, 2005). An especially important perspective emphasizes the role that communities play as "secondary" groups between "state" and "individual" (Durkheim, 1964) and as mediators between microlevels and macrolevels of the political and social processes affecting health and development. The globalization of current public health challenges, and of the HIV/AIDS pandemic specifically, makes it increasingly necessary to understand the role of the receiving "community" as it impacts the individuals and families who shape its social and structural processes (Barnett & Whiteside, 2002; Kawachi, 2003). Public health professionals have long appreciated the complexities of "community" (Drevdahl, 2002), especially in the implementation of *community*-based initiatives. However, programs and policies have often been less than effective when expectations of collaboration, shared goals, abilities, and motivation for collective action do not exist. Thus combined research strategies are needed—both qualitative research, especially ethnographic methods, and quantitative/epidemiological studies—to provide history, context, process, description, and prevalence among these vulnerable groups.

A part of the community is the issue of race, ethnicity, and discrimination on migrant and immigrant health. Latino residents in new receiving communities are more vulnerable to violence than Latinos who reside in areas that have traditionally been the destinations for immigrants from Central and Latin America, with a homicide rate that is nearly 50% higher (9.06 vs. 6.30 per 100,000). A report by Oxfam of Latinos and African Americans in postdisaster New Orleans describes racial tensions that exist between Latinos and African Americans. Whereas 59% of African Americans said they would be comfortable having Latinos in their neighborhoods, only 32% of Latinos said they would be comfortable having African Americans in theirs (Lee, 2008). Barriers to improved racial relations included language, a lack of opportunity for social interaction, and trust, in brief, a lack of familiarity with one another. In surveying our cohort, 47% of the Latino migrants interviewed said that Anglos treated them better than expected, whereas only 22% reported that African Americans treated them better than expected. Racial issues are particularly cogent for new receiving communities such as New Orleans. This has been linked to economic deprivation and linguistic isolation. In areas with established Latino populations, the receiving community is able to assist new immigrants in acclimating to life in the United States as well as finding a job and a safe place to live with, often times, no knowledge of English required. However, in new receiving communities, where there is no protective enclave, Latino immigrants are not only more vulnerable to victimization, but to the anger of current residents perceiving competition for employment. For example, 38% of low-income African Americans felt "strongly" that Latino workers limit job opportunities for them.

PREVENTION IMPLICATIONS

More scientists are pointing toward structural or environmental interventions rather than the individualistic approaches that have been traditionally employed in substance use and HIV/STI prevention. Data from our case study in New Orleans demonstrate the importance of the environment on HIV/STI and drug risk behavior. Socioecological factors clearly increase the risky behaviors of many Latinos in the United States, including poverty, limited education, unemployment, incarceration, inadequate health insurance, language barriers, migration and undocumented status, and limited access to health care. In a meta-analysis of 20 randomized and nonrandomized HIV prevention trial among Latinos, Herbst et al. (2007) point out the need for interventions that are gender specific, non-peer delivered, yet ones that attempt to shape peer norms.

Social network type interventions have been used to shape peer norms. One example of a successful HIV prevention approach was the establishment of new social networks through soccer leagues among Latino farm workers in North Carolina (Rhodes, Montano, Remnitz, Arceo, Bloom, Leichliter, & Bowden, 2006; Rhodes, Zometa, Lindstrom, & Montano, 2008). In our cohort, we found that belonging to a social organization or club was highly protective for both drug use and sex with an FSW, supporting this notion. Structural interventions may also be the most effective. Organista et al. found that condom use with occasional sex partners was predicted by carrying condoms (Organista, Balls Organista, Bola, García de Alba, & Morán, 2000). Interventions that increase condom availability may have an impact.

Interventions for Latinos should include an understanding of traditional cultural norms that embody constructs such as *machismo, familismo, respeto,* and *personalismo* (see Chapter 3 for a critique of the use of these constructs in the literature). Qualitative methods coupled with quantitative methods have great potential to improve investigators' grasp of cultural nuance in context while capturing the distribution of qualitatively derived behaviors (Page, 2005). Clearly there is a need to understand the diversity of cultures and communities within the Latino population (Uribe et al., 2009). Not only do we need to address the diversity of Latino communities, even in a single city, but we need to look beyond individual behavior change initiatives and focus on efforts to reduce vulnerability by conceptualizing immigrant populations in ways that reflect their composition, social dynamics, economic and health status, and permanency.

Several prevention approaches have been suggested for Latino migrants including the use of lay health advisors known as *navegantes,* mobile clinics and outreach programs, provision of bilingual staff at clinics who are informed about the new migrant groups, involvement of local churches, partnering with volunteer organizations, providing education at Latino supermarkets/*tiendas,* and using social networking sites to deliver health messages (Ruiz & Briones-Chavez, 2010). "Intervention cocktails" rather than "one-size-fits-all" interventions are likely needed to address the complexity of risk factors. More evidence-based interventions that are adaptable and address the specific environment and culture are needed.

CONCLUSIONS

Latino migrant men comprise an understudied, vulnerable demographic group at high risk for HIV/STI infection. This risk may be magnified in new receiving communities in which migrants may be isolated from the potentially protective effects of their community. Environmental and contextual factors, particularly social and sexual networks, play an important role in Latino migrants at risk for substance use and HIV/STI risk behavior. The case study of Latino migrants in post-Katrina New Orleans emphasizes how the above factors dynamically related to each other. The literature depicts a pattern of lesser risk that increases over time. However, our data and that of others suggest that the pattern is less contingent on time in a specific place than it is on contextual and environmental factors. A full understanding of cultural, contextual, and social network factors and how they interplay with HIV/STI/substance use risk is key to determining which prevention activities will have the most success.

ACKNOWLEDGMENTS

Thanks to Norine Schmidt, M.P.H., who served as the Program Manager for our two pilot studies for her input and thorough editing of this chapter. Thanks also to Oscar Salinas, M.D., and John Hembling, M.P.H., for their outstanding field work, to Stephanie Kovacs, M.P.H., and Colin Anderson-Smits, M.P.H., for their diligent data analysis, and to Jamie Carpenter for her assistance with the literature search. This chapter is dedicated to the memory of our colleague Raul Magaña who did so much to advance the field of Latino migrant studies.

This work was supported by National Institutes of Health (NIH), National Institute on Drug Abuse (NIDA) Grants 1R21DA030269-01 and R21DA026806. The content is solely the responsibility of the authors and does not necessarily represent the official views of NIDA or the NIH.

REFERENCES

Aguilar-Gaxiola, S., Medina-Mora, M. E., Magana, C. G., Vega, W. A., Alejo-Garcia, C., Quintanar, T. R., et al. (2006). Illicit drug use research in Latin America: Epidemiology service use, and HIV. *Drug and Alcohol Dependence, 84*(1), S85–S93.

Alaniz, M. (2002). Migration, acculturation, displacement: Migratory workers and "substance abuse." *Substance Use & Misuse, 37*(8–10), 1253–1257.

Alegria, M., Canino, G., Shrout, P. E., Woo, M., Duan, N., Vila, D., et al. (2008). Prevalence of mental illness in immigrant and non-immigrant U.S. Latino groups. *The American Journal of Psychiatry, 165*(3), 359–369.

Almeida, J., Molnar, B. E., Kawachi, I., & Subramanian, S. V. (2009). Ethnicity and nativity status as determinants of perceived social support: Testing the concept of familism. *Social Science & Medicine, 68*(10), 1852–1858.

Amaro, H., Whitaker, R., Coffman, G., & Heeren, T. (1990). Acculturation and marijuana and cocaine use: Findings from HHANES 1982–1984. *American Journal of Public Health, 80 Suppl,* 54–60.

Apostolopoulos, Y., Sonmez, S., Kronenfeld, J., Castillo, E., McLendon, L., & Smith, D. (2006). STI/HIV risks for Mexican migrant laborers: Exploratory ethnographies. *Journal of Immigrant and Minority Health, 8*(3), 291–302.

Barnett, T., & Whiteside, A. (1999). HIV/AIDS and development: Case studies and conceptual framework. *European Journal of Development Research, 11,* 200–234.

Barnett, T., & Whiteside, A. (2002). *AIDS in the twenty-first century: Disease and globalization.* New York: Palgrave Macmillan.

Barrington, C., Latkin, C., Sweat, M. D., Moreno, L., Ellen, J., & Kerrigan, D. (2009). Talking the talk, walking the walk: Social network norms, communication patterns, and condom use among the male partners of female sex workers in La Romana, Dominican Republic. *Social Science & Medicine, 68*(11), 2037–2044.

Bettinger, J. A., Adler, N. E., Curriero, F. C., & Ellen, J. M. (2004). Risk perceptions, condom use, and sexually transmitted diseases among adolescent females according to social network position. *Sexually Transmitted Diseases, 31*(9), 575–579.

Bordelon, C. (February 5, 2006). Hispanics bring agency new urgency. *Times-Picayune.*

Bourgois, P., Martinez, A., Kral, A., Edlin, B. R., Schonberg, J., & Ciccarone, D. (2006). Reinterpreting ethnic patterns among white and African American men who inject heroin: a social science of medicine approach. *PLoS Medicine, 3*(10), e452.

Bozon, M., Gayet, C., & Barrientos, J. (2009). A life course approach to patterns and trends in modern Latin American sexual behavior. *Journal of Acquired Immune Deficiency Syndromes, 5*(1), S4–S12.

Bronfman, M., Sejenovich, G., & Uribe, P (1998). Migración y SIDA en México y América Central. Mexico, DF: Angulos del Sida.

Caballero-Hoyos, R., Torres-Lopez, T., Pineda-Lucatero, A., Navarro-Nunez, C., Fosados, R., & Valente, T. W. (2008). Between tradition and change: Condom use with primary sexual partners among Mexican migrants. *AIDS and Behavior, 12*(4), 561–569.

Caplan, S. (2007). Latinos, acculturation, and acculturative stress: A dimensional concept analysis. *Policy, Politics, & Nursing Practice, 8*(2), 93–106.

CDC. (2004). *2003 STD Surveillance Report.* Atlanta, GA: U.S. Department of Health and Human Services.

CDC. (2005). *HIV/AIDS Surveillance Report, 2004.* Retrieved from www.cdc.gov.

CDC. (2008). CDC, HIV/AIDS Surveillance Report, *18*(1).

CDC. (2010). Estimated lifetime risk for diagnosis of HIV infection among Hispanics/Latinos—37 states and Puerto Rico, 2007. *Morbidity and Mortality Weekly Report (MMWR), 59*(40), 1297–1301.

Cherpital, C. J., & Ye, Y. (2008). Drug use and problem drinking associated with primary care and emergency room utilization in the US general population: Data from the 2005 national alcohol survey. *Drug and Alcohol Dependence, 97*(3), 226–230.

Conway, K. P., Swendsen, J. D., Dierker, L., Canino, G., & Merikangas, K. R. (2007). Psychiatric comorbidity and acculturation stress among Puerto Rican substance abusers. *American Journal of Preventive Medicine, 32*(6), S219–S225.

Cook, V. J., Sun, S. J., Tapia, J., Muth, S. Q., Arguello, D. F., Lewis, B. L., et al. (2007). Transmission network analysis in tuberculosis contact investigations. *Journal of Infectious Diseases, 196*(10), 1517–1527.

Decena, C. U., & Shedlin, M. G. (2005). Defining new communities: A challenge for immigrant health. *Papeles de Población, 44*, 214–216.

Decena, C. U., Shedlin, M. G., & Martínez, A. (2006). "Los hombres no mandan aquí": Narrating immigrant genders and sexualities in New York State. *Social Text Journal, 24*(3), 88.

De La Rosa, M. (2002). Acculturation and Latino adolescents substance use: A research agenda for the future. *Substance Use & Misuse, 37*(4), 429–456.

De La Rosa, M. R., Khalsa, J. H., & Rouse, B. A. (1990). Hispanics and illicit drug use: A review of recent findings. *International Journal of the Addictions, 25*(6), 665–691.

Denner, J., Organista, K. C., Dupree, J. D., & Thrush, G. (2005). Predictors of HIV transmission among migrant and marginally housed Latinos. *AIDS Behavior, 9*(2), 201–210.

Deren, S., Shedlin M., Decena C. U., & Mino, M. (2005). Research challenges to the study of HIV/AIDS among migrant and immigrant Hispanic populations in the United States. *Journal of Urban Health: Bulletin of the New York Academy of Medicine, 82*(2), 13–25.

Diaz, R. M., Ayala, G., & Bein, E. (2004). Sexual risk as an outcome of social oppression: Data from a probability sample of Latino gay men in three U.S. cities. *Cultural Diversity & Ethnic Minority Psychology, 10*(3), 255–267.

Doherty, I. A., Padian, N. S., Marlow, C., & Aral, S. O. (2005). Determinants and consequences of sexual networks as they affect the spread of sexually transmitted infections. *Journal of Infectious Diseases, 191*(1), S42–S54.

Doherty, I. A., Shiboski, S., Ellen, J. M., Adimora, A. A., & Padian, N. S. (2006). Sexual bridging socially and over time: A simulation model exploring the relative effects of mixing and concurrency on viral sexually transmitted infection transmission. *Sexually Transmitted Diseases, 33*(6), 368–373.

Dolezal, C., Carballo-Diéguez, A., Nieves-Rosa L., & Diaz F. (2000). Substance use and sexual risk behavior: Understanding their association among four ethnic groups of Latino men who have sex with men. *Journal of Substance Abuse, 11*(4), 323–336.

Donato, K., & Hakimzadeh, S. (January 1, 2006). The changing face of the Gulf Coast: Immigration to Louisiana, Mississippi, and Alabama. *Migration Policy Institute.*

Drevdahl, D. J. (2002). Home and border: The contradictions of community. *Advances in Nursing Science Journal, 24*(3), 8–20.

Dunlap, E., Johnson, B. D., & Morse, E. (2007). Illicit drug markets among New Orleans evacuees before and soon after hurricane Katrina. *Journal of Drug Issues, 37*(4), 981–1006.

Durkheim, E. (1964). *The division of labor in society.* Glencoe, IL: The Free Press.

Eschbach, K., Ostir, G. V., Patel, K. V., Markides, K. S., & Goodwin, J. S. (2004). Neighborhood context and mortality among older Mexican Americans: Is there a barrio advantage? *American Journal of Public Health, 94*(10), 1807–1812.

Ferreira Pinto, J., Ramos, R., & Shedlin, M. G. (1996). Migrant males and female sex workers: HIV/AIDS infection in the US-Mexico border. In S. I. Mishra, R. F. Conner, & J. R. Magaña (Eds.), *AIDS crossing borders: The spread of HIV among migrant Latinos* (pp. 69–85). Boulder, CO: Westview Press.

Fernandez-Kelly, M. P. (1983). Mexican border industrialization, female labor force participation and migration. In J. Nash & M. P. Fernandez-Kelly (Eds.), *Women, men, and the international division of labor* (pp. 205–223). New York: SUNY Press.

Fichtenberg, C. M., Muth, S. Q., Brown, B., Padian, N. S., Glass, T. A., & Ellen, J. M. (2009). Sexual network position and risk of sexually transmitted infections. *Sexually Transmitted Infections, 85*(7), 493–498.

Finch, B., Reanne, F., & Vega, W. (2004). Acculturation and acculturation stress: A social-epidemiological approach to Mexican migrant farmworkers' health 1. *The International Migration Review, 38*(1), 236–263.

Finch, B., & Vega, W. (2003). Acculturation stress, social support, and self-rated health among Latinos in California. *Journal of Immigrant Health, 5*(3), 109–117.

Finch, B. K., Catalano, R. C., Novaco, R. W., & Vega, W. A. (2003). Employment frustration and alcohol abuse/dependence among labor migrants in California. *Journal of Immigrant Health, 5*(4), 181–186.

Foley, E. (2010). Workers rebuilding New Orleans face rampant wage theft. *The Washington Independent.*http://washingtonindependent.com/96411/workers-rebuilding-new-orleans-face-rampant-wage-theft.

Foster, M. (2006). Relocated drug trade fuels murder rate in New Orleans suburb. http://www.washingtonpost.com/wp-dyn/content/article/2006/08/15/AR2006081500753.html.

Fox, N. (2008). Feds bust up heroin ring targeting teens in New Orleans http://www.foxnews. com/story/0,2933,331272,00.html.

Friedman, S. R., Bolyard, M., Mateu-Gelabert, P., Goltzman, P., Pawlowicz, M. P., Singh, D. Z., et al. (2007). Some data-driven reflections on priorities in AIDS network research. *AIDS Behavior, 11*(5), 641–651.

Friedman, S. R., Neaigus, A., Jose, B., Curtis, R., Goldstein, M. F., Sotheran, J. L., et al. (1997). Network and sociohistorical approaches to the HIV epidemic among drug injectors. In L. Sherr, J. Catalan, & B. Hedge (Eds.), *The impact of AIDS: Psychological and social aspects of HIV infection* (pp. 89–113). Chur, Switzerland: Harwood Academic Publishers.

Friedman, S. R., & Reid, G. (2002). The need for dialectical models as shown in the response to the HIV/AIDS epidemic. *International Journal of Sociology, 22,* 177–200.

Friedman, S. R., Rossi, D., & Braine, N. (2009). Theorizing "big events" as a potential risk environment for drug use, drug-related harm and HIV epidemic outbreaks. *International Journal of Drug Policy, 20*(3), 283–291.

Gallo, L. C., Penedo, F. J., Espinosa de los Monteros, K., & Arguelles, W. (2009). Resiliency in the face of disadvantage: Do Hispanic cultural characteristics protect health outcomes? *Journal of Personality and Social Psychology, 7*(6), 1707–1746.

Galvan, F. H., Ortiz, D. J., Martinez, V., & Bing, E. G. (2009). The use of female commercial sex workers' services by Latino day laborers. *Hispanic Journal of Behavioral Science, 31*(4), 553–575.

Gayet, C., et al. (2006) *Men who sell sex—a bridge population between men and women in Mexico: HIV prevalence, sexual practices and condom use: Results from a biological and behavioral survey.* Paper presented at the XVI International AIDS Conference, August 13–18, Toronto, Canada.

Gfroerer, J. C., & Tan, L. L. (2003). Substance use among foreign-born youths in the United States: Does the length of residence matter? *American Journal of Public Health, 93*(11), 1892–1895.

Gillmore, M., Catalano, R. F., Morrison, D., Wells, E., Iritani, B., & Hawkins, D. (1990). Racial differences in acceptability and availability of drugs and early initiation of substance use. *The American Journal of Drug and Alcohol Abuse, 16*(3&4), 185–206.

Hall, H. I., Song, R., Rhodes, P., Prejean, J., An, Q., Lee, L. M., et al. (2008). Estimation of HIV incidence in the United States. *Journal of the American Medical Association (JAMA), 300*(5), 520–529.

Handwerker, W. P. (2002). The construct validity of cultures: Cultural diversity, cultural theory and a method for ethnography. *American Anthropologist, 4*(1), 7.

Herbst, J. H., Kay, L. S., Passin, W. F., Lyles, C. M., Crepaz, N., Marin, B. V., et al. (2007). A systematic review and meta-analysis of behavioral interventions to reduce HIV risk behaviors of Hispanics in the United States and Puerto Rico. *AIDS & Behavior, 11*(1), 25–47.

Herdt, G. (1997). *Sexual cultures and migration in the era of AIDS: Anthropological and demographic perspectives.* Oxford: Claredon Press.

Hersh, R., McPherson, T., & Cook, R. (2002). Substance use in the construction industry: A comparison on assessment methods. *Substance Use & Misuse, 37*(11), 1131–1158.

Hertog, S. (2007). Heterosexual behavior patterns and the spread of HIV/AIDS: The interacting effects of rate of partner change and sexual mixing. *Sexually Transmitted Diseases, 34*(10), 820–828.

Hess, R. F., & McKinney, D. (2007). Fatalism and HIV/AIDS beliefs in rural Mali, West Africa. *Journal of Nursing Scholarship, 39*(2), 113–118.

Ibanez, G. E., Van Oss Marin, B., Villarreal, C., & Gomez, C. A. (2005). Condom use at last sex among unmarried Latino men: An event level analysis. *AIDS Behavior, 9*(4), 433–441.

Inciardi, J. A., Surratt, H. L., Colon, H. M., Chitwood, D. D., & Rivers, J. E. (1999). Drug use and HIV risks among migrant workers on the Delmarva Peninsula. *Substance Use & Misuse, 34*(4&5), 653–666.

International Conference on Auditory Display. (2004). In S. Barrass & P. Vickers (Eds.), *The 10th meeting of the international conference on auditory display (ICAD), Sydney, Australia, July 6–9 2004, Proceedings*. International Community for Auditory Display, 2004.

Johnson, K. (2007). Feds target violent crime in New Orleans. http://www.usatoday.com/news/nation/2007-06-03-new-orleans-crime_N.htm.

Jolly, A. M., & Wylie, J. L. (2002). Gonorrhoea and chlamydia core groups and sexual networks in Manitoba. *Sexually Transmitted Infections, 78*(1), 145–151.

Kaste, M. (2006). New Orleans police see signs of increased crime. http://www.npr.org/templates/story/story.php?storyId=5298876.

Kawachi, I. B., & Berkman, L. F. (2003). Introduction. In I. B. Kawachi & L. F. Birkman (Eds.), *Neighborhoods and health* (pp. 1–19). Oxford: Oxford University Press.

Keeling, M. J., & Eames, K. T. (2005). Networks and epidemic models. *Journal of the Royal Society Interface, 2*(4), 295–307.

Kerani, R. P., Golden, M. R., Whittington, W. L., Handsfield, H. H., Hogben, M., & Holmes, K. K. (2003). Spatial bridges for the importation of gonorrhea and chlamydial infection. *Sexually Transmitted Diseases, 30*(10), 742–749.

Kissinger, P., Kovacs, S., Anderson-Smits, C., Schmidt, N., Salinas, O., Hembling, J., et al. (2012). Patterns and predictors of HIV/STI risk among Latino migrant men in a new receiving community. *AIDS Behavior, 16*(1), 199–213.

Kissinger, P., Liddon, N., Schmidt, N., Curtin, E., Salinas, O., & Narvaez, A. (2008). HIV/STI risk behaviors among Latino migrant workers in New Orleans post-hurricane Katrina disaster. *Sexually Transmitted Diseases, 35*(11), 924–929.

Kochhar, R., Suro, R., & Tafoy, S. (2005). *The New Latino South: The context and consequences of rapid population growth*. Report prepared for the conference held at the Pew Research Center on July 26, 2005.

Kretzschmar, M., & Morris, M. (1996). Measures of concurrency in networks and the spread of infectious disease. *Mathematical Biosciences, 133*(2), 165–195.

Latkin, C. A., & Knowlton, A. R. (2005). Micro-social structural production of HIV risk among injecting drug users. *Social Science and Medicine, 17*(1), S102–S113.

Laumann, E. O., & Youm, Y. (1999). Racial/ethnic group differences in the prevalence of sexually transmitted diseases in the United States: A network explanation. *Sexually Transmitted Diseases, 26*(5), 250–261.

Lee, S. (2008). *Building common ground: How shared attitudes and concerns can create alliances between African-Americans and Latinos in a post-Katrina New Orleans*. New Orleans: Oxfam America.

Leigh, B. C., & Stall, R. (1993). Substance use and risky sexual behavior for exposure to HIV. Issues in methodology, interpretation, and prevention. *American Psychologist, 48*(10), 1035–1045.

Levy, V., Page-Shafer, K., Evans, J., Ruiz, J., Morrow, S., Reardon, J., et al. (2005). HIV-related risk behavior among Hispanic immigrant men in a population-based household survey in low-income neighborhoods of northern California. *Sexually Transmitted Diseases, 32*(8), 487–490.

Louisiana Office of Public Health. (June 30, 2008). *Louisiana HIV/AIDS Surveillance Report*.

Louisiana Public Health Institute (LPHI). (2006). Louisiana Health and Population Survey, Survey Report. Retrieved 11/28/2006, from http://popest.org.

Magis-Rodriguez, C., Gayet, C., Negroni, M., Leyva, R., Bravo-Garcia, E., Uribe, P., et al. (2004). Migration and AIDS in Mexico: An overview based on recent evidence. *Journal of Acquired Immune Deficiency Syndromes, 37*(4), S215–S226.

Magis-Rodriguez, C., Lemp, G., Hernandez, M. T., Sanchez, M. A., Estrada, F., & Bravo-Garcia, E. (2009). Going North: Mexican migrants and their vulnerability to HIV. *Journal of Acquired Immune Deficiency Syndromes, 51*(1), S21–S25.

Martínez-Donate, A., Rangel, M. G., Hovell, M. F., Santibáñez, J., Sipan, C. L., & Izazola, J. A. (2005). HIV infection in mobile populations: The case of Mexican migrants to the United States. *Pan American Journal of Public Health, 17*(1), 26–29.

Morris, C. N., & Ferguson, A. G. (2006). Estimation of the sexual transmission of HIV in Kenya and Uganda on the trans-Africa highway: The continuing role for prevention in high risk groups. *Sexually Transmitted Infections, 82*(5), 368–371.

Morris, M., & Kretzschmar, M. (1997). Concurrent partnerships and the spread of HIV. *AIDS, 11*(5), 641–648.

Morris, M., Kurth, A. E., Hamilton, D. T., Moody, J., & Wakefield, S. (2009). Concurrent partnerships and HIV prevalence disparities by race: Linking science and public health practice. *American Journal of Public Health, 99*(6), 1023–1031.

Neaigus, A., Friedman, S. R., Curtis, R., Des Jarlais, D. C., Furst, R. T., Jose, B., et al. (1994). The relevance of drug injectors' social and risk networks for understanding and preventing HIV infection. *Social Science & Medicine, 38*(1), 67–78.

Nordvik, M. K., Liljeros, F., Osterlund, A., & Herrmann, B. (2007). Spatial bridges and the spread of Chlamydia: The case of a county in Sweden. *Sexually Transmitted Diseases, 34*(1), 47–53.

Nossiter, A. (February 16, 2009). Day laborers easy prey in New Orleans. *New York Times.*

Ojeda, V. D., Patterson, T. L., & Strathdee, S. A. (2008). The influence of perceived risk to health and immigration related characteristics on substance abuse among Latino and other immigrants. *American Journal of Public Health, 98*(5), 862–868.

Organista, K. (2007). Towards a structural-environmental model of risk for HIV and problem drinking in Latino labor migrants: The case of day laborers. *Journal of Ethnic & Cultural Diversity in Social Work, 16*(1/2), 95–125.

Organista, K. C., Balls Organista, P., Garcia de Alba, J. E., Castillo Moran, M. A., & Ureta Carrillo, L. E. (1997). Survey of condom-related beliefs, behaviors, and perceived social norms in Mexican migrant laborers. *Journal of Community Health, 22*(3), 185–198.

Organista, K. C., & Kubo, A. (2005). Pilot survey of HIV risk and contextual problems and issues in Mexican/Latino migrant day laborers. *Journal of Immigrant and Minority Health, 7*(4), 269–281.

Organista, K., Balls Organista, P., Bola, J., García de Alba, G., & Morán, M. (2000). Predictors of condom use in Mexican migrant laborers. *American Journal of Community Psychology, 28*(2), 245–265.

Ortiz-Torres, B., Rapkin, B., Mantell, J., & Tross, S. (2010). *The relationship between transculturation and HIV behaviors among immigrant Latinos in the US.* Unpublished manuscript.

Page, J. B. (2005). The concept of culture: A core issue in health disparities. *Journal of Urban Health, 82*(2&3), 35–43.

Painter, T. (2008). Connecting the dots: When the risks of HIV/STD infection appear high but the burden of infection is not known—the case of male Latino migrants in the Southern United States. *AIDS Behavior, 12*(2), 213–226.

Parrado, E., Flippen, C., & McQuiston, C. (2004). Use of commercial sex workers among Hispanic migrants in North Carolina: Implications for the spread of HIV. *Perspectives on Sexual and Reproductive Health, 36*(4), 150–156.

Paschane, D. M., & Fisher, D. G. (2000). Etiology of limited transmission diseases among drug users: Does recent migration magnify the risk of sharing injection equipment? *Social Science & Medicine, 50*(7–8), 1091–1097.

Passel, J. (2006). *The size and characteristics of the unauthorized migrant population in the U.S.: Estimates based on the March 2005 current population survey.* Washington, DC: Pew Hispanic Center.

Passel, J., & Cohn, D. (2008). *U.S. population projections: 2005–2050.* Washington, DC: Pew Research Center.

Passel, J., & Cohn, D. (2009). *Mexican immigrants: How many come? How many leave?* July 22, 2009 Report. Washington, DC: Pew Hispanic Center.

Patterson, T., et al. (2006, August 13–18). *High prevalence of HIV and sexually transmitted infections among female sex workers associated with injection drug use in two Mexican–U.S. border cities.* Paper presented at the XVI International AIDS Conference, Toronto, Canada.

Paz-Bailey, G., Morales-Miranda, S., Jacobson, J. O., Gupta, S. K., Sabin, K., Mendoza, S., et al. (2009). High rates of STD and sexual risk behaviors among Garifunas in Honduras. *Journal of Acquired Immune Deficiency Syndromes, 51*(1), S26–S34.

Paz-Bailey, G., Teran, S., Levine, W., & Markowitz, L. E. (2004). Syphilis outbreak among Hispanic immigrants in Decatur, Alabama: Association with commercial sex. *Sexually Transmitted Diseases, 31*(1), 20–25.

Perlstein, M. (2010). Investigative Reporter WWLTV. New Orleans.

Pew Hispanic Center. (2010). *Statistical portrait of Hispanics in the United States, 2008.*

Plyer, A., & Ortiz, E. (2010). *Who lives in New Orleans and the metro area now?* New Orleans Community Data Center. Based on 2009 U.S. Census Bureau Data.

Potterat, J. J., Muth, S. Q., Rothenberg, R. B., Zimmerman-Rogers, H., Green, D. L., Taylor, J. E., et al. (2002). Sexual network structure as an indicator of epidemic phase. *Sexually Transmitted Infections, 78*, 152–158.

Potterat, J. J., Rothenberg, R. B., & Muth, S. Q. (1999). Network structural dynamics and infectious disease propagation. *International Journal of STD & AIDS, 10*(3), 182–185.

Poundstone, K. E., Strathdee, S. A., & Celentano, D. D. (2004). The social epidemiology of human immunodeficiency virus/acquired immunodeficiency syndrome. *Epidemiologic Reviews Journal, 26*, 22–35.

Rabito, F. A., Perry, S., Salinas, O., Hembling, J., Schmidt, N., Parsons, P. J., et al. (2010). A longitudinal assessment of occupation, respiratory symptoms, and blood lead levels among Latino day laborers in a non-agricultural setting. *American Journal of Industrial Medicine. 54*(5), 366–374.

Ramirez-Valles, J., Garcia, D., Campbell, R. T., Diaz, R. M., & Heckathorn, D. D. (2008). HIV infection, sexual risk behavior, and substance use among Latino gay and bisexual men and transgender persons. *American Journal of Public Health, 98*(6), 1036–1042.

Ramirez-Valles, J., Heckathorn, D. D., Vázuiz, R., Diaz, R. M., & Campbell, R. T. (2005). From networks to populations: The development and application of respondent-driven sampling among IDUs and Latino gay men. *AIDS and Behavior, 9*(4), 387–402.

Ramos, R., Ferreira-Pinto, J. B., Brouwer, K. C., Ramos, M. E., Lozada, R. M., Firestone-Cruz, M., et al. (2009). A tale of two cities: Social and environmental influences shaping risk factors and protective behaviors in two Mexico–US border cities. *Health & Place, 15*(4), 999–1005.

Rhodes, S. D., Hergenrather, K. C., Montano, J., Remnitz, I., Arceo, R., Bloom, F. R., Leichliter, J., & Bowden, W. P. (2006). Using community-based participatory research to develop an intervention to reduce HIV and STD infections among Latino men. *AIDS Education and Prevention, 18*(5), 375–389.

Rhodes, S. D., Hergenrather, K. C., Zometa, C., Lindstrom, K., & Montaño, J. (2008). Characteristics of immigrant Latino men who utilize formal healthcare services: Findings from the HoMBReS study. *Journal of the National Medical Association, 100*(10), 1177–1185.

Rhodes, T. (2002). The risk environment: A framework for understanding and reducing drug-related harm. *International Journal of Drug Policy, 13*, 85–94.

Rhodes, T. (2009). Risk environments and drug harms: A social science for harm reduction approach. *International Journal of Drug Policy, 20*(3), 193–201.

Rhodes, T., & Simic, M. (2005). Transition and the HIV risk environment. *British Medical Journal, 331*(7510), 220–223.

Rhodes, T., Singer, M., Bourgois, P., Friedman, S. R., & Strathdee, S. A. (2005). The social structural production of HIV risk among injecting drug users. *Social Science & Medicine, 61*(5), 1026–1044.

Rhodes, T., Stimson, G. V., Crofts, N., Ball, A., Dehne, K., & Khodakevich, L. (1999). Drug injecting, rapid HIV spread, and the "risk environment": Implications for assessment and response. *AIDS, 13*(A), S259–S269.

Rosen, C. S., Kuhn, E. R., Greenbaum, M. A., & Drescher, K. D. (2008). Substance abuse related mortality among middle-aged male VA psychiatric patients. *Psychiatric Services, 59*(3), 290–296.

Rothenberg, R. (2001). How a net works: Implications of network structure for the persistence and control of sexually transmitted diseases and HIV. *Sexually Transmitted Diseases, 28*(2), 63–68.

Rothenberg, R. B., Potterat, J. J., Woodhouse, D. E., Muth, S. Q., Darrow, W. W., & Klovdahl, A. S. (1998). Social network dynamics and HIV transmission. *AIDS, 12*(12), 1529–1536.

Rothenberg, R. B., Sterk, C., Toomey, K. E., Potterat, J. J., Johnson, D., Schrader, M., et al. (1998). Using social network and ethnographic tools to evaluate syphilis transmission. *Sexually Transmitted Diseases, 25*(3), 154–160.

Ruiz, M., & Briones-Chavez, C. S. (2010). How to improve the health of undocumented Latino immigrants with HIV in New Orleans: An agenda for action. *Revista Panamericana de Salud Pública, 28*(1), 66–70.

Sanchez, M., et al. (2008). *The effect of migration on HIV high-risk behaviors among Mexican migrants.* Paper presented at the XVII International AIDS Conference, Mexico City.

Seidman, S. B. (1983). Internal cohesion of LS sets in graphs. *Social Networks Journal, 5*(2), 97–107.

Sena, A. C., Hammer, J. P., Wilson, K., Zeveloff, A., & Gamble, J. (2010). Feasibility and acceptability of door-to-door rapid HIV testing among Latino immigrants and their HIV risk factors in North Carolina. *AIDS Patient Care and STDS, 24*(3), 165–173.

Sena, A. C., Muth, S. Q., Heffelfinger, J. D., O'Dowd, J. O., Foust, E., & Leone, P. (2007). Factors and the sociosexual network associated with a syphilis outbreak in rural North Carolina. *Sexually Transmitted Diseases, 34*(5), 280–287.

Shedlin, M. G. (2005). Defining new communities: A challenge for immigrant health. *Papeles de Población, 44*.

Shedlin, M. G., & Shulman, L. (2001). *Qualitative needs assessment of HIV services among Dominican, Mexican and Central American immigrant populations living in the New York City EMA.* Westport, CT: Sociomedical Resource Associates.

Shedlin, M. G., & Shulman, L. (2004). Qualitative needs assessment of HIV services among Dominican, Mexican and Central American immigrant populations living in the New York City area. *AIDS Care, 16*(4), 434–445.

Shihadesh, E., & Barranco, R. (2010). Latino employment and black violence: The unintended consequence of U.S. immigration policy. *Social Forces, 88,* 1393–1420.

Singer, M., Valentin, F., Baer, H., & Jia, Z. (1992). Why does Juan Garcia have a drinking problem? The perspective of critical medical anthropology. *Medical Anthropology, 14*(1), 77–108.

Sorensen, N. N. (2004). *Migrant remittances as a development tool: The Case of Morocco.* Unpublished manuscript, Geneva.

Sparacello, M. (2008). Kenner announces drug bust. http://www.nola.com/news/index. ssf/2008/02/kenner_announces_major_drug_bu.html.

Stephenson, K., & Zelen, M. (1989). Rethinking centrality: Methods and examples. *Social Networks Journal, 11,* 1–37.

Strathdee, S. A., Lozada, R., Pollini, R. A., Brouwer, K. C., Mantsios, A., Abramovitz, D. A., et al. (2008). Individual, social, and environmental influences associated with HIV infection among injection drug users in Tijuana, Mexico. *Journal of Acquired Immune Deficiency Syndromes, 47*(3), 369–376.

Strathdee, S. A., Stachowiak, J. A., Todd, C. S., Al-Delaimy, W. K., Wiebel, W., Hankins, C., et al. (2006). Complex emergencies, HIV, and substance use: No "big easy" solution. *Substance Use & Misuse, 41*(10–12), 1637–1651.

Sweat, M., & Denison, J. (1995). Reducing HIV incidence in developing countries with structural and environmental interventions. *AIDS, 9*(A), S251–S257.

Temple, M. T., Leigh, B. C., & Schafer, J. (1993). Unsafe sexual behavior and alcohol use at the event level: Results of a national survey. *Journal of Acquired Immune Deficiency Syndromes, 6*(4), 393–401.

Tori, C. D. (1989). Homosexuality and illegal residency status in relation to substance abuse and personality traits among Mexican nationals. *Journal of Clinical Psychology, 45*(5), 814–821.

UNAIDS. (2008). *Latin America: AIDS epidemic update regional summary.*

UNAIDS/IOM. (1998). Migration and AIDS. *International Migration, 36*(4), 445–468.

UNAIDS/WHO. (2006). AIDS update: Latin America.

Uribe, C. L., Darrow, W. W., Villanueva, L. P., Obiaja, K. C., Sanchez-Brana, E., & Gladwin, H. (2009). Identifying HIV risk-reduction strategies for Hispanic populations in Broward County. *Annals of Epidemiology, 19*(8), 567–574.

United States Census Bureau. (2006). *American community survey, General characteristics for Orleans Parish, Louisiana.* Retrieved 11/14/2006 from http://www.census.gov/acs/www.

Valdez, A., Cepeda, A., Negi, N. J., & Kaplan, C. (2009). Fumando La Piedra: Emerging patterns of crack use among Latino immigrant day laborers in New Orleans. *Journal of Immigrant and Minority Health, 12*(5), 737–742.

Valente, T. W. (2006). Opinion leader interventions in social networks. *British Medical Journal, 333*(7578), 1082–1083.

Valente, T. W., & Fosados, R. (2006). Diffusion of innovations and network segmentation: The part played by people in promoting health. *Sexually Transmitted Diseases, 33*(7), S23–S31.

Vega, W. A., Kolody, B., Aguilar-Gaxiola, S., Alderete, E., Catalano, R., & Caraveo Anduaga, J. (1998). Lifetime prevalence of DSM-III-R psychiatric disorders among urban and rural Mexican-Americans in California. *Archives of General Psychiatry, 5,* 771–778.

Viadro, C., & Earp, J. A. L. (2000). The sexual behavior of married Mexican immigrant men in North Carolina. *Social Science & Medicine, 50,* 723–735.

Wasserheit, J. N. (1994). Effect of changes in human ecology and behavior on patterns of sexually transmitted diseases, including human immunodeficiency virus infection. *Proceedings of the National Academy of Sciences of the United States, 91*(7), 2430–2435.

Weatherburn, P., Davies, P. M., Hickson, F. C., Hunt, A. J., McManus, T. J., & Coxon, A. P. (1993). No connection between alcohol use and unsafe sex among gay and bisexual men. *AIDS, 7*(1), 115–119.

Wong, W., Tambis, J. A., Hernandez, M., & Chaw, J. (2003). Prevalence of sexually transmitted diseases among Latino immigrant day laborers in an urban setting—San Francisco. *Sexually Transmitted Diseases, 30*(8), 661–663.

Worby, P., & Organista, K. C. (2007). Alcohol use and problem drinking among male Mexican American and Central American immigrant laborers. *Hispanic Journal of Behavioral Science, 29*(4), 413–455.

WWLTV. (2008a). Five arrested in Ponchatoula prescription drug bust. http://www.wwltv. com/topstories/stories/wwl061108mlpontch.20764344.html.

WWLTV. (2008b). Marrero drug bust nets $62,000 in heroin. http://www.wwltv.com/ local/stories/wwl040408tpdrug.31ab6df3.html.

Wylie, J. L., Cabral, T., & Jolly, A. M. (2005). Identification of networks of sexually transmitted infection: A molecular, geographic, and social network analysis. *Journal of Infectious Diseases, 191*(6), 899–906.

Zuckerman, M. (2004). *Behavioral expression and biosocial bases of sensation seeking.* Cambridge: Cambridge University Press.

Section III
Best and Promising HIV Prevention Interventions with Diverse Latino Populations, Locations, and Situations

15 Reducing HIV Sexual Risk for Latino Adolescents

An Ecodevelopmental Perspective

Antonia M. Villarruel,
Vincent Guilamo-Ramos,
and Jose Bauermeister

INTRODUCTION

The structural-environmental context for Latino adolescents is similar to that for all Latinos. It includes poverty, immigration stress, limited resource neighborhoods, and limited access to culturally and linguistically appropriate HIV prevention information and reproductive services. Many Latino adolescents have the added challenge of being in schools characterized by high drop-out rates and substandard instruction, and located in resource-poor neighborhoods. Latino families, particularly parents, are important resources for adolescents. But Latino parents are often burdened by stresses of employment, language barriers, and differences in values and expectations between their home country and new environment. Often, Latino children seem to adapt more quickly and better, resulting in gaps in communication and values between parents and their children.

Latino adolescents are challenged to "fit in" to an environment different from that of their parents' environment while at school, often feeling little parental support to deal with challenges never experienced by their parents. Simultaneously, as adolescents they are at a prime developmental stage in their lives where they have the opportunity to define both present and future goals for themselves. Adolescence provides an opportunity to "try out" different identities, most often as a way to gain acceptance with their peers. With adequate support from parents, teachers, and health providers, adolescents are often open to developing attitudes and skills that will help them achieve their goals. Adolescents who are provided with accurate information have the capacity to make decisions to keep healthy and safe.

In this chapter we describe in detail some of the structural-environmental factors that influence adolescent risk behavior. We utilize an ecodevelopmental framework to present an overview of issues confronting Latino adolescents and their parents specifically related to adolescent sexual risk behavior. In our review of the literature, we focus on strategies that have been developed for Latino adolescents and their parents to address this important health and social challenge. We review existing interventions and programs designed to provide Latino adolescents and parents with the knowledge, skills, and abilities needed to prevent HIV. We identify both strengths and gaps in existing interventions, and identify other strategies at the structural level that can be implemented to support Latino parents and adolescents.

HIV/AIDS RISK PROFILE OF LATINO ADOLESCENTS IN THE UNITED STATES

Despite limited epidemiological data, several factors indicate the importance and urgency of addressing HIV prevention efforts for Latino adolescents. Latino teens aged 13 to 19 years accounted for 19% of AIDS cases among U.S. teens in 2006, which is disproportionately high considering that they represented 17% of the U.S. teen population that same year [Centers for Disease Control and Prevention (CDC), 2006]. This margin is even greater in Latino young adults aged 20 to 24 years who in 2006 represented 18% of the U.S. population but accounted for 23% of AIDS cases (CDC, 2006).

Compared to older age groups, the percentage of AIDS cases in adolescence is lower, due in part to the slow progression of HIV infection to AIDS. The proportion of individuals who progressed from HIV infection to AIDS within 12 months following diagnosis of HIV infection in 2004 was 39% among all persons; however, this proportion was lower (between 19% and 30%) among youth aged 13 to 24 years old (CDC, 2008a). Although the proportion of AIDS cases in this age group is low, the incidence of HIV among 24 to 60 year olds is high, which may be attributable to behaviors learned during adolescence or to HIV exposure and infection during this period, thus increasing the importance of prevention efforts for adolescents.

Young Latino men who have sex with men (MSM) are also at high risk for HIV infection and bear a considerable burden of HIV/AIDS diagnoses among young people in the United States (CDC, 2001, 2008a). Furthermore, whereas white MSM are more likely to be infected during adulthood, Latino MSM are more likely to be infected during adolescence and during the transition to early adulthood (Valleroy et al., 2000). Despite a high risk for contracting HIV, few Latino adolescents are getting tested for the virus—13% for Latinos as compared with 22% for African Americans, and an even fewer 11% for whites (CDC, 2009a). The low rates of testing among Latino adolescents are another indication of the potential underestimation of HIV among Latinos.

Unintended Pregnancies and STDs

Latino adolescents are also disproportionately affected by unintended pregnancies and sexually transmitted diseases (STDs), which further highlight Latino adolescent risk for HIV infection. Rates of teen pregnancy have consistently been high among Latinas. Although there was a 2% drop in the teen birth rate among Latinas in 2007 (81.7/1000), rates in this group are still dramatically higher than rates among white (27.2/1000) and African American teens (64.3/1000) (Hamilton, Martin, & Ventura, 2009). Furthermore, among Latina teens, 52% will become pregnant at least once before they turn 20, compared with 19% of non-Latina whites (National Campaign to Prevent Teen and Unplanned Pregnancy, 2010).

Although comprising only 25% of the sexually active population, adolescents and young adults account for nearly half of new cases of STDs (CDC, 2009b).

Existing data suggest that Latino adolescents are also at high risk for acquiring STDs (CDC, 2009b). The CDC (2008b) reported that although Latinos account for 15% of the U.S. population, they account for 19% of all reported Chlamydia cases. In 2007, rates of gonorrhea and syphilis among Latinos (69.2/100,000; 4.3/100,000) were nearly double that among whites (34.7/100,000; 2.0/100,000) that same year (CDC, 2008b).

Sexual Risk Behaviors

Latino youth engage in sexual risk behaviors that place them at increased risk for unintended pregnancies, STDs, and HIV infection. For example, nearly half of Latino high school students report ever having had sexual intercourse, and the majority (86%) report not using birth control pills to prevent pregnancy during their last sexual intercourse (CDC, 2009a). Latino youth are also less likely to use a condom during last sexual intercourse—45% of sexually active Latino students did not use a condom compared to 36.7% of white students and 37.6% of African American students (CDC, 2009a).

Similarly, the Federal Interagency Forum on Child and Family Statistics (2007) reported that although the percentage of high school students who reported ever having sexual intercourse has declined among non-Latino white and African American students, no significant changes have occurred among Latino students. There also was no significant change among Latino students regarding multiple partners (CDC, 2008c). Furthermore, studies have consistently documented that Latino adolescents report lower condom use than African American or white adolescents (Brener et al., 2002; CDC, 2006; Eaton et al., 2006; Kann et al., 2000; Shlay, McClung, Patnaik, & Douglas, 2004). Data from the Youth Risk Behavior Surveillance System (YRBSS) indicate that Latina females were the least likely among all youth and genders to use a condom at last sexual intercourse (CDC, 2008c). Of additional concern is that Latina teens are more likely than their non-Latina peers to have a partner who is significantly older than them (Marin et al.,2000), a factor that places them at greater risk for early sexual debut and coercive sexual relationships, which in turn can facilitate greater exposure to HIV and other sexually transmitted diseases (Sabatiuk & Flores, 2009).

INDIVIDUAL RISK FACTORS

A number of individual risk factors have been positively associated with risky sexual behavior. A review of antecedents of sexual risk behavior by DiClemente, Salazar, and Crosby (2007) indicates that factors such as impulsivity and sensation seeking, depression, working more than 20 hours per week, and low educational goals or career plans are positively associated with high-risk sexual behaviors. Conversely, self-efficacy to use condoms and negotiate sex, perceived risk of infection, and personal control serve as protective factors against sexual risk behaviors. Among Latinos, common factors including acculturative stress, perceived discrimination, and the influence of traditional gender roles place Latino adolescents at risk for engaging in sexual risk behaviors (Gonzalez, Hendriksen, Collins, Duran, & Safren, 2009). Some of these identified sexual risk factors, including traditional gender roles and family support, may also serve as protective factors for Latino adolescents (Hirsch, Muñoz-Laboy, Nyhus, Yount, & Bauermeister, 2009). These seemingly contradictory findings point to the diversity among Latinos and the need to consider context—including the risk and protective influences of migration and family support.

Substance Abuse, School Completion, and Gang Involvement

Especially during adolescence, sexual risk behaviors do not occur in isolation, but often manifest alongside other risk behaviors. There are several factors that are associated with high sexual risk behavior among adolescents. Some of these factors such as substance use (Prado, Schwartz, et al., 2006), dropping out of high school, and gang involvement are more prevalent among Latino adolescents than their non-Latino counterparts. According to the YRBSS, Latino students were more likely than African American or white students to have used cocaine, heroin, methamphetamine, and/or ecstasy one or more times during their life. Latino students were only slightly less likely (25.3%) than white students (29.9%), and much more likely than African American students (11.1%) to have had five or more drinks of alcohol in a row on one or more of the 30 days preceding the survey (CDC, 2007). According to a study conducted by Shih, Miles, Tucker, Zhou, and D'Amico (2010), Latino students had the highest probability of lifetime and past month substance use, even after accounting for factors such as sex, grade in school, and family structure. Rates did not differ between African American and white students.

Although findings have been inconsistent, the majority of studies have concluded that acculturation is positively associated with substance use among Latino adolescents. Substance use has been found to be positively associated with parent–adolescent conflict (Buchanan & Smokowski, 2009), internalizing/externalizing problems (Buchanan & Smokowski, 2009), parent–child discrepancy in U.S. orientation (Unger, Ritt-Olson, Soto, & Baezconde-Garbanati, 2009), and deterioration of Latino family values, attitudes, and familistic behaviors (Gil, Wagner, & Vega, 2000), all factors that commonly coincide with acculturation among Latino adolescents. Wahl and Eitle (2010) found that the extent of these effects varied based on gender, immigrant generation, and Latino ethnicity.

Conversely, school attendance has been found to reduce adolescent substance use and sexual risk-taking behavior (CDC, 2009c; Kirby, 2004). Being in school acts as a protective factor against many risk behaviors by providing structured time, an environment that discourages unhealthy risk taking, an increased future orientation, and an increased sense of competence and improved communication skills (CDC, 2009c; Kirby, 2004). However, high dropout rates among Latino adolescents put them at an increased risk for sexual risk behavior. In 2005, Latino youth aged 16 to 24 accounted for 41% of all current high school dropouts; however, they accounted for only 17% of the total youth population. In that same year, 23% of Latino youth were not enrolled in school and had not completed high school, compared with 11% of African Americans and 6% of whites (Child Trends Databank, 2005; U.S. Census Bureau, 2005).

Latinos are also disproportionately represented in gangs. In large cities, where almost half of the Hispanic population resides, whites constitute only 11% of gang members, while the remainder are ethnic or racial minorities, including Latino youth (Esbensen, 2000). Gang membership is associated with high-risk behaviors including violence, drug use, and risky sexual intercourse (De La Rosa, Rugh, & Rice, 2006; Gatti, Tremblay, Vitaro, & McDuff, 2005; Gordon et al., 2004; Sanders, Schneiderman, Loken, Lankenau, & Bloom, 2009). Gang members are more likely than nonmembers to engage in high-risk sexual behaviors including having sex at an earlier age, having a greater number of partners, and using sex in exchange for money or drugs (Brooks, Lee, Stover, & Barkley, 2009; Harper & Robinson, 1999). Gang involvement, like other risk factors, is the result of individual decisions and behaviors. However, these behaviors must be viewed within a broader context in order to determine the most effective ways to support adolescents.

STRUCTURAL FACTORS CONTRIBUTING TO HIV RISK AMONG LATINOS

The individual sexual and other risks behaviors for Latino adolescents are strongly influenced by numerous structural factors. Specific structural factors were identified in a comprehensive review of HIV/STD adolescent interventions (DiClemente et al., 2007). Factors such as poverty, community violence and disorganization, and communities with a high percentage of foreign born residents were found to be associated positively with sexual risk behaviors, STDs, and HIV. Structural protective factors for adolescents included community involvement, social support, and school connectedness.

DiClemente and colleagues (2007) highlighted some of the reasons why Latino youth are more vulnerable to HIV infection. For example, Hispanic/Latino families are more likely to be living in poverty than non-Hispanic white families, with over 25% of Hispanic children under age 18 living in poverty (U.S. Census Bureau, 2002). Furthermore, nearly half of all foreign born individuals residing in the United States are Hispanic/Latino, comprising approximately 40% of the total Hispanic population in the United States and 6% of the total U.S. population (U.S. Census Bureau, 2010). Poverty and recent immigration status may further restrict access to education, employment, and social mobility, and diminish the opportunity for Latino families to live in communities with a greater set of resources.

Access to health care is another structural factor that could be protective against HIV infection, but lack of health insurance has been a deterrent for many Latino youth. Latinos are the most uninsured racial/ethnic group in the United States (U.S. Census Bureau, 2003). Being insured, however, does not in itself guarantee access to health care. For example, when asked to provide reasons for not having an HIV test, high-risk minority youth reported a low perception of risk, not having insurance, and never having been offered a test by a health care provider (Peralta, Deeds, Hipszer, & Ghalib, 2007; Rios-Ellis, 2010). Similarly, most teens have never discussed STDs with a health care provider (Grunbaum et al., 2002). Although Latino adolescents are at high risk for HIV infection because they are engaged in risky sexual behaviors, there are a number of structural factors that influence these behaviors. Subsequently, we discuss the use of an organizing framework to facilitate creating environments and opportunities for youth to develop and practice safer sex behaviors.

ECODEVELOPMENTAL THEORY

We used ecodevelopmental theory (Szapocznik & Coatsworth, 1999) as an organizing framework to incorporate the individual, family, and structural interrelationships addressed in this chapter. The basic tenets of this theory propose that understanding risk and protective factors for adolescent behaviors requires knowledge of individual and developmental processes and consideration of the social systems in which they occur. Ecodevelomental theory (Perrino, Gonzalez-Soldevilla,

Pantin, & Szapocznik, 2000) proposes that because the family is the most fundamental system influencing human development, it is an ideal system for influencing adolescent risk and protective behaviors. The family is the major social unit in which values, attitudes, beliefs, and behaviors, including those related to health, are developed and maintained. The critical question becomes the identification of specific family characteristics that impact the development of competencies and responsible behavior in adolescents. Within ecodevelopmental theory, maximizing family factors that can be protective to reduce risky behaviors in adolescents is considered a main priority.

MICROSYSTEM FACTORS—PARENTAL INFLUENCES

Parental influences on adolescent sexual activity can be divided into two categories: family structure variables and family process variables. Family structure variables related to adolescent sexual behavior include low educational levels of parents, low family socioeconomic status, and single parenting. Family process variables such as parent–adolescent communication, parental monitoring and supervision, and parent–adolescent relationship satisfaction are particularly salient for Latino youth given the importance Latino culture places on family solidarity and cohesion (Guilamo-Ramos et al., 2006).

Family Structure Variables

Family structure variables such as socioeconomic status, parental education, household composition, and neighborhood characteristics have been widely studied in relation to adolescent sexual behavior (Browning, Burrington, Leventhal, & Brooks-Gunn, 2008; Miller, Kotchick, Dorsey, Forehand, & Ham, 1998; Ramirez-Valles, Zimmerman, & Newcomb, 1998; Upchurch, Aneshensel, Sucoff, & Levy-Storms, 1999). According to a number of longitudinal studies, youth who reside in families of higher socioeconomic status and whose parents are more educated are more likely to have initiated sexual intercourse at later ages (Miller, Levin, Whitaker, & Xu, 1998; Santelli, Lowry, Brener, & Robin, 2000). Furthermore, youth who live in nonintact families (i.e., single parent households or fathers who are not actively involved in parenting) are more likely to have initiated sexual activity earlier than those living with both biological parents (Lammers, Ireland, Resnick, & Blum, 2000; Santelli et al., 2000). Neighborhood characteristics, such as high rates of residential turnover, poverty, and crime, have also been associated with early sexual debut, low use of contraception, and high teen pregnancy rates (Miller, 2002). Although family structure variables are important, they tend to be less amenable to change and, hence, offer more limited opportunities for direct intervention.

Family Process Variables

The most widely studied family process variable in the literature examining adolescent sexual risk behavior is parenting. Research on the role that parents play in the sexual and reproductive health of their children has tended to focus on three main aspects of parenting: parent–adolescent communication, parental monitoring and supervision, and parent–adolescent relationship quality and satisfaction. Below, we review each of these aspects as they pertain to Latino families.

One factor that has been associated with a range of sexual and reproductive health outcomes and behaviors is communication between parents and adolescents. Most research suggests that Latino parents are less likely to talk to their children about sexual topics, and when they do, the discussions are often initiated after sexual activity has begun [Hutchinson, 2002; Kaiser Family Foundation (KFF), 2006; Zambrana, Cornelius, Boykin, & Lopez, 2004]. However, other studies have also shown that Latino parents do discuss certain sexual topics with their children such as abstinence and the negative consequences of sex (Guilamo-Ramos et al., 2006; Guilamos-Ramos, Jaccard, Dittus, Burns, & Holloway, 2007), though they often have more difficulty talking about topics such as contraception and birth control (Raffaelli & Ontai, 2001; Raffaelli & Green, 2003). Research has also shown a gendered component with parent–adolescent communication in which parents tend to discuss sex more with their daughters than with their sons (Guilamo-Ramos, Jaccard, et al., 2007). See Chapter 16 for an innovative approach to HIV prevention involving the facilitation of sex-related conversations between Latina mothers and daughters. In the section below, we review important aspects of parent–adolescent relationships including the content, context, timing, frequency, and barriers, with attention to parental monitoring and other relationship characteristics.

The content of communication between parents and their children is an important factor to consider in understanding adolescent sexual behavior. Research with Latino parents suggests that they most frequently talk about puberty (Ancheta, Hynes, & Shrier, 2005; O'Sullivan, Meyer-Bahlburg, & Watkins, 2001; Raffaelli & Ontai, 2001), the negative consequences of sexual behavior (Guilamo-Ramos et al., 2006; Guilamo-Ramos, Jaccard, et al., 2007), and about sexual morals, attitudes, and values (Guiamo-Ramos, Jaccard, et al., 2007; Raffaelli & Ontai, 2001; Romo, Lefkowitz, Sigman, & Au, 2002). Studies also suggest that Latino parents have difficulties talking about more technical aspects of sexuality such as birth control and contraception, because they feel they lack the knowledge to discuss such topics or fear that talking might encourage adolescent sexual activity (Guilamo-Ramos et al., 2006; Raffaelli & Green, 2003; Raffaelli & Ontai, 2001). However, as shown in longitudinal studies, parental communication about contraception was associated with less sexual risk-taking with Latino adolescents (Hutchinson, Jemmott, Jemmott, Braverman, & Fong, 2003). As stated previously, discussion of sexual topics in Latino families tends to be more common with daughters than with sons (Guilamo-Ramos, Jaccard, et al., 2007). Although adolescents tend to be aware of this dynamic, studies suggest that they would prefer their parents to deliver the same messages about responsible sexual behavior to both sons and daughters (Guilamo-Ramos et al., 2006; Vexler, 2007).

Context is another important factor to consider in understanding parent–adolescent communication about sex. As noted in a number of studies, greater levels of perceived parental openness, responsiveness, comfort, and confidence in discussions about sexual topics were associated with lower levels of adolescent sexual risk behavior (Dutra, Miller, & Forehand, 1999; Guilamo-Ramos et al., 2006; Halpern-Felsher, Kropp, Boyer, Tschann, & Ellen, 2004). In studies with Latino youth, higher levels of parental self-disclosure were found to be predictive of higher levels of perceived parental openness in conversations about sex (Romo et al., 2002). Furthermore, Latino youth who perceive their parents as being willing to talk about how they dealt with challenging issues when they were teens reported less willingness to engage in sexual intercourse (Guilamo-Ramos, 2010). In studies examining the context of communication, trust between parents and adolescents and perceptions of parental expertise and accessibility were found to be associated with lower levels of adolescent sexual behavior (Guilamo-Ramos et al., 2006; Miller et al., 1998a; Velez-Pastrana et al., 2005). High levels of trust in the parent–adolescent relationship were associated with higher levels of communication about sex and lower levels of adolescent sexual behavior (Guilamo-Ramos et al., 2006).

The timing of communication about sex plays a key role when it comes to adolescent sexual behavior and research suggests that parents should begin talking with their teens simultaneously about sex, love, and relationships before their teens start dating or become sexually active (Guzman et al., 2003; O'Donnell et al., 2006). Studies have found that the onset of dating is a strong predictor of sexual activity (Cavanagh, 2004; Van Oss Marin, Coyle, Gómez, Carvajal, & Kirby 2000; Zimmer-Gembeck, Seibenbruner, & Collins, 2004), underscoring the importance of parents talking with their children before they begin dating relationships. In a study of Latino parents and teens, 47% of teens reported being sexually experienced whereas only 30% of parents thought their teen had had sex (National Campaign to Prevent Teen and Unplanned Pregnancy, 2006). Despite the importance of timing of communication about sex, in the absence of any clear signs of sexual activity, parents often assume their child is not sexually active or underestimate the extent of their teen's sexual activity (Albert, Brown, & Flanigan, 2003; Jaccard, Dittus, & Gordon, 1998).

In addition to timing, the frequency of communication can play an important role in reducing sexual risk. For Latinos, studies have shown that the more often parents talk about sexuality related topics, the more likely it is that adolescents will share similar views with their parents on those topics, suggesting that adolescents do listen to their parents and that greater frequency of communication impacts their sexual decision-making (Guilamo-Ramos et al., 2011). Studies with Latino parents and adolescents have also shown that there is often disagreement about the frequency of communication about sex, with parents reporting a greater frequency of conversations compared with adolescents (Guilamo-Ramos, Jaccard, et al., 2007; National Campaign to Prevent Teen and Unplanned Pregnancy, 2001). This suggests that there may be contextual factors influencing each time parents and teens communicate that may affect how parents and adolescents recall these conversations.

Although parents from all ethnic and racial groups experience difficulties talking with their children about sexuality related topics, numerous studies suggest that Latino parents do not discuss sex as often as other parents (Hutchinson et al., 2003; O'Sullivan et al., 2001). In Latino families, parental discomfort and embarrassment are among the most widely reported barriers to communication about sex (Guilamo-Ramos et al., 2006; Guilamo-Ramos, Jaccard, Dittus, & Collins, 2008; Meneses, Orrell-Valente, Guendelman, Oman, & Irwin, 2006). Generational and cultural differences unique to U.S. Latinos may partially explain why this is the case since many Latino parents were raised in families and cultures with limited or no communication about sex (Guilamo-Ramos et al., 2006; National Campaign to Prevent Teen and Unplanned Pregnancy, 2001).

Parental lack of knowledge about the technical aspects of sex is another barrier to sexual communication (Guilamo-Ramos et al., 2008). In studies with Latinos, many parents reported that they felt they did not have the skills or necessary knowledge to talk about sex with their children (Guilamo-Ramos et al., 2008; O'Sullivan et al., 2001). Parental expectations were found to be an additional barrier to communication among Latino parents, who either felt that talking about sex would encourage their child to become sexually active or that not talking about sex would help them avoid the consequences of being sexually active (Guilamo-Ramos et al., 2006, 2008; Vexler, 2007).

Parental Monitoring and Supervision

Parental monitoring and supervision are aspects of parental processes that have been shown to delay sexual initiation and reduce the risk of teen pregnancy and STDs (Cotton et al., 2004; Rai et al., 2003; Rodgers, 1999). Although there are several definitions of monitoring, Jaccard, Guilamo-Ramos, Bouris, and Dittus (2010) present a framework for effecting monitoring and supervision consisting of three core processes—parental behavioral expectations, parental behavioral monitoring, and parental behavioral inducement and enforcement. Among Latino adolescents, a number of studies have found that higher levels of parental monitoring were associated with higher rates of abstinence and delayed sexual onset (Velez-Pastrana et al., 2005) and lower levels of risky sexual behavior (Borawski, Levers-Landis, Lovegreen, & Trapl, 2003; Kerr, Beck, Shattuck, Kattar, & Uriburu, 2003). Parental monitoring has been shown to protect against teen pregnancy and STDs. However, the ways in which parents acquire knowledge about their teen is also important. Although parental monitoring might be protective, the restrictions often placed on girls in Latino families may result in secrecy about dating and tension between parents and adolescents (Raffaelli & Ontai, 2001).

Parent–Adolescent Relationship Quality and Satisfaction

The quality of the parent–adolescent relationship is an important factor that impacts the effectiveness of parental communication. Evidence suggests that parent–adolescent relationships based on mutual warmth, closeness, and trust are one of the strongest factors protecting youth from early sexual activity and pregnancy (Heinrich et al., 2006; Resnick et al., 1997). Among Latinos, adolescents who reported feeling close to their parents were found to be less likely to initiate sex at an early age (Miller et al., 1998a) and more likely to use contraception consistently and carefully (Velez-Pasterna et al., 2005). A number of studies have also noted high levels of warmth and connectedness between Latino parents and adolescents (Guilamo-Ramos, Dittus, et al., 2007), pointing to Latino cultural values of *familismo* (Sue & Sue, 2003; Cauce & Domenech-Rodriguez, 2002) and *simpatia*, which speaks to the value of keeping relationships between people in the family smooth and flowing (Triandis, Marin, Lisansky, & Betancourt, 1984). Important qualities that have been identified as characterizing a good parent–adolescent relationship include respect for one another, understanding each other's feelings, being able to trust each other, having concern for each other's well-being, and knowing each other (e.g., what each other is like, what each other wants, and what each other likes and dislikes) (Guilamo-Ramos & Bouris, 2008).

In summary, Latino parents play a critical role in supporting adolescents in efforts to prevent the consequences of unprotected intercourse, including sexually transmitted HIV infection. Although much more is known about the influence of parent–adolescent communication as a means for supporting adolescents, parental warmth and closeness, in addition to monitoring and supervision, are other important supportive factors. In this next section, we focus on intervention approaches with Latino adolescents and parents.

SEXUAL RISK REDUCTION INTERVENTIONS FOR LATINO ADOLESCENTS
Adolescent-Focused Interventions

Despite the high risk of unintended pregnancy and HIV/STDs among Latino adolescents, few controlled prevention intervention studies have been conducted with this population. Previous reviews of studies (Jemmott & Jemmott, 2000; Robin et al., 2004) included only one study with a significant proportion of Latino participants, and none had any documented scientific effect on behavioral or biological outcomes. In a search of the published literature, we identified only eight intervention studies from 1999 to 2010 with sexual behavior outcomes that had sizable proportions (25% or more of the sample) of Latino adolescents (Harper, Bangi, Sanchez, Doll, & Pedraza, 2009; Jemmott, Jemmott, Braverman, & Fong, 2005; Kennedy, Mizuno, Hoffman, Baume, & Strand, 2000; Kirby et al., 2004; Lesser, Koniak-Griffin, Huang, Takayanagi, & Cumberland, 2009; Mouttapa et al., 2010; Roye, Perlmutter, Silverman, & Krauss, 2007; Villarruel, Jemmott, & Jemmott, 2006). Five studies directly targeted Latinos (Harper et al., 2009; Lesser et al., 2009; Jemmott et al, 2005; Roye et al., 2007; Villarruel et al., 2006) and four studies implemented interventions that were tailored specifically for Latinos, albeit at varying degrees (see Table 15.1; Harper et al., 2009; Lesser et al., 2009; Roye et al., 2007; Villarruel et al., 2006). The results of these four studies in changing sexual risk behaviors, subsequently discussed, have been mixed.

Harper et al. (2009) implemented a nine-session intervention titled *SHERO* (a female-gendered version of the word *hero*), based on organizational development theory, with Mexican American female adolescents The program addressed cultural norms and gender role expectations specific to Mexican American female adolescents. Efforts, including the use of narrative ethnographic methods, were made to reveal cultural narratives that were either barriers or facilitators to safer sex behaviors. Over the course of a short 2-month follow-up period, participants reported using condoms more often than in the preceding 2 months and planned on using them more frequently in the coming 2 months.

Roye et al. (2007) conducted a theory-based randomized controlled trial of three brief single-session experimental conditions: (1) viewing a video developed for the study, (2) receiving counseling (a protocol adapted from Project Respect), and (3) viewing the video plus receiving counseling. There was also a "usual care" condition. Fifty-five percent of the study population was Latina and specific adaptations were made to nsure that these participants felt represented throughout the program, such as including a Latina actress in the video. At the 3-month follow-up, the women who saw the video and received counseling were significantly more likely to have used a condom at the last intercourse. Although the intervention effects were not sustained at the 12-month follow-up assessment, the findings support the implementation of brief interventions for positively changing condom-use behavior, particularly among Latinas.

Villarruel et al. (2006) conducted a randomized controlled trial testing the efficacy of ¡*Cuídate!* (Take care of yourself!)—a behavioral intervention for Latino adolescents—and found significant long-term (12 months) effects in decreasing sexual risk behavior (e.g., unprotected sexual intercourse, multiple partners) and increasing condom use. The *¡Cuídate!* curriculum, comprising six 60-minute modules, incorporated salient aspects of Latino culture and uses them to frame abstinence and condom use as culturally accepted and effective ways to prevent unwanted pregnancy and STDs, including HIV. For example, the Latino cultural value of *machismo* is often described as a man showing power through strength and control in decision making. Within the curriculum, *machismo* is reframed to emphasize protecting oneself and one's partner through safer sexual behaviors. Based on social cognitive theory and the theories of reasoned action and planned behavior, role play, videos, music, interactive games, and hands-on practice were used to build HIV knowledge, understand the vulnerability to HIV infection, identify attitudes and beliefs about HIV and safer sex, and increase self-efficacy and skills for correct condom use, negotiating abstinence, and negotiating safer sex practices. The *¡Cuídate!* curriculum has been identified by the Centers for Disease Control and Prevention (CDC) as meeting the HIV/AIDS Prevention Research Synthesis criteria for "best evidence" of intervention efficacy (Lyles et al., 2007) and is nationally disseminated through the Diffusion of Evidence Based Interventions (DEBI) Program.

Although most of the interventions were conducted in school or community settings, the study by Lesser et al. (2009) was conducted among specific high-risk Latino youth who are parents. In a culturally rooted randomized controlled trial targeting high-risk adolescent Latino parents, Lesser et al. (2009) found significant long-term (6 months) effects on reducing the proportion of unprotected sexual activity both among males and females in the study. The intervention group received the "Respecting and Protecting Our Relationship" program, a couple-focused 12-hour curriculum; the control group received a brief, 1.5-hour didactic HIV prevention education program. Intervention content included HIV awareness, understanding vulnerability to HIV infection, attitudes and beliefs, disease prevention, condom use skills, and sexual negotiation skills. Facilitation used culturally relevant methods, such as the use of an *espejo* (mirror) process of teaching, such as storytelling, reflection, and guidance. The study found moderating effects in terms of the role of male parental protectiveness (i.e., the father–child emotional attachment that positively influences parental behavior) in improving the effectiveness of the intervention for his female partner, suggesting the value of health promotion programs in building on the strengths of inherent protective tendencies in young couples to support protective health behaviors.

Family-Focused Interventions

Traditionally, one of the most pervasive values among Latinos is the importance of the family. Because the family is such a critical aspect in the lives of Latinos, there is a high reliance on the family for material and emotional support and help (Marin & Marin, 1991). The maximization of family factors that can be protective to reducing risky behaviors in adolescents is a priority within ecodevelopmental theory. Interventions focused on parents to build skills, improve self-efficacy, acquire information, and gain positive parenting practices provide the preparation needed for families to work effectively with adolescents in building healthy sexual behaviors and skills to prevent HIV/AIDS (O'Donnell et al., 2005; Pequegnant & Szapocznik, 2000).

Table 15.1 Interventions Targeting Latino Adolescents

Author, Year	Target Population	Ethnicity	Intervention Name	Type of Setting
Harper et al., 2009	Female adolescents U.S. Midwestern City Mean age: 15.2	100% Mexican American	SHERO	CBO
Lesser et al., 2009	Young parents Los Angeles, CA Mean age (F): 18 Mean age (M): 20	100% Latino Subgroups not mentioned	*Respeto/ Proteger*	CBOs, clinics
Roye et al., 2007	Young women New York City, NY Mean age: 18	45% Latino 55% African American	None	Unknown
Villarruel et al., 2006	Adolescents Philadelphia, PA Mean age: 14.9	81% self-identifying Latinos 85.4% Puerto Rican	¡Cuídate!	After-school

Delivery Method	Session Number	Total Time (hours)	Cultural Values/ Cultural Relevance	Results
Cofacilitator: young females Group Discussion	9	18	Addressed cultural norms and gender role expectations Narrative ethnographic methods used to reveal cultural narratives Discussed cultural-specific pressures to HIV risk behavior	Increase in condom use Decrease in vaginal sex
Facilitator: Espejo (mirror) technique	6	12	Use of an *espejo* (mirror) process of teaching (e.g., storytelling, reflection, guidance) Specifically designed activities integrated traditional or cultural teachings to address relational norms	Reduced proportion of unprotected sex among males and females High male parental protectiveness further decreased unprotected female sex.
Counseling and/or video	1–2	40 min	Video included a Latina actor	Increase Condom use
Facilitator Group discussions	6	8	Familialism and gender-role expectations	Increase in consistent condom use Decrease in sexual intercourse, multiple partners, and days of unprotected intercourse

Parent and family-based sexual risk reduction interventions can be viable alternatives to individual-based interventions (Hutchinson et al., 2003; Miller et al., 1998b). Informative and supportive interventions with both Latino and non-Latino parents have also been shown to help them overcome apprehension and fears of embarrassment when discussing sensitive topics relating to sex by increasing their knowledge, comfort, and discussion frequency of such topics with their children (Baptiste et al., 2006; O'Donnell et al., 2005).

Parent-based interventions can also be used to support and enhance interventions targeting adolescents. Fewer studies have evaluated the impact of these interventions on adolescent sexual behavior. Among those that do, the results have tended to be contradictory (Campero, Walker, Atienzo, & Gutierrez, 2011). Nonetheless, some recent parent-based interventions have shown positive behavioral effects including delaying sexual initiation (Forehand et al., 2007), increasing condom use, and reducing the rate of sexual activity (Dilorio et al., 2006).

The unique dynamics within Latino families suggests that support for the implementation of parent–adolescent interventions is particularly needed. Despite the promise of parent-based approaches aimed at reducing adolescent sexual risk behaviors, there has been less of a focus on how Latino families can help shape the health outcomes and behaviors of Latino adolescents. In an extensive search of the electronic literature published from 1995 through 2010, relatively few interventions targeting Latino parents were identified that included sizable proportions (25% or more) of Latino parents and adolescents (Guilamo-Ramos et al., 2011; Kirby et al., 2004; O'Donnell et al., 2005; O'Donnell, Myint-U, Duran, & Stueve, 2010; Pantin et al., 2009; Prado, Pantin, et al., 2007; Villarruel, Loveland-Cherry, & Ronis, 2010) (Table 15.2).

The study by Kirby et al. (2004) included parents as part of a larger school-based intervention. Newsletters were sent to parents three times a year, and students were encouraged to discuss the newsletters with their parents. Although Latino students in this multilevel intervention were more likely to delay sexual debut and increase condom and contraceptive use, the effects of the parent component on communication and adolescent sexual risk behavior were not reported.

Six of the studies specifically targeted Latino parents as the primary recipients of the intervention (O'Donnell et al., 2005, 2010; Pantin et al., 2009; Prado et al., 2007, Villarruel et al., 2010, Guilamo-Ramos et al., 2011) and four of the studies (Pantin et al., 2007, 2009; Villarruel et al., 2010; Guilamo-Ramos et al., 2011) included Spanish-speaking Latinos in their samples. The study conducted by Pantin et al. (2009) examined the effects of *Familias Unidas*, an intervention consisting of nine 2-hour parent group sessions in which parents were taught the skills and knowledge to effectively raise adolescents in the United States, as well as 10 1-hour facilitator-supervised family visits. Although the intervention had no effect on engagement in sexual activity in the past 90 days, adolescents whose parents were randomly assigned to the *Familias Unidas* intervention were significantly more likely to have used a condom in the past 90 days from the 6-month to 30-month postbaseline assessment when compared with those in the control condition.

Similarly, Prado et al. (2007) conducted a randomized controlled trial testing the efficacy of a parent-centered, ecodevelopmentally based combination of two interventions, *Familias Unidas* and *Parent-Preadolescent Training for HIV Prevention* (PATH). *Familias Unidas* is a Hispanic-specific family-based substance use and sexual risk reduction intervention. Although *PATH* was originally designed for a multicultural sample, it was adapted specifically for use with Hispanics (e.g., including an introduction video using a *telenovela* or Spanish language TV soap opera format.). Adolescents in the experimental group were more likely to use a condom at last intercourse and were significantly less likely to report having contracted sexually transmitted diseases than adolescents in either control condition. Furthermore, the experimental group had higher reports of positive parenting and parent–adolescent communication compared to the control condition. Although condition differences in condom use were not sustained at 3 month follow-up, the intervention does provide support for interventions that target not only adolescents and specific health behaviors, but the entire family and family functioning, especially among Latinos.

The study reported by O'Donnell et al. (2005) tested a parent intervention with Latinos and African Americans based in social development theory, diffusion of innovation theory, and the theory of planned behavior. Three audio CDs were developed for this study that contained information and scenarios about parent–adolescent communication skills. For example, the CDs provided models of how a parent can effectively initiate a conversation about sexual health with their child. The CDs focused on the stories of three families, one black, one Hispanic, and one Caribbean, and demonstrated how discussions progress as children grow older. The CDs were mailed to participants' homes at 10-week intervals. Parents in the intervention group reported an increase in general parent–adolescent communication, increased perceptions of family support, and engagement in fewer lifetime risky behaviors, including having a boyfriend/girlfriend, kissing, hand-holding, and kissing and hugging for a long time. However, sexual intercourse was not reported. This parent intervention provided support for the efficacy of a low-intensity program for both parents and adolescents.

O'Donnell et al. (2010) implemented a similar intervention entitled *Especially for Daughters*, a gender-specific parent–adolescent intervention consisting of audio CDs and grounded in the theory of planned behavior, behavioral learning theory, diffusion of innovation theory, and social development model. At the 3-month follow-up, girls in the intervention reported fewer sexual risks and less alcohol consumption. Parents in the intervention reported greater self-efficacy to address alcohol and sex and more communication on these topics with their daughters.

Villarruel et al. (2010) examined the efficacy of a computer-based intervention, *Cuidalos* (Take care of them), designed to increase parent–adolescent communication among Latinos. The intervention was a modification of an effective small group intervention tested among Mexican parents (Villarruel, Cherry, Cabriales, Ronis, & Zhou, 2008) to a computer-based format. In this randomized controlled trial, parents assigned to receive the two-session, 60-minute intervention reported greater general communication and greater sexual communication at the 3-month follow-up than did parents assigned to the wait-list control condition. Adolescents whose parents received the intervention reported higher sexual communication and greater comfort with communication than did adolescents whose parents were in the wait-list control condition. There were no short-term effects of this intervention on adolescent sexual risk behavior.

In a study of a parent-based intervention, *Families Talking Together,* aimed at delaying sexual intercourse among Latino and African American middle school-aged inner city youth, Guilamo-Ramos et al. (2011) delivered a 30-minute clinic-based intervention focused on effective communication and parenting strategies for reducing adolescent sexual risk behavior that included two follow-up booster calls over the ensuing 5 months. Relative to the control group, statistically significant reduced rates of transitioning to sexual activity and frequency of sexual intercourse

Table 15.2 Interventions Targeting Latino Parents

Author, Year	Target Population	Ethnicity	Intervention Name	Type of Setting
Kirby et al., 2004	20 Schools (9th grade students, including teachers and parents)	28.4% Hispanic 19.6% black 30.2% white 13.5% Asian	*Safer Choices*	High School
O'Donnell et al., 2005	Parents of fifth and sixth graders and their children	Youth: 63.7% black 28.7% Hispanic 7.6% other Parents: 63.8% black 27.7% Hispanic 8.5% other	Saving Sex for Later	Parent's home
O'Donnell et al., 2010	Young adolescent girls and their parents	Youth : 34.3% Latina Parents: 29.1% Latino	*Especially for Daughters*	Parent's home

Delivery Method	Session Number	Total Time (hours)	Cultural Values/ Relevance	Results
Trained teacher (also School Health Promotion Council, student peer resource team, parent newsletters, school-community linkages)	20 (10 in 9th grade, 10 in 10th grade)	Not specified	N/A	Significantly delayed initiation of sex among Hispanics Reduced frequency of sex without a condom Reduced number of sexual partners in last 3 months with whom a condom was not used Increased condom use during last sex among those who had sex in last 3 months Increased contraceptive use among those who had sex in the last 3 months
Audio CDs	3 CDs	Length of audio CDs not specified	A Hispanic family was included as one of three families in the short stories	Increase in general parent-adolescent communication Increased perceptions of family support Engagement in fewer risky behaviors (e.g., having boyfriend/girlfriend, kissed, held hands)
Audio CDs	4 Audio CDs	Length of audio CDs not specified	A Hispanic family was included as one of four families in the role-model stories	Adolescents reported fewer sexual risks and less drinking Parents reported greater self-efficacy to address alcohol and sex and more communication

(*Continued*)

Table 15.2 (Continued)

Author, Year	Target Population	Ethnicity	Intervention Name	Type of Setting
Pantin et al., 2009	Hispanic adolescents and their primary caregivers	56.1% born Hispanic Americans Immigrants: 26.9% Hondurans 20.4% Cuban 16.1% Nicaraguan	Familias Unidas	Not specified
Prado et al., 2007	Hispanic 8th graders and their primary caregivers	40.0% born Hispanic Americans Immigrants: 9.0% Hondurans 40.0% Cuban 25.0% Nicaraguan 22.0% other	Familias Unidas + PATH	Not specified
Villarruel et al., 2010	Latino parents and adolescents	100% Latino 83% of Mexican origin	Cuidalos (Take care of them)	Community agency
Guilamo-Ramos et al., 2011	Mother–adolescent dyads in New York City Adolescents aged 11–14	84.5% Latino 15.5% African American	Families Talking Together	Pediatric clinic

Delivery Method	Session Number	Total Time (hours)	Cultural Values/ Relevance	Results
Hispanic facilitators with at least 5 years of clinical experience working with low-income Hispanic families	9 group sessions 10 family visits	18 hours (group sessions) 10 hours (family visits)	Hispanic-specific cultural issues were integrated into all aspects of the intervention	More likely to have used a condom in the past 90 days from six months to 30 months post-baseline
Hispanic facilitators with at least 5 years of clinical experience working with low-income Hispanic families	15 group sessions 8 family visits 2 parent–adolescent circles	49 hours	Specifically adapted for Hispanics Use of *telenova* in introductory video	More likely to use a condom at last intercourse Less likely to have contracted STDs
Computer-based parent–adolescent "homework" activities	2	60 min	Mnemonics based on the Spanish words *¡Cuídate!* and "DIRAS"	Parents reported greater general communication at 3 month follow-up and greater sexual communication at 3 month follow-up Adolescents reported higher sexual communication and greater comfort with communication
Meeting with social worker Written communication aids Parent–adolescent "homework" activities	1	30 min		Reduced rates of transitioning to sexual activity and frequency of sexual intercourse

were observed. Specifically, they found that sexual activity increased from 6% to 22% for adolescents in the "standard of care" control condition, whereas it remaining at 6% among adolescents in the intervention condition at the 9-month follow-up.

Some elements are common among many of the more successful interventions involving Latino adolescents. These include longer and multifaceted interventions, those that target specific behavior (e.g., condom use), and those that accommodate participant-specific characteristics (e.g., culture, gender, and status as a couple). These findings are consistent with previous studies (Robin et al., 2004; Mullen, Ramirez, Strouse, Hedges, & Sogolow, 2002; Peterson & DiClemente, 2000).

INTERVENTION GAPS AND RECOMMENDATIONS FOR FUTURE RESEARCH

Despite the limited research with Latino adolescents and parents, the body of existing work has significantly contributed to the evidence base of how to work effectively with this group. First, several interventions, both individual and parent-based approaches, have been developed that have demonstrated efficacy in reducing sexual risk behaviors and/or factors that influence those behaviors. Many of these interventions incorporated salient Latino cultural values, including discussion of gender roles (e.g., *machismo/marianismo*) and the importance of family (e.g., *familismo*) in framing sexual decision-making. Second, several interventions have been tested with Spanish-dominant Latino adolescents and parents, a group that has limited access to culturally and linguistic tailored resources. Third, interventions have been conducted in diverse settings including schools, community-based settings, and primary care settings, and these have also represented a diversity of Latino ethnicities. The use of behavioral theories in interventions that have demonstrated efficacy adds to the body of work conducted with other adolescents and efforts to reduce sexual risk behavior.

Despite these important contributions, there are significant gaps in research with Latino adolescent and parents. There have been some studies conducted with high-risk Latino youth, but most have been conducted in school and community settings. Furthermore, the majority of studies have been conducted in a small group format. Interventions need to be developed that incorporate individual approaches and make use of technology, such as smart phone applications, texting, and social media applications, to broaden their reach and appeal for youth. Studies should also be conducted with Latino adolescents who are not in school or who are in the juvenile justice system, because they may be harder to reach through traditional community programs. In addition, despite the rising incidence of HIV among young Latino MSM, there are no interventions that have been developed or tested with this group. Descriptive studies that examine how ecodevelopmental processes and cultural values may be integrated into an MSM-friendly HIV intervention for Latino youth are warranted.

Strategies also need to be tested with Latino youth, including programs aimed at school completion and those that incorporate positive youth development. In addition, there have been a number of interventions developed for white and African American youth that may be applicable to Latino adolescents. There are also a number of strategies available to guide adaptations of efficacious interventions for other populations. These approaches need to be tested to determine if they could be acceptable and could work with Latinos. In addition, there are a number of "home grown" programs developed at the community level that should also be reviewed and strengthened by what we know works in order to promote the use of successful local approaches.

In relation to intervention studies with parents and adolescents, more studies and approaches are needed to find ways to incorporate this important resource for Latino youth. Interventions and programs should be designed and tested with both mothers and fathers, and should focus on developing skills other than solely communication. Importantly, interventions need to be developed in multiple contexts and in ways that increase access to information and programs without increasing burdens of cost and time.

Recommendations for Structural Interventions

Structural interventions are notably absent as an approach to reduce sexual risk behavior among Latino adolescents together. There are several approaches, however, that should be considered. On a more proximal level, comprehensive sex education for adolescents should be available in both school and community settings. Only recently has federal funding been made available for this approach. Past funding policies have supported abstinence-only education, despite the lack of evidence demonstrating the effectiveness of this approach in reducing sexual risk behaviors. In addition to education, access to health care, including reproductive services, should be made available to adolescents. New opt-out testing policies for HIV can be useful in reducing stigma, but providers and policy makers need to be aware of potential barriers, such as requiring parental notification, that may counteract the potential protective effects of early detection. A policy that would facilitate access to education, testing, and health services is to designate youth as a priority and at-risk population for HIV infection. Such a designation by the CDC would facilitate the targeting of prevention interventions.

Another important structural intervention that could be useful in reducing sexual risk behavior would be strategies aimed at keeping adolescents in school, supporting academic achievement and progression, facilitating connections to schools and communities, and providing opportunities for economic gain. These more distal approaches are aimed at providing a context that can support youth with positive expectations regarding the future and the skills needed to succeed (Rotheram-Borus, 2000).

In conclusion, Latino youth are an important resource for society. Their development is an important investment for our nation's future. Despite the many obstacles confronted by Latino youth and their families, there are strengths within the family unit that can be used effectively to protect youth from HIV infection. Resources in the environment can be mobilized to secure this important investment in our future.

REFERENCES

Albert, B., Brown, S., & Flanigan, C. (Eds.) (2003). *14 and younger: The sexual behavior of young adolescents*. Washington, DC: National Campaign to Prevent Teen and Unplanned Pregnancy.

Ancheta, R., Hynes, C., & Shrier, L. A. (2005). Reproductive health education and sexual risk taking among high-risk female adolescents and young adults. *Journal of Pediatric and Adolescent Gynecology, 18*(2), 105–111.

Baptiste, D. R., Bhana, A., Peterson, I., McKay, M., Voisin, D., Bell, C., & Martinez, D. D. (2006). Community collaborative youth-focused HIV/AIDS prevention in South Africa and Trinidad: Preliminary findings. *Journal of Pediatric Psychology, 31*(9), 905–916.

Borawski, E. A., Levers-Landis, C. E., Lovegreen, L. D., & Trapl, E. S. (2003). Parental monitoring, negotiated unsupervised time, and parental trust: The role of perceived parenting practices in adolescent health risk behaviors. *Journal of Adolescent Health, 33*(2), 60–70.

Brener, N., Lowry, R., Kann, L., Kolbe, L., Jansen, R., & Jaffe, H. (2002). Trends in sexual risk behaviors among high school students: United States, 1991–2001. *Morbidity and Mortality Weekly Report, 51*(38), 856–859.

Brooks, R. A., Lee, S., Stover, G. N., & Barkley, T. W. (2009). Sexual risk behaviors of young Latino male urban street gang members: Implications for HIV prevention. *AIDS Education Prevention, 21*(5), 80.

Browning, C. R., Burrington, L. A., Leventhal, T., & Brooks-Gunn, J. (2008). Neighborhood structural inequality, collective efficacy, and sexual risk behavior among urban youth. *Journal of Health and Social Behavior, 49*(3), 269–285.

Buchanan, R. L., & Smokowski, P. R. (2009). Acculturation stress. *Substance Use & Misuse, 44,* 740–762.

Campero, L., Walker, D., Atienzo, E. E., & Gutierrez, J. P. (2011). A quasi-experimental evaluation of parents as sexual health educators resulting in delayed sexual initiation and increased access to condoms. *Journal of Adolescence, 34*(2), 215–223.

Cauce, A. M., & Domenech-Rodriguez, M. (2002). Latino families: Myths and realities. In J. M. Contreras, K.A. Kerns, & A. M. Neal- Barnett (Eds.), *Latino children and families in the United States* (pp. 5–25). Westport, CT: Praeger Press.

Cavanagh, S. E. (2004). The sexual debut of girls in early adolescence: The intersection of race, pubertal timing, and friendship group characteristics. *Journal of Research on Adolescence, 14*(3), 285–312.

Centers for Disease Control and Prevention (CDC). (2001). HIV incidence among young men who have sex with men—seven US cities, 1994–2000. *Morbidity and Mortality Weekly Report (MMWR), 50,* 440–444.

Centers for Disease Control and Prevention (CDC). (2005). *HIV/AIDS Surveillance Report, 2004.* Atlanta: U.S. Department of Health and Human Services, *16,* 1–46.

Centers for Disease Control and Prevention (CDC). (2006). Youth risk behavior surveillance—United States, 2005. Surveillance Summaries, June 9. *Morbidity and Mortality Weekly Report (MMWR) 55* (No. SS–5).

Centers for Disease Control and Prevention (CDC). (2007). Highlights in minority health & health disparities. Retrieved from http://www.cdc.gov/omhd/highlights/2007/HSept07.htm.

Centers for Disease Control and Prevention (CDC). (2008a). HIV/AIDS among youth. Retrieved from http://www.cdc.gov/hiv/resources/factsheets/youth.htm.

Centers for Disease Control and Prevention (CDC). (2008b). *Sexually transmitted disease surveillance, 2007.* Atlanta, GA: U.S. Department of Health and Human Services; December 2008. Retrieved from http://www.cdc.gov/std/stats07/Surv2007FINAL.pdf.

Centers for Disease Control and Prevention (CDC). (2008c). Youth risk behavior surveillance—United States, 2007. Surveillance Summaries, June 6. *Morbidity and Mortality Weekly Repor (MMWR), 57* (No. SS-4).

Centers for Disease Control and Prevention (CDC). (2009a). HIV testing among adolescents. http://www.cdc.gov/healthyyouth/sexualbehaviors/pdf/hivtesting_adolescents.pdf.

Centers for Disease Control and Prevention (CDC). (2009b). *Sexually Transmitted Disease Surveillance, 2008.* Atlanta, GA: U.S. Department of Health and Human Services;

December 2008. Retrieved from http://www.cdc.gov/std/stats08/surv2008-Complete. pdf.

Child Trends Databank. (2005). Dropout rates. Retrieved from http://www.childtrendsdatabank.org/pdf/1_PDF.pdf.

Cotton, S., Mills, L., Succop, P., Biro, F., & Rosenthal, S. (2004). Adolescent girls' perceptions of the timing of their sexual initiation: "Too young" or "just right"? *Journal of Adolescent Health, 34,* 453–458.

De La Rosa, M., Rugh, D., & Rice, C. (2006). An analysis of risk domains associated with drug transitions of active Latino gang members. *Journal of Addictive Diseases, 25*(4), 81–90.

DiClemente, R. J., Salazar, L. F. & Crosby, R. A. (2007). A review of STD/HIV preventive interventions for adolescents: Sustaining effects using an ecological approach. *Journal of Pediatric Psychology, 32*(8), 888–906.

Dilorio, C., Resnicow, K., McCarty, F., De, A. K., Dudley, W. N., Wang, D. T., & Densmore, P. (2006). Keepin' it R.E.A.L.! Results of a mother–adolescent HIV prevention program. *Nursing Research, 55*(1), 43–51.

Dutra, R., Miller, K. S., & Forehand, R. (1999). The process and content of sexual communication with adolescents in two-parent families: Associations with sexual risk-taking behavior. *AIDS and Behavior, 3*(1), 59–66.

Eaton, D. K., Kann, L., Kinchen, S., Ross, J., Hawkins, J., Harris, W. A., Wechsler, H., et al. (2006). Youth risk behavior surveillance—United States, 2005. *Journal of School Health, 76*(7), 353–372.

Esbensen, F. (2000). Preventing adolescent gang involvement. U.S. Department of Justice, Office of Juvenile Justice and Delinquency Prevention. *Juvenile Justice Bulletin.* Retrieved from http://www.ncjrs.gov/pdffiles1/ojjdp/182210.pdf.

Federal Interagency Forum on Child and Family Statistics. (2007). *America's children: Key national indicators of well-being.* Federal Interagency Forum on Child and Family Statistics. Washington, DC: U.S. Government Printing Office.

Forehand, R., Armistead, L., Long, N., Wyckoff, S. C., Kotchick, B. A., Whitaker, D., Miller, K. S., et al. (2007). Efficacy of a parent-based sexual-risk prevention program for African American preadolescents: A randomized controlled trial. *Archives of Pediatric and Adolescent Medicine, 161*(12), 1123–1129.

Gatti, U., Tremblay, R. E., Vitaro, F., & McDuff, P. (2005). Youth gangs, delinquency and drug use: A test of the selection, facilitation, and enhancement hypotheses. *Journal of Child Psychology and Psychiatry, 46*(11), 1178–1190.

Gil, A. G., Wagner, E. F., & Vega, W. A. (2000). Acculturation, familism, and alcohol use among Latino adolescent males: Longitudinal relations. *Journal of Community Psychology, 28,* 443–458.

Gonzalez, J. S., Hendricksen, E. S., Collins, E. M., Durán, R. E., & Safren, S. A. (2009). Latinos and HIV/AIDS: Examining factors related to disparity and identifying opportunities for psychosocial intervention research. *AIDS Behavior, 13*(3), 582–602.

Gordon, R. A., Lahey, B. B., Kawai, E., Loeber, R., Stouthamer-Loeber, M., & Farrington, D. P. (2004). Antisocial behavior and youth gang membership: Selection and socialization. *Criminology, 42*(1), 55–88.

Grunbaum, J., Kann, L., Kinchen, S., Williams, B., Ross, J., Lowry, R., & Kolbe, L. (2002). Youth risk behavior surveillance—United States, 2001. *Morbidity and Mortality Weekly Report (MMWR), 51*(SS-4), 1–68.

Guilamo-Ramos, V. (2010). Dominican and Puerto Rican mother-adolescent communication: Maternal self-disclosure and youth risk intentions. *Hispanic Journal of Behavioral Science, 32*(2), 197–215.

Guilamo-Ramos, V., & Bouris, A. (2008). *Parent-adolescent communication about sex in Latino families: A guide for practitioners.* Washington, DC: The National Campaign to Prevent Teen and Unplanned Pregnancy.

Guilamo-Ramos, V., Bouris, A., Jaccard, J., Gonzalez, B., McCoy, W., & Aranda, D. (2011). A parent-based intervention to reduce sexual risk behavior in early adolescence: Building alliances between physicians, social workers, and parents. *Journal of Adolescent Health, 48*(2), 159–163.

Guilamo-Ramos, V., Dittus, P., Jaccard, J., Goldberg, V., Casillas, E., & Bouris, A. (2006). The content and process of mother-adolescent communication about sex in Latino families. *Social Work Research, 30*(3), 169–181.

Guilamo-Ramos, V., Dittus, P., Jaccard, J., Johansson, M., Bouris, A., & Acosta, N. (2007). Parenting practices among Dominican and Puerto Rican mothers. *Social Work, 52*(1), 17–30.

Guilamo-Ramos, V., Jaccard, J., Dittus, P., Bouris, A., & Holloway, I. (2007). Adolescent expectancies, parent–adolescent communication, and intentions to have sexual intercourse among inner city middle school youth. *Annals of Behavioral Medicine, 34*(1), 56–66.

Guilamo-Ramos, V., Jaccard, J., Dittus, P., & Collins, S. (2008). Parent-adolescent communication about sexual intercourse: An analysis of maternal reluctance to communicate. *Health Psychology, 27*(6), 760–769.

Guzman, B. L., Schlehofer-Sutton, M. M., Villanueva, C. M., Stritto, M. E. D., Casad B. J., & Feria A. (2003). Let's talk about sex: How comfortable discussions about sex impact teen sexual behavior. *Journal of Health Communication, 8*, 583–598.

Halpern-Felsher, B. L., Kropp, R. Y., Boyer, C. B., Tschann, J. M., & Ellen, J. M. (2004). Adolescents' self-efficacy to communicate about sex: Its role in condom attitudes, commitment, and use. *Adolescence, 39*(155), 443–456.

Hamilton, B. E., Martin, J. A., & Ventura, S. J. (2009). Births: Preliminary data for 2007. *National Vital Statistics Reports, 57*(12).

Harper, G. W., Bangi, A. K., Sanchez, B., Doll, M., & Pedraza, A. (2009). A quasi-experimental evaluation of a community-based HIV prevention intervention for Mexican American female adolescents: The Shero's program. *AIDS Education and Prevention, 21*(B), 109–123.

Harper, G. W., & Robinson, W. L. (1999). Pathways to risk among inner-city African American adolescent females: The influence of gang membership. *American Journal of Community Psychology, 27*(3), 383–404.

Henrich, C. C., Brookmeyer, K. A., & Shrier, L. A. (2006). Supportive relationships and sexual risk behavior in adolescence: An ecological transactional approach. *Journal of Pediatric Psychology, 31*(3), 286–296.

Hirsch, J. S., Muñoz-Laboy, M., Nyhus, C. M., Yount, K. M., & Bauermeister, J. A. (2009). They "miss more than anything their normal life back home": Masculinity and extramarital sex among Mexican migrants in Atlanta. *Perspectives in Sexual and Reproductive Health, 41*(1), 23–32.

Hutchinson, M. K. (2002). The influence of sexual risk communication between parents and daughters on sexual risk behaviors. *Family Relations, 51*(3), 238–248.

Hutchinson, M. K., & Cooney, T. M. (1998). Patterns of parent-teen sexual risk communication: Implications for intervention. *Family Relations, 47*(2), 185–194.

Hutchinson, M. K., Jemmott, J. B., III, Jemmott, L. S., Braverman, P., & Fong, G. T. (2003). The role of mother–daughter sexual risk communication in reducing sexual risk behaviors among urban adolescent females: A prospective study. *Journal of Adolescent Health, 33*, 98–107.

Jaccard, J., Dittus, P. J., & Gordon, V.V. (1998). Parent-adolescent congruency in reports of adolescent sexual behavior and in communications about sexual behavior. *Child Development, 69*, 247–261.

Jaccard, J., Guilamo-Ramos, V., Bouris, A., & Dittus, P. (2010). A three-process system of parental monitoring and supervision. In V. Guilamo-Ramos, J. Jaccard, & P. Dittus (Eds.), *Parental monitoring of adolescents: Current perspectives for researchers and practitioners* (pp. 177–203). New York: Columbia University Press.

Jemmott, J. B., III, & Jemmott, L. S. (2000). HIV behavioral interventions for adolescents in community settings. In J. Peterson & R. DiClemente (Eds.), *Handbook of HIV prevention* (pp. 103–127). New York: Kluwer Academic/Plenum Publishers.

Jemmott, J. B., III, Jemmott, L. S., Braverman, P. K., & Fong, G. T. (2005). HIV/STD risk reduction interventions for African American and Latino adolescent girls at an adolescent medicine clinic. *Archives of Pediatrics and Adolescent Medicine, 159*, 440–449.

Kaiser Family Foundation (KFF). (2006). *Sexual health statistics for teenagers and young adults in the United States.* Menlo Park, CA: The Henry J. Kaiser Family Foundation. Retrieved November 21, 2006 from http://www.kff.org/womenshealth/upload/3040-03.pdf.

Kann, L., Kinchen, S. A., Williams, B. I., Ross, J. G., Lowry, R., Grunbaum, J. A., Kolbe, L. J., & State and Local YRBSS coordinators. Youth Risk Behavior Surveillance System. (2000). Youth risk behavior surveillance—United States, 1999. *Morbidity and Mortality Weekly Record, 47*(SS-3), 1–89.

Kennedy, M. G., Mizuno, Y., Hoffman, R., Baume C., & Strand, J. (2000). The effect of tailoring a model HIV prevention program for local adolescent target audiences. *AIDS Education and Prevention, 12*(3), 225–238.

Kerr, M. H., Beck, K., Shattuck, T. D., Kattar, C., & Uriburu, D. (2003). Family involvement, problem and prosocial behavior outcomes of Latino youth. *American Journal of Health Behavior, 27*(Sl1), 55–65.

Kirby, D. B., Baumler, E., Coyle, K., Basen-Engquist K., Parcel G. S., Harrist R., & Banspach, S. W. (2004). The "safer choices" intervention: It's impact on the sexual behaviors of different subgroups of high school students. *Journal of Adolescent Health, 35*, 442–452.

Lammers, C., Ireland, M., Resnick, M., & Blum, R. (2000). Influences on adolescents' decisions to postpone onset of sexual intercourse: A survival analysis of virginity among youths aged 13 to 18 years. *Journal of Adolescent Health, 26*, 42–48

Lesser, J., Koniak-Griffin, D., Huang, R., Sumiko, T., & Comberland, W. G. (2009). Parental protectiveness and unprotected sexual activity among Latino adolescent mothers and fathers. *AIDS Education and Prevention, 21*(B), 88–102.

Lyles, C. M., Kay, L. S., Crepaz, N., Herbst, J. H., Passin, W. F., Kim, A. S., Mullins, M. M., et al. (2007). Best-evidence interventions: Findings from a systematic review of HIV behavioral interventions for US populations at risk, 2000–2004. *American Journal of Public Health, 97*(1), 133–143.

Marín, B. V., Coyle, K. K., Gómez, C. A., Carvajal, S. C., & Kirby, D. B. (2000). Older boyfriends and girlfriends increase risk of sexual initiation in young adolescents. *Journal of Adolescent Health, 27*(6), 409–418.

Marin, G., & Marin, B. V. (1991). *Research with Hispanic populations.* Newbury Park, CA: Sage.

Meneses, L. M., Orrell-Valente, J. K., Guendelman, S. R., Oman, D., & Irwin, C. E. (2006). Racial/ethnic differences in mother-daughter communication about sex. *Journal of Adolescent Health, 39*(1), 128–131.

Miller, B. C. (2002). Family influences on adolescent sexual and contraceptive behavior. *The Journal of Sex Research, 39*(1), 22–26.

Miller K. S., Kotchick, B. A., Dorsey, S., Forehand, R., & Ham, A. Y. (1998a). Family communication about sex: What are parents saying and are their adolescents listening? *Family Planning Perspectives, 30*(5), 218–235.

Miller, K. S., Levin, M. L., Whitaker, D. J., & Xu, X. (1998b). Patterns of condom use among adolescents: The impact of mother–adolescent communication. *American Journal of Public Health, 88*(10), 1542–1544.

Mouttapa, M., Watson, D. W., McCuller, W. J., Reiber, C., Tsai, W., & Plug, M. (2010). HIV prevention among incarcerated male adolescents in an alternative school setting. *Journal of Correctional Health Care, 17,* 27–38.

Mullen, P. D., Ramirez, G., Strouse, D., Hedges, L. V., & Sogolow, E. (2002). Meta-analysis of the effects of behavioral HIV prevention interventions on the sexual risk behavior of sexually experienced adolescents in controlled studies in the United States. *Journal of Acquired Immune Deficiency Syndromes (JAIDS), 30,* s94–s105.

National Campaign to Prevent Teen and Unplanned Pregnancy. (2001). It all starts at home: Hispanic parents speak out on preventing teen pregnancy. A focus group report. Washington, DC: Author.

National Campaign to Prevent Teen and Unplanned Pregnancy. (2006). New survey highlights disconnect between Latino parents and teens in talking about sex. Retrieved from http://www.teenpregnancy.org/press/pdf/Latina_Release_04_06.pdf.

National Campaign to Prevent Teen and Unplanned Pregnancy. (2010). Briefly. . .a national campaign analysis of the 2008 birth rate. Retrieved from http://www.thenationalcampaign.org/resources/pdf/Briefly_2008TBRIncrease.pdf.

O'Donnell, L., Myint, U. A., Duran, R., & Stueve, A. (2010). Especially for daughters: Parent education to address alcohol and sex-related risk taking among urban adolescent girls. *Health Promotion and Practice, 11,* 70S–78S.

O'Donnell, L., Stueve, A., Agronick, G., Wilson-Simmons, R., Duran, R., & Jeanbaptiste, V. (2005). Saving sex for later: An evaluation of a parent education intervention. *Perspectives on Sexual and Reproductive Health, 37*(4), 166–173.

O'Donnell, L., Stueve, A., Wilson-Simmons, R., Dash, K., Agronick, G., & Jean Baptiste, V. (2006). Heterosexual risk behaviors among urban young adolescents. *The Journal of Early Adolescence, 26,* 87–109.

O'Sullivan, L. F., Meyer-Bahlburg, H. F. L., & Watkins, B. X. (2001). Mother-daughter communication about sex among urban African American and Latino families. *Journal of Adolescent Research, 16*(3), 269–292.

Pantin, H., Prado, G., Lopez, B., Huang, S., Tapia, M. I., Schwartz, S. J., Branchini, J., et al. (2009). A randomized controlled trial of Familias Unidas for Hispanic adolescents with behavior problems. *Psychosomatic Medicine, 71*(9), 987–995.

Pequegnant, W., & Szapocznik, J. (2000). The role of families in preventing and adapting to HIV/AIDS: issues and answers. In W. Pequegnat & J. Szapocznik (Eds.), *Working with families in the era of HIV/AIDS* (pp. 3–26), Thousand Oaks, CA: Sage Publications.

Peralta, L., Deeds, B. G., Hipszer, S., & Ghalib, K. (2007). Barriers and facilitators to adolescent HIV testing. *AIDS Patient Care and STDs, 21*(6), 400–410.

Perrino, T., Gonzalez-Soldevilla, A., Pantin, H., & Szapocznik, J. (2000). The role of families in adolescent HIV prevention: A review. *Clinical Child and Family Psychology Review, 3*(2), 81–96.

Peterson, J. L., & DiClemente, R. J. (Eds.) (2000). *Handbook of HIV prevention.* New York: Kluwer Academic/Plenum Publishers.

Prado, G., Pantin, H., Briones, E., Schwartz, S. J., Feaster, D., Huang, S., Szapocznik, J., et al. (2007). A randomized controlled trial of a parent-centered intervention in preventing substance use and HIV risk behaviors in Hispanic adolescents. *Journal of Consulting and Clinical Psychology, 75*(6), 914–926.

Prado, G., Schwartz, S. J., Pattatucci-Aragón, A., Clatts, M., Pantin, H., Fernández, M. I., Szapocznik, J., et al. (2006). The prevention of HIV transmission in Hispanic adolescents. *Drug and Alcohol Dependence, 84*(1), S43–S53.

Raffaelli, M., & Green, S. (2003). Parent-adolescent communication about sex: Retrospective reports by Latino college students. *Journal of Marriage and Family, 65*, 474–481.

Raffaelli, M., & Ontai, L. L. (2001). "She's 16 years old and there's boys calling over to the house": An exploratory study of sexual socialization in Latino families. *Culture, Health, and Sexuality, 3*, 295–310.

Rai, A. A., Stanton, B., Wu, Y., Li, X., Galbraith, J., Cottrell, L., Burns, J., et al. (2003). Relative influences of perceived parental monitoring and perceived peer involvement on adolescent risk behaviors: An analysis of six cross-sectional data sets. *Journal of Adolescent Health, 33*, 108–118.

Ramirez-Valles, J., Zimmerman, M. A., & Newcomb, M. D. (1998). Sexual risk behavior among youth: Modeling the influence of prosocial activities and socioeconomic factors. *Journal of Health and Social Behavior, 39*, 237–253.

Resnick, M. D., Bearman, P. S., Blum, R. W., Bauman, K. E., Harris, K. M., Jones, J., Udry, J. R., et al. (1997). Protecting adolescents from harm: Findings from the national longitudinal study on adolescent health. *Journal of the American Medical Association, 278*(10), 823–832.

Rios-Ellis, B. (2010). Increasing HIV-related knowledge, communication, and testing intentions among Latinos: Protege tu familia: hazte la prueba. *Journal of Health Care for the Poor and Underserved, 21*(3), 148–168.

Robin, L., Dittus, P., Whitaker, D., Crosby, R., Ethier, K., Mezoff, J., Ches, P. H., Miller, K., & Pappas-Deluca, K. (2004). Behavioral interventions to reduce incidence of HIV, STD, and pregnancy among adolescents: A decade in review. *Journal of Adolescent Health, 34*, 3–26.

Rodgers, K. B. (1999). Parenting processes related to sexual risk-taking behaviors of adolescent males and females. *Journal of Marriage and the Family, 61*, 99–109.

Romo, L. F., Lefkowitz, E. S., Sigman, M., & Au, T. K. (2002). A longitudinal study of maternal messages about dating and sexuality and their influence on Latino adolescents. *Journal of Adolescent Health, 31*(1), 59–69.

Rotheram-Borus, M. J. (2000). Expanding the range of interventions to reduce HIV among adolescents. *AIDS, 14*(1), S33–S40.

Roye, C., Perlmutter Silverman, P., & Krauss, B. (2007). A brief, low-cost, theory-based intervention to promote dual method use by black and Latina female adolescents: A randomized controlled trial. *Health Education and Behavior, 34*(4), 608–621.

Sabatiuk, L., & Flores, R. (2009). Toward a common future. Latino teens and adults speak out about teen pregnancy. Washington, DC; National Campaign to Prevent Teen and Unplanned Pregnancy.

Sanders, B., Schneiderman, J. U., Loken, A., Lankenau, S. E., & Bloom, J. J. (2009). Gang youth as a vulnerable population for nursing intervention. *Public Health Nursing, 26*(4), 346–352.

Santelli J. S., Lowry, R., Brener N. D., & Robin L. (2000). Adolescent sexual behavior: Estimates and trends from four nationally representative surveys. *Family Planning Perspectives, 32*, 156–165.

Shih, R. A., Miles, J. N., Tucker, J. S., Zhou, A. J., & D'Amico, E. J. (2010). Racial/ethnic differences in adolescent substance use: Mediation by individual, family, and school factors. *Journal of Studies on Alcohol and Drugs, 71*(5), 640–651.

Shlay J. C., McClung, M. W., Patnaik, J. L., & Douglas, J. M., Jr. (2004). Comparison of sexually transmitted disease prevalence by reported level of condom use among patients attending an urban sexually transmitted disease clinic. *Sexually Transmitted Diseases, 31*(3), 160.

Sue, D. W., & Sue, D. (2003). *Counseling the culturally diverse: Theory and practice* (4th ed.). Hoboken, NJ: John Wiley.

Szapocznik, J., & Coatsworth, J. D. (1999). An ecodevelopmental framework for organizing the influences on drug abuse: An ecodevelopmental model for risk and prevention. In M. Glantz & C.R. Hertel (Eds.), *Drug abuse: Origins and interventions* (pp. 331–366), Washington, DC: American Psychological Association.

Triandis, H. C., Marin, G., Lisansky, J., & Betancourt, H. (1984). Simpatía as a cultural script of Hispanics. *Journal of Personality and Social Psychology, 47*(6), 1363–1375.

Unger, J. B., Ritt-Olson, A., Soto, D. W., & Baezconde-Garbanati, L. (2009). Parent-child acculturation discrepancies as a risk factor for substance use among Hispanic adolescents in Southern California. *Journal of Immigrant Minority Health, 11,* 149–157.

Upchurch, D. M., Aneshensel, C. S., Sucoff, C. A., & Levy-Storms, L. (1999). Neighborhood and family contexts of adolescent sexual activity. *Journal of Marriage and the Family, 61,* 920–933.

U. S. Census Bureau. (2002). US Hispanic population: 2002. Retrieved from http://www.census.gov/population/www/socdemo/hispanic/ho02.html.

U.S. Census Bureau. (2003). Health insurance coverage in the United States: 2002. Retrieved from http://www.census.gov/prod/2003pubs/p60-223.pdf.

U.S. Census Bureau. (2005). School enrollment—social and economic characteristics of students: October 2005. Retrieved from http://www.census.gov/population/www/socdemo/school/cps2005.html.

U.S. Census Bureau. (2010). Race and Hispanic origin of the foreign-born population in the United States: 2007. Retrieved from http://www.census.gov/prod/2010pubs/acs-11.pdf.

Valleroy, L. A., MacKellar, D. A., Karon, J. M., Rosen, D. H., McFarland, W., Shehan, D. A., Janssen, R. S., et al. (2000). HIV prevalence and associated risks in young men who have sex with men. *Journal of the American Medical Association, 284*(2), 198–204.

Van Oss Marín, B., Coyle, K. K., Gómez, C. A., Carvajal, S. C., & Kirby, D. B. (2000). Older boyfriends and girlfriends increase risk of sexual initiation in young adolescents. *Journal of Adolescent Health, 27*(6), 409–418.

Vélez-Pastrana, M. C., González-Rodríguez, R. A., & Borges-Hernández, A. (2005). Family functioning and early onset of sexual intercourse in Latino adolescents. *Adolescence, 40*(160), 777–791.

Vexler, E. J. (2007). *Voices heard: Latino adults and teens speak up about teen pregnancy.* Washington, DC: The National Campaign to Prevent Teen Pregnancy.

Villarruel, A. M., Cherry, C. L., Cabriales, E. G., Ronis, D. L., & Zhou, Y. (2008). A parent-adolescent intervention to increase sexual risk communication: Results of a randomized controlled trial. *AIDS Education and Prevention, 20*(5), 371–383.

Villarruel, A. M., Jemmott, J. B., III, & Jemmott, L. S. (2006). A randomized controlled trial testing an HIV prevention intervention for Latino youth. *Archives of Pediatrics & Adolescent Medicine, 160*(8), 772–777.

Villarruel, A. M., Loveland-Cherry, C. J., & Ronis, D. L. (2010). Testing the efficacy of a computer-based parent–adolescent sexual communication intervention for Latino parents. *Family Relations, 59*(5), 533–543.

Wahl, A. M., & Eitle, T. M. (2010). Gender, acculturation and alcohol use among Latina/o adolescents: A multi-ethnic comparison. *Journal of Immigrant and Minority Health, 12*(2), 153–165.

Zambrana, R. E., Cornelius, L. J., Boykin, S. S., & Lopez, D. S. (2004). Latinas and HIV/AIDS risk factors: Implications for harm reduction strategies. *Research and Practice, 94*(7), 1152–1158.

Zimmer-Gembeck, M. J., Seibenbruner, J., & Collins, W. A. (2004). A prospective study of intraindividual and peer influences on adolescents' heterosexual romantic and sexual behavior. *Archives of Sexual Behavior, 33*(4), 381–394.

16 Improving Latina Intergenerational Family-Based Communication to Decrease HIV and Other Sexual Risks

Britt Rios-Ellis

Madre es el nombre de Dios que vive en los labios y el corazón de todos los niños.
Mother is synonymous with the word "God," which lives on the lips and in the hearts of all children.

INTRODUCTION

Although Latino cultural characteristics have been recognized as key to the health and welfare of diverse Hispanic communities, few HIV/AIDS interventions integrate positive cultural attributes so as to work from a foundation of assets versus deficits. The *Rompe el Silencio* [Break the Silence] intervention was informed by findings from eight focus groups with Latina mothers and female adolescents combined with important Latino cultural concepts such as *familismo* (familism, the importance of family and family unity) and *respeto* (respect for elder family members and persons of authority) to develop an HIV prevention pilot intervention seeking to improve both sexual risk knowledge and communication within the family as well as with sex partners.

Furthermore, the potential role of the mother within the Latino family to educate and foster an environment wherein culturally congruent open communication regarding sexual risk can take place within the home has not been sufficiently explored. Little has happened within the past 15 to 20 years to address the capacity of mothers and women to serve as change agents not only to mitigate the risky sexual realities of their children and alter the immediate structures of family environment and the cultural structures that confine communication norms, but also to address the risk that frequently occurs within their own often monogamous, long-term heterosexual relationships. As we begin to enter the fourth decade of the HIV/AIDS pandemic, it is crucial that HIV/AIDS prevention efforts are grounded in a framework that addresses the multiple contexts of risk women experience beyond their stereotypic roles as "mothers" or "whores" (Caravano, 1991; Amaro,

1995), while simultaneously acknowledging and maximizing the potential that cultural expectations of motherhood can provide to both underserved women and their families.

Rompe El Silencio [Breaking the Silence] corresponds to the structural-environmental model proposed by Organista and colleagues in Chapter 1 in several ways primarily because it addresses the risk experienced by Latinas not within an individual behavioral intervention paradigm but rather through a lens that acknowledges that risk experiences occur through diverse and dynamic contexts and within the immediate environment of family. For much too long government-sponsored interventions have focused on behavior change as if risk behaviors occurred under highly controlled conditions and that the dynamic contexts wherein risk takes place can be altered by the individual. Although we all know that behavior is much more complex, few interventions address the complexities of familism and its collectivist nature. The lack of available resources is particularly limited for immigrant populations, due to both the xenophobic attitudes that lead to public policy and the lack of culturally and linguistically congruent health care professionals. Therefore, within the structured environment of the family, given the immediate lack of resources, the cultural asset of *familismo* can be honed to incorporate culturally sanctioned communication patterns and practices that reinforce sexual risk-reduction communication and respond to HIV risk.

When addressing immigrant Latina risk in particular, and among families wherein children raised in the United States hold values closer to mainstream U.S. adolescent culture while their parents maintain those of their countries of origin, the dynamic interplay of culture and language is tenuous at best. As both generations of Latinas respond to the corresponding cultured communication structures that define their respective environments, the home and the family represent the one common environment wherein the adaptation of communication patterns that address sexual risk can be nurtured. Latino immigrant populations resiliently manage a myriad of stressful *environmental factors* that include documentation status (often mixed in families with some members being "legal" and others deprived of basic human protection and rights); separation from the tightly knit nexus of social support so often found in communities of origin versus American individualistic values and behaviors; economic difficulties (which often contribute to adolescents having to leave school to contribute to the family's well-being); female economic, social, and transportation dependency; lack of education and health care access; and workforce inequity, to name a few. *Individual factors* include psychological distress related to differing expectations in childrearing and lack of education and skills needed to address their adolescent's risk here in the United States; gender-based expectations that differ from those held in by mainstream U.S. culture; psychological stress related to domestic violence; experience of gender-based and class-based discrimination; and depression and lack of sexual negotiation skills and authority to mandate safer sex expectations once the knowledge deficit is filled.

In response to these risks adult Latinas often learn that sex is an obligation or duty owed to their male partners and that their closeness to their partners is paramount to their successful adaptation to the United States given all the other problems they must confront. They learn that to discuss or initiate condom use would be to imply a crucial lack of *confianza* [trust] and cast doubt on the sanctity of their relationship and their own chastity and fidelity. Due to their dependence on men for economic survival, and often transportation and language translation, women learn to *aguantar* [endure, put up with] and lower their expectations of male behavior, often leading to different expectations placed on their male and female children, thus exacerbating the risk for the younger generation. Adolescent Latinas engage in sexual risk with few outlets for information because mere inquiry might be deemed a sign of sexual activity that could bring shame or *vergüenza* to their families. The expectations they face are quite different from those experienced by their parents and the disconnect between generations does not facilitate the potential use of cultural factors such as *familismo* and *respeto*. To optimize the use of *familismo*, *respeto*, and *confianza*, *Rompe El Silencio* builds on communication strategies such as role play and condom negotiation while integrating cultural structures and values into the intervention. This provides the adult and adolescent female dyad with culturally and linguistically sanctioned opportunities to discuss and negotiate sexual risk within the contexts of their lives and expectations as Latinas living in the United States while creating the intergeneration support mechanisms with the potential to sustain HIV/AIDS knowledge, interest, and dialogue not only among women, but among all family members within the individual's immediate environment being the family. By utilizing Latino assets as opposed to the deficit or "pobrecito" [poor thing] model, we can optimize the recognition of the importance of Latinos cultural values within the family in addressing the immediate environment and heightening recognition of cultural strengths within the xenophobic and discriminatory environment currently experienced by many Latinos in the United States.

The current surveillance practice of including "heterosexual" cases into overall HIV and AIDS numbers reinforces the aforementioned viewpoint to a certain extent. If a woman tests positive for HIV she is not included as a "heterosexual" case until the status of her partner can be verified. Although understanding the behaviors of men who have sex with men and women (MSMW) is crucial to better targeting HIV prevention efforts, a woman deserves to have her case count from her individual risk factor. Until her partners' case can be confirmed, her case will continue to be listed as "risk unreported/unknown." Furthermore, heterosexual risk is often referred to as "high-risk heterosexual contact," and may not accurately describe the risk for many HIV-positive Latinas who were in monogamous relationships and had sexual histories with only one partner. These surveillance practices underplay women's risk, particularly minority immigrant women who may be somewhat linguistically isolated, uninsured or underinsured, and dependent on their male partners for economic survival, transportation, and negotiation and maneuvering within larger society (see Chapter 4 for a full discussion of gendered HIV risk for Latinas).

Rompe el Silencio (hereafter RES), funded by the USDHHS Office on Women's Health, was designed to incorporate an intergenerational approach to: increase HIV/AIDS female-driven family-based communication among Latina adult and adolescent dyads, address gender-specific control of the particular contexts of HIV risk that Latinas face, and reinforce cultural protective factors and communication strategies. To culturally sanction dialogue regarding sexual risk, RES included joint group discussions and cultural- and gender-congruent activities to facilitate interfamilial sexual health-related communication, and to promote support and understanding of the importance of risk-reduction efforts. Fifty Latina female family dyads from Los Angeles County participated in the pilot intervention.

BACKGROUND

Latinos continue to represent a growing proportion of those diagnosed with AIDS increasing from 15% in 1985 to 21% in 2008 (Kaiser Family Foundation, 2010).

In 2004, the Kaiser Family Foundation reported that at least half of all new HIV infections were estimated to occur among those under the age of 25, with Latina/o adolescents at especially high risk (Rios, 2005). According to the CDC (2008), 70% of Latinos report having had sex and compared to their non-Latino white counterparts, Latino adolescents in grades 9 to 12 reported a higher prevalence of sexual intercourse (52% vs. 43.7%), respectively, and greater likelihood of having four or more partners by the 12th grade. A recent study of HIV risk among African American, Hispanic, and white adolescents found that Latino adolescents were at greater risk for sex without a condom (Bartlett, Buck, & Shattell, 2008). Moreover, in a recent comparative study of HIV-positive and HIV-negative Latinas in Los Angeles, the HIV risk behavior profile was found to be very similar, with HIV-positive Latinas less likely to report recent unprotected sex compared to their HIV-negative counterparts (Rice, Green, Santos, Lester, & Rotheram-Borus, 2010). These findings suggest that prevention efforts targeting Latinas need to amplify their focus by moving beyond the traditional targeting of those who have engaged only in "high-risk heterosexual sex" because many Latinas may not know the sexual histories of their partners and may not have the HIV prevention education or cultural or gender power base necessary to enforce protected sex within their relationships.

Latinos bear a disproportionately high burden of HIV/AIDS and their risk results from a myriad of complex and dynamic institutional, socioeconomic, and cultural factors (Rios-Ellis, 2006), some of which include acculturation, traditional family dynamics, patterns of parent–adolescent communication, and gender roles. To effectively address HIV/AIDS risk among Latino adolescents, an intergenerational approach that facilitates family support for healthy sexual development is essential. The need for effective HIV/AIDS interventions is underscored by the fact that by 2025, 25% of all U.S. adolescents will be Latino (The National Campaign to Prevent Teen and Unplanned Pregnancy, 2008).

Acculturation

Acculturation is a broadly defined term used to explain the processes immigrants may undergo when adopting cultural values and norms of a new country, and is often measured with instruments detailing contextual use of language, immigrant status, amount of time lived in the United States, social norms and social support, values, and generational evolutions. Studies examining the role of acculturation on sexual risk taking and HIV infection among Latinos have yielded mixed results. Although some have found acculturation to be strongly associated with healthier behaviors (van Servellen, Chang, & Lombardi, 2002), others have reported disparate results (Adam, McGuire, Walsh, Basta, & LeCroy, 2005; Kaplan, Erickson, & Juarez-Reyes, 2002; Ebin et al., 2001). Despite indications in the literature that acculturation may increase sexual risk among Latinos, there are also aspects of traditional Latino culture such as gender role expectations that have the potential to increase risk, particularly among newer female immigrants.

Gender Roles

Research has demonstrated that the strongly defined gender roles supported by traditional Latino culture can lead to expectations for appropriate male and female sexual behavior and thus are important in understanding Latino sexual risk behavior (Logan, Cole, & Leukefeld, 2002). Studies have also documented that manifestations of traditional gender roles such as *machismo* (negative male characteristics that can include violence, overbearing control, and sexual aggression) and *marianismo* (female characteristics such as being sexually chaste, passive, and not discussing sexual topics) may contribute to HIV risk, and have been linked to unprotected sexual behavior and multiple sexual partners (Villarruel, Jemmott, Jemmott, & Ronis, 2004; Flores-Ortiz, 2004).

Culture, religion, and gender often interact in ways that limit clear communication and result in the dichotomization of sexually chaste women as "good" and sexually active women as "bad" or promiscuous (Mark & Miller, 1986). Within the context of Latina risk, careful evaluation of perceived or actual inability to communicate effectively about sex and sexual risk, combined with culturally and gender-sanctioned sexual pressure from male partners, may add to the risk of girls experiencing unwanted sexual encounters or unprotected sex (Blythe, Fortenberry, M'Hamed, Tu, & Orr, 2006). Studies of older inner-city Latinos have shown that women were less likely to have had sex with a condom and to report *machismo* and lack of perceived HIV risk as prospective barriers to condom use (Hillman, 2008). It should be noted that although *machismo* is often perceived as a negative and oppressive male trait wielded against women, the potential for a positive *machismo*-oriented framework wherein expectations of males to use condoms and remain faithful so as to protect their partners and families should not go without mention.

Traditional Family Dynamics

As in many cultures, a great deal of information regarding health and behavior is learned within the family and *familismo*, a cultural value emphasizing the strength of family unity and an individual's sense of family attachment, is a significant tenet across Latino subpopulations (Jacobs, 2008). *Familismo* is more pronounced within Latino cultures, where individualism is less valued, and family unity is often perceived as critical to successful adaptation and advancement in the United States. *Respeto* or respect for one's elder relatives and persons of authority is also highly valued within traditional Latino families. Due to the importance and relevance of *familismo* and *respeto* within Latino families and communities, parents who are able to effectively educate and communicate with their children regarding sexual risk have the potential to positively impact the sexual health behaviors of their offspring.

A pilot study implemented in Chicago, Illinois, similar to the current study, incorporated 34 intergenerational pairs to assess parent communication about sex and its effects on sexual risk taking, demonstrated findings parallel to those in the literature reviewed above. Results revealed that African American and Latino parents engaged in fewer conversations about sex with their teens than did white parents. Pilot findings illuminate the importance of family-based interventions to improve parent–adolescent communication about sex and risky sexual behavior (Wilson & Donnenberg, 2004).

Studies have shown that Latino parents play a major role in forming both adolescent sexual attitudes and contraceptive behaviors (East, 1998; Prado et al., 2007; Bourdeau, Thomas, & Long, 2008; Burgess, Dziegielewski, & Green, 2005), and that these types of intergenerational interventions are crucial in influencing communication between dyads. Wilson and Donnenberg (2004) found that the quality, as opposed to frequency, of mother–daughter interactions was protective against sexual risk among white, African American, and Hispanic adolescent females.

Romo, Lefkowitz, Sigman, and Au (2002) found this to be particularly true among Hispanic adolescent females. Furthermore, parent–child communication, specifically that between mothers and daughters, has proven to reduce sexual risk behaviors among adolescent girls (Teitelman, Ratcliffe, & Cederbaum, 2008). Additionally, there is some evidence to indicate that less frequent sexual risk communication between adolescent females and their parents translates into fewer discussions with partners about STIs, HIV/AIDS, and condom use, and contributes to lower self-efficacy in sexual risk negotiation and the ability to refuse an unsafe sexual encounter (DiClemente et al., 2001).

Studies have also shown that Latino parents experience difficulty discussing sexuality and contraception with their children (Sangi-Haghpeykar, Horth, & Poindexter, 2001), or view sexual health as a topic that should not be discussed due to cultural traditions and beliefs. Shame or *vergüenza* (embarrassment) can be a major barrier among Latinas to open communication about sex with family members and sex partners (Bourdeau et al., 2008).

Research has also demonstrated generational similarities and differences among Mexican women regarding their perspectives of male–female relationships and marriage. Whereas older women valued *respeto* and obligation within their marriages, younger Latinas tended to prefer companionate marriage and valued *confianza* (trust) within theirs (Hirsch, Higgins, Bentley, & Nathanson, 2002). Although women of different generations viewed their relationships and expectations of such quite distinctly, both generations were found to be reluctant to acknowledge infidelity of, or to suggest the use of condoms to, their male partners. Despite the traditional conservatism of many Latino families, *familismo* remains a largely untapped and unmeasured resource for HIV/AIDS prevention targeting Latino youth and families.

The purpose of this community-based participatory research study was to reduce HIV infection among U.S.-based Latina intergenerational dyads of female family members by developing and testing a culturally based intervention to assist Latinas in decreasing barriers to HIV/AIDS communication within the family and across generations. Exploratory research questions included the following: Can an intervention be created to increase HIV knowledge, the number of conversations about sexual risk among mother–daughter dyads, as well as comfort with such conversations among Latina intergenerational family dyads with diverse cultural expectations, histories, and experiences? Also, can *familismo* and other cultural values be successfully integrated into HIV education and prevention for female family dyads to increase sexual risk-related dialogue and prevention?

METHODS
Research Design

Mixed research methods were used beginning with formative focus groups of Latinas of diverse age groups and language abilities and preferences (Spanish and English) to inform the development, implementation, and evaluation of a cross-generational intervention. The pilot intervention was tested using pretest, posttest, and 1-month follow-up intervals in a noncontrol convenience sample design. Due to the limited funding time span, the follow-up was limited to 30 days. The project was conducted in three stages: formative focus groups, development of the intervention, and pilot implementation and evaluation.

All project materials, instrumentation, and educational curriculum were first developed in Spanish and reviewed by a Pan-Latino, bilingual/bicultural project group to ensure the universality of the Spanish as well as ease of participant comprehension. The materials were then translated to English and any discrepancies vetted until universal agreement was reached by the project team. Project materials and procedures received approval from the California State University Long Beach Institutional Review Board.

QUALITATIVE METHODS
Focus Group Participants

Formative focus group participants ranged in age from 12 to 91. The majority was born in Mexico (53%, $n = 35$), followed by El Salvador, Guatemala, Puerto Rico, or the Dominican Republic (10.5%, $n = 7$), while the remainder were born in the United States (36.5%, $n = 24$), with approximately half of them (18%, $n = 12$) reporting that one or both their parents were born in Mexico. English was the preferred language of communication among the adolescent participants, whereas the older participants were more often Spanish monolingual or had a strong preference for Spanish.

Focus Group Procedures

In an effort to understand different perceptions, attitudes, and behaviors and how they are influenced by Latino cultural practices and values, and affected by socioeconomic status, immigration experiences, and gender inequities, focus groups with diverse age groups of Latinas were held. Eight 2-hour age-specific focus groups were held with 66 Latina women and adolescents. These groups provided the project team with the opportunity to explore and garner information regarding the nexus of knowledge, behaviors, and cultural values, as well as valuable information regarding a culturally relevant intervention design (Barker & Rich, 1992; Rios-Ellis et al., 2008).

Discussion points included HIV risk within the Latino community, differences in gender roles and their effects on HIV/AIDS risk, knowledge regarding risk, family-based sexual risk communication, and challenges to dialogue. More specifically, among other questions participants were asked the following: "What are the differences between Latino male and female roles and how do these affect HIV/AIDS risk?," "What were the messages you received about sexuality from your family?," and "What are the difficulties or barriers that parents have when they want to talk with their children about sex?" Participants were also asked to recommend methods for effective HIV prevention targeting Latinas of different ages and strategies for increasing sexual health communication across generations within the Latino family.

Project staff worked in collaboration with *promotoras de salud* [peer health educators] to recruit participants by posting flyers in the East Los Angeles Women's Center and AltaMed (two collaborating community-based organizations that provide health services to Latino families), and through word of mouth. To facilitate conversation and increase our understanding of the age, gender, and culturally related dynamics of sexual risk communication between the intergenerational female dyads, three focus groups were held with adolescent groups, ages 12 to 15, and 16 to 19, and four focus groups with women 20 to 35, 35 to 50, and 51 and older. To gain and integrate additional insight specific to HIV risk context, an additional focus group was held with HIV-positive Latinas ages 40 to 65 ($N = 7$). The adult groups were invariably held in Spanish, whereas the focus groups with youth were held predominantly in English.

Although the focus group recruiting materials specified that the discussions were to be held in Spanish or English and participants were recruited using language-based criteria, several participants interchanged languages, which often resulted in a bilingual dialogue. The same bilingual/bicultural moderator presided over all group meetings and was assisted by two bilingual/bicultural research assistants. Transcripts were developed by a bilingual court-reporting service and checked for accuracy by project staff.

Analysis of Qualitative Data

Using a Grounded Theory approach (Strauss & Corbin, 1988), transcripts were then substantively coded for prominent themes and concepts to guide the development of a thematic categorical matrix by two bilingual project staff. Maintaining an emic approach, subsequent thematic categories were allowed to emerge during deliberations of the focus group findings and matrix development among project staff present throughout the focus groups and the two staff involved in transcript analyses. Discrepancies in coding were flagged and deliberated until the coders reached agreement. In addition, as substantive coding led to the emergence of themes and concepts, memoing was also conducted within the matrix structure to further define ideas and potential relationships and conceptualizations regarding themes and concepts and their potential for integration into the intervention (Glaser, 1998). The intervention developed was informed by the following key concepts garnered from the adolescent and adult focus groups as described below.

FOCUS GROUP RESULTS
Adolescents

Focus group adolescents perceived themselves and their communities at very low risk for HIV infection, but did report a lack of information regarding Latinos who do not fall into, or perceive themselves as part of, the high-risk groups of men who have sex with men (MSM) and injection drug users (IDUs). Although participants perceived themselves at fairly low risk, they acknowledged unequal gender role expectations in their relationships such as low expectations of male fidelity. Adolescent participants said that their parents use mixed messages by promoting negative perceptions about sexuality and double standards that support traditional gender norms. They reported receiving vague and general warnings such as "be careful," "don't get pregnant," or "don't do 'it'," but not specific information that they could use to avoid sex or pregnancy.

When they say "Don't do IT!" what they keep telling us is really not to get pregnant or have sex but they don't tell us how not to get pregnant. We have to learn from our friends because I can't even think of asking my dad and if I ask my mom she will think that I am already having sex.

As illustrated, participants reported fear of suspicion as being a significant barrier to communicating with their parents about sex because their mothers would then believe that their daughters were sexually active. Furthermore, adolescent participants stated that they probably would not trust the information they received from their parents because the adolescents did not believe that their parents were credible sources of needed information. In addition, talking with one's parents about sex would cause embarrassment for both the parent and the adolescent. Less than one-third (7 out of 23) of adolescent focus group participants had discussed sex with their parents. Adolescents reported that their parents felt that sex education was handled in the school setting and should be limited to the biological explanations related to pregnancy and childbearing. They reported "Wishing that their parents would understand that they didn't receive all of the information they needed from school." The adolescents talked about the need to be trusted, supported, and understood by their parents, and wished parents would be more open-minded. Participants stated that they wished that their parents would make the first move in communication and that they really hoped that the intervention would give their parents confidence to "make the first move." Participants nodded emphatically when one exclaimed, "Tell them to come to us. We shouldn't have to go to them."

Female participants of all ages emphatically agreed that the culturally held images of women dramatically increased HIV and STI risk. In general, adolescent Latinas saw themselves portrayed in the media as poor, hard working, and struggling. They reported that the virgin–whore dichotomy portrayed two very limiting manifestations of Latinas and that neither applied to their contextual realities. Participants stated that they were expected to be either "caliente" or hot and sexy or calm and submissive, and that these roles left the male partner in firm control and able to do "whatever they want." "I don't want to be seen as invisible but at the same time I don't want people to think I am a whore." Another stated, "Either Latinas are hot and erotic and portrayed as loose and ready for sex or we are passive and have no say about anything that happens sexually. There is no in-between for us and most of us want to be somewhere in the middle." Participants acknowledged that many Latinas perceived their partners as faithful even when faced with the contrary, and also acknowledged the benefits of having a boyfriend both in terms of increasing popularity and self-esteem.

Focus group adolescent participants suggested that we initiate HIV prevention education in middle school "before it is too late" through the use of small gender-specific classes so as to encourage dialogue. Although adolescent participants did recommend same-gender, family-based classes to challenge cultural taboos regarding females and sexual risk-related knowledge and communication, they also counseled us to separate mothers and daughters for particular intervention elements in order to avoid potential judgments and/or reactions that could inhibit comfort levels. That is, after each generation had the opportunity to voice its opinions and experiences with their peers, both generations could then be brought into a common space to share each groups' viewpoints. Adolescents reported wanting to learn about condoms and STIs, as well as activities to illustrate how to increase their self-esteem and confidence levels. Interestingly, the adolescent participants requested similar activities for their adult counterparts so that their mothers and aunts could increase their self-confidence and initiate sexual health-related dialogue within the home and family setting.

Adults

Focus group dialogue from Latina adults reflected a deep sense of worry about adolescent sexuality and the difficulties they experienced discussing sexual issues with both their partners and children. They also spoke of the need to target younger aged adolescent "before it is too late." The Latina adults discussed cultural expectations related to having to *aguantar* or "put up with" the Latino male's infidelity, machismo, and reluctance to use condoms. Some adults reported using fear-based tactics when discussing sex with their children to make up for their lack of knowledge and better sexual communication skills. These tactics were exemplified by one participant telling her son, "If you have sex with too many women your penis will fall off" to prevent him from being promiscuous. Overall, the adults felt more comfortable engaging in dialogue with smaller children due to the ability to avoid sexually explicit conversations. Adult participants emphatically and repeatedly reported not having the communication skills or knowledge necessary to prepare their adolescent girls for sexual risk-taking.

When discussing their personal sexual risk several adult participants described sex as a *deber* (duty) as opposed to a *placer* (pleasure). They talked about fulfilling their male partner's expectations and not having much of an opinion regarding whether they wanted sex on any given occasion. The older participants in long-term relationships were more apt to perceive dialogue about both sexual risk and sexual pleasure with their partners as a daunting task. For some women, engaging in sexual risk dialogue with their children was often perceived as easier to do than with their partners because patterns of communication have been formed over long periods of time. Furthermore, the power of *familismo* to incite communication needed to protect their children is a strong motivator among the adult participants regardless of their comfort levels.

Latina adults also spoke of the restrictions religious expectations placed on them in terms of both fertility and condom use. The youth and adult Latinas recommended a small-group educational session format that incorporated multiple generations of family members. Furthermore, both generations recommended that the environment be open, safe, and free of both cultural and religious expectations so as to increase their ability to engage in sexually related dialogue free from embarrassment. In terms of intervention materials and exercises, both age groups wanted to learn more about condoms and to receive more Spanish language materials. When asked what each generation asked of the other regarding communication, the adults asked for their children's respect and patience, and the youth asked that their parents listen, understand, and trust them.

QUANTITATIVE METHODS
Intervention Participants

Intervention participants were recruited by three distinct Latino family-focused community-based organizations located in the Los Angeles County area. Recruitment methods included outreach within each organization's community programs, the distribution of flyers and presentations at community events (i.e., health fairs), and word of mouth. Those interested in participating were screened using the following eligibility criteria: females of Latino/Hispanic origin aged 12 and older, family dyads consisting of more than one generation, and residents of Los Angeles County. Informed consent was collected for all participants aged 18 years or older and parental consent and assent were collected for adolescents under the age of 18.

Four groups of family dyads participated in the pilot intervention for a total of 50 family dyads consisting of 50 adult participants and 56 adolescent participants.

The dyads were comprised of a mother with one or more daughter(s). A small number ($n = 3$) also included a niece. Participants were predominantly of Mexican origin ($n = 105$, 99%). All U.S.-born adolescent participants ($N = 50$) reported that one or both parents were born in Mexico with the exception of one participant with mixed Latino heritage.

Intervention Procedures

The development of the *Rompe el Silencio* was based heavily on participant recommendations from the focus group sessions, and on a combination of elements derived from many of the important social cognitive theories currently in use in HIV prevention (Fishbein et al., 2001), including social cognitive theory (Bandura, 1986), the theory of planned behavior (Ajzen, 1991), and the information-motivation-behavioral skills model (Fisher & Fisher, 1996). The theoretical perspective used (Rhodes & Malotte, 1996) recognizes that risk behavior is influenced at multiple levels and is significantly influenced by (1) behavioral beliefs, (2) normative beliefs, (3) social support structures, and (4) personal/environmental barriers and facilitators (including information, risk perception, and skills). These four elements are mediated by the action of cultural influences, such as appropriate gender roles and the importance of family, and personal history factors. Thus, factors such as "familismo," "confianza," and "respeto," described in the Latino Health Communications Model (Karliner, Edmonds Crewe, Pacheco, & Cruz-Gonzalez, 1998; Rios-Ellis, 2010), were used throughout the intervention through communication and interactive exercises designed to support the positive cultural characteristics that influence resiliency among Latinos. An emphasis was placed on creating a culturally and linguistically relevant milieu wherein sexual communication was sanctioned and Latina mother/daughter and aunt/niece dyads would feel comfortable dialoguing more openly and frequently about sexual health. Based on focus group findings, the intervention content was designed to increase (1) knowledge of sexual risk, (2) recognition of cultural factors that impact risk, (3) parent–adolescent communication about sex, and (4) skills and self-efficacy in risk reduction.

The *Rompe el Silencio* intervention was conducted by bilingual, bicultural facilitators in Spanish and English and each participant received a $20 gift card for their participation. The intervention is conducted in two sessions totaling 8 hours, including an introduction and two educational modules per session. See Table 16.1 for a content description of each module and see Table 16.2 for demographic characteristics of the participants.

Session 1, which deals with understanding communication and the history of sexual dialogue and education within the two generations that have often spent their formative years in very different environments, provides an opportunity for adults and youth to understand and communicate each others' formative contexts. Session 1 is designed to facilitate and sanction sexual risk-related dialogue within the female family dyads. Although many differences exist between the generations, the activities and discussion topics were designed to encourage communication, to facilitate dialogue regarding sexual health between the family dyads and intergenerational groups, and to promote mutual support for risk-reduction efforts. Session 2 activities are designed to facilitate discussion of HIV and general sexual health-related topics, beginning with less sensitive topics and later discussing those of a more sensitive nature.

Table 16.1 *Rompe el Silencio*: Break the Silence Intervention Content

---

Session 1

Module 1—Welcome and Discussion of Sexual Values

Agenda/Lecture Content	Activity
Introduction to Project	*Individual introductions*
	Review session objectives and guidelines for working together
Development of Sexual Values	*Full Group Discussion to Introduce Topic of Sexuality*
	Questions for the Group: *Where do our values about sexuality come from? What messages do you receive about sex from others?*
Definition of Sex and Sexuality	Lecture—Objective: increase participants' understanding of sexuality beyond sex
	Activity—Separate Adult and Adolescent Groups
	Objective: understand each group's experience and concerns regarding communication about sexuality in the family
	Questions for Adults: *What could your parents have done differently to help you understand sexuality? How do you think your children would answer this question?*
	Questions for Adolescents: *What would you like your parents to do to help you understand sexuality? What would you like to learn about?*

Module 2—Communication in the Family

Agenda/Lecture Content	Activity
Importance of Communication about Sex in the Family	*Full Group Discussion*
	Objective: to increase participants' understanding of the impact of communication about sexuality in the family
	Question: *Why talk about sexuality?*
Perceptions in Latino Culture about Sex	Lecture—Qualitative data used to address the impact of perceptions in Latino culture on sexuality and communication about sex
Communication Barriers in the Family	*Full Group Discussion*
	Question: *How can we open communication about sexuality in the family?*
Communication Styles	Lecture on ineffective communication and strategies to improve communication
	Role Plays—Individual Volunteer Activity
	Mother–Daughter scenarios
	Activity—Separate Adult and Adolescent Groups
	"Between Mothers and Daughters"—Discussion of life goals

Table 16.1 (Continued)

Session 2

Module 3—HIV and STIs

Agenda/Lecture Content	Activity
Review of Session 1	Lecture
Latinos and HIV and Risks for Latina Women	Lecture—Demonstration of current data on HIV and Latinos to dispel myths about low risk within monogamous relationships and personalize risk for Latinas
Reproductive Anatomy	Lecture—Teaching women about their bodies and functions
	Family Dyad Joint Activity: Reproductive Anatomy Worksheet
	Objective: encourage family dyad communication about reproductive functions
HIV and AIDS	Lecture
	Full Group Discussion
	Objective: to address myths in Latino culture about HIV/AIDS
	Question: *What have you heard about HIV/AIDS?*
HIV Risk Factors	Lecture—Risk factors discussed with a focus on gender-based risk, heterosexual risk, and unknown risk with male partners (MSM and MSW)
STIs	Lecture
STI Risk Factors	Lecture—Risk factors discussed with a focus on gender-based risk, heterosexual risk, and unknown risk with male partners

Module 4—HIV/STI Prevention

Agenda/Lecture Content	Activity
Risk Reduction	Lecture—Discussion of strategies to reduce sexual risk
	Full Group Discussion
	Question: *How can we protect ourselves against HIV and STIs?*
Challenges to Using Condoms	Lecture—Discussion of barriers to condom use with an emphasis on partner-specific barriers and strategies to address those barriers
	Family Dyad Joint Activity: Condom Placement and Practice
	Objective: to build self-efficacy with condom use and promote communication about risk reduction within the family dyads

(Continued)

Table 16.1 (Continued)

Module 4—HIV/STI Prevention (Continued)

Agenda/Lecture Content	Activity
Talking about Condoms	Lecture—Strategies for discussing condom use with a partner
	Family Dyad Joint Role Play
	Getting Your Partner to Use a Condom—How to Say NO!
	Activity—Adult and Adolescent Pairs
	La Conquista—The older female tries to convince her younger counterpart to have sex without a condom
Sexual Assault	Lecture
Closing	*Family Dyad Joint Activity: Promises and Values*
	Participants identify strategies to improve future communication about sex within their family
	Presentation of Certificates

Analysis of Quantitative Data

Data were collected from participants using self- and *promotores*-administered pre- and immediate postintervention surveys. Approximately 1 month later a bilingual research assistant contacted the participants to conduct a follow-up survey with the same questions as the immediate postintervention survey. Participant HIV risk and prevention knowledge were measured using a scale consisting of seven

Table 16.2 Intervention Participant Characteristics

Demographic Characteristics	Adults n = 44	Adolescents n = 49
Age range	32–56	12–20
Mean age	40.70	14.76
Birth place		
U.S.	0	43 (87.8%)
Mexico	43 (97.7%)	6 (12.2%)
El Salvador	1 (2.3%)	0
Range of year in the United States	1–35	12–17
Mean length of time in the United States	18.86	15.25
Languages spoken		
English only	1 (2.3%)	1 (2.0%)
Spanish only	36 (81.8%)	1 (2.0%)
Both English and Spanish	7 (15.9%)	47 (95.9%)
Language "most comfortable" speaking		
English	1 (2.3%)	17 (34.7%)
Spanish	41 (93.2%)	3 (6.1%)
Both English and Spanish	2 (4.5%)	29 (59.2%)

true–false (Carey, Morrison-Beedy, & Johnson, 1997) and three multiple choice items in the preintervention, postintervention, and follow-up surveys. One-tailed paired *t*-tests were conducted for both groups to assess change in HIV knowledge score between preintervention and 1 month postintervention as determined by the total number of correct responses. Furthermore, one-tailed paired *t*-tests were used to measure changes in frequency of sexual risk communication as well as diversity of sexual risk-related topics discussed between preintervention and 1-month follow-up. Analyses were limited to those who completed all points of the intervention.

QUANTITATIVE RESULTS

Participant attendance varied for the intervention sessions: 34 adults/41 adolescents attended both sessions, 6 adults/7 youth did not return for the second session, and 10 adults/8 adolescents attended only the second session.

Significant preintervention to postintervention changes in HIV knowledge were found using one-tailed paired *t*-tests conducted in both age groups with significant increases in the percentage of correct responses observed for both adults, $t = 7.661$ (valid $n = 44$, $p < 0.0001$), and for adolescents, $t = 7.558$ (valid $n = 49$, $p < 0.0001$). A one-tailed *t*-test demonstrated a significant difference in HIV/AIDS-related knowledge between the two age groups within the generational dyads ($t = 4.103$, $p < 0.0001$), with the correlation coefficient 0.0408 (one-tailed $p = 0.002$) indicating that the adolescent females on average scored below their older counterparts despite the significant positive correlation observed between their scores.

One of the major components of the evaluation was to determine whether the 8-hour intervention would result in sustained increases in sexual risk-related communication between the female dyad after the intervention was completed. To address this objective, communication about sex between members in family dyads was assessed in the preintervention and 1-month follow-up surveys by asking participants to estimate the number of times they talked in the past month about sex with their other-generation partner (respectively, mother/aunt or daughter(s)/niece). A significant pre- to follow-up increase in the reported number of conversations was observed in both age groups. The paired *t*-statistic for the adult group was 4.004 (valid $n = 39$, one-tailed $p < 0.0001$) and for the adolescent group, $t = 2.779$ (valid $n = 38$, $p = 0.004$). More specifically, the dyads experienced a 160% increase in sexually related discussions from 4.174 at pretest to 6.696 at follow-up survey (adults, $n = 23$, $t = 4.075$, $p < 0.001$; adolescents, $n = 22$, $t = 3.78$, $p < 0.001$), and 58% (23 of 40) of youth reported talking to their mothers about sex with less restraint than they did prior to the intervention. Adult comfort to discuss sexually related topics increased significantly ($n = 41$, $t = 5.799$, $p < 0.0001$).

To assess differences in family and partner-focused communication, four questions addressing sexual communication comfort level were asked: whether the person feels comfortable when talking about sex and risk with (1) family and (2) partner (if applicable) and whether there are certain things about sex that the person cannot talk about to her (3) family and (4) partner (if applicable). Responses were assessed using a five-point scale with 1 = "totally disagree," 5 = "totally agree," and 3 = "neutral/unsure." The average of these four responses for each individual was used as the outcome variable. One-tailed paired *t*-tests for adults and separately for adolescents were conducted, comparing preintervention scores with follow-up scores. The tests were first conducted for all adults for whom the data were available

($n = 41$, $t = -5.799$, $p < 0.0001$) as well as for all adolescents ($n = 39$, $t = -1.447$, $p = 0.078$). Then the sample was reduced by removing those adults and adolescents who did not attend day 1 of the intervention when the tools for increasing communication comfort were discussed. For the adults ($n = 32$), $t = -5.283$, $p < 0.0001$, and for the adolescents ($n = 34$), $t = -0.905$, $p = 0.186$, results showed that there was a significant increase in communication comfort level from preintervention to follow-up for the adult participants (in the full sample as well as the reduced sample). However, for the adolescents no differences in communication comfort level were found.

DISCUSSION

This project, designed to increase both comfort with, and number of, sexual risk-related conversations within the family was successful in that activities and content provided the participants with a safe and culturally sanctioned environment wherein they were able to utilize increases in HIV/AIDS knowledge, healthy intentions, and move toward increases in intergenerational dialogue about risk. Findings clearly demonstrated a sustained increase in both comfort engaging in sexual communication and the frequency of sexual health-related communication among the adult participants. Although adolescent comfort levels did not increase from preintervention to follow-up, both adolescents and adults were engaging in dialogue about sexual matters with increased frequency and breadth of topic following the intervention. That adolescents did not evidence increased comfort in communication warrants speculation and further research. It could be very meaningful for culturally relevant Latino sexuality research to discern between the effects of cultural norms and the adolescent period of development on comfort with family-based sexual dialogue. This knowledge would enable researchers and interventionists to hone in on key nuances for effective program development targeting Latinos. The nonsignificance of adolescent comfort with sexual risk-related dialogue may also be an effect of the limited 30-day follow-up period in that insufficient time had passed for adolescents to become comfortable engaging in sexuality related dialogue with their parents.

One adolescent reported that the intervention had helped her realize that the lack of sex education and knowledge among older Latina family members had resulted in a domino effect leading to younger generations lacking the information needed to feel comfortable talking about sex with their families, friends, and partners. The fact that adult participants reported a significantly higher increase in sexual communication comfort levels when compared to their adolescent family members may indicate that participation in the intervention may help curb this trend. Although comfort levels in discussing topics of a sensitive nature did significantly increase among adolescents, these findings did not affect who initiated the conversation within the dyad. This signifies that despite a lack of comfort, adolescents were dialoguing about sexual matters with equal frequency when compared to their adult counterparts. This increase in frequency would have been less probable without changes in maternal reactions to sensitive topics. The saying or *dicho*, "de eso no se habla" or "of this one shouldn't speak," appears to have been diminished by the family-based sexual communications dynamic thus directly impacting expectations that define communication patterns within the structural environment of the immediate family.

Utilizing a mix of qualitative and quantitative methods provided a rich opportunity to initiate dialogue and better understand the contextual differences that Latinas, on diverse points on the spectrum of developmental and transculturative processes, experience when attempting to communicate effectively to mitigate sexual risk. These qualitative data and subsequent intervention findings (Table 16.3) allowed us to recognize how diverse life experiences, cultural expectations, and language use play a role in actual HIV/AIDS risk and understanding how to mitigate this risk among diverse generations within one family. Most adolescents developed their understanding of sexual risk within the United States where they spend their formative developmental years. However, the culturally based sexual expectations set by parental norms are quite different from those adolescents experience within their communities and school settings. Furthermore, immigrant parents, due to their lack of education and related sex and basic HIV/AIDS education, often relegate their power to communicate about sexual risk to the school setting wherein curriculum is designed without consideration of the cultural norms of either immigrant parents or students.

Latina immigrant mothers and their daughters, who may have immigrated during their childhood, have formed their ability to communicate about sex through very

Table 16.3 Intervention Findings

Question/Test	Adults	Adolescents	Adults vs. Adolescents
HIV knowledge/correct responses on pre- and postintervention surveys	$n = 44$ $t = 7.661^{***}$ $p < 0.0001$	$n = 49$ $t = 7.558^{***}$ $p < 0.0001$	
HIV knowledge/comparing percentages of correct responses on the posttest			$n = 49$ $t = 4.103^{***}$ $p < 0.0001$
HIV knowledge/correlation for adults' vs. adolescents' scores on the posttest			$n = 49$ $t = 0.408^{*}$ $p = 0.002$
Sex-related communication/number of conversations in pre- and follow-up surveys	$n = 39$ $t = 4.004^{***}$ $p < 0.0001$	$n = 38$ $t = 2.779^{*}$ $p = 0.004$	
Sex-related communication/number of topics addressed in conversations in pre- and follow-up surveys	$n = 23$ $t = 4.075^{**}$ $p < 0.001$	$n = 22$ $t = 3.78^{**}$ $p < 0.001$	
Sex-related communication comfort level/ pre- and follow-up average responses for the full sample	$n = 41$ $t = -5.799^{***}$ $p < 0.0001$	$n = 39$ $t = -1.447^{\dagger}$ $p = 0.078$	
Sex-related communication comfort level/ pre- and follow-up averaged responses (reduced model excluding those who did not attend day 1)	$n = 32$ $t = -5.283^{***}$ $p < 0.0001$	$n = 34$ $t = -0.905$ $p = 0.186$	

$^{\dagger}p < 0.10$, $^{*}p < 0.01$, $^{**}p < 0.001$, $^{***}p < 0.0001$.

different linguistic, cultural, educational, and experiential frameworks. Furthermore, youth in our study expressed a paucity of sexual communication strategies when attempting to talk with their parents, and noted that because their parents were not reliable sources of sexual risk-related information, the effort would yield little result. Using the Latino Health Communications (Belief) Model, developed by the Center for Hispanic Health Promotion (now the Institute of Hispanic Health) at the National Council of La Raza (Karliner, Edmonds Crewe, Pacheco, & Cruz-Gonzalez, 1998; Arroyo & Thompson, 2011), facilitated the incorporation of several cultural value-based assets to reinforce positive cultural characteristics or cultural structures such as *familismo, respeto, confianza*, and *personalismo*. These were seen as key to reinforcing positive cultural characteristics that buttress both cultural pride and resiliency and to enhancing intergenerational communication skills and strategies. By understanding cultural characteristics, such as *familismo*, as Latino community assets, and *respeto* and *confianza* as key values needed to maintain effective family-based communication, the intervention was able to reframe communication with norms that were both culturally congruent and acceptable to both mother and daughter.

One intervention activity, *La Conquista* [The Conquest], exemplifies the way in which gender roles and culturally bound knowledge and experiences can be shared to demonstrate how existing knowledge between the generations can challenge the oft-held beliefs of adolescents that their mothers cannot accurately describe the contexts of sexual risk in modern United States' society. In this exercise, the older female counterpart (usually mother and sometimes aunt) is asked to role play as if she is a male trying to convince her younger counterpart to have sex without using condoms. As much as this exercise provokes humor, it also results in a great deal of reflection as the younger females often give up and concede to the wishes of their older counterparts. Upon conclusion of the exercise the two generations are asked to reflect on the process. Just as the youth realize that they were too easily convinced, their older counterparts often report, "If it was that easy for me to convince her to have sex without using a condom, there is no doubt in my mind that it will be much easier for her boyfriend to do so. This means that I really need to improve my sexual communication and education skills and help her gain the knowledge, confidence, and skills she needs to defend herself and her wishes so that she is not putting herself at sexual risk." These reflections acknowledge the ability of Latina participants of both generations to alter the cultural structures that confine communication dynamics surrounding sexuality, thus enabling the immediate family environment to honor traditional values while facilitating a more comprehensive and contemporary response to the dynamic contexts of HIV risk.

Study Limitations

There are several marked limitations that merit discussion. First, due to the geographic limitations combined with the subpopulation Mexican majority, these results may not be transferable to other Latina dyads. Because our results are based on a small, nonrandom, convenience sample of intergenerational Latinas in Los Angeles County, they do not constitute a representative sample of Latinas at risk for HIV outside of their geographic region. In addition, participant attendance in the intervention was inconsistent. We were also limited to a certain extent by inconsistent participation with some pairs attending only the first day and the others arriving halfway through the intervention on the second day. This occurred despite the fact that the intervention was clearly advertised as a 2-day class held on specific dates and at scheduled times. From the perspective of a new community-based project attempting to address the needs of a group of underserved and often uninsured Latina women and their daughters, we did not think it appropriate to turn away participants given the fact that they had often gone to great lengths to arrive at the location of the guided educational session (*charla*). New arrivals were most often individuals invited by participants who attended the first session, and had not gone through the registration process put in place by our community collaborators who conducted outreach for the intervention. Despite this increase of participants through word of mouth, partial attendance in the intervention required omission of these family dyads in the final data analysis. Furthermore, given the short duration of the study, long-term changes in participant knowledge, intention, and risk were not measured beyond the 30-day follow up telephone interview. Lastly, the data were self-reported and as such are subject to participant recall bias.

CONCLUSIONS AND RECOMMENDATIONS FOR FUTURE APPLICATIONS

Despite its limitations, this formative data collection and intervention process highlights several important elements when working with Latina intergenerational dyads and with mother–daughter dyads in particular. The formative data collection period was integral to our understanding of the distinct cultures of the mothers and the daughters, as well as our ability to integrate messages and strategies that resonated with the contextual realities wherein both groups experience HIV and sexual health risk situations. While including important concepts from behavioral theories, such as perceived self-efficacy and behavioral beliefs, and by integrating cultural strengths, we were able to address Latina-specific contextual risk factors and give credence to characteristics of culturally related resiliency such as *familismo, confianza* and *respeto*, without vilifying or stereotyping behavioral manifestations such as *marianismo* and *machismo*. Given that Latino immigrants demonstrate fairly positive health outcomes on a number of indicators, despite an overwhelming lack of access to health care and insurance and low socioeconomic status, the incorporation of cultural values and strategies as fundamental intervention components could add to the resiliency and overall well-being of Latino communities throughout the United States. Throughout each module, culturally relevant constructs were discussed and *dichos* (common sayings) and Latino-specific beliefs incorporated throughout the curriculum (e.g., *Ojos que no ven-corazón que no siente; Donde fuego hubo cenizas quedan; Cuando el río suena, agua lleva; La palabra es plata, el silencio oro.*). [Eyes that don't see—A heart that doesn't feel; Where there was fire ash remains; A river that makes noise carries water; Words are silver but silence is golden.]

Despite the difference in the findings between the generational groups regarding sexual communication comfort level, the increase in reported number of conversations about sex in both groups demonstrates promise in developing HIV risk communication in Latino families, while building HIV/AIDS knowledge specific to the dynamic contexts of the risks Latinas face in the United States. The intervention provided us with the opportunity to frame the skills and strategies needed to engage Latina intergenerational family members into culturally and linguistically relevant HIV/AIDS prevention messages and dialogue. The formative data collection and intervention process facilitated the development of an understanding of the intergenerational differences and similarities regarding HIV risk perceptions and relate them to the expectations and aspirations of women living in families. Involving Latino community-based partners and community members was the key to ensuring that these prevention efforts both resonated and reflected the contextual experience of HIV risk for Latina Angelinos.

An additional drawback of this intervention is its sole focus on women and female adolescents. Although women-centered programs are important and essential, the continual reliance on females as the sole change agents within relationships that are often sexually dominated by males increases the responsibility placed on women and girls, and implicitly minimizes expectations of preventive male behavior. Within the oppressive and xenophobic environment experienced by many Latinos overall and immigrants in particular, low expectations of male behavior have the potential to increase internalized sexism, racism, hopelessness, and despair, therefore contributing to an attitude that does not reinforce male preventive behaviors. Furthermore, these expectations coupled with gender-exclusive intervention methods exacerbate the gender imbalance and weaken the potential reinforcement to be had through the employment of positive cultural characteristics such as *familismo*. The incorporation of males in the intervention would enable the curriculum to address machismo in a positive light because men could learn how to "protect" their partner(s)' and family's sexual health.

Male involvement in the sex communication intervention would have the potential to benefit women and girls in several ways, particularly given the fact that marriage has been acknowledged as the most influential HIV risk factor in Mexico among women (Pan American Health Organization, 2001). Male involvement may also facilitate more frequent and consistent participation on behalf of women and girls who have dominant male partners or fathers who do not allow for sexual risk education given the cultural limitations of womanhood. If *familismo* could be incorporated to its full potential, participation could be viewed as a family, as opposed to female, priority.

Despite its limitations, *Rompe el Silencio* afforded the opportunity to create both an environment and support mechanisms to reinforce sexual health communication and risk-prevention strategies that were based on both female generations' experiences and HIV risk context. By framing HIV/AIDS risk among Latinas within a cultural assets framework, we were able to create an environment that fostered open sexual risk dialogue while employing and reinforcing cultural assets such as *familismo, respeto,* and *confianza.* The intervention facilitated dialogue whereby Latina family-based intergenerational dyads could model new communication and risk-reduction strategies and bring the skills and knowledge back into the safety and security of their homes, thus provoking greater dialogue around topics that have been interpreted as taboo within Latino cultures overall.

ACKNOWLEDGMENTS

This chapter was authored by Dr. Britt Rios-Ellis with editorial assistance from Dr. Mara Bird, Dr. Lilia Espinoza, Dr. Selena Nguyen-Rodriguez, and Nina Smallwood. Several individuals including Ana Carolina Canjura, Melawhy Garcia, Dr. Kevin Malotte, and Dr. Olga Korosteleva assisted with project and research design and the analyses of results presented in this chapter. The author and research team remain indebted to the *promotores de salud* and Latina participants who readily gave of their time and insight to make this project a reality.

REFERENCES

Adam, M. B., McGuire, J. K., Walsh, M., Basta, J., & LeCroy, C. (2005). Acculturation as a predictor of the onset of sexual intercourse among Hispanic and white teens. *Archives of Pediatric & Adolescent Medicine, 159*(3), 261–265.

Ajzen, I. (1991). The theory of planned behavior. *Organizational Behavior and Human Decision Processes, 50,* 179–211.

Amaro, H. (1995). Love, sex and power. Considering women's realities in HIV prevention. *American Psychologist, 50*(6), 437–447.

Arroyo, L. E., & Thompson, N. (2011). *Latino health beliefs: A guide for health care professionals.* National Council of La Raza Institute for Hispanic Health. Unpublished report.

Bandura, A. (1986). *Social foundations of thought and action: A social cognitive theory.* Englewood Cliffs, NJ: Prentice-Hall.

Barker, G., & Rich, S. (1992). Influences on adolescent sexuality in Nigeria and Kenya: Findings from recent focus-group discussions. *Studies in Family Planning, 23,* 199–210.

Bartlett, R., Buck, R., & Shattell, M. M. (2008). Risk and protection for HIV/AIDS in African-American, Hispanic, and white adolescents. *Journal of the National Black Nurses Association, 19*(1), 19–25.

Blythe, M. J., Fortenberry, J. D., M'Hamed, T., Tu, W., & Orr, D. P. (2006). Incidence and correlates of unwanted sex in relationships of middle and late adolescent women. *Archives of Pediatric and Adolescent Medicine, 160,* 591–595.

Bourdeau, B., Thomas, V. K., & Long, J. K. (2008). Latino sexual styles: Developing a nuanced understanding of risk. *Journal of Sex Research, 45*(1), 71–81.

Burgess, V., Dziegielewski, S. F., & Green, C. E. (2005). Improving comfort about sex communication between parents and their adolescents: Practice-based research within a teen sexuality group. *Brief Treatment and Crisis Intervention, 5*(4), 379–390.

Carey, M., Morrison-Beedy, D., & Johnson B. (1997). The HIV-knowledge questionnaire. *AIDS & Behavior, 1*(1), 61–74.

Carovano, K. (1991). More than mothers and whores: Redefining the AIDS prevention needs of women. *International Journal of Health Services, 21*(1), 131–142.

Centers for Disease Control and Prevention. (2008). Youth risk behavior surveillance—United States, 2007. *Morbidity and Mortality Weekly Report, 57*(SS-4), 1–24, 101.

DiClemente, R. J., Wingood, G. M., Crosby, R., Cobb, B. K., Harrington, K., & Davies, S. L. (2001). Parent-adolescent communication and sexual risk behaviors among African American adolescent females. *Journal of Pediatrics, 139*(3), 407–412.

East, P. L. (1998). Racial and ethnic differences in girl's sexual, marital, and birth expectations. *Journal of Marriage and the Family, 60,* 150–162.

Ebin, V. J., Sneed, C. D., Morisky, D. E., Rotheram-Borus, M. J., Magnusson, A. M., & Malotte, C. K. (2001). Acculturation and interrelationships between problem and health-promoting behaviors among Latino adolescents. *Journal of Adolescent Health, 28,* 62–72.

Fishbein, M., Triandis, H. C., Kanfer, F. H., Becker, M., Middlestadt, S. E., & Eichler, A. (2001). Factors influencing behavior and behavior change. In A. Baum, T. A. Revenson, & J. E. Singer (Eds.), *Handbook of health psychology* (pp. 3–17). Mahwah, NJ: Lawrence Erlbaum Associates.

Fisher, J. D., & Fisher, W. A. (1996). The information-motivation-behavioral skills model of AIDS risk behavior change: Empirical support and application. In S. Oskamp & S. C. Thompson (Eds.), *Understanding and preventing HIV risk behavior: Safer sex and drug use* (pp. 100–127). Thousand Oaks, CA: Sage Publications.

Flores-Ortiz, Y. (2004). Domestic violence in Chicana/o families. In *The handbook of Chicana/o psychology and mental health* (pp. 267–284). Mahwah, NJ: Lawrence Erlbaum Associates Publishers. Retrieved April 13, 2009, from PsycINFO database.

Glaser, B. G. (1998). *Doing grounded theory-issues and discussions.* Mill Valley, CA: Sociology Press.

Hayes-Baustista, D. (2004). *La nueva California: Latinos in the golden state.* Berkeley, CA: University of California Press.

Hillman, J. (2008). Knowledge, attitudes, and experience regarding HIV/AIDS among older adult inner-city Latinos. *International Journal of Aging and Human Development, 66*(3), 243–257.

Jacobs, R. J. (2008). A theory-based collaborative approach to HIV/AIDS prevention in Latino youth. *Journal for Specialists in Pediatric Nursing, 13*(2), 126–129.

Kaiser Family Foundation. (2004). *HIV/AIDS policy fact sheet: The HIV/AIDS epidemic in the U.S.* (Publication No. 3029-03). Washington, DC: Kaiser Family Foundation

Kaiser Family Foundation. (2008). *HIV/AIDS Policy Fact Sheet.* (Report #6007-08.) Washington, DC: Kaiser Family Foundation.

Kaplan, C. P., Erickson, P. I., & Juarez-Reyes, M. (2002). Acculturation, gender role orientation, and reproductive risk-taking behavior among Latina adolescent family planning clients. *Journal of Adolescent Research, 17,* 103–121.

Karliner, S., Edmonds Crewe, S., Pacheco, H., & Cruz-Gonzalez, Y. (1998). *Latino health beliefs: A guide for health care professionals.* Washington, DC: Center for Health Promotion.

Logan, T., Cole, J., & Leukefeld, C. (2002). Women, sex, and HIV: Social and contextual factors, meta-analysis of published interventions, and implications for practice and research. *Psychological Bulletin, 128*(6), 851–885.

Mark, M. M., & Miller, M. L. (1986). The effects of sexual permissiveness, target gender, subject gender, and attitude toward women on social perception: In search of the double standard. *Sex Roles, 15*(5/6), 311–322.

National Council of La Raza. (2009). *Updated Latino health communications model.* Washington, DC.

Pan American Health Organization. (2001). Fact Sheet: Gender and HIV/AIDS. http://www.paho.org/english/hdp/hdw/GenderandHIVFactSheetI.pdf.

Prado, G., Pantin, H., Briones, E., Schwartz, S. J., Feaster, D., Huang, S., et al. (2007). A randomized controlled trial of a parent-centered intervention in preventing substance use and HIV risk behaviors in Hispanic adolescents. *Journal of Consulting and Clinical Psychology, 75*(6), 914–926.

Rhodes, F., & Malotte, C. K. (1996). HIV risk interventions for active drug users: Experience and prospects. In S. Oskamp & S. Thompson (Eds.), *Understanding and preventing HIV risk behavior: Safer sex and drug use* (pp. 207–236). Thousand Oaks, CA: Sage Publications.

Rice, E., Green, S., Santos, K., Lester, P., & Rotheram-Borus, M. J. (2010). A lifetime of low-risk behaviors among HIV-positive Latinas in Los Angeles. *Journal of Immigrant and Minority Health, 12*(6), 875–881.

Rios, E. A. (2005). *Las olvidadas/The forgotten ones: Latinas and the HIV/AIDS epidemic.* Washington, DC: Hispanic Federation.

Rios-Ellis, B. (2006). *Redefining HIV/AIDS for Latinos: A promising new paradigm for addressing HIV/AIDS in the Hispanic community.* Washington, DC: White Paper published by the National Council of La Raza.

Rios-Ellis, B., Frates, J., Hoyt D'Anna, L., Dwyer, M., Ugarte, C., & Lopez-Zetina, J. (2008). Addressing the need for access to culturally and linguistically appropriate HIV/AIDS prevention for Latinos. *Journal of Immigrant and Minority Health, 10,* 445–460.

Rios-Ellis, B. (2010). The Latino health communications model: Understanding keys to creating meaningful provider patient dialogue. Kaiser Permanente, November 2010. Presentation made to executive management network.

Romo, L. F., Lefkowitz, E. S., Sigman, M., & Au, T. K. (2002). A longitudinal study of maternal messages about dating and sexuality and their influence on Latino adolescents. *Journal of Adolescent Health, 31*(1), 59–69.

Sangi-Haghpeykar, H., Horth, F., & Poindexter, A. N. (2001). Condom use among sterilized andnonsterilized Hispanic women. *Sexually Transmitted Diseases, 28,* 546–551.

Strauss, A., & Corbin, J. (1988). *Basis of qualitative research: Grounded theory procedures and techniques* (2nd ed.). Thousand Oaks, CA: Sage Publishing.

Teitelman, A. M., Ratcliffe, S. J., & Cederbaum, J. A. (2008). Parent-adolescent communication about sexual pressure, maternal norms about relationship power, and STI/HIV protective behaviors of minority urban girls. *Journal of the American Psychiatric Nurses Association, 14*(1), 50–60.

The National Campaign to Prevent Teen and Unplanned Pregnancy. (2008, 12/9/08). *An overview of Latina teen pregnancy and birth rates* from http://www.thenationalcampaign. org/espanol/PDF/latino_overview.pdf.

van Servellen, G., Chang, B., & Lombardi, E. (2002). Acculturation, socioeconomic vulnerability, and quality of life in Spanish-speaking and bilingual Latino HIV-infected men and women. *Western Journal of Nursing Research, 24*(3), 246–263.

Villarruel, A. M., Jemmott, J. B., III, Jemmott, L. S., & Ronis, D. L. (2004). Predictors of sexual intercourse and condom use intentions among Spanish-dominant Latino youth: A test of the planned behavior theory. *Nursing Research, 53*(3), 172–181.

Wilson, H. W., & Donnenberg, C. (2004). Quality of parent communication about sex and its relationship to risky sexual behavior among youth in psychiatric care: A pilot study. *Journal of Child Psychology and Psychiatry, 45*(2), 387–395.

17 The Landscape of Latina HIV Prevention Interventions and Their Implementation

Cultural Sensitivity in Community-Based Organizations

Miriam Y. Vega and Lina Cherfas

INTRODUCTION

The United States is at a sociocultural crossroads with demographic shifts that are rapidly changing the public health landscape, placing current models of HIV prevention at risk of becoming irrelevant or counterproductive, unless we address new realities. On July 13, 2010, the White House unveiled the National AIDS Strategy for the United States (The White House Office of National AIDS Policy, 2010). The strategy is meant to be a clear, action-driven roadmap for addressing the HIV epidemic in the United States. It aims to lower the HIV incidence rate by 25% by 2015 and increase by 90% the proportion of people living with HIV who know their serostatus. With cultural shifts, new demands on public health practitioners, new culturally salient delivery modes, techniques, and tactics need to be implemented if we are to meet the goals set forth in the National AIDS Strategy.

Between 1999 and 2004, Latinas with heterosexually acquired HIV dramatically increased by 4.5% (Espinoza, Hall, Hardnett, Selik, Qiang, et al., 2007). In the United States a growing proportion of heterosexually acquired HIV infections occurs in women and in persons of color (Espinoza et al., 2007) and most HIV infections in women in the United States are heterosexually acquired (Hadler, 2001). Gender inequalities, socioeconomic disadvantage, violence, substance abuse, and nonculturally responsive and salient prevention messages and programmatic responses (i.e., interventions) to the epidemic have been identified as factors that increase the risk of HIV in Latinas (Peragallo, DeForge, O'Campo, Lee, & Kim, 2005). If the goals set by the National AIDS Strategy are to be met, these sociocultural realities need to be addressed.

As Organista et al. note in the opening chapter of this volume, there is a need for community and culture-based interventions that situate individual risk behavior within a structural environmental model. This chapter will serve as a review of the HIV prevention landscape in regard to Latinas, rooted in both the experience of community-based organizations (CBOs) as implementers of interventions and

Latino-specific cultural scripts and values, providing concrete examples of HIV prevention programs as currently delivered in the field. We highlight and deconstruct four HIV prevention interventions, as recently implemented by CBOs in different parts of the United States, into surface and deep-level cultural considerations. Engaging with the structural and environmental contexts of HIV risk, the interventions addressed barriers to participation, took women out of their often-constrained social roles, promoted local activism, and engaged participants in conversations about migration and transnational identity as Latinas. By taking into account surface and deep level characteristics, these interventions worked to address structural, environmental, and individual level factors influencing HIV risk among Latinas.

The chapter ends by addressing future opportunities as well as structural barriers by looking at microbicides and preexposure prophylaxis (PReP), interventions that may place protection in the female's control. The chapter also considers treatment as a community, structured intervention. We discuss how CBOs will have a continuing role even in these biomedical approaches. Their embeddedness in the community places them in a unique position to address the structural and environmental factors involved in HIV transmission.

The need for community-based HIV prevention programs that are culturally specific, appropriate, and responsive is well recognized (Minkler & Wallerstein, 1997), but at the same time, in accordance with the Institute of Medicine (2003), the Centers for Disease Control and Prevention (CDC) recommends that health departments and CBOs implement evidence-based behavioral interventions (Collins, Harshbarger, Sawyer, & Hamdallah, 2006) that are often designed and validated on populations different from those currently most needy. Unfortunately, as the rate of Latinas with heterosexually acquired HIV increases, of those interventions labeled by the CDC as effective, only three are culturally specific to Latinos overall and only one is specific to Latinas (CDC, 2003). Furthermore, the National AIDS Strategy proposes to increase knowledge of serostatus and decrease the incidence rate through increased use of evidence-based HIV prevention interventions in a more targeted fashion to address the epidemic in communities most heavily impacted. This approach presupposes the existence and common availability of HIV interventions both culturally responsive to Latinas, as well as evidence-based, setting up tension between recognized local community needs, national strategies, and funding mandates. Nonetheless, community-based efforts, with established public sector relationships and depth of grassroots experience, can be marshaled as an effective tool in aiding HIV prevention efforts, particularly those related to the National AIDS Strategy and Latinas.

THE BEDROCK: CULTURAL SENSITIVITY AND THEORETICAL CONSIDERATIONS

Health interventions adapted to an ethnic group's cultural context are more likely to increase an intervention's external validity (Bernal, Bonilla, & Bellido, 1995). Interventions need to be culturally sensitive and targeted toward specific populations, because individuals tend to adhere to and benefit from interventions congruent with their beliefs, narratives, and frames of reference (Sue, 1998). There are two dimensions of cultural sensitivity that public health intervention developers, adapters, and implementers tend to apply: surface structure and deep structure (Resnicow, Baranowski, Ahluwalia, & Braithwaite, 1999). Surface structure is the extent to which interventions match social, behavioral, and appearance aspects of target populations. The components of surface structure include intervention materials, messages, channels, settings, and recruitment strategies that match characteristics of target populations. Addressing surface structure involves matching intervention materials and messages to observable, "superficial" characteristics of a target population (e.g., using people, places, language, music, food, locations, and clothing familiar to, and preferred by, the target audience). Deep structure recognizes that cultural, social, historical, and environmental variables influence health behaviors, and values ethnic and cultural differences in perceptions of disease prevention. Deep structure addresses values, norms, and interpersonal scripts that go beyond language and phenotypic similarity by deconstructing and incorporating cultural, social, and interpersonal scripts that impact the adoption of behaviors. Addressing deep cultural structures can include acknowledging concepts of time, gender roles, physical distance (how far apart should people stand) to greetings upon meeting (handshakes versus kisses on the cheek), and other forms of nonverbal communication. These are cultural structures that are not ostensibly immediately noticeable (such as gender and race) but instead require an understanding of what is considered normative. While addressing surface structure increases receptivity to or acceptance of messages, deep structure increases salience. The extent to which HIV prevention can address both surface and deep structural cultural dimensions determines the likelihood that participants will come, stay, and consequently change behaviors, with subsequent overall increases in serostatus awareness and decreases in HIV incidence rates.

Cultural values, which can enhance the salience of an intervention, are the bases for the specific norms and scripts that tell people what is appropriate in situations (Markus & Kitayama, 1994) and are at the root of cultural sensitivity, both in terms of surface structure and deep structure. Although there are important sociodemographic differences among Latino subgroups according to country of origin, educational attainment, and acculturation level, there is agreement about a number of shared cultural values (Marin, 1989; Taylor, 1996). Cultural values that denote certain interpersonal scripts need to be properly understood, addressed, and applied for interventions to be acceptable and salient to Latinas. For example, *personalismo* (Marin, 1989) is often defined as "formal friendliness," placing emphasis on personal aspects of a relationship. This importance of personal relationships may lead Latinos to value and seek out CBOs for primary care and guidance. Furthermore, a strong sense of collectivism (Markus & Kitayama, 1994) in Latino communities, which reflects the importance assigned to friends and family members who may provide companionship and help solve personal problems, can be harnessed to enhance skills building sessions in group-level interventions. *Familismo,* reflecting high value on social support from and a strong sense of loyalty/reciprocity to an in-group, which typically consists of both the nuclear and extended family, but may include close friends, co-workers, and social networks in cohesive communities (Cervantes & Castro, 1985), can drive high program retention rates. There is the interpersonal script of *comadrismo,* a term derived from *madre* (mother), commonly used by Latinas to describe relationships of trust and mutual support among women, denoting co-motherhood and godmother status (Preloran, Browner, & Lieber, 2001). Lastly, a key Latino value is *respeto,* prescribing deference to individuals holding high prestige in society (Marin & Triandis, 1985), including medical doctors and the elderly. Such deference can influence how prevention messages are received, delivered, and framed. Cultural values can be used to motivate individual behaviors and to develop and market interventions. However, these values are not always protective and can have negative consequences (Abel & Chambers, 2002). Arguably, *familismo* and *respeto* can encourage silence about issues such as domestic violence, unprotected sex outside marriage, and abuse (but see Ellis-Rios' efforts to promote sex-related communication between mothers and daughters in Chapter 16).

There are also cultural values that delineate gender roles. Machismo entails the man being strong, a protector of wife and family, and sexually experienced (Galanti, 2003). It is expected that such men have multiple partners before and even after marriage and this may increase Latinas' risk for acquiring HIV (Sabogal & Catania, 1996). The complement of machismo is marianismo, with submission of women to men as a significant component (Galanti, 2003). This produces a double standard whereby Latinas may be categorized as either good mothers or bad women who are sexually available and experienced (Galanti, 2003). Marianismo implies that the most important values for women are chastity, motherhood, self-sacrifice, and care-taking (Galanti, 2003). Although it could be argued that *machismo* and *marianismo* enhance HIV risk for Latinas, these values can also have positive aspects— deep cultural values of caregiving, motherhood, and protection can be molded to motivating messages making health screenings salient. Needless to say, not all Latinos subscribe to all of these cultural values, but for those who do, the impetus is to harness their positive aspects to ensure that interventions will be culturally appropriate, acceptable, and effective with Latinos (see Carrillo's critique of these constructs in Chapter 3). This begs the question of what aspects of an intervention make it culturally appropriate and salient.

In a systematic review (Herbst, Kay, Passin, Lyles, Crepaz, et al., 2007) examining the efficacy of 20 HIV behavioral interventions through 2006 designed to reduce HIV risk behaviors or incidence of sexually transmitted diseases (STDs) among Latinos residing in the United States or Puerto Rico, researchers found that interventions successful in reducing the odds of any sex risk behavior included the following elements: used nonpeer deliverers; included four or more intervention sessions; taught condom use or problem-solving skills; and addressed barriers to condom use, sexual abstinence, or peer norms. Furthermore, Herbst et al. (2007) found that interventions that specifically addressed the cultural value of *machismo* or those developed through ethnographic interviews about cultural norms were more successful. Such a review highlights the need to address surface cultural considerations that make interventions acceptable (i.e., number of sessions, nonpeer deliverers) and deep cultural considerations that make interventions salient (i.e., enhance skills sets, address *machismo* and other values). Interestingly, what made the interventions acceptable was the use of nonpeer facilitators. This may be related to the value of *respeto;* those interventions were made salient with facilitators seen as high in professional status. But what does this mean in terms of peers and the possible use of *personalismo* and *comadrismo* to be culturally sensitive?

Any review of Latina-centered interventions would be remiss if it ignored *promotoras*. Promotoras (lay community educators or community health workers) are peers, community leaders, and social gatekeepers who build bridges between communities and agencies. The *promotora* model is a popular method for reaching vulnerable populations. *Promotoras* have disseminated information on diabetes, nutrition, maternity, child health, smoking cessation, and HIV/AIDS. In the United States, *promotoras* have been used largely in Latino communities in the West and Southwest (more rural areas). Past research has identified at least five roles taken on by *promotoras*: educator, case manager, role model, program facilitator, and advocate (Cherrington, Ayala, Amick, Scarinci, Allison, et al., 2008). Chapter 16 describes the integration of *promotoras* in an intervention to increase communication about sex and HIV between Latina mothers and daughters. In addition, Rhodes et al. (2007) in a systematic review of lay health advisor approaches with Latino communities found that they also help with recruitment and data collection. In a review of 58 studies, published from 1980 to November 2008, Viswanathan et al. (2010) found limited evidence for behavior change, but stronger evidence that community health workers can increase appropriate health care utilization for some interventions. In looking at interventions (Elder, Ayala, Slymen, Arredondo, & Campbell, 2009) meant to enhance nutrition, in which tailored Spanish print materials were compared to materials plus *promotoras*, researchers found that use of *promotoras* resulted in significant initial behavior change, but tailored materials were instrumental in continued behavior change. The use of *promotoras* may be a culturally sensitive way to increase "receptivity to" or "acceptance of" recruitment and HIV prevention messages whereas other methods may enhance the salience of interventions. Two key strengths of *promotoras* that should not be overlooked are that they educate providers about the community's health needs and provide feedback about the cultural relevancy of interventions (Witmer, 1995), while building community capacity.

In addition to cultural characteristics, interventions targeting Latinos must take into account relevant sociopolitical contexts of their clients' lives. One characteristic is immigration and transnational identity. About 40% of Latinos living in the United States are foreign born (Grieco, 2009), and many others have strong ties to the countries of origin of their parents, through relatives and trade links. Recent immigrants encounter many obstacles to HIV prevention, among other health issues: precarious employment status, lack of health insurance, language and cultural barriers to accessing care, lack of education about preventive health, and growing stigma against undocumented Latinos. As with other immigrant groups, Latinos balance not only languages, but also the cultural values (deep structures) of the United States and those of their countries of origin. In cases of repeated migration and transnationalism (interactions linking people across the borders of nations), this balancing act further intensifies, as exemplified by the constant state of cultural flux experienced by Puerto Ricans, alternately residing on the island and in New York City, or Mexican migrants as discussed by Carrillo in Chapter 3.

Many Latinos are marginalized due to undocumented immigration status; the full impact of recent increases in rates of deportations has yet to be recorded. Undocumented status is a factor in HIV transmission in that it enhances legal and economic dependence of undocumented sexual partners on documented spouses, as well as contributing to rates of sex work by undocumented immigrants. Latino families are often divided among undocumented members (usually parents) and documented members (usually children), which furthers the challenges of CBOs in providing interventions that include, for example, linkages to other social services, many of which require proof of legal residence for eligibility. Interventions targeting women face the task of surmounting gender-based vulnerability in the context of migration, documentation, and trans-nationalism.

Employment of surface structure characteristics (Spanish language materials, bilingual facilitators, and nonpeer facilitators) and deep structure characteristics (health belief theory, tailored materials) increases the acceptance and salience of interventions targeting Latinos, but a closer and more methodical review is needed to develop a functional model that describes which characteristics are best utilized in a given intervention.

THE CURRENT LANDSCAPE OF EVIDENCE-BASED HIV PREVENTION TARGETING LATINAS

Funders of public health interventions increasingly require implementation of evidence-based, effective behavioral interventions. An effective intervention must be published in peer-reviewed journals, with a rigorous study design consisting of longitudinal and control arm designs with large enough data sets (Lyles, 2006). CBOs do not have the technical capability, resources, or research focus to establish homegrown interventions as effective. This inadvertently forces many CBOs to offer interventions already identified as behaviorally effective, but not culturally specific/sensitive to the Latino communities they serve.

In 1999, the CDC developed a *Compendium of HIV Prevention Interventions with Evidence of Effectiveness* to highlight science-based interventions effective for HIV prevention that demonstrated evidence of effectiveness in reducing sex and drug-related risk behaviors or improving health outcomes. The 2009 *Compendium* included 69 evidence-based HIV behavioral interventions (individual, group, and community level), the majority of which were originally conducted in the early to mid-1990s. Forty-one of these interventions are catalogued as best evidence and 28 as promising evidence. There were a total of seven "best evidence" interventions including Latinos as a target population (Connect, *Cuídate, Modelo de Intervención Psicomédica*, Project Safe, Sisters Saving Sisters, Voices/*Voces*, and Women's Health Project) and only one "promising evidence" intervention targeting Latinos (*SEPA*). SEPA is the only intervention specifically for Latinas. Thus, of these eight compendium interventions that originally had Latinos included in their studies, only three were culturally specific to Latinos overall and only one was specific to Latinas.

In 2002, the CDC implemented the Diffusion of Effective Behavioral Interventions (DEBI) project, designed to bring science-based HIV prevention interventions to community-based service providers and state and local health departments (Collins et al., 2006). These interventions were packaged by the CDC, along with trainings and capacity building assistance, so they can be implemented with fidelity (Collins et al., 2006). As of July 2009, there were 23 DEBI interventions with a growing inventory (Stallworth, Andía, Burgess, Alvarez, & Collins, 2009). Three interventions designed specifically for Latinos are included: *Cuídate, Modelo de Intervención Psicomédica* (MIP), and *Salud, Educacion, Prevencion y Autocuidado* (SEPA). *Cuídate* targets youth, *MIP* targets injection drug users, and *SEPA*, a six-session, small group, skill-building intervention, originally conducted in Chicago, Illinois, between 1999 and 2001, is the only one that specifically targets heterosexual adult Latinas.

Because the majority of these DEBI interventions did not originally focus on Latinos and Latino culture with any specificity, they typically have to be adapted by CBOs who wish to implement an intervention targeting Latinas. Often, attempts at adapting programs consider only surface structure modifications, hiring ethnically matched staff, and modifying videos or pictures to show ethnically similar individuals. Thus, from the beginning of the DEBI Project, there has been a challenge to meet the needs of the diverse Latina populations at risk for HIV/AIDS. The central challenges of disseminating and implementing DEBIs include goodness of fit with the community served, recruitment and retention of participants, and staff turnover

(Vega, 2009; Veniegas, Kao, Rosales, & Arellanes, 2009). Issues surrounding "goodness of fit" imply the need to adjust to the realities of surface and deep structural considerations while maintaining fidelity. There is little doubt that unofficially "effective" interventions are seeded throughout the national landscape of community-based organizations and these can provide us with useful insights.

OUT IN THE FIELD: IMPLEMENTATION HIGHLIGHTS OF LATINA-CENTERED INTERVENTIONS

Community-based organizations, usually in partnership with researchers, funders, and government agencies, are developing innovative homegrown interventions or adapting existing "approved" HIV prevention programs for Latinas. A well-known adaptation is the American Red Cross basic HIV course for Latinos. The American Red Cross adapted its original course, in English, by addressing the two cultural sensitivity dimensions: they translated into Spanish (surface structure) and based it on the popular education philosophy of Brazilian educator Paulo Freire, emphasizing *plática* or dialogue (deep structure). The *plática* as a learning method encourages exchange of experiences within a group to empower members. The Red Cross also addressed deep structures such as customs, family relationships, spirituality, sexuality, and health beliefs of Latinos.

This section highlights four CBO programs that translated community-led ideas into local interventions for Latinas: (1) a replication and extension of an effective intervention that was originally Latina centered, (2) an adaptation of a DEBI project intervention originally for African American women, (3) a homegrown intervention, and (4) a hybrid intervention consisting of an adapted DEBI joined with a homegrown intervention. These four intervention types are typical of how CBOs operationalize interventions in order to address the needs of Latinas and recruit and retain Latinas outside of academic settings, while striving to meet funder requirements or do without funding.

The manner in which a CBO functions, including its goals, modes of agency operation, relationship with the community, and intervention development and implementation, expresses its cultural values. CBOs often focus on serving a particular subpopulation, such as immigrants from a particular region, and thus intimately knowing the cultural characteristics of that group becomes part of the CBO's self-definition. Because cultural values and processes are shared, CBOs can draw on them to select and develop salient interventions and appropriate recruitment strategies. Each of the highlighted programs attempts to address both surface and deep cultural dimensions and features a blended facilitation format, a space for *pláticas* and testimonials, and the provision of Spanish-language materials specific to the local population. These examples reflect a rich diversity of programs in terms of geography, populations of Latinas served, and sponsoring organizations.

Replication and Extension Highlight

From 2007 through 2010, the Latino Commission on AIDS (The Commission) implemented in New York City, as a replication and extension, *Latinas Por La Salud* (LPLS) [Latinas for Health], an intensive 12-session HIV prevention intervention for high-risk Latinas. LPLS was developed by Dr. Hortensia Amaro and colleagues from Northeastern University with financial support from the Massachusetts Department of Public Health (Amaro, Raj, Reed, & Cranston, 2002). The curriculum was originally developed to build upon a community-based intervention of home-based "Safety Net parties" implemented in Massachusetts in the 1990s; these one-session interventions, however, were not sufficient to address the varied social and cultural structures that affect women's responses to HIV/AIDS. Firmly rooted in an awareness of the social determinants of HIV risk, the LPLS curriculum includes safer sex negotiation and sexuality education as well as the identification of social factors increasing a Latina's risk for HIV. Impressively, the sessions covered culture, immigration and life in the United States, how to use condoms, condom negotiation, sexually transmitted diseases, domestic violence, self-esteem, economics and future planning, community building, substance use, and a celebration of sexuality. There was also a graduation ceremony. Participants were offered HIV testing and were referred, according to needs, to a broad range of local social services.

At the time that the Commission selected and implemented LPLS (funded by the Pfizer Foundation) there were no Latina-centered interventions in the DEBI project. In terms of replication, of particular interest was whether this type of curriculum was attractive to recent immigrants from Mexico, South America, and the Caribbean. The Commission's implementation extended the original research by incorporating enhanced sessions on key cultural topics. After feedback from the first cohort, the Commission extended information on STDs and condom use, and added a second session on domestic violence. Because sessions on these topics became *pláticas*, they were extended. Facilitators added an extra session focused solely on domestic violence in which women could further *desahorgase* (literally to "un-drown" oneself, but referring to testimonial-based catharsis in a supportive environment). Many of the cohorts went on shopping trips to a local condom selling store to further build sexual confidence, enhance group bonding, and provide concrete skills-building support to each other.

The LPLS groups were facilitated by two bilingual Latinas: one MPH/MSW level director and one HIV-positive Latina from the community. This blended facilitation style combined aspects of *comadrismo*—the lay "CHW"/*promotora* facilitator as a community representative, with *respeto*—the highly educated "expert" facilitator as a representative of the medical establishment. By also having an HIV-positive facilitator the cultural value of *personalismo* was made instrumental. Onsite childcare was also provided to the women, acknowledging Latina childrearing and care roles, and reducing barriers to attendance.

Fourteen cohorts, each consisting of between 6 and 21 participants, completed the intervention. In all, 183 graduated from the program. Thirteen participants (7.2%) reported having been born in the United States; of the rest, 42.7% reported living in the United States for 10 years or less. Residence of 10 years or fewer is commonly considered an indicator of recent immigrant status (Finch & Vega, 2003). All the women considered themselves Hispanic or Latina, with a plurality (45%) indicating they were Mexican and 28% Dominican. Furthermore, 19.6% indicated not knowing their race, and 67.2% selected no racial identifier. Racial categories as commonly defined in surveys may not be relevant to Latinas. This finding is similar to that reported by past surveys on racial and ethnic identification of Latinos. A 2006 Pew Hispanic Center survey found that 48% of Hispanic adults generally describe themselves by their country of origin first.

According to process and outcome monitoring data, LPLS was an effective strategy for reaching the target population with HIV/STD prevention messages. The main form of risk reduction examined in the measures—condom use—became more acceptable and more widely practiced by participants after their participation in the intervention. There was a significant increase in the use of condoms with main partners during vaginal intercourse from baseline to postperiod and the mean difference in frequency of condom use with the main partner after controlling for confounders. The increase in frequency of condom use score was primarily linear (see Figure 17.1), meaning that the women not only continued to use condoms but that condom use increased months after the end of the program. Participants also reported a greater ability to negotiate condom use. In addition, participants demonstrated increased knowledge about HIV, STDs, and condom use; improved attitudes toward condom use; and increased self-esteem and decreased loneliness. Participants reported in postintervention surveys that they appreciated the opportunity to come together in mutual support for the duration of the cohorts, and some expressed a wish to continue meeting after the conclusion of LPLS. That is, group participation may have been an important element contributing to the success of the intervention. One participant noted, "it is not the same to learn from a book or school than among women." Another asked, "Is there a way for the group to stay together and meet again?"

In this CBO replication and extension of an already-evaluated (non-DEBI) Latina-centered intervention, surface and deep structure Latina cultural considerations were addressed. Surface intervention components included facilitation by bilingual Latina women and Spanish language materials. These aspects made it easier to participate in the intervention. The blended facilitation style that allowed for the cultural values of *respeto* and *personalismo* to be manifested made the intervention more deeply salient and engaging for the women. Furthermore, the *comadrismo* engendered by the use of *pláticas*, extra sessions on specific matters of concern to the group (i.e., domestic violence), and the field trip to the condom-carrying store created enhanced saliency. Lastly, provision of childcare made LPLS acceptable to the women by removing an often-cited participation barrier. The supportive environment was instrumental in the program's high retention rate (183 graduates of 204 enrolled overall), which is an unusual achievement for a program of such length (i.e., 13 sessions) and intensity. When both surface and deep cultural dimensions are addressed, recruitment, retention, and behavior changes are made possible.

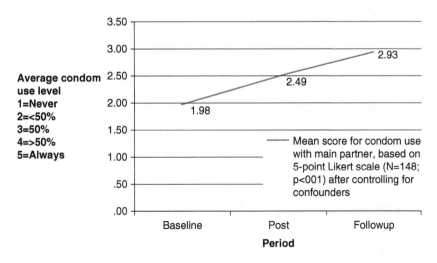

FIGURE 17.1 Frequency of condom use by period in the Latinas Por La Salud Intervention.

DEBI Adaptation Highlight

Adaptation, which is particularly necessary to ensure intervention relevance for Latinas, entails modifying key characteristics, activities, and delivery methods without contradicting core elements, theory, or internal logic of an intervention (McKleroy, Galbraith, Cummings, Jones, Harshbarger, et al., 2006). As reviewed above, the DEBI project, as a direct CDC funding mechanism, poses a conundrum to Latina-serving CBOs because of its lack of interventions that target Latinas. As one of the few female-specific group-level skills-building interventions within the DEBI project, SISTA (Sisters Informing Sisters about Topics on AIDS) has been widely implemented by Latina-serving organizations, although the intervention was originally created specifically for African American women (DiClemente & Wingood, 1995). Five peer-led group sessions are conducted that focus on ethnic and gender pride, HIV knowledge, and skills training around sexual risk-reduction behaviors and decision making. Even if the SISTA intervention addresses specific Latina risk determinants, English materials may need to be translated to Spanish before implementation. Thus, there is an immediate need for CBOs to engage surface structure adaptations before delving into any deep structure adaptations.

Puerto Rico CoNCRA (Community Network for Clinical Research on AIDS) is a community-based clinic in San Juan, Puerto Rico, established in 1990 that implements multiple HIV prevention and treatment programs. From 2004 through 2008, CoNCRA adapted and implemented SISTA for its local target population of high-risk Puerto Rican women ages 18–29 years. First, CoNCRA implemented *Amigas* (friends) as a loose translation of the SISTA intervention that entailed some surface cultural adaptations (i.e., the use of Spanish language songs instead of the poems by African American authors presented in the original intervention) but retained the original five-group session structure of SISTA. Realizing that such a surface level adaptation was not sufficient, in particular at retaining the women, CoNCRA implemented a further adaptation, called *ALAS*, literally "wings," but actually an acronym for Amigas Luchando Antes el SIDA (friends fighting against AIDS), to address specific deep structure cultural needs.

ALAS included additional opportunities for participants to deconstruct their identity as a Puerto Rican/Latina woman, and made the major structural change of providing the intervention as a one-time 3-day retreat, or *campamento*, rather than a five-session intervention spread over several weeks, as SISTA was originally implemented. By holding a retreat, the women were to bond more closely with other women, learn from each other, and most importantly stay for the whole intervention. There were a total of 10 *ALAS* cohorts/retreats. The retreats were held at a *parador* or local country inns that are meant to give individuals a sense of the beauty of the island in a low-cost but charming (all inclusive) hotel alternative. *ALAS* was facilitated by bilingual women: one peer and another female with Masters level education. Interestingly, *ALAS* also included a male staff member who could participate in role plays, allowing the women to have a realistic setting for developing assertiveness and communication skills with a male. In doing so, *ALAS*, allowed the women to tackle head-on *machisimo* and *marianismo*, rallied by a supportive group of females. Although most of the participants in *ALAS* were born in Puerto Rico, 35.7% were born elsewhere, mostly the mainland United States. One of the emphases of the adaptation was the salience of an identity alternately described as Puerto Rican, Caribbean, Latina, and Hispanic, which emerged in discussions of and challenges to the word "Latina" with the participants. This was an important deep cultural adaptation for both the participants born in Puerto Rico and off the island. This identity aspect—migration and transnationalism—is an important cultural consideration that CoNCRA added to SISTA.

The retreat format of *ALAS* was shown to be an effective adaptation in achieving the desired outcomes as well as in improving recruitment and retention rates. A process and outcome monitoring review of the interventions, conducted in collaboration between CoNCRA and the Latino Commission on AIDS, found that intention to use condoms in the future increased from baseline to postsurvey conducted 3 months after the intervention ended; *ALAS* was also successful in decreasing the number of participants' potentially high-risk sexual relations without condoms. In addition, ALAS participants demonstrated a statistically significant increase in HIV/AIDS knowledge scores between baseline and postsurvey. Reported control over condom use increased significantly between baseline and postsurvey.

CoNCRA's experience with *ALAS* and *Amigas* demonstrates how cultural dimensions are considered and can be operationalized. The retreat format of *ALAS* allowed the participants a respite from their daily activities as caregivers, and a chance to come together in a supportive environment, a chance for *desahogarse*, as they went through the intervention. The women were more likely to stay for the entire intervention because they saw it as a pleasant retreat away from home, rather than an added responsibility of weekly group sessions in the midst of weekly activities. This surface cultural adaptation was the key in recruiting and retaining Latinas in an intervention not originally targeting them. The deep cultural adaptations, including discussions focusing on migration, transnationalism, and Latina identity, allowed for the intervention's increased salience. Given the exceptional short-term and intermediate outcomes that *ALAS* produced, this promising adaptation warrants further, rigorous evaluation to assess additional outcomes and long-term impacts, as well as support for homegrown efforts.

Homegrown Prevention Interventions for Latinas

A "homegrown" intervention is developed locally in close collaboration with an at-risk population in the communities served by an organization. Many homegrown interventions are developed organically: as CBOs look to provide prevention services they refine their practice over many years, and may eventually "standardize" the practice into curricula or intervention manuals. Homegrown interventions are usually prized for their cultural and linguistic competency and local community relevance. Some homegrown interventions are replicated by other organizations, although most remain standard practices only in the CBOs in which they were originally developed (Dworkin, Pinto, Hunter, Rapkin, & Ramien, 2008).

Mujeres Unidas Contra el SIDA (Mujeres) is a CBO in San Antonio, Texas, founded in 1994 as a bilingual and bicultural support group primarily serving Mexican-American Latinas infected and/or affected by HIV and lacking a support system. Many women came together to form and develop Mujeres as a response to the HIV crisis in the 1990s and the needs of their families, both in the United States and abroad (Interview with Yolanda Escobar, 2010).

One of the organization's main interventions is the *Pláticas* program, which is truly organic in its origins: in the mid-1990s, when the organization was starting a support group, Mujeres staff who conducted community presentations always brought along an HIV-positive woman from the community to co-facilitate.

This gave the co-facilitators an opportunity to tell their story of learning their status and living as an HIV-positive Latina and to develop their public speaking skills. As a next step, the women received more in-depth training, which covered HIV 101, mental health, STDs, how to find support when supporting others, and how to become "Madrinas" (Godmothers). The *madrinas* held *pláticas*, or small group sessions, in the community with approximately five women each. These groups were social in nature, with *madrinas* making the decision about the appropriate time to introduce HIV information into each group's discussion. The *pláticas* took place mainly in participants' homes, but also in CBOs, schools, hairdressing classes, and other venues representing core activities in the community. The reach of the groups expanded by word of mouth, reminiscent of "Tupperware Parties." Approximately—four to six *madrinas* at a given time, compensated with rotating stipends, facilitated the program and helped develop both its content and reach. The *Pláticas* program engendered an offshoot intergenerational initiative, upon request of the participants, in which women and their teenage daughters met in small group settings to acquire the skills to openly discuss HIV, STDs, drug use, and initiation of sex.

The program was funded by the Pfizer Foundation for 3 years, during which time it reached at least 200 participants per year; participants demonstrated an increase in knowledge about HIV (the main outcome of interest). In other years, the program was not consistently evaluated due to lack of funding. The majority of participants were second- and third-generation Mexican American women. Many of the participants were so-called "damas de la casa" (housewives), who initially had a very low perception of HIV risk and did not use condoms. The *pláticas* were a way to come together, to learn in a mutually supportive environment, and to *desahogarse*. The program closed in 2009 due to loss of funding after 12 years in existence.

The *Pláticas* program, as originated and implemented by Mujeres, used a form of the community health worker or *promotora* approach. One of the key aspects of its longevity was the support provided to the *madrinas* (as *promotoras*) by a program coordinator who was qualified as an MSW/registered nurse. This was a much needed resource of self-care for the *madrinas*, all of whom were infected or affected by HIV, particularly when they provided support to newly diagnosed women. As such, *Pláticas* provided a space for them to engage in *comadrismo* while enjoying the credibility and support associated with the mental health professional, or *respeto*. When considering different program options, Mujeres decided that the DEBIs would not work for its target population, because no DEBI had been developed with a Mexican American population, and even those adapted to a Spanish-speaking audience do not use Mexican American idioms and do not include Mexican American characters in role-play scenarios. It would be too much of a burden for Mujeres to adapt a DEBI, and Mujeres did not want to compromise its commitment to addressing local needs by implementing a DEBI that would not be a cultural fit. In growing their own Latinas initiative, Mujeres capitalized on *comadrismo* and *respeto*, as well as the support group atmosphere to *desahogar* that allowed participants a space for reflection and self-care. As a homegrown initiative, *Pláticas* was foremost a community-based, local intervention relevant to the community and flexible to its needs.

Hybrid: Homegrown plus DEBI

The last intervention that we will highlight is a hybrid approach combining a DEBI—in this case SISTA—with a long-standing homegrown intervention.

This hybrid intervention is a unique approach not just in its goals (explicitly including building community leadership), but also in its intentional use of the DEBI curriculum to bolster a homegrown intervention.

Voces Latinas [Latina Voices] is a CBO in Queens, New York City, that began in 2003 as a series of community forums and conferences, allowing immigrant Latinas a space to speak out about conditions in their lives placing them at high risk for HIV, including documentation status, cultural norms, domestic violence, alcohol and substance abuse, and isolation. Voces Latinas developed into an organization offering a variety of services to Latinas (interview with Nathaly Rubio-Torio, 2010). In 2007, Voces Latinas started the "Promotoras Leadership and Advocacy Program" (Promotoras) for high-risk clients who had progressed through other services offered by the organization and who felt empowered to become involved in their community as a way of continuing their healing and giving back.

Promotoras, more commonly used in southwestern and rural regions, were seen by local stakeholders as an important component of any HIV intervention targeting Latinas, lending credibility and empowering a Latina community in Queens that is expanding rapidly. The promotoras go through a rigorous recruitment process: they are nominated by senior promotoras, interviewed, and oriented regarding a 1-year program commitment once accepted. This commitment involves 12–14 weeks of training, following the Promotoras curriculum developed by Voces Latinas, as well as doing community events and outreach alongside staff and other promotoras. The curriculum has three major components: HIV prevention, domestic violence prevention, and advocacy/community mobilization. Once trained, promotoras conduct outreach in the community to identify other women at risk. They reach out to their social networks and visit local businesses to leave condoms and informational baskets. The promotoras help Voces Latinas stay in touch with the community's emerging Latina population. Approximately 20% of new Voces Latinas clients are identified through this outreach.

The program also involves the promotoras in numerous community activities, from advocacy days in Albany, New York, to presentations in community forums, and cofacilitation of some of the organization's support groups together with the professional staff members. Senior promotoras help cofacilitate parts of the Promotoras training by incorporating their field outreach expertise. Voces Latinas employs the same hybrid of comadrismo and respeto noted in the facilitation styles of the programs reviewed above. The promotoras do not receive any financial compensation for their efforts; they do this work out of commitment to the community and as a way to receive further experience and training. All of the promotoras are immigrant, monolingual Spanish-speaking Latinas who appreciate this chance at exposure to community work in practice. Most (approximately seven of nine current promotoras) have been in the United States for under 10 years (Finch & Vega, 2003). A total of 15 promotoras have been through the program thus far, with nine still acting in that capacity. Many of the women are affected by HIV, and some of the past promotoras have been HIV positive.

In 2010, Voces Latinas collaborated with another New York City organization to coimplement the SISTA intervention with their clients. Voces Latinas decided on a unique hybrid of the programs: the clients who participate in SISTA, as adapted for Latinas, throughout the cycle will be given the opportunity to graduate into the Promotoras training program. The combination of SISTA and Promotoras is meant to serve two purposes: first, retention in SISTA is expected to be high because of potential graduation to Promotoras and assumption of a leadership role in the community; and for the *Promotoras* program, the SISTA component is meant to add content on HIV and condom use as well as to start the group on its conversation, to be carried out throughout the rest of the year-long *Promotoras* training, about what their roles can be in HIV prevention.

Outcomes are not yet available for this hybrid (homegrown plus DEBI) initiative, because it recently started. It will be of interest to learn from the experiences of this hybrid approach that encompasses many of the characteristics of the other interventions described here: combining *respeto* with *comadrismo* to achieve a facilitation style that resonates with the community, building the skills of lay community health workers to reach deep into the Latina community, creating a supportive group learning environment (*desahogarse*), and incorporating an evidence-based intervention (SISTA). Other characteristics that are part of Voces Latinas' approach are less present in the other interventions reviewed: incorporating a strong emphasis on leadership and advocacy in the form of community mobilization (*abogar*), and utilizing an evidence-based intervention as a complement to an existing, successful homegrown approach.

Comparison and Review of the Highlighted Interventions from the Field

All highlighted interventions address surface and deep cultural dimensions (see Table 17.1 for a summary of their characteristics). All have a blended facilitation model involving a member of the community and a "professional." This approach is a combination of *comadrismo* and *respeto*, recognizing the importance of experiential credibility, particularly when dealing with sensitive health issues, as well as the finding that "professionals" are accorded respect that is useful in an intervention. A *promotora* is part of the in-group and thus also invokes the value of *personalismo*. The peer is a broker and the professional is a transmitter of formal service and information. As a result, Latinas were taught through support and information in a value-laden manner ways to make healthy personal decisions.

Many of the women in the highlighted interventions are immigrants or transnationals who have undergone physical and emotional journeys. The interventions, in their deep structure cultural considerations, have allowed women to grow through expression of life histories to a supportive group—to *desahorgarse* and thus to both alleviate some of the psychological burden as well as validate themselves. The women were allowed to give testimonials. The women's roles as *damas de la casa* were also recognized and the interventions created spaces where scripts of being tied to the house and caregiving could be disrupted. Women were pampered and literally taken out of their personal environments. This goes further than most *promotora* approaches by incorporating both surface and deep cultural and interpersonal scripts.

Some evidence is available showing the effectiveness of these approaches in reaching Latinas with HIV prevention messages and influencing their risk behaviors. Because the Commission and CoNCRA were implementing interventions that were designated as "proven effective" and packaged, there is much more outcome monitoring data available. The two CBOs implementing homegrown interventions have collected substantial process data but outcome data are pending. This pending data status speaks to the need for more funds directed at evaluating culturally appropriate homegrown interventions.

Table 17.1 Surface and Deep Structure Cultural Considerations across Differing Types of Highlighted Interventions

	Participants	*Surface*	*Deep*
Adaptation of SISTA	Puerto Rican, transnational	• Bilingual facilitators • Spanish language materials • Retreat	• Blended facilitators • Focus on identification and transnationalism • Concrete skills enhancement: use of males in the retreat.
Replication of Latinas por la Salud	Mainly Mexican and Dominican Recent immigrants	• Bilingual facilitators • Spanish language materials • Childcare provided	• Blended facilitators • Additional session on domestic violence • Focus on identification and transnationalism • Graduation • Concrete skills enhancement: Field trip to condom store
Homegrown: *Pláticas*	Second- and third-generation Mexican American	• Bilingual facilitators • Spanish language materials • Held in venues frequented by the community	• Blended facilitators • Intergenerational component • Organic in nature
Homegrown plus EBI: *Promotoras* plus SISTA	Recent immigrants from various countries in Latin America	• Monolingual Spanish facilitators • Spanish language materials • Field trips to Albany • Sponsored conference attendance	• Blended facilitators • Session on domestic violence and being an advocate • Graduation • Hands-on outreach experience in the community

ON THE HORIZON, SOWING THE SEEDS OF LATINA-SPECIFIC HIV PREVENTION

In his review of the National AIDS Strategy, Holtgrave (2010) challenged researchers to deliberate about fundamental research questions that need to be rapidly investigated as an essential precursor to addressing the goals expressed within the new strategy. Although existing prevention tools have had a significant positive impact on controlling the severity of the epidemic, an urgent need remains for new prevention options if we are to promote health and reduce the social impact of HIV in the United States. We need to apply an integrated concept as well as a broader view of "social medicine" to our National AIDS Strategy. Increasingly, emphasis on biomedical and behavioral interventions delivered in tandem will help to ensure that the tools for combating HIV at our disposal are maximized, and that our social and medical efforts work in conjunction rather than at odds. A number of promising biomedical strategies to consider in ongoing prevention efforts are on the horizon, and will likely change the sociomedical landscape of HIV prevention and treatment efforts.

Microbicides

Many women, because of limited economic options and gender inequality, cannot reliably negotiate sexual encounters, leaving them vulnerable to unwanted pregnancy and sexually transmitted infections, including HIV. Women often cannot control if or when condoms are used by their male partners even after participating in prevention interventions. Women need prevention tools that they can decide to use on their own. Microbicides, the application of vaginal gels containing antiretroviral drugs to prevent HIV transmission during sex, have often been heralded as such a potential tool. In fact, researchers have developed a mathematical model that shows that if even a small proportion of women in lower income countries used a 60% efficacious microbicide in half the sexual encounters in which condoms are not used, 2.5 million HIV infections could be averted over 3 years (Culter & Justman, 2008). Researchers (Karim, Karim, Frohlich, Grobler, Baxter, et al., 2010) testing a vaginal microbicide with an antiretroviral (ARV) drug called tenofovir reported its use before and after sex was significantly more protective against HIV infection than a placebo gel among women at high risk of HIV. Specifically, there were 39% fewer HIV infections among women who used tenofovir gel before and after sex than among those who used the placebo gel.

Researchers, policy makers, and advocates argue that vaginal microbicides might offer women control over HIV prevention, including through covert use (Bentley, Morrow, Fullem, Chesney, Horton, et al., 2000). Covert use, however, could bring added mistrust and physical danger, expose male partners to microbicides without their knowledge, and elicit questions about whether covert use is really empowering (Woodsong, 2004). Although many would agree with the goal of increasing women's power and autonomy in sexual health decision-making, women may resent having to assume sole responsibility for using microbicides. Microbicides could become another example of women taking on the burden for protection. The use of microbicides, currently hailed as a great step toward protection against HIV, may be scripted by women for its contraceptive use (Morrow et al., 2007). The use of microbicides by Latinas and by women in general will be scripted and contextualized by their current relationship, sexual norms, socioeconomic status, other health concerns, and cultural values. Encouraging Latinas to utilize such a preventive measure would still entail increasing awareness, knowledge, and perceived benefits along with empowering them.

PrEP

With an effective vaccine still years away, there is mounting evidence that antiretroviral drugs may be able to play an important role in reducing the risk of HIV infection (Denton, Estes, & Sun, 2008). An effective daily preventative treatment could help address the urgent need for female-controlled prevention methods and, when combined with existing prevention measures, help reduce new HIV infections among men and women at high risk. Researchers are investigating a promising approach called oral preexposure prophylaxis (PrEP), which involves daily use of an ARV tablet. A safety trial (Peterson, Taylor, Roddy, Belai, Phillips, et al., 2007) of tenofovir for HIV prevention among young women showed PrEP with tenofovir was both safe and acceptable for use by HIV-negative women. Other research (Paltiel, Freedberg, & Scott, 2009) has shown that in a cohort with a mean age of 34 years, PrEP reduced lifetime HIV infection risk from 44% to 25% and increased average life expectancy from 39.9 to 40.7 years; PrEP could be a cost-effective option for younger or higher-risk populations. Even if effective, Latinas would have to be educated about the benefits and use of PrEP. Furthermore, there is the potential for risk disinhibition or sexual risk compensation (Guest, Shattuck, Johnson, Akumatey, Kekawo, et al., 2008) and Latinas do have high rates of other sexually transmitted diseases (CDC, 2007). Thus, culturally sensitive counseling and other educational sessions would still be of importance as a complementary preventative practice alongside PrEP.

Treatment as Prevention

Treatment as prevention is a term increasingly used to describe HIV prevention methods that use antiretroviral treatment with HIV-positive individuals to decrease the chance of HIV transmission. In 2008, a group of Swiss scientists produced the first ever consensus statement that asserted that an HIV-positive person who is taking effective antiretroviral therapy, has an undetectable viral load, and is free from STDs has a negligible risk of infecting others with the virus (Vernazza, Hirschel, Bernasconi, & Flepp, 2008). Although HIV treatment can significantly reduce infectiousness if taken as prescribed, it cannot eliminate the transmission risk completely. Thus, treatment as prevention on a public health level does need to be complemented with medication education, condom use, and adherence strategies that are culturally sensitive. It needs to be noted that even though there has been a decline in overall AIDS mortality, the number of deaths from AIDS among Latinos has remained relatively stable since the beginning of the new millennium (CDC, 2010), signaling that access to care remains a major barrier, particularly when Latinos have low insurance rates and there are HIV medication waiting lists across many U.S. states. Only with increased access to treatment for HIV-positive Latinos overall can treatment as prevention become an option for this group.

CONCLUDING THOUGHTS

It is imperative to understand not only the social, cultural, and political conditions of sexual practice and associated risk of HIV transmission for Latinas, but also the programmatic response to the epidemic. Interventions must be culturally sensitive and focus on empowering and supporting communities. Community-based organizations have a front-line role in prevention activities and as such they are key partners in the National AIDS Strategy (The White House, 2010). The highlighted interventions from the field exemplify that communities can and do respond to the threat of HIV and can do more if supported and funded.

Although the CDC has identified a limited number of evidence-based interventions (EBIs) for Latinas, there remains an urgent need to develop additional culturally appropriate EBIs for various subpopulations of Latinas. There is an inherent tension between the need for clear standardized effective interventions and the need to avoid rigid applications to the detriment of tailoring interventions to populations and settings. Funding agencies should consider continued and increased development, evaluation, and funding of homegrown culturally sensitive programs for Latinas. The highlighted interventions show the importance of acknowledging and building on community responses, instead of relying on externally validated, "one size fits all" interventions.

Promising biomedical approaches are on the horizon that need to be coupled with community-based approaches and with increased access to care. There is a need for a combined systems approach to prevention so that there are multiple access points and multiple intervention types targeting Latinas—both structural and individual behavioral interventions that are both salient and acceptable. There is a need for a public health model to arise that acknowledges that different social-cultural environments require different prevention responses that take account of the cultural and eschew narrowly validated, generic interventions. Interventions that address surface, as well as deep cultural dimensions need to be considered an essential element of any National AIDS Strategy implementation plan addressing Latina HIV prevention needs.

REFERENCES

Abel, E., & Chambers, K. B. (2002). Factors that influence vulnerability to STDS and HIV/AIDS among Hispanic women. *Health Care for Women International, 25,* 761–780.

Amaro, H., Raj, A., Reed, E., & Cranston, K. (2002). Implementation and long-term outcomes of two HIV intervention programs for Latinas. *Health Promotion Practice, 3,* 245–254.

Bentley, M., Morrow, K. M., Fullem, A., Chesney, M. A., Horton, S. D., Rosenberg, Z., & Mayer, K. H. (2000). Acceptability of a novel vaginal microbicide during a safety trial among low-risk women. *Family Planning Perspective, 32,* 184–188.

Bernal, G., Bonilla, J., & Bellido, C. (1995). Ecological validity and cultural sensitivity for outcome research: Issues for the cultural adaptation and development of psychosocial treatments with Hispanics. *Journal of Abnormal Child Psychology, 23,* 67–82.

Centers for Disease Control and Prevention. (2007). *Sexually transmitted disease surveillance, 2006.* Atlanta, GA: U.S. Department of Health and Human Services.

Centers for Disease Control and Prevention. (2009). *Compendium of evidence-based interventions.* http://www.cdc.gov/hiv/topics/research/prs/evidence-based-interventions.htm.

Centers for Disease Control and Prevention. (2010). *HIV/AIDS surveillance report 2008,* Volume 20. Atlanta, GA: U.S. Department of Health and Human Services.

Cervantes, R. C., & Castro, F. G. (1985). Stress, coping, and Mexican American mental health: A systematic review. *Hispanic Journal of Behavioral Sciences, 1,* 1–73.

Cherrington, A., Ayala, G., Amick, H., Scarinci, I., Allison, J., & Corbie-Smith, G. (2008). Applying the community health worker model to diabetes management: Using mixed methods to assess implementation and effectiveness. *Journal of Health Care for Poor and Underserved, 19,* 1044–1059.

Collins, C., Harshbarger, C., Sawyer, R., & Hamdallah, M. (2006). The diffusion of effective behavioral interventions project: Development, implementation, and lessons learned. *AIDS Education and Prevention, 18*(A), 5–20.

Cutler, B., & Justman, J. (2008). Vaginal microbicides and the prevention of HIV transmission. *Lancet Infectious Diseases, 8,* 685–697.

Das, M., Chu, P. L., Santos, G-M., Scheer, S., Vittinghoff, E., McFarland, W., & Colfax, G. N. (2010). Decreases in community viral load are accompanied by reductions in new HIV infections in San Francisco. *PLoS One, 5*(6), e11068.

Denton, P. W., Estes, J. D., Sun, Z., et al. (2008). Antiretroviral pre-exposure prophylaxis prevents vaginal transmission of HIV-1 in humanized BLT mice. *PLoS Medicine, 5*(1), e16.

DiClemente, R. J., & Wingood, G. M. (1995). A randomized controlled trial of an HIV sexual risk-reduction intervention for young African-American women. *Journal of the American Medical Association, 274,* 1271–1276.

Dworkin, S. L., Pinto, R. M., Hunter, J., Rapkin, B., & Remien, R. H. (2008). Keeping the spirit of community partnerships alive in the scale up of HIV/AIDS prevention: Critical reflections on the roll out of DEBI (diffusion of effective behavioral interventions). *American Journal of Community Psychology, 42,* 51–59.

Elder, J. P., Ayala, G. X., Slymen, D. J., Arredondo, E. M., & Campbell, N. R. (2009). Evaluating psychosocial and behavioral mechanism of change on a tailored communication intervention. *Health Education and Behavior, 36,* 366–380.

Espinoza, L., Hall, I., Hardnett, F., Selik, R. M., Qiang, L., & Lee, L. M. (2007). Characteristics of persons with heterosexually acquired HIV infection, United States 1999–2004. *American Journal of Public Health, 97,* 144–149.

Finch, B. K., & Vega, W. A. (2003). Acculturation stress, social support, and self-rated health among Latinos in California. *Journal of Immigrant Health, 5,* 109–117.

Galanti, G. (2003). The Hispanic family and male–female relationships: An overview. *Journal of Transcultural Nursing, 14,* 180–185.

Grieco, E. M. (2009). Race and Hispanic origin of the foreign-born population in the United States: 2007. *Race and American Community Survey Results, ACS-II.* Washington, DC: U.S. Census Bureau.

Groff, J. Y., Mullen, P. D., Byrd, T., Shelton, A. J., Lees, E., & Goode, J. (2000). Decision making, beliefs, and attitudes toward hysterectomy: A focus group study with medically underserved women in Texas. *Journal of Women's Health & Gender-Based Medicine, 9,* 39–50.

Guest, G., Dominick, S., Johnson, L., Akumatey, B., Kekawo, C., Essie, E., Chen, P-L., & MacQueen, K. M. (2008). Changes in sexual risk behavior among participants in a PrEP HIV prevention trial. *Sexually Transmitted Diseases, 35,* 1002–1008.

Hadler, S. L., Smith, D. K., Moore, J. S., & Holmberg, S. D. (2001). HIV infection in women in the United States: Status at the millennium. *Journal of the American Medical Association (JAMA), 285,* 1186–1192.

Herbst, J. H., Kay, L. S., Passin, W. F., Lyles, C. M., Crepaz, N., Marín, B. V., & the HIV/AIDS Prevention Research Synthesis (PRS) Team. (2007). A systematic review and meta-analysis of behavioral interventions to reduce HIV risk behaviors of Hispanics in the United States and Puerto Rico. *AIDS Behavior, 11,* 25–47.

Holtgrave, D. (2010). On the epidemiologic and economic importance of the national AIDS strategy for the United States. *Journal of AIDS, 14,* 493–503.

Institute of Medicine. (2003). *The future of the public's health in the 21st century.* Washington, DC: National Academy Press.

Karim, Q. A., Karim, S. A., Frohlich, J. A., Grobler, A. G., Baxter, C., Mansoor, L. E., Kharsany, A. B. M., et al. (2010). Effectiveness and safety of tenofovir gel, an antiretroviral microbicide, for the prevention of HIV infection in women. *Science, 329,* 1168–1174.

Lyles, C. M., Crepaz, N., Herbst, J. H., Kay, L. S., & the HIV/AIDS Prevention Research Synthesis Team. (2006). Evidence- based HIV behavioral prevention from the perspective of CDC's HIV/AIDS Prevention Research Synthesis Team. *AIDS Education and Prevention, 18*(A), 21–31.

Lyles, M. C., Kay, L. S., Crepaz, N., Herbst, J. H., Passin, W. F., Kim, A. S., Rama, S. M., et al. (2007). Best-evidence interventions: Findings from a systematic review of HIV behavioral interventions for US populations at high risk, 2000–2004. *American Journal of Public Health, 97*(1), 133–143.

Marin, G. (1989). AIDS prevention among Hispanics: Needs, risk behaviors, and cultural values. *Public Health Reports, 104*(5), 411–415.

Marin, G., & Triandis, H. C. (1985). Allocentrism as an important characteristic of the behavior of Latin American and Hispanics. In R. Diaz (Ed.), *Cross-cultural and national studies in social psychology* (pp. 85–104). Amsterdam: Elsevier Science Publishers.

Markus, H., & Kitayama, S. (1991). Culture and the self: Implications for cognition, emotion, and motivation. *Psychological Review, 98*, 224–253.

Markus, H., & Kitayama, S. (1994). The cultural construction of self and emotion: Implications for social behavior. In H. R. Markus (Ed.), *Emotion and culture: Empirical studies of mutual influence* (pp. 89–130). Washington, DC: American Psychological Association.

Mckleroy, V. S., Galbraith, J., Cummings, B., Jones, P., Harshbarger, C., Collins, C., et al. (2006). Adapting evidence-based behavioral interventions for new settings and target populations. *AIDS Education and Prevention, 18*(A), 59–73.

Mier, N., Ory, M. G., & Medina, A. A. (2010). Anatomy of culturally sensitive interventions promoting nutrition and exercise in Hispanics: A critical examination of existing literature. *Health Promotion Practice, 11*, 541–554.

Minkler, M., & Wallerstein, N. (1997). Improving health through community organizing and community building. In K. Glanz, F. M. Lewis, & B. Rimer, (Eds.), *Health behavior and health education* (pp. 241–269). San Francisco, CA: Jossey-Bass Publishers.

Morrow, K. M., et al (2007). Willingness to use microbicides is affected by the importance of product characteristics, use parameters and protective properties. *Journal of AIDS, 45*, 93–101.

Paltiel, A. D., Freedberg, K. A., Scott, C. A., Schackman, B. R., Losina, E., Wang, B., Seage, G. R., et al. (2009). HIV pre-exposure prophylaxis (PrEP) in the United States: Impact on lifetime infection risk, clinical outcomes, and cost-effectiveness. *Clinical Infectious Diseases, 48*, 806–815.

Peragallo, N. (1996). Latino women and AIDS risk. *Public Health Nursing, 13*, 217–222.

Peragallo, N. P., DeForge, B., O'Campo, P., Lee, S., Kim, Y. J., Cianelli, R., & Ferrer, L. (2005). A randomized clinical trial of an HIV risk reduction intervention among low-income Latina women. *Nursing Research, 54*(2), 108–118.

Peterson, L., Taylor, D., Roddy, R., et al. (2007). Tenofovir disoproxil fumarate for prevention of HIV infection in women: A phase 2, double-blind, randomized, placebo-controlled trial. *PLoS Clinical Trials, 2*(5), e27.

Pew Hispanic Center. (2007). The 2006 national survey of Latinos. Washington, DC.

Preloran, H. M., Browner, C. H., & Lieber, E. (2001). Strategies for motivating Latino couples' participation in qualitative health research and their effects on sample construction. *American Journal of Public Health, 91*, 1832–1841.

Ramos, I. N., May, M., & Ramos, K. (2001). Environmental health training of Promotoras in Colonias along the Texas-Mexico border. *American Journal of Public Health, 91*, 568–570.

Resnicow, K., Baranowski, T., Ahluwalia, J. S., & Braithwaite, R. L. (1999). Cultural sensitivity in public health: Defined and demystified. *Ethnicity & Disease, 9*, 10–21.

Reynoso-Vallejo, H. (2009). Support group for Latino caregivers of dementia elders: Cultural humility and cultural competence. *Ageing International, 34*, 67–78.

Rhodes, S. D., Foley, K. L., Zometa, C. S., & Bloom, F. R. (2007). Lay health advisor interventions among Hispanics/Latinos a qualitative systematic review. *American Journal of Preventive Medicine, 33*, 418–427.

Rosenstock, I. M. (1966). "Why people use health services." *Milbank Memorial Fund Quarterly, 44,* 94–127.

Sabogal, F., & Catania, A. (1996). HIV risk factors, condom use and HIV antibody testing among heterosexual Hispanics: The national AIDS behavioral surveys. *Hispanic Journal of Behavioral Sciences, 18,* 367–391.

Schlickau, J. M., & Wilson, M. E. (2005). Breastfeeding as health-promoting behaviour for Hispanic women: Literature review. *Journal of Advanced Nursing, 52,* 200–210.

Stallworth, J. M., Andía, J. F., Burgess, R., Alvarez, M. E., & Collins, C. (2009). Diffusion of effective behavioral interventions and Hispanic/Latino populations. *AIDS Education and Prevention, 21*(5), 152–163.

Sue, S. (1998). In search of cultural competence in psychotherapy and counseling. *American Psychologist, 53,* 440–448.

Taylor, J. M. (1996). Cultural stories: Latina and Portuguese daughters and mothers. In B. J. R. Leadbeater & N. Way (Eds.), *Urban girls: Resisting stereotypes, creating identities* (pp.117–131). New York: New York University Press.

Vega, M. Y. (2009). The CHANGE approach to capacity building assistance. *AIDS Education and Prevention, 21,* 137–151.

Veniegas, R. C., Uyen, H. K., Rosales, R., & Arellanes, M. (2009). HIV prevention technology transfer: Challenges and strategies in the real world. *American Journal of Public Health, 99,* S124–S130.

Vernazza, P., Hirschel, B., Bernasconi, E., & Flepp, M. (2008). Les personnes séropositives ne souffrant d'aucune autre MST et suivant un traitement antirétroviral efficace ne transmettent pas le VIH par voie sexuelle. *Bulletin des Médecins Suisses, 9,* 5.

Viswanathan, M., Kraschnewski, J. L., Nishikawa, B., Morgan, L. C., Honeycutt, A. A., Thieda, P., Lohr, K. N., et al. (2010). Outcomes and costs of community health worker interventions: A systematic review. *Medical Care, 48,* 792–808.

White House Office of National AIDS Policy. (2010). *National HIV/AIDS strategy for the United States.* Washington, DC: White House, July 13, 2010.

Witmer, A. (1995). Community health workers: Integral members of the health care work force. *American Journal of Public Health, 85,* 1055–1058.

Woodsong, C. (2004). Covert use of topical microbicides: Implications for acceptability and use. *Perspectives in Sexual Reproductive Health, 36,* 127–131.

18 Interventions to Prevent HIV and Other Sexually Transmitted Diseases among Latino Migrants

Thomas M. Painter, Kurt C. Organista,
Scott D. Rhodes, and
Fernando M. Sañudo

INTRODUCTION

Our chapter begins with an overview of sociodemographic characteristics of Latino migrants in the United States and the features of their mobile livelihoods that can affect their vulnerability to infection by HIV and other sexually transmitted diseases (STDs), and their access to prevention, care, and treatment services. We summarize findings from studies of HIV/STD risk factors and infection among Latino migrants and emphasize the need for interventions to prevent infection among them. We describe two approaches for developing HIV/STD prevention interventions for Latino migrants: adapting evidence-based interventions designed for nonmigrants for use with Latino migrants and developing interventions specifically for Latino migrants. We illustrate the latter approach by describing three interventions that several chapter co-authors helped to develop, deliver, and evaluate. Fernando Sañudo describes *Tres Hombres Sin Fronteras* for male Latino farmworkers in San Diego County, California; Kurt Organista describes a pilot intervention for male migrant Latino day laborers in Berkeley, California; and Scott Rhodes describes *HoMBReS*, an intervention for recent immigrant Latino males in central rural North Carolina. To our knowledge, these are the only HIV/STD prevention interventions for Latino migrants or recent immigrants that have been evaluated for efficacy and described in published reports. For each intervention, we describe the perceived need leading to its creation, how it was developed, and its content and delivery, summarize reported evidence of its efficacy, and describe factors that the intervention codevelopers and their community partners believe contributed to the success of their intervention projects. We conclude by considering the common and differentiating characteristics of the interventions and the implications for HIV/STD prevention efforts among Latino migrants.

Our review of HIV/STD risks and infection among Latino migrants describes structural, situational, and behavioral factors that can affect migrants' risk of infection. During the development of several of the interventions we describe, participants also expressed concerns about broader socioeconomic factors that affected their lives and livelihoods: obtaining gainful employment, housing, health care, and food. Although the three interventions do not address these broader factors directly, we stress in our discussion that approaches to HIV/STD prevention for Latino migrants must do more than focus on individual actions that affect their infection risks. Greater attention must be given to clarifying and *influencing* the mechanisms and processes that link migrants' circumstances to their ability to manage HIV/STD risks. The *HoMBReS* intervention, described by Scott Rhodes, draws on social networks that occur among immigrant Latino soccer players, and represents a welcome step in this direction. More interventions of this kind are needed to influence the social environments within which migrants seek their livelihoods and cope with HIV/STD infection risks to themselves, their sex partners, and their families.

LATINO MIGRANTS IN THE UNITED STATES

Latino migrants are those foreign-born, often undocumented Latino men and women who seek employment opportunities by traveling periodically between their countries of origin in Latin America and the United States. Many find jobs as day laborers or service workers in urban and suburban areas, or as farmworkers and laborers in agroprocessing and other industries in rural areas. By contrast, Latino immigrants, many of whom may do the same kind of work, travel to the United States with the intention of settling permanently (Organista et al., 2004). Although the two terms are often used interchangeably, we focus on those Latinos who, like migrants in other world areas, engage in mobile livelihoods to exploit transnational action spaces in order to obtain the resources they and their families need for their well-being (López, 2007; Massey et al., 2005; Newland, 2009; Painter, 1996, 1999; Portes & Walton, 1981; Sassen, 1988; UNDP, 2009).

There are no accurate figures on the number of Latino migrants in the United States. By early 2009, however, 80% (8.9 million) of the estimated 11.1 million foreign-born, undocumented persons in the United States were from Mexico (6.7 million) or other Latin American countries (2.3 million) (Passel & Cohn, 2010). This figure of approximately 9 million may serve as a crude proxy measure of the number of Latino migrants and recent immigrants in the United States, who may account for as much as 20% of all Latinos in this country (Passel & Cohn, 2008). However, this estimate may be too low. Undocumented persons may be undercounted in census-based figures. Moreover, this estimate does not include migrants who are in the United States legally with H2A visas and who work largely in agriculture and related industries. Crop workers—documented or undocumented—number 1.3–2.6 million (D. Carroll, U.S. Department of Labor, personal communication, March 31, 2009), and nearly 80% are Latinos (U.S. Department of Labor, 2005).

Nearly half of all Latinos in the United States live in California and Texas (U.S. Census, 2007), but their numbers in states that have not been traditional Latino destinations have increased rapidly. In Alabama, Arkansas, Georgia, North Carolina, South Carolina, and Tennessee, for example, Latinos accounted for less than 1% of state populations in 1990, but increased by an average of nearly 600% by 2007 (U.S. Census, 1990, 2007). Contributing factors included strong economic growth in the South, saturated urban labor markets in traditional, western Latino destination states, and stricter enforcement of federal regulations by the U.S. Immigration and Customs Enforcement in border states, resulting in a shift of undocumented Latino migrants to the Southeast and Midwest (Kandel & Parrado, 2004; Kochhar et al., 2005).

Many Latino migrants are adult males who are single or married but are unaccompanied by their spouses. Compared to documented Latino immigrants and native-born Latino populations in the United States, undocumented Latino migrants are younger (aged 18–44) and less educated (nearly one-third have less than a ninth-grade education). They are more likely to be employed (with a labor force participation rate of 93%), but to work in low-wage jobs with average yearly incomes of $27,400 per family ($12,000 per person), to live in poverty (27% of adults fall below 100% of the Federal poverty line), and to have no health insurance (59%) (Passel, 2005; Passel & Cohen, 2010). Many of the jobs performed by Latino migrants require minimal skills and education, and provide few if any benefits or prospects for advancement and stability (Kochhar, 2005).

SEARCHING FOR OPPORTUNITIES AND FINDING RISKS: FACTORS THAT AFFECT LATINO MIGRANTS' VULNERABILITY TO HIV/STD INFECTION AND ACCESS TO PREVENTION, TREATMENT, AND CARE
Structural and Situational Factors

Studies have described structural and situational factors that can increase the vulnerability of Latino migrants and their sex partners to HIV or STD infection (Organista et al., 2004; Organista, 2007) and other health-related problems (Lara et al., 2005). These factors include low wages; poverty; unemployment and underemployment; substandard housing; homelessness; constant mobility; lack of health insurance; undocumented status and the associated risks and fears of discovery, detention, and deportation. Additional factors that can contribute to Latino migrants' vulnerability to HIV/STDs include social and geographic isolation (Sanchez et al., 2004); loneliness (Muñoz-Laboy et al., 2009); disrupted family relationships (Hirsch et al., 2002, 2007, 2009; Organista, 2007); attenuated or missing family- or community-based social controls on potential risk behaviors; residence and socializing in areas—urban apartment complexes or rural agricultural camps—where men far outnumber women (Grzywacz et al., 2004; Hirsch et al., 2002; Kochhar et al., 2005; Parrado et al., 2004), and where alcohol consumption (which may lead to binge drinking) (Organista, 2007), drug use (Apostolopoulos et al., 2006; Inciardi et al., 1999), and transactional sexual contacts are easily available, risky diversions. The effects on potential HIV/STD risk behaviors of this displacement and the desperation (*desesperación*) or depression that may occur (Apostolopoulos et al., 2006; Organista, 2007) may be amplified among those migrants who travel to the South and the Midwest where Latino communities are more recent and where social support and sexual networks found in states with larger, well-established, Latino populations are underdeveloped (Apostolopoulos et al., 2006; Frasca, 2009; Hirsch & Yount, 2001; Menjívar, 2000; Painter, 2008; Vega et al., 1991). The limited education and English-language proficiency of many Latino migrants and, increasingly, limited or no Spanish proficiency among migrants from indigenous populations (e.g., *Mixtecs, Zapotecs*) in southern Mexico and Central America (Cornelius et al., 2007) may exacerbate the potentially poor fit between these newcomers and mainstream American society.

Factors such as these may also contribute to inadequate knowledge and erroneous beliefs about HIV/STD transmission and prevention, low levels of perceived infection risks, and a lack of information about care and treatment options

(Organista et al., 1997, 2006; Parrado et al., 2004). This in turn may negatively affect their ability to take protective actions. Acculturation by Latino migrants to American society, whether measured by language use or length of residence in the United States, has an ambiguous relationship with HIV/STD risks. Studies have reported that greater exposure to the dominant culture may be associated with actions that can increase (Galvan et al., 2008; Hernandez et al., 2007; Paz-Bailey, 2004; Sanchez et al., 2008) or decrease (Parrado et al., 2004; Viadro & Earp, 2000) migrants' risks of infection.

Concerns about discrimination by health care providers, the effects of HIV/AIDS-related stigma, fear of seeking HIV testing and possible involuntary serostatus disclosure, and the risks of having their undocumented status discovered, can create additional barriers to Latino migrants' participation in health-related services (Espinoza et al., 2008; Hirsch, 2003; Rajabiun et al., 2008; Sanchez et al., 2004). Restrictive immigration policies at various levels may also discourage or bar their participation in needed services. The result may be untreated or poorly-treated STDs, low rates of HIV and STD testing and non-receipt of test results, and late presentation for HIV testing when migrants are more likely to be symptomatic for AIDS (Aranda-Naranjo et al., 2000; Kullgren, 2003; Levy et al., 2005, 2007; Solorio et al., 2004).

Behavioral Factors

Numerous behavioral studies have described actions by Latino migrants that can increase their HIV/STD risks. These include frequent, often unprotected sex with female sex workers (Apostolopoulos, 2006; Organista et al., 2004; Painter et al., 2011; Parrado et al., 2004; Viadro & Earp, 2000), unprotected sex by several men with the same female sex worker (Apostolopoulos, 2006; Paz-Bailey et al., 2004; Magaña, 1991; Viadro & Earp, 2000), sex with other males who may or may not be sex workers (Carrillo, 2002; Organista et al., 2004; Painter et al., 2011; Sanchez et al., 2008), unprotected sex with their wives and other regular female sex partners in the United States and in their countries of origin (Organista & Kubo, 2005; Rangel et al., 2006), and multiple sex partners. The heavy consumption of alcohol, particularly beer (Muñoz-Laboy et al., 2009; Organista, 2007; Shedlin et al., 2005), marijuana, crack cocaine, and methamphetamine use (Hernández et al., 2009; Inciardi, 1999; Magis-Rodriguez et al., 2004) and, less frequently, injection drug use (Painter, 2008), and therapeutic self-injection of antibiotics and vitamins with shared needles or by injectionists whose needles and syringes may be unclean (Lafferty, 1991; Lafferty et al., 1990–1991; McVea, 1997) can also increase Latino migrants' HIV/STD risks. Although some studies have described relatively high rates of condom use or more consistent condom use by male Latino migrants with female sex workers (Kissinger et al., 2012; Muñoz-Laboy et al., 2009; Parrado et al., 2004; Sanchez et al., 2008; Viadro & Earp, 2000), condom use may decline as migrants get to know their commercial sex partners better (Muñoz-Laboy et al., 2009; Parrado et al., 2004; Sanchez et al., 2008; Viadro & Earp, 2000).

Migrants as Potential Bridge Populations

For many Latino migrants, the search for opportunities in the United States entails periodic travel between areas that have been affected differently by HIV/AIDS. The estimated adult HIV prevalence in Mexico (0.3%), the source of most Latino migrants in the United States, is half that of adults in this country (CENSIDA, 2003; Magis-Rodriguez et al., 2004). The cyclical movement of Latino migrant men between their countries of origin and U.S. destinations where HIV/STD prevalence rates are higher, and where factors such as those described above can increase their likelihood of engaging in risk behaviors, may contribute to the spread of HIV infection to migrants' wives and other sex partners in their home communities. Furthermore, the men's female sex partners in their countries of origin may have limited ability to practice safe sex during the migrants' return visits (Hirsch et al., 2002 2007). In Mexico, there is accumulating evidence that HIV infection is spreading due to the effects of the migratory process. Initially associated primarily with urban male-to-male sex and drug use in border areas, HIV/AIDS in Mexico is becoming increasingly rural and heterosexual in nature (Bastos et al., 2008; Bronfman et al., 1998; CONASIDA, 2000; Del Rio & Sepúlveda, 2002; Gayet et al., 2000; Magis-Rodriguez et al., 2004; Sowell et al., 2008). One-third of all reported AIDS cases in Mexico may be from states that send large numbers of migrants to the United States (Sanchez et al., 2004).

HIV/STD INFECTION AMONG LATINO MIGRANTS

Surveillance-based information does not report HIV/STD infections or risk factors that affect migrants. Consequently, current understandings concerning HIV/STD infection among Latino migrants are based largely on findings from locally focused studies that may include small numbers of nonrandomly selected migrants. These studies, some of which were conducted nearly two decades ago, have reported HIV infection rates that vary from none [e.g., 0.0% in North Carolina (CDC, 1988), California (Martinez-Donate et al., 2005; Ruiz et al., 1997; Sanchez et al., 2004), and Louisiana (Kissinger et al., 2012)] to low or moderately low [0.1% in California (Hernandez et al., 2007); 0.6%, 0.9%, and 1.8%, respectively, in California (Hernandez et al., 2005, 2007, 2008); and 0.47% in Texas (Varela-Ramirez et al., 2005)], to relatively high estimates [e.g., 12% in the Delaware, Maryland, Virginia (DelMarVa) Peninsula (Inciardi et al., 1999) and 14% in South Carolina (Jones et al., 1991)]. Reported rates of other STDs among Latino migrants also vary considerably (Brammeier et al., 2008; Hernandez et al., 2007; Kissinger et al., 2008, 2012; Paz-Bailey et al., 2004; Wong et al., 2003).

More recent studies describe low HIV infection rates among Latino migrants, but continue to describe frequent actions that can increase their HIV/STD infection risks (Brammeier et al., 2008; Martinez-Donate et al., 2005; Hernandez et al., 2007; Kissinger et al., 2012; Sanchez et al., 2004). Furthermore, evidence suggests that migrants and recent immigrants, including Latinos, who are infected with HIV, are more likely to have been infected in the United States than in their countries of origin (Harawa et al., 2002; Levy et al., 2007; Los Angeles Department of Health Services, 2000). These seemingly contradictory findings require further study. Although Latino migrants are often described as having limited HIV-related knowledge, some migrant men may be engaging in protective actions, and as noted above, high rates of condom use with female sex workers have been reported by some studies (Kissinger et al., 2012; Parrado et al., 2004; Viadro & Earp, 2000). It is also possible that the migrants' sexual networks have low rates of infection - so far.

In summary, Latino migrants in the United States constitute a large population that is vulnerable to HIV/STD infection. Furthermore, there is growing evidence that male Latino migrants are linking populations with low levels of HIV infection

355

Interventions to Prevent HIV and Other Sexually Transmitted Diseases among Latino Migrants in some of their home communities with populations having higher HIV prevalence in the United States. There is an urgent need for culturally appropriate, effective HIV/STD prevention interventions for Latino migrants. But what prevention resources are currently available for migrants? We consider these points next.

HIV/STD PREVENTION FOR LATINO MIGRANTS

There are two kinds of evidence-based behavioral interventions for HIV/STD prevention among Latino migrants, be they farmworkers or urban-based migrant workers: interventions that were initially developed for nonmigrants and subsequently adapted for use with migrants and interventions developed specifically for migrants.

Adapted Interventions

Most evidence-based HIV/STD prevention interventions that are currently delivered by community-based organizations and health departments to at-risk populations in the United States are disseminated with support from the Centers for Disease Control and Prevention (CDC). However, before dissemination can occur, the CDC must assess interventions for the strength of evidence concerning reported efficacy and the rigor of evaluation design (http://www.cdc.gov/hiv/topics/research/prs/tiers-of-evidence.htm), and include those that pass muster in the *Compendium of Evidence-Based HIV Prevention Interventions* (http://www.cdc.gov/hiv/topics/research/prs/evidence-based-interventions.htm). Based on a review of HIV prevention needs, interventions listed in the *Compendium* are selected for packaging (http://www.cdc.gov/hiv/topics/prev_prog/rep/) and are eventually disseminated to service providers with CDC support through the Diffusion of Effective Behavioral Interventions (DEBI) project (http://www.effectiveinterventions.org/en/AboutDebi.aspx). In addition, some evidence-based interventions may be packaged and made available independently of the CDC process. It may take several years for an efficacious intervention to be packaged and disseminated. None of the 69 evidence-based interventions listed in CDC's 2009 *Compendium* were designed for migrants. In an effort to fill this gap, some interventions that were designed for nonmigrants have been adapted with CDC support for use with migrants. However, the adaptation process requires additional time because of the need to adjust existing interventions for new populations and, in the case of Latino migrants, ensure that adaptations are responsive to Latino values and norms and are translated into Spanish. Currently two evidence-based behavioral HIV prevention interventions have been adapted for potential use with Latino migrants. The English-language Popular Opinion Leader intervention to reduce HIV risk behaviors among gay men (http://www.cdc.gov/hiv/topics/prev_prog/rep/packages/pol.htm) has been adapted as the Young Latino *Promotores* intervention for young migrant Latino men who have sex with men. When assessed using preintervention and postintervention measures, participants in the adapted intervention reported a reduction in sexual risk behaviors (Somerville et al., 2006). The English-language Safety Counts intervention, designed to reduce drug-related and sexually-related risk actions among out-of-treatment, active injection and noninjection drug users (http://www.effectiveinterventions.org/en/Interventions/SafetyCounts.aspx), has been adapted for use with out-of-treatment drug-using Latino migrant farmworkers

(Anderson, 2006; Scott & Wascher-Tavares, 2008), but its efficacy or effectiveness has not been evaluated. In addition, preliminary work is underway to adapt the Voices/*Voces* intervention (http://www.effectiveinterventions.org/en/Interventions/ VOICES.aspx) to increase condom use and reduce incident STDs among heterosexual African American and Latino men and women who visit STD clinics for use with Latino migrant farmworkers (Ricky Wascher-Tavares, personal communication, October 12, 2010). However, the availability of these adaptations for Latino migrants is extremely limited. The Young *Promotores* intervention was delivered to Latino migrant farmworkers in San Diego County, California, from 2005 to 2007, but is no longer available in that locality due to funding limitations (Fernando Sañudo, personal communication, June 18, 2010). Pending finalization, Safety Counts is being delivered to Latino migrant workers on a pilot basis in several states (Jonny Andia, personal communication, June 18, 2010; Ricky Wascher-Tavares, personal communication, September 30, 2010).

Interventions Developed Specifically for Latino Migrants

We are aware of only three HIV/STD prevention interventions that have been developed specifically for Latino migrants or recent immigrants for which some evidence of efficacy has been reported. Mishra and Conner (1996) developed *Tres Hombres Sin Fronteras* (Three Men without Borders) in the early 1990s for Mexican farmworkers, and delivered and assessed it twice in northern San Diego County, California, between 1991 and 1995 (Mishra & Conner, 1996; Mishra, Sañudo, & Conner, 2004). In 2003, Organista et al. (2006) developed and delivered a pilot intervention for Mexican migrant day laborers in Berkeley, California. Also beginning in 2003, Rhodes et al. (2009) developed and delivered *HoMBReS* (*Hombres Manteniendo Bienestar y Relaciones Saludables*—Men Maintaining Wellbeing and Healthy Relationships) for recent immigrant Latino (largely Mexican) male farm and construction workers in Chatham and Lee Counties in rural central North Carolina. A systematic review and meta-analysis of published behavioral HIV prevention interventions for Hispanics/Latinos by Herbst et al. in 2007 included both versions of *Tres Hombres Sin Fronteras* (Mishra & Conner, 1996; Mishra, Sañudo, & Conner, 2004), based on reported evidence of increased condom use by the male participants with female sex workers. Sañudo's subsequent analysis (1999) confirmed the intervention's efficacy. The meta-analysis also noted that the Organista et al. (2006) pilot intervention had provided significant preintervention to postintervention changes in participants' sex risk behaviors. However, neither the farmworker nor the day laborer intervention reported evidence of efficacy that was sufficiently strong to be included in the CDC *Compendium*. Very recently (August 2011), the *HoMBReS* intervention was added to the *Compendium* as an evidence-based community-level intervention (http://www.cdc.gov/hiv/topics/research/ prs/resources/factsheets/hombres.htm), the first such intervention to be listed for recent Latino immigrants.

For each of these interventions, we describe the perceived need leading to its creation, how it was developed, and its content and delivery, we summarize evidence of its efficacy when delivered, and we describe factors that the codevelopers believe contributed to the success of their intervention projects. Table 18.1 provides additional information on the features of the interventions' participants, intervention delivery, evaluation methods, and outcomes.

TRES HOMBRES SIN FRONTERAS
Need Meets Opportunity: HIV Prevention among Latino Migrant Farmworkers in San Diego County, California

The Vista Community Clinic in northern San Diego County, California, has served low-income residents and nearly 25,000 mostly Mexican agricultural workers since 1972. During this time, local growers frequently brought their male workers to the clinic to be treated for STDs. The men often stated that they believed they had been infected by female sex workers. Despite efforts by clinic staff to provide condoms to the workers, recurring reports of infections suggested limited condom use by the men. To address this problem, the clinic initiated educational outreach at farmworkers' workplaces in 1987. These efforts were modest, however, due to limited funding, and farmworkers continued to be diagnosed with STDs. The clinic's staff realized that more was needed. In the early 1990s, researchers from the University of California, Irvine, were looking for a community partner to help implement and evaluate an HIV/STD prevention intervention they had developed for male Latino farmworkers. The four-session intervention, *Tres Hombres Sin Fronteras*, was an innovative approach for the United States in that it used Spanish language *fotonovelas* (photo story books) and a *radionovela* (a multipart radio series or soap opera). Both *novela* formats are widely used in Latin America, require little or no reading, and may be effective for educating low-literacy Spanish speakers about HIV/STD prevention (Magaña et al., 1990; Conner, 1990).

A partnership was formed to deliver and evaluate *Tres Hombres*. Clinic staff helped the researchers gain entrée to the farmworker communities, familiarize them with the men's living and working conditions, and identify and address potential challenges to delivering and evaluating the intervention. The study partners also conducted formative research to clarify the acceptability of the study to the farmworkers and identify issues of particular concern to them. These issues included housing, food, employment, accessing health care, and HIV/AIDS.

The *Tres Hombres Sin Fronteras* Intervention

The intervention aimed to positively affect the Latino migrant farmworkers' HIV knowledge and attitudes concerning HIV/STD prevention and increase their perceptions of personal vulnerability to HIV infection and condom use with female sex workers. It was based on principles of the Health Belief Model (Rosenstock, 1960), the Theory of Reasoned Action (Fishbein & Ajzen, 1975), and Cognitive-Social Learning Theory (Bandura, 1977). The *Tres Hombres Sin Fronteras fotonovela* depicted the stories of three men, Marco, Sergio, and Victor, who had left their families in Mexico to do farm work in the United States (Figure 18.1). After arriving in the United States, they find themselves exposed to the harsh realities of life in agricultural campsites and separation from families and friends. All of the men meet female sex workers, and each makes different decisions concerning sex with the women. Victor does not have sex with them for fear of contracting HIV and infecting his wife in Mexico. Marco has sex with sex workers, but uses a condom. Sergio also has sex with sex workers, but he refuses to use condoms, contracts HIV, and both his wife and infant eventually become infected. The *fotonovela* described modes of HIV transmission and prevention methods. In a second *fotonovela, Marco Aprende Como Protegerse* (Marco learns how to protect himself), a sex worker teaches Marco about the importance of condom use and illustrates correct usage. The *fotonovela* also contained six packaged condoms. The intervention's *radionovela* component

TRES HOMBRES SIN FRONTERAS

¡GRATIS!   Una Fotonovela Diferente

¡¡PROTÉGETE!!

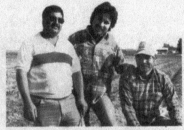
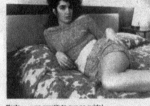

Marco, Sergio y Víctor — tres hombres que salen de su pueblo en busca de oportunidades, ¡¡se encuentran peligros!!

Karla — ¡una prostituta que se cuida!

FIGURE 18.1 *Tres Hombres Sin Fronteras.* Provided with permission by the Northwest Communities' Education Center, Public Radio KDNA 91.9 FM, Granger, Washington; image quality enhanced by Susie Childrey.

was based on the *Tres Hombres fotonovela,* and included fifteen 5-minute segments, three to four of which were played during each intervention session.

During Session 1, participants received the *fotonovelas,* discussed the information they received, and asked questions of the facilitator. The session clarified the difference between AIDS and HIV, explained how the immune system combats diseases and infections, and described the prevalence of HIV/AIDS at the local, national, and global levels. At the end of all sessions, participants were asked to consider what they had learned and how it related to the situations of the men in the *Tres Hombres fotonovela.* Session 2 described the bodily fluids that can transmit HIV, how HIV is and is not transmitted, and typical symptoms of persons who are diagnosed with AIDS. During Session 3, the participants reviewed and discussed the *Marco Aprende fotonovela.* The facilitator showed the men how to check a condom package for the expiration date, how to open it without damaging the condom, and demonstrated the correct application of a condom on a plastic penis model. The participants took turns demonstrating the correct application of the condom to the model to their peers, while outreach workers observed and provided feedback. Session 4 provided information on HIV testing, the meaning of negative and positive test results, and resources available to persons who test as HIV positive. The facilitator ended the session with a review of all intervention topics.

Delivering the Intervention

The intervention results described here are based on Sañudo's (1999) reanalysis of data from the 1994–1996 study by Mishra, Sañudo, and Conner (2004). During the study, clinic outreach workers delivered the Spanish-language *Tres Hombres Sin Fronteras* as four once-weekly sessions of about 2 hours each to farmworkers at agricultural campsites in northern San Diego County. The sites were randomized to receive *Tres Hombres* (10 campsites comprising 142 men) or the comparison condition (10 sites with 144 men). Clinic outreach workers visited comparison participants weekly to hold discussion sessions on nutrition, first aid, and other topics unrelated to HIV. All of the participants were from Mexico.

Intervention Effects

An assessment conducted 1 month after the men received *Tres Hombres Sin Fronteras* indicated that intervention participants had greater HIV-related knowledge than comparison participants. Participants in both study conditions reported slight increases in sex with female sex workers, either in the United States or Mexico. However, among those who reported no condom use prior to the baseline assessment, more intervention than comparison participants who reported sex with sex workers during the 1-month follow-up period also reported using condoms. Table 18.1 provides additional information about the participants and the delivery and evaluation of the intervention.

Conclusions

The *Tres Hombres Sin Fronteras* study demonstrated that an HIV prevention intervention designed for Latino migrant farmworkers that uses familiar Spanish-language formats—*fotonovelas* and *radionovelas*—to depict farmworkers in circumstances similar to those of intervention participants, and who encounter similar dilemmas concerning HIV/STD risks, can contribute to improved HIV/STD-related knowledge and risk-reducing actions. The following factors contributed to the project's success:

- A trusting relationship between university researchers and clinic staff.
- The willingness of the researchers to spend considerable time with clinic staff in the field and experience the challenges of working with migrant populations.
- The direct involvement of clinic staff members in the development and implementation of the intervention and the evaluation design.
- An excellent relationship between clinic staff members and the migrant farmworkers in the study, based on the clinic's reputation for providing quality health care.
- Formative research conducted by the researchers with clinic staff to pilot test all components of the intervention and evaluation.
- The use of *fotonovelas* and *radionovelas* to provide important health information to low-literacy Latino farm workers.
- The theoretical grounding of the *Tres Hombres Sin Fronteras* intervention.

A PILOT HIV PREVENTION INTERVENTION FOR LATINO MIGRANT DAY LABORERS
Migrant Day Laborers and HIV Risks in Berkeley, California

Concerned about the use of female sex workers by male Latino day laborers in Berkeley, California, and reports of binge drinking and STD infections among the men, the HIV Planning Committee of the city's HIV/AIDS Program included this population in its prevention activities beginning in 2000. Before moving ahead, however, the Program's leadership needed more information about risk factors that affected day laborers. Following a presentation on his work with Latino migrants, Kurt Organista was asked to conduct a risk survey. During the fall of 2001, he and the program's staff surveyed 120 men concerning their sexual, alcohol, and substance use behaviors, psychosocial problems, circumstantial factors that could affect their HIV risks, and their condom-related beliefs, knowledge, and behaviors (Organista & Kubo, 2005). The survey results confirmed the Committee's concerns that the men knew little about proper condom use. It also revealed that they were primarily concerned about the effects on their lives of having too little work and money. Based on the survey results, Organista conducted a pilot HIV prevention activity to determine the feasibility of delivering a group intervention to Latino migrant day laborers, sharing the survey results with the men and discussing the implications for HIV prevention, and learning about how their lives as day laborers affected their HIV risks. A focus group provided additional information on risk factors that affected the men.

Intervention Development

The intervention addressed the men's cultural needs, limited education, and their status in the United States as undocumented, oppressed, stigmatized individuals who are often subject to discrimination. It incorporated aspects of the Health Belief Model (Glanz et al., 1997), which posits that individuals will take protective actions if they are aware of the risks, possess needed risk-reduction skills, and feel confident that their skills will be effective. However, Organista and colleagues wanted to avoid a situation in which health educators delivered elements of the model didactically, thereby duplicating the dynamics of oppression that can affect vulnerable populations such as migrants. They believed the intervention needed to facilitate participants' critical thinking about problems and their efforts to identify solutions rather than imposing specialized knowledge on them (e.g., concerning HIV transmission and prevention).

Inspired by Paulo Freire's model of popular participatory education (Freire, 1970), the intervention used a problem-solving focus and, drawing on principles described by Wallerstein (1992), stressed the use of culturally appropriate approaches rather than written materials. These approaches included the use of story and visual triggers to prompt discussions among intervention participants. The story trigger was a vignette about a migrant day laborer who had come to the San Francisco Bay Area, intending to earn and send money back home, only to confront too little work, loneliness, isolation, feelings of failure, and to succumb to problem drinking and unprotected sex. Intervention participants were asked to react to the vignette— did it seem familiar, and what could the person in the story have done to reduce his risk of HIV infection? Cards from the Loteria game, which is popular throughout Latin America, were adapted as posters for use as visual discussion triggers. The poster-sized cards with their tarot-like images included, among others, El Borracho (the drunk), which shows a Mexican man, hunched over and intoxicated, La Muerte (death), depicting the Grim Reaper, and La Escalera (the ladder), symbolizing progress. Additional poster-size loteria-like cards were developed to illustrate the HIV risk factors described by the men during the risk survey and the focus group. These cards included, for example, La Prostituta (the prostitute) and

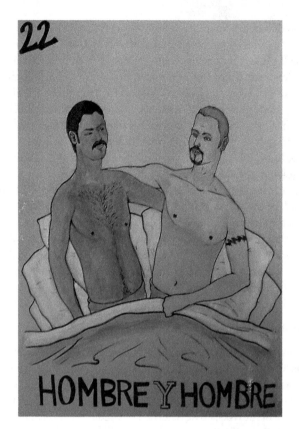

FIGURE 18.2 *Hombre y hombre* (male to male sex). Prepared by Ari Haytin and provided with permission by Kurt C. Organista.

Sexo entre Hombres (sex between men), to prompt discussions about this taboo topic (Figure 18.2).

The intervention included three 2-hour group sessions delivered during 1 week in order to be responsive to the men's mobility and unpredictable work schedules. It also aimed to foster social cohesion and facilitate their efforts to discuss personal, sexual, and other risk-related matters. Session 1 elicited descriptions of the men's experiences as day laborers and the HIV risks they encountered, why they migrated to the United States, and the obstacles they faced. It also gave the facilitators an opportunity to assess the men's HIV/AIDS awareness by having them react to the risk-related images on the large *loteria* cards. During Session 2, a staff member from the clinic in which the intervention was delivered provided HIV/AIDS-related information, and the men used bananas to practice correct application of condoms. The day laborer vignette was used to facilitate discussion about HIV risks that the men had heard about and experienced. Session 3 reviewed all of the HIV risk scenarios previously described by participants. The men were asked to describe different ways of reducing those risks, to assess how realistic their prevention strategies were, to consider several back-up strategies, and to provide feedback on the sessions.

Delivery of the Pilot Intervention

The intervention was conducted during the spring of 2003 at a Berkeley community health clinic that provides outpatient care to residents from diverse socioeconomic circumstances and is trusted by migrants. The clinic was located near a spot where day laborers gathered to seek construction jobs. Outreach workers from the city's HIV/AIDS Program contacted potential participants, screened them for eligibility, and on the day of the first group session, accompanied them to the clinic. The sessions were delivered in Spanish by Organista and a male Latino MPH student. An outreach worker observed and recorded the sessions, and debriefed the facilitators. The intervention was delivered to 23 day laborers in two different groups over a 3-week period.

Intervention Effects

An assessment conducted 1 month after the intervention indicated that relative to results of the baseline assessment, participants' knowledge about correct condom use improved and more of them reported always carrying condoms. They reported having less sex in general and less unprotected sex with various female partners, including sex workers. Table 18.1 provides additional information about the participants and the delivery and evaluation of the intervention.

Intervention Features and Processes

The vignette and the large *loteria* cards stimulated participants' discussion of sensitive issues. Giving the men an opportunity to assess how realistic their prevention strategies were and encouraging them to consider back-up strategies were useful. One participant, for example, who had been in the United States for less than 6 months, suggested that abstinence would be an effective HIV prevention strategy. Several other men who had been in the country longer challenged him, strongly suggesting that he carry and use condoms. They explained that they had relied on abstinence initially, but it eventually failed them. When asked what about the intervention was helpful to them, some participants described the idea of having back-up prevention strategies; others simply enjoyed having an opportunity to learn with their peers. The observer's debriefings made it possible to adjust intervention delivery as needed. The review of qualitative data confirmed earlier risk survey findings that the most frequently mentioned concern was the men's inability to earn money, frequently resulting in a state of *desesperación*. They frequently described the connection between their difficult circumstances, their feelings, and falling into *vicios* (vices): problem drinking, occasional illicit drug use, and risky sex.

Conclusions

The pilot activity demonstrated the feasibility of developing and delivering a brief HIV/STD prevention intervention to male Latino migrant day laborers. The following factors contributed to the success of the pilot activity:

- The city's HIV/AIDS Planning Committee's decision to do something about HIV risks that affected day laborers, and program leadership willing to focus resources on a population that is frequently neglected.
- Effective collaboration between the Committee, the HIVAIDS Program, and researchers.
- Formative work to identify ideas and approaches for the intervention.
- A theoretical framework that combined elements from models for health promotion and empowering marginalized, oppressed individuals to better

understand the causes of their vulnerability to HIV risks and develop possible solutions.

- The creative use of components from Latino popular culture to engage participants and elicit discussions of risk factors.

HOMBRES—AN HIV/STD PREVENTION INTERVENTION FOR RECENT IMMIGRANT LATINO MEN IN RURAL NORTH CAROLINA
A Rapidly Growing Latino Population in Need of Resources for HIV and STD Prevention

North Carolina is one of several southern states that have experienced a rapid growth of Latino populations. From 1990 to 2007, the number of Latinos living in the state increased by more than 700% (U.S. Census 1990, 2007). North Carolina is also part of a region of the United States that has some of the higher AIDS and STD case rates in the country (CDC, 2006, 2007). In light of the rapid increase in Latino populations, a partnership of community members and researchers was increasingly concerned with the capacity of the local service delivery system to address the health needs of Latinos in rural communities. The partnership had used community-based participatory research (CBPR) earlier (Parker et al., 1998) to address the health needs of African American faith communities, and had begun exploring the use of CBPR to clarify these issues among Latinos. To do this, partnership members collaborated with the *Liga Hispana de Fútbol de North Carolina* (the North Carolina Hispanic Soccer League), a multicounty soccer league with more than 1800 male Latino immigrant members. The partnership focused on male soccer players because Latino communities in rural North Carolina were disproportionately male, a pattern that is gradually changing as men bring and create families of their own (Southern State Directors Work Group, 2008). Furthermore, the soccer players had repeatedly asked the league leadership for information about the signs of HIV and STDs and available health resources.

Developing an Approach for HIV/STD Prevention

The soccer league leadership worked with the partnership members to design and conduct focus groups with team members and analyze the results (Cashman et al., 2008). This formative research identified the need to prioritize immigrant Latino men's sexual health. Specific issues included their limited knowledge about HIV, STDs, and prevention; inconsistent condom use; sex with multiple partners; use of sex workers; alcohol use prior to sexual intercourse; barriers to accessing health care; the role of masculinity in influencing risk behaviors; and the importance of using an approach for HIV/STD prevention that incorporated the social networks that occur among soccer league members (Knipper et al., 2007; Rhodes et al., 2007). The partnership identified prevention priorities that included increasing the men's awareness of the magnitude of HIV/STD infection in general and among Latinos in the United States and North Carolina; providing them with HIV and STD-related information, including types of infections, modes of transmission, signs and symptoms, and local options for testing, care, and treatment; increasing their condom-related skills, self-efficacy, and use; and their use of available sexual health care services. The partnership also wanted the intervention to support soccer team members' HIV/STD prevention efforts by reinforcing positive aspects and reframing the negative aspects of what it means to be a Latino man. Finally, the partnership wanted the intervention to tap into natural helping processes that occur within Latino communities and to identify and train natural helpers to play more broadly supportive roles for health promotion (Eng et al., 2009).

The *HoMBReS* Intervention

To address their priorities, the partnership developed, implemented, and evaluated *HoMBReS* [*Hombres Manteniendo Bienestar y Relaciones Saludables* (Men Maintaining Wellbeing and Health Relationships)], an HIV/STD prevention intervention for heterosexually active soccer league members. *HoMBReS* aimed to increase the men's use of condoms and participation in HIV/STD-related services. A partnership subgroup developed intervention activities for review by the entire partnership to ensure that the intervention was based on the men's lived experiences and sound prevention science. Two theories fit with the desired approach: social cognitive theory (Bandura, 1986) and popular participatory education (Freire, 1970, 1973; Wallerstein, 1994). These theoretical foundations provided a framework for raising Latino men's consciousness about the impact of HIV and STDs through critical reflection, the development of skills and self-efficacy for protective actions such as condom use, and social support for reducing risk behaviors and addressing health-compromising norms and values.

Preparing Soccer Team Members to Deliver *HoMBReS* to Their Teammates

Recently-arrived Latino male soccer league members were selected by their team mates to be trained as lay health advisors to deliver *HoMBReS* (Rhodes et al., 2006). Because bilingual, bicultural services are not commonly available in rural North Carolina, the men needed to have some English-language skills to help their non-English-speaking teammates communicate with non-Spanish-speaking service providers. The Latino community was familiar with *promotoras de salud*, a term used for female lay health workers who work with Latino populations, but wanted to describe their health advisors in a way that did not have a possible feminine connotation. They also wanted to better reflect the kind of support the *HoMBReS* lay health advisors were expected to provide to their teammates and the community: informational, material, and emotional support, and practical guidance on how to "navigate" the U.S. health care system and obtain needed resources. As a result, the *HoMBReS* lay health advisors were called *Navegantes* (Navigators). The *Navegantes* were trained by a Spanish-speaking Latino male who was well-versed in the *HoMBReS* intervention and health behavior theory and the design of the planned evaluation study, and was an effective facilitator. Like many men in the community, he had come to North Carolina as an undocumented immigrant to work on farms, in poultry processing, and construction, and eventually received his green card. The training included four sessions, totaling 16 hours over two consecutive weekends. It included four modules, was designed as a comprehensive guide for trainers, and contained triggers to facilitate discussion during the training sessions. The sessions were both didactic and interactive, using activity-based components to build rapport and trust of the *Navegantes* by the persons who would receive *HoMBReS*. Module 1 explained the background and purpose of *HoMBReS*, described the impact of HIV and STDs

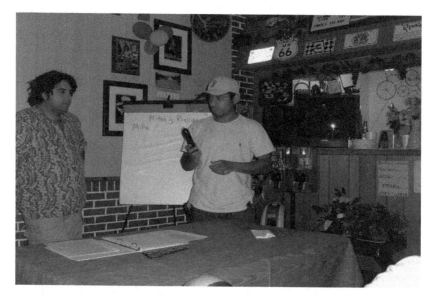

FIGURE 18.3 *HoMBReS*—teaching correct condom use. Provided by Scott D. Rhodes with permission of Wake Forest University, Winston Salem, North Carolina.

among Latinos in the United States and North Carolina, and the *Navegantes'* roles and responsibilities. Module 2 focused on sexual health, HIV, STDs, and their prevention, covered symptoms and treatment of common STDs, and distinguished myths from realities. It also provided *Navegantes* with opportunities to develop skills for correct condom use and techniques for teaching others (Figure 18.3). Module 3 taught effective communication techniques, how to reframe health-compromising social norms and expectations about being a man, and how to serve as community advocates. Module 4 explained the value of evaluating *HoMBReS* and the evaluation process.

Training *Navegantes* to Deliver *HoMBReS*

The *Navegantes* training was delivered to 15 men from October 2003 to March 2007. After their training, each *Navegante* worked with his teammates and other Latino community members for 18 months. The *Navegantes* discussed health in general and sexual risks, provided information about resources for dealing with individual sexual problems, helped participants locate sources of free condoms, distributed condoms and demonstrated correct condom using a penis model, and referred participants and other community members to local organizations and health departments for additional information and HIV and STD testing. The *Navegantes* were also trained to confront sociocultural barriers to sexual health, such as *machismo*. Rather than conducting formal intervention activities, the *Navegantes* offered guidance and support to their teammates and community members. Men in the comparison condition received the intervention after the *HoMBReS* participants completed their 18-month follow-up assessment.

Intervention Effects

Eighteen months after the *Navegantes* training, men in the 15 soccer teams who received *HoMBReS* had significantly higher levels of knowledge about HIV/STD transmission and prevention and self-efficacy for condom use than men from the 15 soccer teams who did not receive the intervention (Rhodes et al., 2009). *HoMBReS* participants were 2.3 times more likely than comparison participants to report consistent condom use with sex partners during the past 30 days and 2.5 times more likely to have been tested for HIV. Qualitative data from the *Navegantes'* monthly activity logs provided details on the intervention delivery process (Vissman et al., 2009) and demonstrated that although the *Navegantes* frequently worked with other teammates, nearly half of their interactions were with nonteam members, suggesting their potentially broader reach in the Latino community. Table 18.1 provides additional information about the participants and the delivery and evaluation of the intervention.

Conclusions

The following factors contributed to the success of the *HoMBReS* project:

- Latino men from the community identified HIV and STDs as important issues.
- Community trust and respect were built and nurtured by the partnership members.
- The partnership process ensured equitable participation by all community partners throughout—from identifying health-related priorities to the development and delivery of the intervention, analysis, and interpretation of the evaluation results to determine intervention efficacy, and the eventual dissemination of the evaluation findings.
- The partnership collected formative data that informed the design of the intervention and evaluation study, ensuring that the content of *HoMBReS* and the procedures used to collect assessment data broadly reflected the perspectives and priorities of the community rather than only those of the researchers.
- The study team reflected the local community—foreign-born Spanish-speaking males having similar immigration histories—and the team was committed to the activity's success.
- The *Navegantes* training sessions were provided in community locations and at times of day (e.g., Friday evenings and Sunday mornings) that were easily accessible to participants.

DISCUSSION

Despite the large number of Latino migrants who live and work in urban and rural areas of the United States, and whose circumstances and actions may place them and their sex partners in this country and in their countries of origin at risk of HIV/STD infection, very few evidence-based prevention interventions have been developed or adapted for this diverse population, and fewer still are being delivered. *Tres Hombres Sin Fronteras* for Latino migrant farmworkers is not being delivered due to funding constraints. The potential efficacy of the pilot intervention for Latino migrant day laborers needs to be more rigorously evaluated before it can be considered for broader use, and so it too is not being delivered to Latino migrants. This is unfortunate, given that the number of urban-based Latino migrants is probably several times the number of those who work in agricultural occupations. Of the three interventions we have described, only *HoMBReS* has been delivered by a service provider organization (a CBO) to immigrant Latino men for a period of time. Coverage is limited to a few counties in central North Carolina, but plans are underway to package and make the intervention more broadly available. Although the availability of these interventions remains limited, they share several features in common. These features and the interventions' varying levels of success suggest that future HIV/STD prevention efforts for Latino migrants would be well-advised to give them serious consideration.

The interventions were developed in response to concerns by communities and service provider organizations about the HIV/STD risks that affect Latino migrants. Formative research was used to identify and clarify the risks of infection and identify feasible, acceptable approaches to prevention and intervention assessment. All of the interventions were delivered in Spanish, using approaches that were responsive to the migrants' frequently low educational and literacy levels. They all incorporated elements of Latino popular culture or social organization—*fotonovelas* and *radionovelas*, *loteria* game cards, and soccer teams. The use of these culturally appropriate elements engaged participants' interest and attention, and may have contributed to their increased HIV/STD-related knowledge, perceptions of infection risks, and HIV/STD-protective actions. Two of the three interventions were delivered relatively rapidly, using no more than four sessions during 1 to 4 weeks. These delivery formats facilitated participation by migrants whose lives and livelihoods are mobile, and, as a consequence, may be hard to reach.

All of the interventions incorporated elements of social-behavioral theories, and two interventions used elements of empowerment theories to address the migrants' typically precarious socioeconomic and legal circumstances. Incorporating empowerment principles in prevention interventions for Latino migrants may complement the use of sociobehavioral theories by supporting migrants' efforts to better understand how broader structural factors can affect their vulnerability to HIV/STD infection and their ability to prevent infection. The development, delivery, and assessment of the interventions were facilitated by effective partnerships of researchers, health care providers, other local organizations, and members of the migrant communities. The interventions were delivered through local organizations that were trusted by migrants—community health clinics and soccer teams—and were made available to participants at locations (migrant camps, clinics, community venues) and times that facilitated migrants' participation.

All of the interventions were developed for and delivered to men. This focus on male Latino migrants is extremely important, given the demographic profile of Latino migrants and recent immigrants, the greater autonomy that men enjoy relative to women as actors in Latino value systems and gender interactions, and their potential role as a bridge population for the transnational spread of HIV and STD infection. Nevertheless, there is a need to develop HIV/STD prevention interventions for women, who represent a gradually increasing proportion of Latino migrants and recent immigrants in the United States, and for interventions that include both male Latino migrants and their sex partners.

The formative and process data that were collected during the development of *Tres Hombres Sin Fronteras* and the migrant day laborer interventions revealed the salience of the men's concerns about their difficult socioeconomic circumstances. The co-authors of this chapter are keenly aware of how these circumstances can shape Latino migrants' HIV/STD risks and protective actions, and the interventions integrated a degree of critical reflection on these issues by their participants. Nevertheless, the interventions do not address these broader structural issues directly. This suggests the limitations of approaches to HIV/STD prevention for Latino migrants that focus solely or largely on changing knowledge, attitudes, and actions of individuals when broader circumstances and processes shape their actions. Greater attention must be given, first, to clarifying the mechanisms and processes that link broader structural and situational factors with migrants' HIV/STD risks and protective actions and, second, to developing, implementing, and assessing concrete strategies to influence these factors in HIV/STD prevention efforts (Organista et al., this volume, Chapter 1; Painter, 2008; Worby & Organista, 2007).

Surveillance-based information could better support efforts to improve understandings concerning mobility-related factors that affect Latino migrants' HIV/STD risks. Data could be collected and reported, for example, on migrants' country of origin, length of time and mobility in the United States, number of return trips to their countries of origin, urban or rural residence, prior residence in other states, place and circumstances of probable HIV/STD infection, whether single, partnered, or married, and if married, whether accompanied by a spouse, and describe sexual contacts more varied than those currently listed in risk factor hierarchies. The meta-analysis of behavioral HIV prevention interventions for Latinos (Herbst et al., 2007) referred to earlier identified intervention characteristics that were associated with greater efficacy. These features included delivery to males or females separately, no use of peer outreach or peer intervention deliverers, the use of four or more sessions, the use of problem-solving activities, discussion of barriers to condom use or sexual abstinence, opportunities for participants to practice condom use skills, and changes to peer norms to encourage risk-reducing actions. Although the interventions we have described included many of these features, there were several notable differences. The *HoMBReS* intervention effectively used peers for outreach and intervention delivery. Furthermore, although two interventions included no more than four sessions, *HoMBReS* used a longer, continuous 18-month period of exposure during which the *Navegantes* worked with soccer teammates and other community members on a range of issues relative to HIV/STD prevention and health promotion more generally. These differences may reflect, in part, the long-term partnership that *HoMBReS* researchers and community members have developed, thereby creating the basis for effective peer-based outreach and delivery. The use of peer-based *Navegantes* and social relationships of which they are a part, and the reinforcement during *Navegante* training of their potential as natural helpers, illustrates how an HIV/STD prevention intervention can usefully tap into social networks that exist among Latino migrants. To date, the potential for using Latino migrants' social support networks to affect shared understandings, values, and norms for purposes of HIV/STD prevention and health promotion has received very little attention by researchers or prevention initiatives (Painter, 2004, 2008).

The diversity of features and approaches that were used by the three Latino migrant interventions suggests that working with Latinos who are migrants creates needs and corresponding opportunities to use a variety of innovative approaches as long as they reflect a solid understanding of and are responsive to the circumstances and actions that increase migrants' vulnerability to HIV/STD infection. Given the severe shortage of effective, culturally appropriate prevention interventions for Latino migrants, there is an urgent need for the development, assessment, and dissemination of interventions for the many Latino migrants who live, work, socialize, and have sex in rural and urban areas of the United States.

Table 18.1 Three HIV/STD Prevention Interventions for Latino Migrants

	Interventions and Evaluation Features		
	Tres Hombres Sin Fronteras *Sañudo (1999)*	*Day Laborer Pilot Intervention* Organista et al. (2006)	HoMBReS *Rhodes et al. (2009)*
Intervention			
Target population	Male Latino migrant farmworkers, >18 years of age.	Male Latino migrant day laborers, ≥18 years of age.	Male Latino immigrant farm and construction workers who were soccer league members, ≥ 18 years of age.
Type	Small group	Small group	Community level
Evaluation			
Location	North San Diego County, California	Berkeley, California	Chatham and Lee Counties, North Carolina
Format of intervention delivery when evaluated	Four weekly 2-hour sessions delivered to groups of 8 to 15 farmworkers at agricultural worksites.	Three 2-hour sessions delivered to two groups of men during a single week each at a city health clinic.	15 lay health advisors (*Navegantes*) trained during four 4-hour sessions over two consecutive weekends. *Navegantes* provided HIV/STD prevention information to soccer teammates and community members, served as opinion leaders to change participants' health-compromising attitudes and norms concerning sexual health and what it means to be a Latino man, served as community advocates to health service agencies and for improved service delivery.

Sociodemographic characteristics of participants	100% of 286 participants were from Mexico; the mean ages of intervention and comparison participants = 24 and 23 years, respectively; 52.9% and 61.1% were single, 43.5% and 38.9% were married; 64.7% and 73.7% had ≥6 years of education; nearly 90% of men in both conditions read and spoke Spanish only; 65.9% and 47.8% were in United States for the first time.	70% of 23 participants were from Mexico; others were from Central American countries; the mean age = 34 years; 48% were married, 39% were single, 3% were divorced; predominantly monolingual Spanish speakers; average time in United States = 4 years; 78% earned $100–$400 per week, the remainder earned less than $100 per week. Nearly half of the earnings were sent to men's families in their countries of origin.	66% of 15 lay health advisors were from Mexico; others were from Central American countries; the mean age = 31.5 years; 70% were married.	61% of 222 participants were from Mexico; others were from Central American countries; mean age = 29.8 years (18–71 years); 53% were accompanied by their wife, partner, or girlfriend; 53% had completed ≤8 years of education; 70% were employed year-round; 69% had estimated annual salaries ≤$21,000; the mean length of time in the United States = 8.8 years; all self-identified as heterosexual; six reported sex with men during the past year.
Deliverer	Six Spanish/English-speaking (bilingual) Latino health educators/outreach workers.	Two bilingual Latino facilitators.		One bilingual Latino trained lay health advisors; met with them as a group at least monthly to support their intervention activities, facilitate discussions of challenges and successes, and solve problems.

(Continued)

Table 18.1 [Continued]

	Interventions and Evaluation Features		
	Tres Hombres Sin Fronteras *Sañudo (1999)*	Day Laborer Pilot Intervention *Organista et al. (2006)*	HoMBReS *Rhodes et al. (2009)*
Delivery language	Spanish	Spanish	Spanish
Evaluation design, types of outcomes assessed, and data collection points	Concurrent comparison group. Random assignment of agricultural campsites to concurrent intervention (10 sites) or comparison (10 sites) conditions; behavioral outcomes and HIV-related knowledge assessed at baseline and 4 weeks after intervention.	Preintervention and postintervention assessment without comparison condition. Behavioral outcomes and HIV-related knowledge assessed at baseline and 1 month after the intervention.	Quasiexperimental. Fifteen soccer teams were randomly selected from the southern region of the soccer league for the intervention condition; 15 teams were randomly selected from the northern region of the soccer league for the comparison condition in which participants were offered the intervention after the collection of 18-month follow-up data. Differences in sociodemographic characteristics of intervention and comparison participants were not statistically significant. Behavioral and other outcomes were assessed at baseline and 18 months after the intervention.
Retention	61% of 286 men completed the baseline and 1-month follow-up assessments.	74% of 23 men who started the intervention completed all sessions; 48% completed the 1-month follow-up assessment.	81% of 222 participants who completed the baseline assessment completed the 18-month follow-up assessment.
Sample at time of baseline assessment	286 Latino males: 142 in the intervention condition; 144 in the comparison condition.	23 Latino males; intervention was delivered to two groups of 12 and 13 men, respectively.	222 Latino males: 108 in the intervention condition; 114 in the delayed intervention condition.

| Principal outcomes | At 1-month follow-up: percentages of men reporting sex with a sex worker increased from 24% to 28% and from 24% to 29% in the intervention and comparison conditions, respectively; among men who reported no condom use prior to baseline and who had sex with sex workers in the United States by the follow-up assessment, 62% of the intervention participants and 0% of the comparison participants reported condom use; 23% of the intervention participants and 4% of the comparison participants who had sex with sex workers in Mexico used condoms. | At 1-month follow-up: the percentage of men responding correctly to condom use questions nearly doubled; the percentage of men who reported sex with one or more female sex partners, with or without condoms, declined from 73% to 33%; the percentage of men who reported sex with sex workers, with or without condoms, declined from 30% to zero; the percentage of men who always carried condoms increased from 43% to 83%; those who never carried condoms decreased from 26% to zero; the percentage of men who reported sex with one or more female partners without using condoms decreased from 43% to zero; the percentage of men who reported not using condoms during sex with one-time only partners, regular partners, or female sex workers, respectively, decreased from 21% to zero. | At 18-month follow-up, relative to delayed intervention participants, intervention participants reported greater HIV transmission and prevention-related knowledge (unadjusted analysis, 74.1% vs. 43.5%; $p < 0.001$), greater condom use self-efficacy (unadjusted analysis, 55.6% vs. 38.2%; $p < 0.01$), more consistent condom use during the prior 30 days (unadjusted analysis, 65.6% vs. 41.3%; $p < 0.001$), any condom use [adjusted odds ratio (AOR) = 2.3; 95% confidence internal (CI) = 1.2–4.3], and HIV testing (AOR = 2.5; CI = 1.5–4.3). Differences between intervention and delayed intervention participants' adherence to masculine norms and mastery of life's circumstances were not significant. |

DISCLAIMER

The findings and conclusions in this chapter are those of the authors and do not necessarily represent the views of the Centers for Disease Control and Prevention.

REFERENCES

Anderson, C. A. (2006). *Final report to the Centers for Disease Control and Prevention on adapting Safety Counts for migrant workers who use drugs.* Tucson, AZ: Border Health Foundation.

Apostolopoulos, Y., Somnez, S., Kronenfeld, J., Castillo, E., McLendon, L., & Smith, D. (2006). STI/HIV risks for Mexican migrant laborers: Exploratory ethnographies. *Journal of Immigrant and Minority Health, 8,* 291–302.

Aranda-Naranjo, B., Gaskins, S., Bustamente, L., Lopez, L. C., & Rodriguiz, J. (2000). La desesperación: Migrant and seasonal farm workers living with HIV/AIDS. *Journal of the Association of Nurses in AIDS Care, 11*(2), 22–28.

Bandura, A. (1977). *Social learning theory.* Englewood Cliffs, NJ: Prentice-Hall.

Bandura, A. (1986). *Social foundations of thought and action: A social cognitive theory.* Englewood Cliffs, NJ: Prentice-Hall.

Bastos, F. I., Cáceres, C., Galvão, J., Veras, M. A., & Castilho, E. A. (2008). AIDS in Latin America: Assessing the current status of the epidemic and the ongoing response. *International Journal of Epidemiology, 37,* 729–737.

Brammeier, M., Chow, J. M., Samuel, M. C., Organista, K. C., Miller, J., & Bolan, G. (2008). Sexually transmitted diseases and risk behaviors among California farmworkers: Results from a population-based survey. *The Journal of Rural Health, 24*(3), 279–284.

Bronfman, M., Sejenovich, G., & Uribe, P. (1998). *Migración y SIDA en México y América Central.* Mexico City: Ángulos del SIDA and CONASIDA [Consejo Nacional para la prevención y Control del VIH/SIDA].

Carrillo, H. (2002). *The night is young: Sexuality in Mexico in the time of AIDS.* Chicago, IL: University of Chicago Press.

Cashman, S. B., Adeky, S., Allen, A., Corburn, J., Israel, B. A., Montaño, J., et al. (2008). Analyzing and interpreting data with communities. In M. Minkler & N. Wallerstein (Eds.), *Community-based participatory research for health: From process to outcomes* (2 ed., pp. 285–302). San Francisco, CA: Jossey-Bass.

CDC (Centers for Disease Control and Prevention). (1988). Epidemiologic notes and reports: HIV seroprevalence in migrant and seasonal farmworkers—North Carolina, 1987. *Morbidity and Mortality Weekly Report, 37,* 517–519.

CDC. (2006). AIDS cases, by geographic area of residence and metropolitan statistical area of residence, 2004. *HIV/AIDS surveillance supplemental report 2006, 12*(2), 1–65. Atlanta, GA: Centers for Disease Control and Prevention, Division of STD Prevention. Also available at http://www.cdc.gov/hiv/topics/surveillance/resources/reports/2006supp_vol12no2/default.htm. Accessed September 30, 2008.

CDC. (2007). *Sexually transmitted disease surveillance 2006.* Atlanta, GA: Centers for Disease Control and Prevention, Division of STD Prevention, November. Available at http://www.cdc.gov/std/stats/toc2006.htm. Accessed September 26, 2008.

CENSIDA. (2003). *Epidemiología del VIH/SIDA en México en el año 2003.* Mexico, D.F.: Centro Nacional para la prevención y control del VIH/SIDA, Secretaría de Salud. 01 noviembre. Available at http://www.salud.gob.mx/conasida/estadis/pre2003.pdf. Accessed November 10, 2006.

CONASIDA. (2000). *El SIDA en México en el año 2000*. Mexico, D.F.: Centro Nacional para la prevención y control del VIH/SIDA. Available at http://www.ssa.gob.mx/conasida. Accessed November 10, 2006.

Conner, R. F. (1990). *AIDS prevention with Hispanic farm workers:* A formative evaluation. Report to the California Community Foundation, Los Angeles, California.

Cornelius, W. A., Fitzgerald, D. S., & Fisher, P. W. (Eds.) (2007). *Mayan journeys: The new migration from Yucatán to the United States*. La Jolla, CA: Center for Comparative Immigration Studies, University of California, San Diego.

Del Rio, C., & Sepúlveda, J. (2002). AIDS in Mexico: Lessons learned and implications for developing countries. *AIDS, 16,* 1445–1457.

Eng, E., Rhodes, S. D., & Parker, E. (2009). Natural helper models to enhance a community's health and competence. In R. J. DiClemente, R. A. Crosby, & M. C. Kegler (Eds.), *Emerging theories in health promotion practice and research* (2nd ed., pp. 303–330). San Francisco, CA: Jossey-Bass.

Espinoza, L., Hall, H. I., Selik, R. M., & Hu, X. (2008). Characteristics of HIV infection among Hispanics, United States 2003–2006. *Journal of Acquired Immune Deficiency Syndromes, 49,* 94–101.

Fishbein, M., & Ajzen, I. (1975). *Beliefs, attitudes, intention, and behavior: An introduction to theory and research*. Reading, MA: Addison-Wesley.

Frasca, T. (2009). *Shaping the new response: HIV/AIDS & Latinos in the Deep South*. New York: The Latino Commission on AIDS. Available at http://www.latinoaids.org/programs/southproject/docs/DeepSouthReportWeb.pdf. Accessed February 11, 2009.

Freire, P. (1970). *Pedagogy of the oppressed* (Ramos, M. B., Trans.). New York: Continuum.

Freire, P. (1973). *Education for critical consciousness*. New York: Seabury Press.

Galvan, F. H., Ortiz, D. J., Martinez, V., & Bing, E. G. (2008). Sexual solicitation of Latino male day laborers by other men. *Salud Pública de México, 50,* 439–446.

Gayet, C., Magis-Rodriguez, C., & Bronfman, M. P. (2000). Aspectos conceptuales sobre la relación entre la migración y el SIDA en México. *Enfermedades Infecciosas y Microbiologicas, 20,* 134–140.

Glanz, K., Marcus Lewis, F., & Rimer, B. K. (Eds.). (1997). *Health behavior and health education: Theory research and practice* (2nd ed.). San Francisco, CA: Jossey-Bass.

Grzywacz, J. G., Quandt, S. A., Early, J. T., Tapia, J., Graham, C. N., & Arcury, T. A. (2004). *Leaving family for work: Ambivalence & mental health among migrant Latino farmworkers*. Working Paper 04-01, Center for Latino Health Research, Department of Family and Community Medicine. Winston-Salem, NC: Wake Forest University School of Medicine.

Harawa, N. T., Bingham, T. A., Cochran, S. D., Greenland, S., & Cunningham, W. E. (2002). HIV prevalence among foreign- and US-born clients of public STD clinics. *American Journal of Public Health, 92,* 1958–1963.

Herbst, J. H., Kay, L. S., Passin, W. F., Lyles, C. M., Crepaz, N., & Marin, B. V. for the HIV/AIDS Prevention Research Synthesis (PRS) Team. (2007). A systematic review and meta-analysis of behavioral interventions to reduce HIV risk behaviors of Hispanics in the United States and Puerto Rico. *AIDS and Behavior, 11,* 25–47.

Hernández, M. T., Sanchez, M., Aoki, B., Ruiz, J., Bravo Garcia, E., Samuel, M., & Lemp, G. (2007). *Epidemiology of HIV and sexually transmitted infections among Mexican migrants in California. Los Angeles, California*. 14th Conference on Retroviruses and Opportunistic Infections, Los Angeles, California, February 25–27, 2007. Abstract no. 965. Available at http://www.retroconference.org/2007/Abstracts/29358.htm. Accessed April 3, 2009.

Hernández, M. T., Sanchez, M. A., Ayala, L., Magis-Rodríguez, C., Ruiz, J. D., Samuel, M. C., Aoki, B. K., Garza, A. H., & Lemp, G. F. (2009). Methamphetamine and cocaine use among Mexican migrants in California: The California-Mexico Epidemiological Surveillance Pilot. *AIDS Education & Prevention, 21*(5, Suppl 1), 34–44.

Hernández, M. T., Sanchez, M. A., Ayala, L. A., Magis-Rodriguez, C., Ruiz, J. D., Samuel, M. D., Lemp, G. F., & Drake, M. V. (2008). *Mexican migrants in California and methamphetamines: The California–Mexico Epidemiological Surveillance Pilot (CMESP).* XVII International AIDS Conference, Mexico City, August 3–8, 2008. Available at http://www.aids2008.org/Pag/Abstracts.aspx?AID=3914. Accessed April 3, 2009.

Hernández, M. T., Sanchez, M. A., Ruiz, J. D., Samuel, M. C., Magis, C., Drake, M. V., & Lemp, G. F. (2005). *High STI rates and risk behaviors among Mexican migrants in California.* National HIV Prevention Conference, Atlanta, Georgia, June 12–15. Abstract No. M3-B0202. Available at http://www.aegis.org/conferences/nhivpc/2005/M3-B0202.html. Accessed April 3, 2009.

Hirsch, J. S. (2003). *A courtship after marriage: Sexuality and love in Mexican transnational families.* Berkeley: University of California Press.

Hirsch, J. S., Higgins, J., Bentley, M. E., & Nathanson, C. A. (2002). The social constructions of sexuality: Marital infidelity and sexually transmitted disease—HIV risk in a Mexican migrant community. *American Journal of Public Health, 92*, 1227–1237.

Hirsch, J. S., Meneses, S., Thompson, B., Negroni, M., Pelcastre, B., & del Rio, C. (2007). The inevitability of infidelity: Sexual reputation, social geographies, and marital HIV risk in rural Mexico. *American Journal of Public Health, 97*(6), 886–996.

Hirsch, J. S., Muñoz-Laboy, M., Nyhus, C. M., Yount, K. M., & Bauermeister, J. A. (2009). "Because he misses his normal life back home": Masculinity and sexual behavior among Mexican migrants in Atlanta, Georgia. *Perspectives on Sexual and Reproductive Health, 41*(1), 23–32.

Hirsch, J. S., & Yount, K. M. (2001). *"Because he misses his normal life back home": Social and cultural influences on Mexican migrants' and HIV risk behaviors.* 2001 Meeting of the American Anthropological Association, Washington, DC, November 28–December 2.

Inciardi, J. A., Surrat, H. L., Colon, H. M., Chitwood, D. D., & Rivers, J. E. (1999). Drug use and HIV risks among migrant workers on the DelMarVa Peninsula. *Substance Use & Abuse, 34*, 653–666.

Jones, J. L., Rion, P., Hollis, S., Longshore, S., Leverette, W. B., & Ziff, L. (1991). HIV related characteristics of migrant workers in rural South Carolina. *Southern Medical Journal, 84*, 1088–1090.

Kandel, W., & Parrado, E. A. (2004). Hispanics in the American south and the transformation of the poultry industry. In D. D. Arreola (Ed.), *Hispanic spaces, Latino places: Community and cultural diversity in contemporary America* (pp. 255–276). Austin: University of Texas Press.

Kissinger, P., Kovacs, S., Anderson-Smits, C., Schmidt, N., Salinas, O., Hembling, J., Beaulieu, A., Longfellow, L., Liddon, N., Rice, J., & Shedlin, M. (2012). Patterns and predictors of HIV/STI risk among Latino migrant men in a new receiving community. *AIDS and Behavior, 16*(1), 199–213.

Kissinger, P., Liddon, N., Schmidt, N., Curtin, E., Salinas, O., & Narvaez, A. (2008). HIV/STI risk behaviors among Latino migrants in New Orleans post-hurricane Katrina disaster. *Sexually Transmitted Diseases, 35*, 924–929.

Knipper, E., Rhodes, S. D., Lindstrom, K., Bloom, F. R., Leichliter, J. S., & Montano, J. (2007). Condom use among heterosexual immigrant Latino men in the southeastern United States. *AIDS Education and Prevention, 19*(5), 436–447.

Kochhar, R. (2005). Latino labor report, 2004: More jobs for new immigrants but at lower wages. Washington, DC: Pew Hispanic Center. Available at http://pewhispanic.org/files/reports/45.pdf. Accessed April 3, 2009.

Kochhar, R., Suro, R., & Tafoya, S. (2005). *The new Latino South: The context and consequences of rapid population growth. Report.* Washington, DC: PEW Hispanic Center. Available at http://pewhispanic.org/files/reports/50.pdf. Accessed April 3, 2009.

Kullgren, J. (2003). Restrictions on undocumented immigrants' access to health services: The public health implications of welfare reform. *American Journal of Public Health, 80,* S54–S60.

Lafferty, J. (1991). Self-injection and needle sharing among migrant farmworkers. *American Journal of Public Health, 81,* 221.

Lafferty, J., Foulk, D., & Ryan, R. (1990–91). Needle sharing for the use of therapeutic drugs as a potential AIDS risk behavior among migrant Hispanic farmworkers in the Eastern stream. *International Quarterly of Community Health Education, 11,* 135–143.

Lara, M., Gamboa, C., Kahramanian M. I., Morales, L. S., & Bautista, D. E. (2005). Acculturation and Latino health in the United States: A review of the literature and its sociopolitical context. *Annual Review of Public Health, 26,* 367–397.

Levy, V., Page-Shafer, K., Evans, J., Ruiz, J., Morrow, S., Reardon, J., Lynch, M., Raymond, H. F., Klausner, J. D., Facer, M., Molitor, F., Allen, B., Ajufo, B. G., Ferrero, D., Sanford, G. B., McFarland, W., & HeyMan Study Team. (2005). HIV-related risk behavior among Hispanic immigrant men in a population-based household survey in low-income neighborhoods of northern California. *Sexually Transmitted Diseases, 32*(8), 487–490.

Levy, V., Prentiss, D., Balmas, G., Chen, S., Israelski, D., Katzenstein, D., & Page-Shafer, K. (2007). Factors in the delayed HIV presentation of immigrants in northern California: Implications for voluntary counseling and testing programs. *Journal of Immigrant and Minority Health, 9*(1), 49–54.

Lopez, A. A. (2007). *The farmworkers' journey.* Berkeley: University of California Press.

Los Angeles County Department of Health Services. (2000). *HIV epidemiology program:* An epidemiological profile of HIV and AIDS in Los Angeles County. Los Angeles, CA: Los Angeles Department of Health Services.

Magaña, J. R. (1991). "Sex, drugs and HIV: An ethnographic approach." *Social Science and Medicine, 33,* 5–9.

Magaña, J. R., Conner, R. F., Mishra, S. I., & Lewis, M. A. (1990). An *AIDS prevention program for Hispanic/Latino farmworkers.* Annual meeting of the American Public Health Association, New York, September 30–October 4.

Magis-Rodriguez, C., Gayet, C., Negroni, M., Leyva, R., Bravo-Garcia, E., Uribe, P., & Bronfman, M. (2004). Migration and AIDS in Mexico. An overview based on recent evidence. *Journal of Acquired Immune Deficiency Syndromes, 37,* S215–S226.

Martinez-Donate, A. P., Rangel, M. G., Hovell, M. F., Santibanez, J., Sipan, C. L., & Izáosla, J. A. (2005). HIV infection in mobile populations: The case of Mexican migrants in the United States. *Pan American Journal of Public Health, 17*(1), 26–29.

Massey, D. D., Arango, J., Hugo, G., Kouaouci, A., Pellegrino, A., & Taylor, J. E. (2005). *Worlds in motion: Understanding international migration at the end of the millennium.* Oxford and New York: Oxford University Press.

McVea, K. L. S. P. (1997). Lay injection practices among migrant farmworkers in the age of AIDS: Evolution of biomedical folk practices. *Social Science and Medicine, 45,* 91–98.

Menjívar, C. (2000). *Fragmented ties: Salvadoran immigrant networks in America.* Berkeley: University of California Press.

Mishra, S. I., & Conner, R. F. (1996). Evaluation of an HIV prevention program among Latino farmworkers. In S. I. Mishra, R. F. Conner, & J. R. Magaña (Eds.), *AIDS crossing borders: The spread of HIV among Migrant Latinos* (pp. 157–181). Boulder, CO: Westview Press.

Mishra, S. I., Conner, R. F., & Magaña, J. R. (1996). Migrant workers in the United States: A profile from the fields. In S. I. Mishra, R. F. Conner, & J. R. Magaña (Eds.), *AIDS crossing borders: The spread of HIV among migrant Latinos* (pp. 3–24). Boulder, CO: Westview Press.

Mishra, S. I., Sañudo, F., & Conner, R. F. (2004). Collaborative research toward HIV prevention among migrant farmworkers. In B. P. Bowser, S. I. Mishra, C. J. Reback, & G. F. Lemp (Eds.), *Preventing AIDS: Community-science collaborations* (pp. 69–95). Binghamton, NY: Haworth Press.

Muñoz-Laboy, M., Hirsch, J. S., & Quipse-Lazaro, A. (2009). Loneliness as a sexual risk factor for male Mexican migrant workers. *American Journal of Public Health, 99,* 1–9.

Newland, K. (2009). *Circular migration and human development.* Human Development Research Paper 2009/42. New York: United Nations Development Programme.

Organista, K. C. (2007). Towards a structural-environmental model of risk for HIV and problem drinking in Latino labor migrants: The case of day laborers. *Journal of Ethnic and Cultural Diversity in Social Work, 16,* 95–125.

Organista, K. C., Alvarado, N., Balbutin-Burnham, A., Worby, P., & Martinez, S. (2006). An exploratory study of HIV prevention with Mexican/Latino migrant day laborers. *Journal of HIV/AIDS and Social Services, 5*(2), 89–114.

Organista, K. C., Balls Organista, P., Garcia de Alba, G., Castillo Moran, M., & Ureta Carillo, L. (1997). Survey of condom-related beliefs, behaviors, and perceived social norms in Mexican migrant laborers. *Journal of Community Health, 22,* 185–198.

Organista, K. C., Carillo, H., & Ayala, G. (2004). HIV prevention with Mexican migrants: Review, critique, and recommendations. *Journal of Acquired Immune Deficiency Syndromes, 37,* S227–S239.

Organista, K. C., & Kubo, A. (2005). Pilot survey of HIV risk and contextual problems and issues in Mexican/Latino migrant day laborers. *Journal of Immigrant Health, 7*(4), 269–281.

Painter, T. M. (1996). Space, time and rural-urban linkages in Africa. Notes for a geography of livelihoods. *African Rural and Urban Studies, 3*(1), 79–98.

Painter, T. M. (1999). Livelihood mobility and AIDS prevention in West Africa: Challenges and opportunities for social scientists. In C. Becker, J-P. Dozon, C. Obbo, & M. Touré (Eds.), *Vivre et penser le sida en Afrique/Experiencing and understanding AIDS in Africa* (pp. 645–665). Paris: Karthala, IRD; Dakar: CODESRIA.

Painter, T. M. (2004). *A missing link? Migrants' social support networks as a potential resource for increasing migrants' participation in HIV/STD-related and other health care services.* Presentation at the 17th Annual East Coast Migrant Stream Forum, St. Petersburg, Florida, October 21–23.

Painter, T. M. (2008). Connecting the dots: When the risks of HIV/STD infection appear high but the burden of infection is not known—the case of male Latino migrants in the southern United States. *AIDS and Behavior, 12,* 213–226.

Painter, T. M., Schulden, J. D., Song, B., Valverde, E., Borman, M. A., Monroe-Spencer, K., Bautista, G., Saleheen, H., Voetsch, A., & Heffelfinger, J. D. (2011). *HIV testing histories and risk factors reported by migrants tested for HIV by three CBOs.* 2011 National HIV Prevention Conference, Atlanta, Georgia, August 14–17, 2011. Abstract no. 1287.

Parker, E. A., Eng, E., Laraia, B., Ammerman, A., Dodds, J., Margolis, L., et al. (1998). Coalition building for prevention: Lessons learned from the North Carolina community-based public health initiative. *Journal of Public Health Management and Practice, 4*(2), 25–36.

Parrado, E. A., Flippen, C. A., & McQuiston, C. (2004). Use of commercial sex workers among Hispanic migrants in North Carolina: Implications for the diffusion of HIV. *Perspectives on Sexual and Reproductive Health, 36,* 150–156.

Passel, J. S. (2005). *Unauthorized migrants: Numbers and characteristics.* Washington, DC: Pew Hispanic Center, June 14. Available at http://pewhispanic.org/files/reports/46.pdf. Accessed April 3, 2009.

Passel, J. S., & Cohn, D. (2008). *Trends in unauthorized immigration: Undocumented inflow now trails legal inflow.* Washington, DC: Pew Hispanic Center, October 2008. Available at http://pewhispanic.org/files/reports/94.pdf. Accessed April 3, 2009.

Passel, J. S., & Cohn, D. (2010). *U.S. unauthorized immigration flows are down sharply since mid-decade.* Washington, DC: Pew Hispanic Center, September 1. Available at http://pewhispanic.org/reports/report.php?ReportID=126. Accessed December 8, 2010.

Paz-Bailey, G., Teran, S., Levine, W., & Markowitz, L. E. (2004). Syphilis outbreak among Hispanic immigrants in Decatur, Alabama. *Sexually Transmitted Diseases, 31,* 20–25.

Portes, A., & Walton, J. (1981). *Labor, class, and the international system.* New York: Academic Press.

Rajabiun, S., Rumptz, M. H., Felizzola, J., Frye, A., Relf, M., Yu, G., & Cunningham, W. W. (2008). The impact of acculturation on Latinos' perceived barriers to HIV primary care. *Ethnicity & Disease, 18,* 403–408.

Rangel, M. G., Martínez-Donate, A. P., Hovell, M. F., Santibáñez, J., Sipan, C. L., & Izazola-Licea, J. A. (2006). Prevalence of risk factors for HIV infection among Mexican migrants and immigrants: Probability survey in the north border of Mexico. *Salud Pública de México, 48,* 3–12.

Rhodes, S. D., Eng, E., Hergenrather, K. C., Remnitz, I. M., Arceo, R., Montano, J., et al. (2007). Exploring Latino men's HIV risk using community-based participatory research. *American Journal of Health Behavior, 31*(2), 146–158.

Rhodes, S. D., Hergenrather, K. C., Bloom, F. R., Leichliter, J. S., & Montaño, J. (2009). Outcomes from a community-based, participatory lay health advisor HIV/STD prevention intervention for recently arrived immigrant Latino men in rural North Carolina, USA. *AIDS Education & Prevention, 21*(5), 103–108.

Rhodes, S. D., Hergenrather, K. C., Montano, J., Remnitz, I. M., Arceo, R., Bloom, F. R., Leichliter, J. S., & Bowden, W. P. (2006). Using community-based participatory research to develop an intervention to reduce HIV and STD infections among Latino men. *AIDS Education and Prevention, 18*(5), 375–389.

Rosenstock, I. M. (1960). What research in motivation suggests for public health. *American Journal of Public Health, 50,* 295–301.

Ruiz J. D., Da Valle, L., Junghkeit, M., Mobed, K., & Lopez, R. (1997). *Seroprevalence of HIV and syphilis and assessment of risk behaviors among migrant and seasonal farmworkers in Northern California.* Sacramento, CA: Office of AIDS, California Department of Health Services.

Sanchez, M. A., Hernández, M. T., Vera, A., Magis Rodriguez, C., Ruiz, J. D., Drake, M. V., & Lemp, G. F. (2008). *The effect of migration on HIV high-risk behaviors among Mexican migrants.* 2008 International AIDS Conference, Mexico City, August 3–8, 2008. Abstract no. TUAD0203. Available at http://www.aids2008.org/Pag/Abstracts.aspx?SID=282&AID=15433. Accessed April 3, 2009.

Sanchez, M. A., Lemp, G. F., Magis-Rodríguez, C., Bravo-García, E., Carter, S., & Ruiz, J. D. (2004). The epidemiology of HIV among Mexican migrants and recent immigrants in California and Mexico. *Journal of Acquired Immune Deficiency Syndromes, 37*(4), S204–S214.

Sañudo, F. M. (1999). *The effects of a culturally appropriate HIV intervention on Mexican farmworkers' knowledge, attitudes, and condom use behavior.* Unpublished master's thesis. San Diego, CA: Department of Public Health, San Diego State University.

Sassen, S. (1988). *The mobility of labor and capital. A study in international investment and labor flow.* Cambridge: Cambridge University Press.

Scott, S., & Wascher-Tavares, R. (2008*). Safety Counts for migrant farmworkers: A cognitive-behavioral intervention to reduce HIV/hepatitis risks among migrant farmworkers who use drugs.* Draft Program Manual. Tucson and Atlanta: Border Health Foundation and Centers for Disease Control and Prevention.

Shedlin, M. G., Decena, C. U., & Oliver-Velez, D. (2005). Initial acculturation and HIV risk among new Hispanic immigrants. *Journal of the National Medical Association, 97,* 32S–37S.

Solorio, M. R., Currier, J., & Cunningham, W. (2004). HIV health care services for Mexican migrants. *Journal of Acquired Immune Deficiency Syndromes, 37,* S240–S251.

Somerville, G. G., Diaz, S., Davis, S., Coleman, K. D., & Taveras, S. (2006). Adapting the popular opinion leader intervention for Latino young migrant men who have sex with men. *AIDS Education and Prevention, 18*(A), 37–148.

Southern State Directors Work Group. (2008). *Southern States Manifesto: Update 2008. HIV/AIDS and sexually transmitted diseases in the South.* Birmingham, AL: Southern AIDS Coalition.

Sowell, R. L., Holtz, C. S., & Velasquez, G. (2008). HIV infection returning to Mexico with migrant workers: An exploratory study. *Journal of the Association of Nurses in AIDS Care, 19,* 267–282.

UNDP. (2009). Human Development Report 2009. *Overcoming barriers: Human mobility and development.* New York: United Nations Development Programme.

U.S. Census. (1990). Table DP-1, *General population and housing characteristics, 1990 census of population and housing,* Summary Tape File 1 (100% Data). Washington, DC: U.S. Bureau of the Census, 1990. Available at http://factfinder.census.gov. Accessed September 25, 2008.

U.S. Census. (2007). Table DP-1, *General demographic characteristics, 2007 population estimates.* Washington, DC: U.S. Bureau of the Census, July 1, 2007. Available at http://factfinder.census.gov. Accessed September 25, 2008.

U.S. Department of Labor. (2005). *Findings from the national agricultural workers survey (NAWS) 2001–2002.* Research Report No. 9. Washington, DC: U.S. Department of Labor, Office of the Assistant Secretary for Policy, Office of Programmatic Policy. March. Available at http://www.doleta.gov/agworker/report9/naws_rpt9.pdf. Accessed April 3, 2009.

Varela-Ramirez, A., Mejia, A., Garcia, D., Bader, J., & Aguilera, R. J. (2005). HIV infection and risk behavior of Hispanic farm workers at the west Texas-Mexico border. *Ethnicity & Disease, 15*(4 Suppl 5), S5–92–96.

Vega, W. A., Kolody, B., Valle, R., & Weir, J. (1991). Social networks, social support, and their relationship to depression among Mexican women. *Human Organization, 50,* 154–162.

Viadro, C. I., & Earp, J. A. L. (2000). The sexual behavior of married Mexican immigrant men in North Carolina. *Social Science & Medicine, 50,* 723–735.

Vissman, A. T., Eng, E., Aronson, R. E., Bloom, F. R., Leichliter, J. S., Montaño, J., & Rhodes, S. D. (2009). What do men who serve as lay health advisors really do?: Immigrant Latino men share their experiences as *Navegantes* to prevent HIV. *AIDS Education and Prevention, 21*(3), 220–232.

Wallerstein, N. (1992). Health and safety education for workers with low-literacy or limited-English skills. *American Journal of Internal Medicine, 22*(5), 751–765.

Wallerstein, N. (1994). Empowerment education applied to youth. In A. C. Matiella (Ed.), *The multicultural challenge in health education* (pp. 153–176). Santa Cruz, CA: ETR Associates.

Wong, G., Tambis, J. A., Hernandez, M. T., Chaw, J. K., & Klausner, J. D. (2003). Prevalence of sexually transmitted diseases among Latino immigrant day laborers in an urban setting—San Francisco. *Sexually Transmitted Diseases, 30,* 661–663.

Worby, P., & Organista, K. C. (2007). Alcohol use and problem drinking among male Mexican and Central American immigrant laborers: A review of the literature. *Hispanic Journal of Behavioral Sciences, 29,* 413–455.

19 HIV Prevention Interventions with Puerto Rican Injection Drug Users

Lisa de Saxe Zerden, Luz Marilis López, and Lena Lundgren

INTRODUCTION

As previous chapters have discussed, HIV/AIDS knows no geographic or human boundaries. Socially marginalized groups disenfranchised by health inequalities, poverty, and lack of access to resources continue to be impacted most by the transmission of HIV through injection drug use (IDU) and high-risk sexual behaviors (National Institute on Allergy and Infectious Disease, 2008; National Institute of Drug Abuse, 2003). Through the sharing of contaminated needles and syringes, and other paraphernalia such as cotton swabs, water, and cookers, injection drug users (IDUs) are at increased risk of both developing HIV/AIDS and contracting blood-borne viruses, primarily the hepatitis C virus (HCV) and other sexually transmitted infections (Palmateer, Kimber, Hickman, Jutchinson, Rhodes, & Goldberg, 2010). It is estimated that there are 15.9 million IDUs worldwide (Mathers, Degenhardt, Phillips, Wiessing, Hickman, & Strathdee, 2008). In the United States, as of 2005, injection drug use accounted for about 20% of all HIV infections and HCV infections (Centers for Disease Control and Prevention, 2007).

Although the HIV/AIDS epidemic is not uniformly distributed throughout the United States, AIDS prevalence among Latinos is clustered in areas with high concentration of Latino residents such as California, Texas, Florida, and several of the Northeast and mid-Atlantic states—areas with the highest predominance of Puerto Ricans. The Commonwealth of Puerto Rico, an unincorporated U.S. territory populated by approximately 4 million people, roughly the size of Connecticut, is considered an HIV/AIDS epicenter within the Western Hemisphere (U.S. Department of Health and Human Services, 2007) (see Chapter 13 for more discussion on this topic). HIV/AIDS infection rates in the Caribbean are among the highest in the world, second only to those in Sub-Saharan Africa (World Bank, 2001; UNAIDS, 2010). It is estimated that the prevalence rate of adults living with HIV/AIDS globally is 0.8%, compared to 5.2% in Sub-Saharan Africa and 0.8% in the Caribbean (UNAIDS,2010; The Kaiser Family Foundation, 2009). In the Caribbean, AIDS is one of the leading causes of death among those aged 25–44 years and IDU has been noted as the key factor in HIV/AIDS transmission in Puerto Rico and Bermuda specifically (The Kaiser Family Foundation, 2009).

For Latinos, rates of HIV/AIDS, behavioral risk factors, and mode of transmission differ by country of birth (Montoya, Bell, Richard, Carlson, & Trevino, 1999; Centers for Disease Control and Prevention, 2005; The Kaiser Family Foundation, 2008a). First, with respect to AIDS rates in the United States, Latinos born on the mainland accounted for 34% of the estimated AIDS cases among Latinos in 2006, followed by Latinos born in Puerto Rico and those born Mexico; the latter two groups accounted for 17%, respectively (The Kaiser Family Foundation, 2008a). Second, in terms of mode of transmission, Latinos born in Puerto Rico are more likely to contract HIV as a result of injecting drugs (Centers for Disease Control and Prevention, 2005) (see Chapter 13 for an interesting focus on serodiscordant heterosexual Puerto Rican couples). Also, Puerto Ricans have the worst overall health outcomes compared to other Latino ethnic groups in the United States (Hajat, Lucas, & Kingston, 2000; Delgado, 2007) and evidence has shown that Puerto Ricans are more susceptible to increased infection of HIV and other blood-borne pathogens (Colón et al., 2001).

More than half of all AIDS cases among Puerto Ricans have been attributed to IDU (Deren, Kang, Colón, & Robles, 2007a) and it has been estimated that approximately 40% of Puerto Rican women have been infected as a result of sexual contact with a male injection drug user (Latino Commission on AIDS, 2004). The alarming rate of IDU in Puerto Rico and among Puerto Ricans who migrate to the U.S. mainland requires comprehensive HIV prevention strategies that are developed to respond to increasing HIV/AIDS vulnerability of Puerto Rican IDUs, their sexual partners, and what this means for Puerto Rican transnationality. Increased HIV/AIDS risk factors are predicated on complex internal and external conditions related to acculturative stress, comorbidity associated with substance abuse (e.g., mental illness, homelessness, employment, and incarceration histories), prevalence of drugs including the type and what practices are commonly used as the route of administration—all factors connected to behavioral and social norms deeply rooted within the island, and among Puerto Ricans diasporic communities living stateside.

This chapter reviews existing research to identify key socioeconomic and cultural factors that need to be acknowledged when developing HIV prevention efforts aimed at Puerto Rican IDUs. Second, it provides specific recommendations with respect to how to improve HIV prevention strategies aimed at Puerto Rican IDUs specifically. This chapter connects well to the structural-environmental (SE) model of HIV risk and prevention given its emphasis on contextualizing HIV risk based on individual, behavioral, and structural factors. The SE model applies well with Puerto Rican IDUs because it is not simply a model for risk behaviors but also of resiliency, prevention, and positive change. In social work, this is known as a strengths perspective rather than a deficit focus. Although rates of IDU and HIV are alarming among Puerto Ricans in comparison to other groups of Latinos, and especially so on the island, this chapter describes how community-led prevention efforts are being conducted in order to reduce stigma and bring about positive change in getting community members to understand the impact of HIV/AIDS and substance abuse as not just an individual's deficit but rather a community-wide problem requiring structural intervention.

PUERTO RICO'S UNIQUE POLITICAL STATUS

The Commonwealth of Puerto Rico is rich in history and traditions. Its unique political status makes Puerto Rico a "Commonwealth"—a term that allows for a simultaneous form of self-government on local matters but lacks sovereignty and independence in other arenas including defense, currency, external relations with other nations, highway and road infrastructure, postal service, and social welfare policies including social security and welfare—domains that fall within the jurisdiction of the U.S. federal government (Puerto Rico Federal Affairs Administration, 2008). Although Puerto Rico can raise its own flag, has drafted its own Constitution, and uses Spanish as the official language, Puerto Ricans cannot be elected to the U.S. House of Representatives or Senate or vote for the U.S. president,[1] and their congressional representative has no voting privileges (Bea & Garret, 2010).

Historically, under President Theodore Roosevelt, Congress passed the Jones–Shafroth Act in 1917, which granted Puerto Ricans U.S. citizenship and established Puerto Rico as an "organized but unincorporated" territory of the United States (Presidential Task Force, 2005, p. 3). In 1950, the Puerto Rican Federal Regulations Act (also known as Public Law 600) was passed allowing Puerto Rico the right to establish their own constitution for internal affairs "on matters of purely local concern" (p. 8). The implications for public health have resulted in a fragmented and decentralized system of care wherein funding and access to health care has been limited in comparison to health services available in the mainland United States.

Although Puerto Ricans currently comprise the second largest Hispanic subgroup in the United States (U.S. Census Bureau, 2006; Tucker et al., 2010), they continually report the worst health status and highest prevalence of several acute and chronic health conditions, when compared with other Hispanic subgroups and non-Hispanic whites (Tucker et al., 2010). Limited educational and employment opportunities, high rates of poverty among Puerto Ricans on the island and mainland, political disenfranchisement, and a legacy of historical trauma continue to shape the context in which IDUs function.

Recently, the U.S. Department of Health and Human Services announced that the Centers for Disease Control and Prevention (CDC) awarded funding for 94 projects totaling $42.5 million to state, tribal, local, and territorial health departments to improve their ability to provide public health services through the Affordable Care Act. However, the Puerto Rico Department of Health was the recipient of only one $200,000 award of federal monies in order to improve the quality and effectiveness of health services offered on the island (U.S. Department of Health and Human Services, 2009).

Unique Migratory Patterns

Because Puerto Ricans are U.S. citizens and passport holders, their travel to and from Puerto Rico is done with relative ease in comparison to other Latino groups who face increasingly stringent immigration laws, visa requirements, national quotas, and financial obstacles (Deren et al., 2003a; Acevedo, 2004). A unique type of migratory patterns common among Puerto Ricans is known as *circular migration*, used to describe a revolving door relationship that often exists for many Puerto Ricans between the island and the mainland United States. Duany (1996, 2002) utilizes a "flying bus" metaphor whereas Deren et al. (2003a) uses an "air bridge" to illustrate these unique migration patterns of Puerto Ricans from Puerto Rico to the mainland, particularly in the northeast corridor of the United States. This migratory pattern is also described by Duany (2002) as a part of the Puerto Rican national identity:

Diasporic communities are an integral part of the Puerto Rican nation because they continue to be linked to the Island by an intense circular movement of people, identities, and practices, as well as capital, technology and commodities. Hence, the Puerto Rican nation is no longer restricted to the Island but instead is constituted by two distinct yet closely intertwined fragments: that of Puerto Rico itself and that of the diasporic communities settled in the continental U.S. (p. 5)

Literature on Puerto Rican migratory patterns has measured circular migration in various ways, often leading to varied outcomes. Although some researchers have attempted to measure these migration patterns as length of stay, by the frequency of trips between Puerto Rico and the U.S. mainland, by familial connections, or by time spent in each location over a lifetime, a clear consensus of how best to measure and understand what circular migration means is still under debate. The lack of a cohesive definition has contributed to what Godoy, Carvalho, Hexner, and Jenkins (2002) consider the "polemic about the causes and consequences of circular migration" for Puerto Ricans (p.26). Hence, depending on the researcher and the particular facet of Puerto Rican migration being researched, consequences of circular migration vary both positively and negatively.

Duany (2002) theorizes that circular migration erodes conventional definitions of citizenship and national identity. There are significant benefits of this kind of movement including a strong sense of pride and attachment to Puerto Rico even while living in the United States for decades. Similarly, circular migration allows Puerto Rican to combine various sources of social support and human capital in both locations, an approach that can be seen as a survival strategy in order to maximize employment opportunities and financial resources, among other supports. More problematic views of circular migration suggest it weakens Puerto Rican human capital and job stability, increases family disruption, and may contribute to Puerto Rican's high rates of divorce[2] (Godoy et al., 2002; Riviera-Batiz & Santiago, 1996). This lack of permanence limits job opportunities and pushes circular migrants toward unskilled service jobs because they do not stay long enough to develop additional skills via employment or educational opportunities (Duany, 2002).

The status of Puerto Ricans in the United States has been deeply entrenched in racism, discrimination, and a minority status similar to what other communities of color in the United States have experienced. High rates of poverty, persistently so for Puerto Ricans living stateside, female-headed households (Baker, 2002), substandard living conditions, and "discriminatory mechanisms embedded in the labor market" have further affected the Puerto Rican identity and the minority status of Puerto Ricans in the mainland United States (Pimentel, 2008, p. 231).

A major limitation of Puerto Rican migration research is that there are few large, reliable databases detailing the specific features of circular migration. Due to Puerto Rico's unique status, Puerto Rican movement patterns are not as scrupulously documented and recorded as are statistics on the migratory patterns of other Latino immigrant groups. Although labor and employment seem to be a major motivator for migration between the United States, the island, and back again, little is known about the patterns of movement among the most vulnerable populations including IDUs and those living with HIV/AIDS, or how such movement contributes to the initiation of drug use in the first place.

Today, some consider Puerto Rico a stateless nation that has not assimilated into mainstream mainland U.S. society despite citizenship for Puerto Rican residents since 1917 and nearly a century of U.S. domination (Duany, 1996, 2002). Although U.S. federal involvement and massive migration of Puerto Ricans to the U.S. mainland have resulted in a diasporic community integral to the Puerto Rican

The Role of Acculturation Theory and Measurement

An understanding of acculturation theory is necessary as it addresses individual and social factors relating to the acculturative markers of Puerto Ricans in a more comprehensive manner. However, utilizing acculturation as a concept in assessing the health of Latinos, particularly their patterns of substance use and HIV risks, is a complex matter due to variations in how acculturation has been previously conceptualized and measured.

A large number of research studies have identified a positive association between Latino substance abuse and acculturation to U.S. society (Gil, Wagner, & Vega, 2000; Ortega, Rosenheck, Alegría, & Desai, 2000). Acculturation-related factors such as nativity, length of time in the U.S. mainland, familial factors, and other migration patterns differ between Puerto Ricans and other Latino groups; these are important factors to consider as social and environmental conditions that put IDUs at risk for increased HIV infection (Singer et al., 2005).

As Cortés, Deren, Andía, Colón, Robles, and Kang (2003) explain, examining the role of acculturation is pertinent in that substance abuse may emerge as a coping mechanism to mitigate the stresses immigrants/migrants encounter during the process of adaptation to different sociocultural systems, a particularly salient point given the minority status of Puerto Ricans in the mainland United States. The authors state: "Among IDUs, moving to a culture with different norms with regard to risky injection behaviors (e.g., sharing needles) may have an impact on injection-related risk" (p. 198). Existing literature focusing on drug use and the acculturation processes of Puerto Ricans has measured acculturation in varying ways that do not take into account the complexities of biculturalism (Cortés et al., 2003; Lara et al., 2005) or the vulnerabilities associated specifically with an IDU population such as cooccurring conditions including infections related to STI and HCV, as well as homelessness, incarceration histories, and unemployment.

Measurements of Acculturation and Substance Abuse

Research by Warner, Valdez, Vega, de la Rosa, Turner, and Canino (2006) highlight the inclusion of "culture change" in current Latino substance abuse research, and show that acculturative markers have consistently been found to be positively associated with substance abuse (Gil et al., 2000; Ortega et al., 2000). However, the majority of scales have been "tested with non-probability samples of Mexican Americans, often first generation immigrants residing in primarily California or Texas" (Yamada, Valle, Barrio, & Jeste, 2006, p. 544). A review of existing acculturation measurements identified a dearth of measurements and definitions specific to Puerto Ricans or acculturating substance abusing populations.

Recommendations to improve existing measurements include more uniform proxy measures of the acculturation process and the improvement in the operationalization of such factors (Cabassa, 2003). Most importantly, the context in which populations experience acculturation needs to be taken into account. Although limitations exist, current measures demonstrate that it is possible to find reasonable levels of reliability and concurrent validity when looking at the acculturative experiences of specific populations. In addition, existing measures and variables can be used to create more comprehensive measures of acculturation appropriate for Puerto Ricans.

Even though there is a debate about how best to measure migratory patterns and acculturation of Puerto Ricans, existing research also points to the importance of acknowledging these factors when developing any type of public health HIV prevention effort. By understanding the specific acculturative influences of Puerto Ricans and, specifically, Puerto Rican IDUs, service providers can make prevention and treatment programs more effective.

ARE PUERTO RICAN IDUS ON THE MAINLAND AT GREATER RISK FOR HIV COMPARED TO THOSE ON THE ISLAND OF PUERTO RICO?

Research on Puerto Ricans IDUs has revealed different type and levels of HIV/AIDS risk behaviors associated with where they reside. However, the majority of research points to higher levels of HIV risky activities associated with IDUs living in Puerto Rico in comparison to those living in the mainland United States. For example, Deren et al. (2003a) studied Puerto Rican IDUs in New York and Puerto Rico who had a history of injecting drugs in the geographic location opposite to where data were collected. Results indicated that the sample of Puerto Rican IDUs in New York was significantly less likely to report sharing injection equipment (10% vs. 37%, respectively) compared to the sample in Puerto Rico. Additionally, 52% of the New York sample was also significantly less likely to have injected heroin and cocaine in the past month as compared to 90% of the sample in Puerto Rico. The authors also note that IDUs who had recently moved to New York city, "a location with lower levels of injection-related risk behaviors and more tools available for risk reduction," demonstrated higher levels of risk behaviors in comparison to other Puerto Rican IDUs in New York (Deren et al., 2003a, p. 814). However, a limitation of this study is that the classification of migration groups does not fully take into account the circular migration patterns as previously discussed.

Similar findings have been demonstrated by a mixed-methods study of 800 IDUs in Harlem, New York, and 400 IDUs in Bayamón, Puerto Rico (Deren et al., 2003b). Although high levels of HIV risk behaviors in both communities were present, significantly higher levels of injection-related risk behaviors were reported among those in Puerto Rico. In this study, the frequency of IDU in the past 30 days was 183 times for those in Puerto Rico compared to 76 times among the New York sample, and nearly 80% of the sample in Puerto Rico had used "shooting galleries" (localities in which IDUs inject drugs) compared to 23% of the New York sample (Deren et al., 2003b). Furthermore, the sharing of any drug paraphernalia was about five times higher among the participants in Puerto Rico (34%) compared to those in Harlem (7%) (Deren et al., 2003b). These findings reiterate those of Colón et al. (2001) whose earlier study also found that the mean frequency of injection among those in Puerto Rico was significantly higher in comparison to Puerto Rican IDUs residing in New York.

Delgado et al. (2008) focused on needle sharing activities for two groups of Puerto Rican IDUs within the United States: those born in the United States ($n = 69$; 34.5% of the sample) and those born in Puerto Rico ($n = 131$; 65.0% of the sample).[3] Findings indicate that born in the United States was significantly associated with an increased likelihood of sharing needles (Delgado et al., 2008). Given that these findings contradict the higher risk typically found among island IDUs, researchers used focus groups to interpret these findings. The researchers suggest that "cultural differences between the two groups in both the interpretation of questions or willingness to provide information may be the result of this finding rather than actual differences in HIV risky behaviors" (Delgado et al., 2008, p. 89). Such findings reinforce the need for a more comprehensive understanding of culture and addictive behaviors, as well as acculturation theories, and the migration patterns particularly among Puerto Rican IDUs.

Rates and Type of Drugs Used by Puerto Rican IDUs

IDUs in Puerto Rico use heroin, cocaine, and often "speedball," which is a mix of heroin and cocaine, as a common drug of choice (Colón et al., 2001; Finlinson, Colón, Robles, & Soto-López, 2006). In a study of drug users in San Juan, Puerto Rico, participants reported pre-IDU histories of cocaine and heroin use through nasal administration at similar rates, 88% versus 82%, respectively. The average age of initiation for snorting cocaine was 17 years old and 18.4 years for the first age of heroin use (Finlinson et al., 2006). The combination of drugs was used to modulate the "high" or "down" effects of the primary drug, cocaine or heroin.

The mixing of different substances can bring additional drug risk behaviors for IDUs. In recent years there have been reports of the combined use of heroin or speedball with "*anestesia de caballo*" (horse anesthesia), known as xylazine, a veterinary analgesic sedative used by some Puerto Rican drug users on the island (Rodriguez et al., 2008). This combination has been associated with negative health consequences for IDUs, including severe open skin ulcers and abscess wounds at the injection sites on the body (Rodriguez et al., 2008). There might be an association with the use of xyalzine and higher risks for HIV/AIDS infection due to the IDUs having open ulcers and the possibility of being in contact with HIV-infected blood while injecting themselves or others.

In another dual city study, Puerto Rican IDUs on the island compared to Puerto Ricans IDUs in New York were significantly more likely to report using more shooting galleries (29% vs. 4%, respectively) as well as the sharing of drug paraphernalia (67% vs. 29%) (Deren et al., 2007a). Another HIV and STI risk behavior for Puerto Rican IDUs is that they often use syringes to measure the water to be poured into cookers and to draw drug solutions from the cookers as a group during episodes of drug sharing (Finlinson, Colón, López, Robles, & Cant, 2005). Initially, clean needles could be contaminated with blood residue or other toxic materials. The types of drug combinations and the sharing of drug paraphernalia present serious public health concerns for Puerto Rican IDUs.

Puerto Rican IDU and Rates of Needle Sharing

For IDUs, Friedman Curtis, Neaigus, Jose, and Des Jarlis (1999) and Sherman, Latkin, and Gielen (2001) emphasize social action by highlighting the influence of social networks on IDUs. The act of injecting drugs is typically a social exchange wherein users buy and inject drugs together. In some instances, IDUs who decide not to share injection drug equipment are viewed negatively by friends, relatives, and sexual partners who view this decision as a lack of trust or comradeship. Structurally, these decisions are complicated by larger forces that contribute to engaging in drug use and sexual risk behaviors that put Puerto Ricans at risk for HIV/AIDS.

Because the act of needle sharing is almost always a social behavior requiring the participation of two or more IDUs, it is paramount to understand the social bonding and cultural values embedded in drug use and needle sharing behaviors among Puerto Rican IDUs. A study by Andía, Deren, Robles, Kang, and Cólon (2008) evidenced higher rates of sharing drug paraphernalia and also exhibited more peer norms encouraging HIV risky behaviors. Based on these findings, Puerto Rican IDUs residing in Puerto Rico appeared to normalize sharing more frequently among peers and seemed to object less to HIV risk behaviors [e.g., believing it is okay to "share injecting paraphernalia" (p. 255), pooling money for drugs, and injecting in galleries]. Prevention programs to reduce needle sharing need to take into account the different kinds of risk norms as well as other demographic factors that place Puerto Rican IDUs at increased risk for HIV/AIDS and related infections.

HIV RISK AND DEMOGRAPHIC CHARACTERISTICS
Gender

A number of studies have been conducted on gender differences in HIV risky behaviors among Latino/a IDUs (Fitzgerald, 2008) and have identified that women drug users are at particular high risk of contracting HIV (Evans et al., 2003; Delgado et al., 2008; Johnson, Yep, Brems, Theno, & Fisher, 2002). Unger, Kipke, De Rosa, Hyde, Ritt-Olson, and Montgomery (2006) explain gendered needle sharing as a possible consequence of unequal partner dynamics within platonic or romantic relationships. Within the context of romantic relations, these researchers posit that the "refusal to share needles might be interpreted as a lack of trust or intimacy," which can particularly affect young women with male partners who may be especially "un-empowered to insist on clean needles if they are dependent on the partner to provide them with instrumental support such as money, a place to stay, or protection on the streets" (p. 1609). In the context of Latino machismo, this is a reality not unrealistic to many female substance users (Amaro & Raj, 2000). Furthermore, mental illness such as depression and PTSD, gendered power struggles in relationship dynamics, and previous histories of abuse are several factors that interfere with treatment completion among Latina women (Amaro et al., 2004; Amaro & Raj, 2000).

Age

Dual-site studies have revealed differentiating results in how age is associated with HIV/AIDS risk behaviors for Puerto Rican IDUs. Lundgren, Amodeo, and Chassler (2005) concluded that IDUs who were older were more likely to share needles. Similarly, another dual-site study of Puerto Rican IDUs in Puerto Rico and Massachusetts found significant differences in mean age of first injection drug use by location. For example, the mean age of first injection among the sample in Puerto Rico (20.8 years) was approximately 2 years less than the mean age of the sample in western Massachusetts (22.4 years), indicating that IDUs in Puerto Rico began using injection drugs at an earlier age than those living in the mainland United States (López, Zerden, Fitzgerald, & Lundgren, 2008). Although the authors are unsure why this trend exists, they posit fewer educational and labor opportunities as a plausible explanation for earlier experimentation and drug initiation.

Homelessness

In a review of the needs and scientific opportunities for research on substance abuse among Latino adults, Amaro, Arévalo, Gonzalez, Szapocznik, and Iguchi (2006) note that the "Hispanic homeless" are more likely to share needles than those who do not identify as homeless (p. 65). In several of the studies reviewed here, homelessness was a common demographic characteristic. Almost half (44%) of the sample of Lundgren et al. (2005) of 507 IDUs in Massachusetts identified themselves as homeless. Mino, Deren, and Kang (2006) also found higher rates of homelessness among Puerto Rican IDUs in New York who identified themselves as migrants compared to those who identified themselves as nonmigrants. However, López et al. (2008) did not find homelessness to be significantly related to Puerto Rican IDUs rates of hepatitis C, STDs, or positive HIV status, a surprising finding given that homeless IDUs present additional social and health complexities. The authors hypothesize that being an IDU is risk enough regardless of whether an individual identifies as homeless or not.

Cooccurring Disorders: Mental Illness and Substance Abuse

Psychiatric comorbidity is common among substance abusers and has been associated with worse treatment prognosis and more health, employment, and social problems (McLellan, Luborsky, Woody, O'Brien, & Druley, 1983; Rounsaville & Kleber, 1985; Friedmann, Lemon, Anderson, & Stein; 2003; Dixon, 1999; Grant, Stinson, Dawson, Chou, Dufour, Compton, et al., 2004).

There is accumulating evidence that psychiatric symptoms are positively associated with needle sharing. For example, in a methadone-treated population, Metzger, Woody, De Philippis, McLellan, O'Brien, and Platt (1991) found a strong association between psychiatric symptoms and needle sharing, with subjects who had shared needles in the preceding 6 months evidencing significantly more depression, anxiety, and symptoms of other psychiatric conditions. In studying over 500 male and female street IDUs, Johnson et al. (2002) found that people who share needles had higher levels of depression than nonsharers. Finally, a study that examined the relationship between mental health symptoms, drug treatment use, and needle sharing among a sample of 507 IDUs in the state of Massachusetts (including Puerto Ricans, African Americans, and whites) identified anxiety as significantly and positively associated with needle sharing (Lundgren et al., 2005). In this study the prescribed use of psychotropic medications was significantly and negatively associated with needle-sharing behaviors, which suggests mental health treatment can possibly reduce HIV risk behaviors among Puerto Rican IDUs.

It should be noted that a number of studies of Puerto Rican IDUs have not identified mental health status as associated with needle sharing. However, the issue of mental health needs to be considered when exploring HIV prevention strategies for Puerto Rican IDUs given the high rates of comorbidity between substance abuse and mental health. To provide effective addiction treatment for addicted individuals, mental health needs to be of paramount concern.

Incarceration Histories

Among IDUs, a discussion of incarceration is particularly salient when considering the involvement of the criminal justice system in drug-related offenses. The incarceration of IDUs has been shown to have major implications for individual prisoners and public health, more generally due to the transmission of infections during incarceration periods (Wood et al., 2005; Kang et al., 2005). HIV risky behaviors during incarceration include needle sharing among IDUs (Desai, Latta, Spaulding, Rich, &

Flanigan, 2002; Muller, Stark, Guggenoos-Holzman, Wirth, & Beinzle, 1995), as well as the sharing of needles and other equipment for tattoos, and unprotected sexual contact between men (Kang et al., 2005; Desai et al., 2002). See chapter 12 by Comfort and colleagues for an extended discussion of HIV risk in incarcerated Latinos, including Puerto Ricans.

Among a dual-site sample of Puerto Rican IDUs in Massachusetts and Puerto Rico, a history of having ever been incarcerated was significantly associated with having shared needles in the past 6 months and also having ever shared needles with someone who is HIV positive (Zerden, 2009). These findings support research by Kang et al. (2005) whose comparative study of Puerto Rican IDUs in New York and Puerto Rico found needle sharing while in prison occurred in both locales but was more prevalent in Puerto Rico. Specifically, the overwhelming majority of both New York and Puerto Rico inmates within their sample who injected drugs during their last incarceration period admitted to sharing needles and other equipment while inside correctional facilities almost always (100% in New York vs. 97%, Puerto Rico) (Kang et al., 2005). In addition, IDUs living in Puerto Rico were more likely to use shooting galleries[4] prior to incarceration (77% vs. 20%) and to share syringes (22% vs. 8%) and other injection equipment (47% vs. 21%) (Kang et al., 2005).

Rates of incarceration were found to be equally high for López et al. (2008). In their study the overwhelming majority of sample participants in both locales had been previously incarcerated. Despite high rates of incarceration in both locales, there were significant differences between sample locations. IDUs residing in Puerto Rico had significant higher rates of overall incarceration (84.2%) compared to their counterparts residing in western Massachusetts (74.3%).

SOCIOLOGICAL, DEMOGRAPHIC AND CULTURAL FACTORS ASSOCIATED WITH HIV RISK BEHAVIORS OF PUERTO RICAN IDUs

In summary, the research studies above highlight Puerto Rican drug user groups that are at particular risk for HIV and other blood-borne infections. This includes those on the Island of Puerto Rico, those with a recent history of using drugs in Puerto Rico, women, those with long histories of drug use, those who are homeless, those with comorbid disorders, and those with criminal justice histories. In addition, some studies indicate that for Puerto Rican IDUs in Puerto Rico, needle sharing is a normative behavior, further placing them at increased risk of contracting HIV/AIDS and passing it on to those they share drugs with, their sexual partners, and their families.

Findings by Zerden (2009) illustrate that drug use severity was positively associated with increased HIV risk. Puerto Rican IDUs who use more frequently and have overdosed in the past year were more likely to have shared needles in the past 6 months and to have ever shared needles with someone who is HIV positive. Finding such as these indicate that those with the most pervasive, chronic forms of addiction are the most at risk for the health consequences associated with IDU. Despite the fact that these individuals are most in need of various medical and social interventions, they are the ones most often neglected and ignored.

Second, this review suggests that HIV prevention strategies targeting Puerto Ricans need to account for and be structured around the unique migratory patterns and acculturation histories of Puerto Ricans. Below are recommendations for improved HIV prevention efforts within this population.

PROGRAMMATIC RECOMMENDATIONS

Given the alarming rates of injection drug use among Puerto Ricans, comprehensive HIV prevention, drug abuse treatment, community-based outreach, HIV testing and counseling, coupled with HIV treatment are needed. These recommendations are supported by the National Institute Drug Abuse (2008). However, the research on HIV prevention among syringe using drug users points to one program model as uniquely effective.

Specifically, public health officials, scientists, practitioners, and research have shown that one of the most effective and evidence-based strategies to reduce HIV/AIDS risk among injection drug-abusing populations is through needle exchange programs, also known as syringe exchange programs (NEPs/SEPs) (Tempalski, Friedman, Keem, Cooper, & Friedman, 2007; Palmateer et al., 2010). NEPs/SEPs have been highly effective in reducing HIV transmission among drug-abusing populations (Centers for Disease Control and Prevention, 2007; Downing et al., 2005). The United States government has not been supportive of NEPs/SEPs.[5,6] In 2009 the federal government briefly lifted a 20-year ban giving states the option to use federal funds toward NEP/SEP programming. Although a largely symbolic gesture given that no additional funding was allocated for NEP programming, this was viewed as a step toward evidence-based HIV/AIDS prevention particularly impacting IDUs. However, as of December 2011, Congress once again prohibited the use of federal funds for syringe exchange programs (Hudson, 2011). The reinstatement of the funding ban is particularly troubling for Puerto Rican IDUs given their alarming rates of injection drug use. For this population, having easy access to needles provided in a nonstigmatized manner can significantly reduce needle sharing and other HIV risky behavior both stateside and on the island. As of December 2010, the Puerto Rico Department of Health confirmed that there are currently four officially registered NEP/SEP in Puerto Rico (personal communication, December 14, 2010). However, a longitudinal study of syringe acquisition of Puerto Rican IDUs in New York and Puerto Rico shed light on one program in particular and its limitations (Finlinson et al., 2006). For example, the program offered few NEP/SEP sites, operated only a fewer days a week, for fewer hours, and had a more strict exchange policy whereby NEP/SEP consumers were usually given half as many clean, new needles for what they exchanged. In Puerto Rico, private sellers tended to be a more common way for IDUs to acquire syringes than through NEPs/SEPs (Finlinson et al., 2006). Clearly these are inadequate situations on both the island and mainland.

In addition to the need for Puerto Rico to develop more NEP/SEPs, and increase access to needle-exchange services for Puerto Rican IDUs, this chapter provides the following program and policy recommendations.

Increase Access to Addiction Treatment and Mental Health Services

It is critical that addiction treatment services, including medications for opiate dependence be made available to Puerto Rican IDUs both on the island and the mainland United States. Medications such as Methadone, Suboxone, and Subutex have been found to significantly reduce both opiate dependence and also HIV risks related to drug injection. A health concern that needs to be addressed is the combined use of Xylazine and heroin on the island, which not only results in the reduced effectiveness of medications but also in increased health risks.

The literature review indicates high levels of comorbid substance abuse and psychiatric needs among the population of Puerto Rican IDUs, with higher levels of needle sharing found among this population. Therefore, it is critical that a combination of addiction treatment and mental health services be provided. Robles et al. (2003) suggest that Puerto Rico has significantly fewer drug treatment and health services available for substance users compared to those available in New York, and that seeking treatment has been cited as a reason for Puerto Rico migration among IDUs (Deren et al., 2003a). However, a comparative analysis looking at these services (or lack thereof) is currently nascent in comparing service availability and utilization rates among Puerto Rican IDUs residing in Puerto Rico and stateside.

Provide HIV Prevention Services and Addiction Treatment with Staff Who Share Similar Cultural and Ethnic Make Up of Consumers

The effect of having similar cultural and ethnic make-up of staff and consumers is explained well by Delgado (2007) who asserts: "the benefits of having Latino staff go beyond provisions of quality services, and extend to good public relations and an increased likelihood of grounding services within the context of what the community believes it wants and needs" (p. 81–82). HIV prevention and treatment programs that hire Puerto Rican personnel among all levels of the staff hierarchy—from those working on the ground to administration—who have experienced such movement, or are sensitive to circular migratory patterns, will greatly increase understanding among consumers and providers as discussed honestly and openly by service providers. For this to be beneficial for Puerto Rican IDUs, Puerto Rican Spanish should be used and adapted in client interactions. Another unique lens can be the discussion between staff and consumers who have lived in both locales, as this opens the dialogue about migration and sheds light on the differences, hardships, and benefits of life in both locations.

Agencies can continually conduct cultural competency trainings regarding their client population, and identify Puerto Rican stakeholders within the community who can assist in the translation of specific cultural nuances. This includes participation at local and international conferences and establishing partnerships with agencies in Puerto Rico and the mainland United States that work with similar client populations. Having a personal contact in either locale can be vital in offering migrating IDUs treatment away from their current residence. This is of particular importance, especially if Puerto Rican IDUs need to remove themselves from their current social network but still want to be among others who share their cultural and ethnic make-up. Another approach includes partnerships with research teams and academia that utilize and emphasize the importance of community-based participatory research methods to conduct research and future needs assessments for this population.

Develop Service Delivery Models Specific to Puerto Rican IDUs

For community-based organizations to best serve Puerto Rican IDUs, both in Puerto Rico and in the mainland United States, these organizations must build coalitions with other agencies, creating collaborations with referring agencies to work together, and enhance a sense of community, rather than shunning people with substance abuse issues from the communities in which they live. Given that people who have acquired HIV/AIDS by injection drug use experience a double burden, or are "doubly stigmatized—for being HIV-positive and for being 'addicts,'" it is fundamental that communities' most vulnerable groups are not further disenfranchised (Tempalski et al., 2007, p. 1251). However, participation in the community should be extended to consumers as well.

An example of how this strategy can be implemented has been demonstrated by López et al. (2008) who describe how a community agency in Puerto Rico utilizes Delgado's (2007) Capacity Enhancement Model to involve consumers in a project that requires teamwork and participatory action. Through a peer-led educational theater group that writes plays and then performs vignettes in public venues as a means of educating audience members on substance abuse, HIV risk, and their own personal experiences, participants in Puerto Rico provided an educational and inspirational learning opportunity for community members surrounding these issues. This is a prime example of how consumers and community workers can partner together to enhance community capacity, build self-esteem and confidence among IDUs, as well as demystify common misconceptions about persons with HIV/AIDS and substance abuse. Although López et al. (2008) recognize further research is needed to apply this prevention model to Puerto Ricans in other geographic, socioeconomic, and cultural contexts, it demonstrates a promising example of how this work is currently being conducted in Puerto Rico.

The play features program participants who develop the script based on their own stories. For example, there is usually someone playing a drug user, a sex worker, a homeless person, who prior to being on the streets was a high school teacher, and an HIV+ group member. During the performance it seems that the audience is watching fictional characters but at the end of the play, each of the "actors" reveals this is their own stories and they were playing themselves. They encourage a dialogue and have a question and answer period to increase awareness and reduce the stigma commonly associated with homelessness, addiction, and HIV/AIDS. Plays have been performed at clinics, health fairs, high schools, and community events and have served as a powerful educational tool.

Another suggestion is for current service providers in Puerto Rico to offer integrative services so that consumers could apply a convenient "one-stop shopping" approach to where they go for services. This includes an agency that provides substance abuse treatment, HIV testing, and counseling, as well as other health services, employment, and housing services. In addition, participants could receive help in applying for public assistance programs for which they are eligible and potentially offer family services simultaneously.

Increase Federal Funding for Services Proven to Be Effective

An increase in federal funding for HIV prevention services and addiction treatment targeting Puerto Rican IDUs specifically is essential. Funding from government agencies such as the Substance Abuse Mental Health Services Administration (SAMHSA) and the CDC, among others is one of the most powerful ways Puerto Rican IDUs can be effectively targeted.

For example, although the population difference between the Island of Puerto Rico and Massachusetts is only about 2.5 million people, in terms of overall SAMHSA HIV/AIDS funding in fiscal year 2007, Massachusetts received over $6 million dollars more in federal dollars compared to Puerto Rico (The Kaiser Family Foundation, 2008b). In terms of HIV/AIDS prevention, Puerto Rico received no federal funds whereas Massachusetts was awarded over half a million dollars. Similar disparities are found for HIV/AIDS treatment funds as well (The Kaiser Family Foundation, 2008b). Discrepancies in these rates of funding place agencies in Puerto Rico at a disadvantage that equates to less information, access, training, and technical assistance. This matters greatly given that federal grants offer agencies several components in addition to money to provide services. This includes materials on evidence-based practices, recent literature, technical assistance in data collection, and assistance with forms and administrative tools to collect data, monitor progress with reporting requirements, and opportunities to participate in conferences and other networking forums. Although agencies are able to coordinate these facets of a program on their own, federal infrastructure is undoubtedly a powerful mechanism to organize a program's capabilities.

In October 2010, the National AIDS Fund (NAF) announced HIV/AIDS prevention grant opportunities specifically to support community-based organizations in Puerto Rico to implement HIV/AIDS prevention programs and services. The goal of this funding was to award 7–10 grants of $30,000 each by the end of 2010 in order to bolster the capacity of community-based organizations for prevention services including but not limited to NEPs/SEPs, risk-reduction counseling, groups, HIV testing and counseling, peer-based outreach, community education, and community level interventions to reduce stigma (National Minority AIDS Council, 2010). While this is a step in the right direction, alone, it is not adequate to address the severity of Puerto Rico's AIDS crisis.

Lastly for practitioners, a harm reduction approach is fundamental to working with Puerto Rican IDUs. Instead of exclusively focusing on abstinence, the adoption of harm reduction programming allows practitioners to view substance abuse along a continuum and start where the client is at, a seminal perspective in social work practice. The implementation of harm reduction practice into work with Puerto Rican IDUs may serve as a constructive and realistic approach to helping consumers reduce HIV risk and substance use.

PHILOSOPHICAL SHIFT IN DRUG POLICY AND TREATMENT OF ADDICTION

Furthermore, those with chronic and persistent drug use are most at risk for acquiring HIV/AIDS, yet national, state, and local response to drug abuse is not universally understood within a medical model. Instead, addiction is *still* most commonly viewed behaviorally, as an individual's poor decision or as a result of moral failings and not as a disease.

It is critical that substance abuse is universally understood to be a major public health concern with structural-environmental determinants as argued in Chapter 1 of this book. Current prevention and treatment policies and program are insufficient. For example, the National Institute of Drug Abuse (2008) estimates that drug abuse costs the United States more than $484 billion per year, or several times that of other chronic conditions such as diabetes ($131.7 billion) or even cancer ($171.6 billion). However, despite the prevalence of substance abuse within our society, addiction is not universally understood to be a chronic disease that has hereditary, environmental, neurological, and biological components. Until a philosophical shift occurs and our country understands substance abuse, cooccurring mental health, and substance abusing conditions, treatment for IDUs will continue to be inadequate, because they do not address the root of the problem. Addiction needs to be treated for what it is: a disease that requires behavioral, medical, and social interventions instead of punitive action such as incarceration. In addition, more treatment approaches and evidence-based interventions need to be translated to Spanish, culturally adapted, and made available to Puerto Rican substance users.

RESEARCH OPPORTUNITIES AND FUTURE DIRECTION

Given recent changes in federal policy regarding needle exchange, new research studies need to be developed documenting facilitators and barriers to expanding such services to IDUs, particularly Puerto Rican IDUs both on the island of Puerto Rico and in the mainland United States. It is important that these studies include both qualitative and quantitative methods to better identify the cultural perspectives on drug use, needle sharing, and needle exchange from the perspective of IDUs and service providers. Furthermore, more prevalence-focused research is needed on the troubling findings regarding the combined use of Xylazine and heroin in Puerto Rico.

A review of research on drug treatment services for the Latino population describes several key areas in need of further research and points to the overall need to (1) address the specific drug treatment needs of the Latino community, including understanding community context, and particularly to examine differences among Latino groups by country of origin (Alegría et al., 2006), and (2) focus on integrated care models and system, provider, and client-level barriers to staying in care. Finally, research studies need to be developed testing the effectiveness of adapting existing evidence-based treatments for comorbid mental health and substance abuse disorders for Puerto Rican IDUs.

CONCLUSIONS

Puerto Rico faces several challenges in that there are fewer resources and the IDU population on the island engages in more frequent HIV risk behaviors. These findings highlight the need to supply Puerto Rico not only with additional funds but also with specialized technological and institutional support to enhance current substance abuse and HIV prevention services. This includes the continuing effort to produce prevention materials in Spanish as well as provide translated program manuals and standards that can be easily implemented and adapted by agency staff in Puerto Rico. Efforts to further enhance Puerto Rico's capacity for treatment and services include supporting existing drug treatment facilities and procuring additional funds so that people with substance abuse problems have options to treatment services.

Considering the lack of political power Puerto Rican representatives have in Congress due to a lack of voting rights and the demonstrated need in terms of high-risk HIV/AIDS behaviors, overall high HIV/AIDS rates, and drug use rates in Puerto Rico, federal funding for HIV prevention services appropriated exclusively for Puerto Rico is of critical concern. Research continually demonstrates the connection Puerto Rican IDUs have with the mainland United States. With frequent movement and circular migration, IDU and overall HIV/AIDS risk on the island of Puerto Rico need to be recognized as public health priorities with serious social, health, and economic ramifications that extend beyond the island itself.

NOTES

1. This applies to Puerto Ricans living on the island. Puerto Ricans living in the U.S. mainland can vote after 1 year of living stateside.
2. This is based on a crude divorce rate—the number of divorces per 1000. Puerto Rico's crude divorce rate is among the highest in North America at 3.67 (United Nations Statistics Division, 2005).
3. The sample does not equal 100% due to the fact that one respondent in this study (0.5%) reported being born in a country other than the U.S. mainland or Puerto Rico. This respondent was excluded in the analysis.
4. Although shooting galleries can be a variety of dwellings, both abandoned and occupied, the term is used on the street as a place where illegal drugs may be obtained, prepared, and taken by injection, often with equipment provided on the premises.
5. A common concern opponents had against NEPs is that they sanctioned drug use and would attract criminal activity to neighbourhoods with operating NEPs. However, neither of these issues has been scientifically validated to substantiate such claims.
6. Three of the four NEP/SEPs in Puerto Rico are located in the San Juan Metropolitan area and the fourth is located in Ponce, the second largest city in Puerto Rico. This leaves a significant portion of the island without access to NEP/SEPs.

REFERENCES

Acevedo, G. (2004). Neither here nor there: Puerto Rican circular migration. *Journal of Immigrant and Refugee Services, 2(1–2)*, p. 69–85.

Alegría, M., Page, B. J., Hansen, H., Cauce, A. M., Robles, R., Blanco, C., Cortés, D. E., Amaro, H., Morales, A., & Berry, P. (2006). Improving drug treatment services for Hispanics: Research gaps and scientific opportunities. *Drug and Alcohol Dependence, 84(1)*, 76–84.

Amaro, H., Arévalo, S., Gonzalez, G., Szapocznik, J., & Iguchi, M. Y. (2006). Needs and scientific opportunities for research on substance abuse treatment among Hispanic adults. *Drug and Alcohol Dependence, 84(1)*, 64–75.

Amaro, H., McGraw, S., Larson, M. J., López, L., Nieves, R., & Marshall, B. (2004). Boston consortium of services for families in recovery: A trauma-informed intervention model for women's alcohol and drug addiction treatment. *Alcoholism Treatment Quarterly, 22(3/4)*, 95–119.

Amaro, H., & Raj, A. (2000). On the margin: Power and women's HIV risk reduction strategies. *Sex Roles, 42(7/8)*, 723–749.

Andía, J. F., Deren, S., Robles, R. R., Kang, S. Y., & Colón, H. M. (2008). Peer norms and sharing of injection paraphernalia among Puerto Rican injection drug users in New York and Puerto Rico. *AIDS Education and Prevention, 20(3)*, 249–257.

Baker, S. S. (2002). *Understanding mainland Puerto Rican poverty.* Philadelphia: Temple University Press.

Bea, K., & Garret, S. (2010). *Political status of Puerto Rico: Options for congress.* (Congressional Research Service Report, No. 7-5700). Washington, DC: U.S. Government Printing Office.

Bluthenthal, R. N., Ridgeway, G., Schell, T., Anderson, R., Flynn, N. M., & Kra, A. H. (2007). Examination of the association between syringe exchange program (SEP) dispensation policy and SEP client-level syringe coverage among injection drug users. *Addiction Rand Research Report, 102*, 638–646.

Cabassa, L. J. (2003). Measuring acculturation: Where we are and where we need to go. *Hispanic Journal of Behavioral Sciences, 25(2)*, 127–146.

Centers for Disease Control and Prevention [CDC]. (2005b). *HIV/AIDS surveillance report; volume 16*. Atlanta, GA: Department of Health and Human Services, Centers for Disease Control and Prevention.

Centers for Disease Control and Prevention [CDC]. (2007). Syringe exchange programs: December 2005. Retrieved December 3, 2011, from http://www.cdc.gov/idu/facts/aed_idu_syr.pdf.

Colón, H. M., Robles, R. R., Deren, S., Sahai, H., Finlinson, A. H., Andía, J., Cruz, M. A., Kang, S. Y., & Oliver-Vélez, D. (2001). Between-city variation in frequency of injection among Puerto Rican injection drug users: East Harlem, New York, and Bayamón, Puerto Rico. *Journal of Acquired Immune Deficiency Syndromes, 27*(4), 405–413.

Cortés, D. E., Deren, S., Andía, J., Colón, H., Robles, R., & Kang, S. Y. (2003). The use of the Puerto Rican biculturality scale with Puerto Rican drug users in New York & Puerto Rico. *Journal of Psychoactive Drugs, 35*(2), 197–207.

Delgado, M. (2007). *Social work with Latinos: A cultural assets paradigm*. New York: Oxford University Press.

Delgado, M., Lundgren, L. M., Deshpande, A., Lonsdale, J., & Purington, T. (2008). The association between acculturation and needle sharing among Puerto Rican injection drug users. *Evaluation & Program Planning, 30*(1), 83–91.

Deren, S., Kang, S. Y., Colón, H. M., Andía, J. F., Robles, R. R., Oliver-Velez, D., & Finlinson, A. (2003a). Migration and HIV risk behaviors: Puerto Rican drug injectors in New York City and Puerto Rico. *American Journal of Public Health, 93*(5), 812–816.

Deren, S., Kang, S. Y., Colón, H., & Robles R. (2007a). The Puerto Rico–New York airbridge for drug users: Description and relationship to HIV risk behaviors. *Journal of Urban Health: Bulletin of the New York Academy of Medicine, 84*(2), 243–254.

Deren, S., Kang, S. Y., Colón, H., & Robles, R. R. (2007b). Predictors of injection drug use cessation among Puerto Rican drug injectors in New York and Puerto Rico. *American Journal of Drug and Alcohol Abuse, 33*(2), 291–299.

Deren, S., Kang, S. Y., Rapkin, B., Robles, R., Andía, J. F., & Colón, H. M. (2003b). The utility of the PRECEDE model in predicting HIV risk behaviors among Puerto Rican injection drug users. *AIDS and Behavior, 7*(4), 405–412.

Deren, S., Oliver-Velez, D., Finlinson, A., Robles, R., Andía, J., Colón, M., Kang, S. Y., & Shedlin, M. (2003c). Integrating qualitative and quantitative methods: Comparing HIV-related risk behaviors among Puerto Rican drug users in Puerto Rico and New York. *Substance Use and Misuse, 38*, 1–24.

Deren, S., Strauss, S., Kang. S. Y., Colon, H. M., & Robles, R. R. (2008). Sex risk behaviors of drug users: A dual site study of predictors over time. *AIDS Education and Prevention, 20*(4), 325–337.

Desai, A. A., Latta, E. T., Spaulding, A., Rich, J. D., & Flanigan, P. T. (2002). The importance of routine HIV testing in the incarcerated population: The Rhode Island experience. *AIDS Education and Prevention, 14*(B), 45–52.

Dixon, L. (1999). Dual diagnosis of substance abuse in schizophrenia: Prevalence and impact on outcomes. *Schizophrenia Research, 25*, S93–S100.

Downing, M., Riess, T. H., Vernon, K., Mulia, N., Hollinquest, M., McKnight, C., & DesJarlais, D. C. (2005). What's community got to do with it? Implementation models of syringe exchange programs. *AIDS Education and Prevention, 17*(1), 68–78.

Duany, J. (1996). Imagining the Puerto Rican nation: Recent works on cultural identity. *Latin American Research Review, 31*(3), 248–267.

Duany, J. (2002). *The Puerto Rican nation on the move*. Chapel Hill: The University of North Carolina Press.

Evans, J. L., Hahn, J. A., Page-Shafer, K., Lum, P. J., Stein, E. S., Davidson, P. J., & Moss, A. R. (2003). Gender differences in sexual and injection risk behavior among active young injection drug users in San Francisco (the UFO study). *Journal of Urban Health, 80*(1), 137–146.

Finlinson, H. A., Colon, H. M., Lopez, M. S., Robles, R. R., & Cant, J. G. (2005). Injecting shared drugs: An observational study of the process of drug acquisition, preparation, and injection by Puerto Rican drug users. *Journal of Psychoactive Drugs, 37*, 37–49.

Finlinson, A, Colon, H., Robles, R., & Soto-Lopez, M. (2006). An exploratory qualitative study of polydrug use histories among recently initiated injection drug users in San Juan, Puerto Rico. *Substance Use & Misuse, 41*, 915–935.

Fitzgerald, T. (2008). HIV/AIDS risk reduction health service utilization among injection drug using women. *Dissertation Abstract International* (UMI No. AAT 3298632). Retrieved December 1, 2009, from Dissertations and Theses Abstract.

Friedman, S. R., Curtis, R., Neaigus, A., Jose, B., & Des Jarlis, D. C. (1999). *Social networks, drug injectors' lives, and HIV/AIDS.* New York: Kluwer Academic/Plenum Publishers.

Friedmann, P. D., Lemon, S. C., Anderson, B. J., & Stein, M. D. (2003). Predictors of follow-up health status in the drug abuse treatment outcome study (DATOS). *Drug and Alcohol Dependence, 69*(3), 243–251.

Gil, A. G., Wagner, E. F., & Vega, W. A. (2000). Acculturation, familismo, and alcohol use among Latino adolescent males: Longitudinal relations. *Journal of Community Psychology, 28*, 443–458.

Godoy, R., Carvalho, I., Hexner, J. T., & Jenkins, G. P. (2002). *Puerto Rican migration: An assessment of quantitative studies.* Waltham, MA: Sustainable International Development Programs at the Heller School for Social Policy & Management, Brandeis University.

Grant, D. F., Stinson, F. S., Dawson, D. A., Chou, S. P., Dufour, M. C., Compton, W., et al. (2004). Prevalence and co-occurrence of substance use disorders and independent mood and anxiety disorders: Results from the epidemiologic survey on alcohol and related conditions. *Archives of General Psychiatry, 61*, 807–816.

Hajat, A., Lucas, J., & Kington, R. (2000). *Health outcomes among Hispanic subgroups: United States 1992–1995.* Hyatsville: National Center for Health Statistics.

Hudson, Z. (2011). Congress's Holiday Message to People Who Use Drugs: Drop Dead. Retrieved December 26, 2011 from http://blog.soros.org/2011/12/congresss-holiday-message-to-people-who-use-drugs-drop-dead/.

Johnson, M. E., Yep, M. J., Brems, C., Theno, S. A., & Fisher, D. G. (2002). Relationship among gender, depression and needle sharing in a sample of injection drug users. *Psychology of Addictive Medicine, 16*(4), 338–341.

Kaiser Family Foundation, The [KFF]. (2008a). *HIV/AIDS policy brief: Latinos & HIV/AIDS.* Washington, DC: The Henry J. Kaiser Family Foundation.

Kaiser Family Foundation, The [KFF]. (2008b). Puerto Rico: Substance abuse and mental health services administration (SAMHSA) HIV/AIDS funding, FY2007. Retrieved November 14, 2008, from http://www.statehealthfacts.kff.org/profileind.jsp?cat=11&sub=125&rgn=23.

Kaiser Family Foundation, The [KFF]. (2009). HIV/AIDS policy fact sheet: The HIV/AIDS epidemic in the Caribbean. Retrieved January 3, 2011, from http://www.kff.org/hivaids/upload/7505-06.pdf.

Kang, S. Y., Deren, S., Andía, J., Colón, H. M., Robles, R., & Oliver-Velez, D. (2005). HIV transmission behaviors in jail/prison among Puerto Rican drug injectors in New York and Puerto Rico. *AIDS and Behavior, 9*(3), 377–387.

Lara, M., Gamboa, C., Kahramanian, M. I., Morales, L. S., & Hayes Bautista, D. E. (2005). Acculturation and Latino health in the United States: A review of the literature and its sociopolitical context. *Annual Review of Public Health, 26*, 367–397.

Latino Commission on AIDS. (2004). Key facts: Latinas and HIV/AIDS. Latino AIDS awareness day/día nacional Latino por la concientización del SIDA. Retrieved September 14, 2008, from http://www.galaei.org/pdfs/Latinas%20Women%20and%20HIV%20-percent20english.pdf.

López, L., Zerden, L. D., Fitzgerald, T., & Lundgren, L. (2008). Puerto Rican injection drug users: Prevention implications in Massachusetts and Puerto Rico. *Evaluation and Program Planning, 31*(1), 64–73.

Lundgren, L., Amodeo, M., & Chassler, D. (2005). Mental health status, drug treatment use, and needle-sharing among injection drug users. *AIDS: Prevention and Education, 17*(6), 525–539.

Mathers, B. M., Degenhardt, L., Phillips, B., Wiessing, L., Hickman, M., & Strathdee, S. (2008). Global epidemiology of injecting drug use and HIV among people who inject drugs: A systematic review. *Lancet, 372*, 1733–1745.

McLellan, A. T., Luborsky, L., Woody, G. E., Druley, K. A., & O'Brien, C. P. (1983). Predicting response to alcohol and drug abuse treatments: Role of psychiatric severity. *Archives of General Psychiatry, 40*, 620–625.

Metzger, D., Woody, G., Philippis, D. E., McLellan, A. T., O'Brien, C. P., & Platt, J. J. (1991). Risk factors for needle sharing among methadone-treated patients. *American Journal of Psychiatry, 148*, 636–640.

Mino, M., Deren, S., & Kang, S. Y. (2006). Social support & HIV-related injection risk among Puerto Rican migrant & non-migrant injection drug users recruited in New York City. *AIDS Education & Prevention, 18*(1), 81–90.

Montoya, I. D., Bell, D. C., Richard, A. J., Carlson, J. W., & Trevino, R. A. (1999). Estimated HIV risk among Hispanics in a national sample of drug users. *Journal of Acquired Immune Deficiency Syndromes, 21*(1), 42–50.

Muller, M., Stark, K., Guggenoos-Holzman, I., Wirth, D., & Beinzle, U. (1995). Imprisonment: A risk factor for HIV infection counteracting behavior and prevention programs for intravenous drug users. *AIDS, 9*, 183–190.

National Institute of Allergy and Infectious Disease [NIAID]. (2008). *HIV Infection in minority populations.* Retrieved November 1, 2008, from http://www.niaid.nih.gov/factsheets/Minor.htm.

National Institute of Drug Abuse [NIDA]. (2003). *Drug use among racial/ethnic minorities, revised.* (National Institute on Drug Abuse and National Institute of Health Publication No. NIH Publication No. 03-3888). Bethesda, MD: NIDA.

National Institute of Drug Abuse [NIDA]. (2008). *NIDA InfoFacts: Drug abuse and the link to HIV/AIDS and other infectious diseases.* Retrieved October 27, 2008, from http://www.nida.nih.gov/infofacts/DrugAbuse.html.

National Minority AIDS Council. (October 21, 2010). National AIDS fund request for proposals Puerto Rico HIV/AIDS prevention grant opportunity 2010. Retrieved from http://www.nmac.org/index/news-app/story.502/title.national-aids-fund-rfp-supports-hiv-aids-prevention-in-puerto-rico.

Ortega, A. N., Rosenheck, R., Alegría, M., & Desai, R. A. (2000). Acculturation and the lifetime risk of psychiatric and substance use disorders among Hispanics. *Journal of Nervous and Mental Disorders, 188*, 728–735.

Palmateer, N., Kimber, J., Hickman, J., Hutchinson, S., Rhodes, T., & Goldberg, D. (2010). Evidence for the effectiveness of sterile injecting equipment provision in preventing hepatitis C and human immunodeficiency virus transmission among injecting drug users: A review of reviews. *Addictions, 105*(5), 844–859.

Pimentel, F. (2008). Poverty, culture and social capital in Puerto Rican urban communities. *Centro Journal, XX*(1), 231–245.

Presidential Task Force. (2005). *Report by the President's task force on Puerto Rico's status.* Washington, DC: U.S. Government Printing Office.

Puerto Rico Department of Health, Personal Communication, December 14, 2010.

Puerto Rico Federal Affairs Administration. (2008). *Puerto Rico facts and history.* Retrieved September 10, 2008, from http://www.prfaa.com/aboutpr.asp?id=30.

Rivera-Batiz, F., & Santiago, C. (1996). *Island paradox: Puerto Rico in the 1990s.* New York: Russell Sage Foundation.

Robles, R. M., Matos, T. D., Colón, H. M., Deren, S., Reyes, J. C., Andía, J. F., & Marrero, A. (2003). Determinants of health care use among Puerto Rican injection drug users in Puerto Rico and in New York City. *Clinical Infectious Diseases Journal, 37*(5), 392–403.

Rodriguez, N., Vidot Vargas, J., Panelli, J., Colon, H., Ritchie, B., & Yamamura, Y. (2008). GC-MS confirmation of xylazine (rompun), a veterinary sedative in exchanged needles. *Drug and Alcohol Dependence, 96,* 290–293.

Roundaville, B. J., & Kleber, H. D. (1985). Untreated opiate addicts: How do they differ from those seeking treatment? *Archive of General Psychiatry, 42*(11), 1072–1077.

Sherman, S. G., Latkin, C. A., & Gielen, A. C. (2001). Social factors related to syringe sharing among injecting partners: A focus on gender. *Substance Use & Misuse, 36*(14), 2113–2136.

Singer, M., Stopka, T., Shaw, S., Santelices, C., Buchanan, D., Teng, W., Khooshnood, K., & Heimer, R. (2005). Lessons from the field: From research to application in the fight against AIDS among injection drug users in three New England cities. *Human Organization, 64*(2), 179–191.

Tempalski, B., Friedman, R., Keem, M., Cooper, H., & Friedman, S. R. (2005). NIMBY localism and national inequitable exclusion alliances: The case of syringe exchange programs in the United States. *Geoforum, 38,* 1250–1263.

Tucker, K., Mattei, J., Noel, S. E., Collado, B. M., Mendez, J., Nelson, J., et al. (2010). The Boston Puerto Rican health study, a longitudinal cohort study on health disparities in Puerto Rican adults: Challenges and opportunities. *BMC Public Health, 10,* 107–119.

UNAIDS, the Joint United Nations Program on HIV/AIDS. (2010). Global Report: Caribbean Fact Sheet. Retrieved December 26, 2011 from http://www.unaids.org/documents/20101123_FS_carib_em_en.pdf.

Unger, J. B., Kipke, M. D., De Rosa, C. J., Hyde, J., Ritt-Olson, A., & Montgomery, S. (2006). Needle sharing among young IV drug users and their social network members: The influence of the injection partner's characteristics on HIV risk behavior. *Addictive Behaviors, 31,* 1607–1618.

United Nations Statistics Division. (2005). Divorces and crude divorce rates by urban/rural residence: 2000–2004. Retrieved January 3, 2011 from http://unstats.un.org/unsd/demographic/products/dyb/DYB2004/Table25.pdf.

U.S. Census Bureau. (2006). American community survey: ACS demographic and housing estimates. Retrieved January 10, 2011 from http://factfinder.census.gov/servlet/ADPTable?-geo_id=01000US&-qr_name=ACS_2006_EST_G00_DP5&-ds_name=ACS_20 06_EST_G00_.

U.S. Department of Health and Human Services [USDHHS]. (2007). Resolutions on HIV Puerto Rico emergency. Retrieved January 2, 2011 from http://m.aids.gov/feature/federal-resources/policies/pacha/resolutions/puerto-rico/#.

U.S. Department of Health and Human Services [USDHHS]. (2009). Sebelius announces $42.5 million for public health improvement programs through the Affordable Care Act. Retrieved January 3, 2011, from http://www.hhs.gov/news/ press/2010pres/09/20100920a.html.

Warner, L. A., Valdez, A., Vega, W.A., de la Rosa, M., Turner, J. R., & Canino, G. (2006). Hispanic drug abuse in an evolving cultural context: An agenda for research. *Drug and Alcohol Dependence, 84*(1), 8–16.

Wood, E., Li, K., Small, W., Montaner, J. S., Schechter, M. T., & Kerr, T. (2005). Recent incarceration independently associated with syringe sharing by injection drug users. *Public Health Reports, 120*(March–April 2005), 150–157.

World Bank. (2001). *HIV/AIDS in the Caribbean: Issues and options, volume 52*. Washington, DC: The World Bank. Retrieved from http://books.google.com/books?id=XqRj2xdFaa QC&pg=PA5&lpg=PA5&dq=world+bank+puerto+rico+aids&source=bl&ots=4At3s_ 5G-A&sig=sS198yKvx7gIvbEkiPvIc2KWG7I&hl=en&ei=JKD1TIHAGsSp8Ab9A#v=o nepage&q=world%20bank%20puerto%20rico%20aids&f=false.

Yamada, A. M., Valle, R., Barrio, C., & Jeste, D. (2006). Selecting an acculturation measure for use with Latino older adults. *Research on Aging, 28*(5), 519–561.

Zerden, L. D. (2009). Acculturation and needle sharing: A dual-site study of Puerto Rican injection drug users. *Dissertation Abstract International* (UMI No. AAT 3357802). Retrieved October 9, 2010, from Dissertations and Theses Abstract.

Index